Textbook of Pharmaceutical Chemistry

Textbook of Pharmaceutical Chemistry

Mathew George
M. Pharm., Ph.D., FAGE

Lincy Joseph
M. Pharm., Ph.D., FAGE

Viva Books

New Delhi | Mumbai | Chennai | Kolkata | Bengaluru | Hyderabad | Kochi | Guwahati

Publisher's note

First Published 2009
Reprinted 2016, 2018

Viva Books Private Limited

- 4737/23, Ansari Road, Daryaganj, New Delhi 110 002
  Tel. 42242200, 23258325, 23283121, Email: vivadelhi@vivagroupindia.net
- 76, Service Industries, Shirvane, Sector 1, Nerul, Navi Mumbai 400 706
  Tel. 27721273, 27721274, Email: vivamumbai@vivagroupindia.net
- Megh Towers, Old No. 307, New No. 165, Poonamallee High Road, Maduravoyal
  Chennai 600 095 Tel. 23780991, 23780992, Email: vivachennai@vivagroupindia.net
- B-103, Jindal Towers, 21/1A/3 Darga Road, Kolkata 700 017
  Tel. 22816713, Email: vivakolkata@vivagroupindia.net
- 7, GF, Sovereign Park Aptts., 56-58, K. R. Road, Basavanagudi, Bengaluru 560 004
  Tel. 26607409, Email: vivabangalore@vivagroupindia.net
- 101-102, Moghal Marc Apartments, 3-4-637 to 641, Narayanguda, Hyderabad 500 029
  Tel. 27564481, Email: vivahyderabad@vivagroupindia.net
- First Floor, Beevi Towers, SRM Road, Kaloor, Kochi 682 018
  Tel. 0484-2403055, 2403056, Email: vivakochi@vivagroupindia.net
- 232, GNB Road, Beside UCO Bank, Silpukhuri, Guwahati 781 003
  Tel. 0361-2666386, Email: vivaguwahati@vivagroupindia.net

www.vivagroupindia.com

ISBN: 978-81-309-1260-8

Published by Vinod Vasishtha for Viva Books Private Limited, 4737/23 Ansari Road, Daryaganj, New Delhi 110 002.

Printed and bound in India by Replika Press Pvt. Ltd.

Dedicated to our
children and parents

Contents

Preface

Pharmaceutical chemistry has seen enormous growth in the past decade. A huge amount of information is available in the field of Advanced Organic Chemistry. We are happy to present Textbook of Pharmaceutical Chemistry to the readers. We have taken great care to discuss each and every topic with clarity and simplicity. We feel indebted to various authors on the subject whose books, and articles in journals and periodicals have been consulted for compiling this textbook. Many topics have been incorporated with the aim of meeting the needs and interests of undergraduate and graduate pharmacy courses according to the syllabi of various Indian universities. We hope students can grasp the subject easily and quickly.

We thank Prof. N. Udupa, Principal, Manipal Academy of Higher Education 'Cops', Manipal, for writing the foreword for this textbook. We are thankful to Prof. K.K. Sreenivasan, Head, Department of Pharmaceutical Chemistry, 'MAHE' 'Cops', Manipal, for his constant encouragement and moral support. We extend our thanks to Mr. Sandeep Bakshi, Chancellor, Jaipur National University, Jaipur and all our Department Colleagues and friends for their cooperation in bringing this book in its present form. We are thankful to the Health Minister of Kerala Ms. P.K. Sreemathy Teacher for unveiling this textbook. The authors are extremely thankful to their family members for the constant encouragement.

We welcome valuable criticism and suggestions from the readers.

Mathew George
Lincy Mathew

Foreword

I am happy that Prof. Mathew George and Prof. Lincy Joseph have undertaken the task of writing a book of Advanced Pharmaceutical Organic Chemistry. Though several books written by foreign and Indian authors are available, this book, written in simple language and catering to the need of pharmacy students, will definitely be accepted by the students wholeheartedly. The redeeming feature of this book is lucid and methodical presentation of complicated chemical reactions and a good number of pharmaceutical applications in each category of reactions.

The book contains information that is relevant to the syllabi prescribed by the universities of Tamil Nadu, Kerala, Andhra Pradesh and Karnataka.

Prof. Mathew and Prof. Lincy are experienced teachers in the pharmacy field and have rendered valuable service to the profession of pharmacy by publishing this book. I am sure students will derive immense benefit from this publication.

Dr. N. Udupa
Principal & Professor
Manipal College of Pharmaceutical Sciences,
Manipal

1

Heterocyclic Chemistry

INTRODUCTION

Heterocyclic Chemistry is an integral part of Organic chemistry, which deals heterocyclic compounds and are widely distributed in nature. Heterocyclic compounds which contain Carbon and minimum one hetero atom.

NOMENCLATURE

Hantzsch-Widman System

This Nomenclature system specifies the ring size and the nature, type and position(s) of the hetero atom(s).

(i) Combination of prefix with stem

The prefix indicate the heteroatoms present in the heterocyclic systems. Prefixes for different heteroatoms are presented in the following table

Table 1

Heteroatom	*Symbol*	*Prefix*
Oxygen	O	Oxa
Sulfur	S	Thia
Selenium	Se	Selena
Tellurium	Te	Tellura
Nitrogen	N	Aza
Phosphorus	P	Phospha
Arsenic	As	Arsa
Antimony	Sb	Stiba
Bismuth	Bi	Bisma
Silicon	Si	Sila
Germanium	Ge	Germa
Tin	Sn	Stanna
Lead	Pb	Plumba
Boron	B	Bora
Mercury	Hg	Mercura

Stems are used to indicate the size of ring, saturation or unsaturation in heteromonocyclic systems and are summerized as follows;

Table 2

Ring Size	*Unsaturation*	*Saturation*
Three membered	-irene	-irane
Four membered	-ete	-etane
Five membered	-ole	-olane
Six membered	-ine	-ane/inane
Seven membered	-epine	-epane
Eight membered	-ocine	-ocane
Nine membered	-onine	-onane
Ten membered	-ecine	-ecane

Few exceptions are there; like trivial names eg: pyrrole, pyrazole, imidazole, pyridine, pyridazine, pyrimidine etc. have been permitted over systemic names by IUPAC. Classical examples for above stated information are given below.

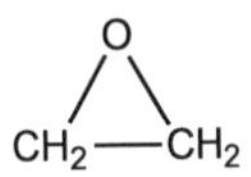

Oxa + irane = Oxirane

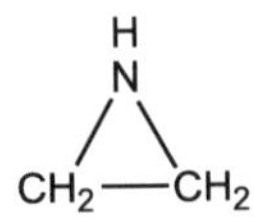

Aza + iridine = Aziridine

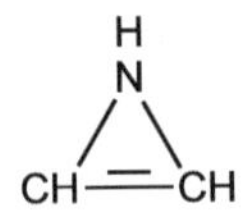

Aza + irine = Azirine

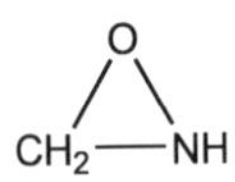

Oxa + aza + iridine = Oxaziridine

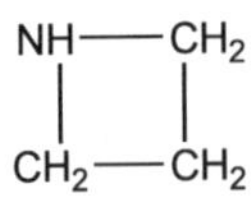

Aza + etidine = Azetidine

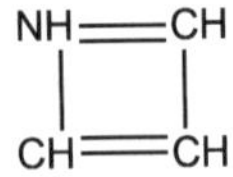

Aza + ete = Azete

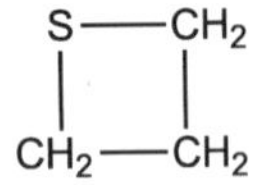

Thia + etane = Thietane

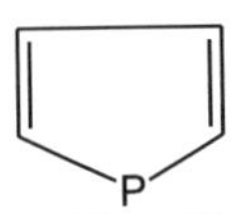

Phospha + Ole = Phosphole

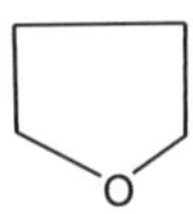

Oxa + Olane = Oxolane

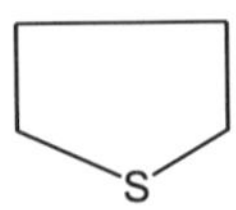

Thia + Olane = Thiolane

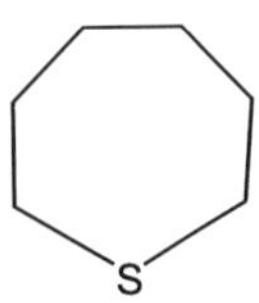

Thia + epane = Thiepane

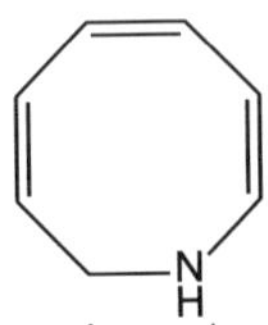

Aza + epine = Azepine

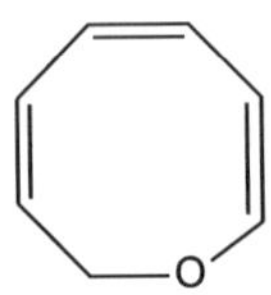

Oxa + epine = Oxepine

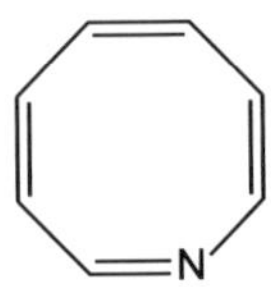

Aza + Ocxine = Azocine

(ii) Presence of identical heteroatoms

When two or more heteroatoms of same type are present in a ring, prefixes like di, tri, tetra ....etc. are placed before prefix of considered heteroatom for example;

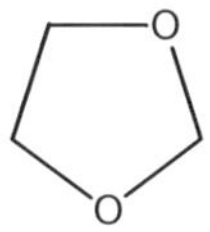
1,3-Dixolane

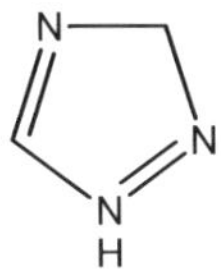
1,2,4-Triazole

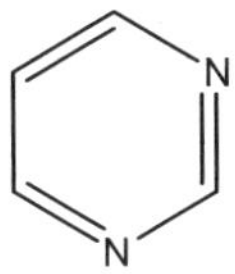
1,3-Diazine = Pyrimidine (Trivial name)

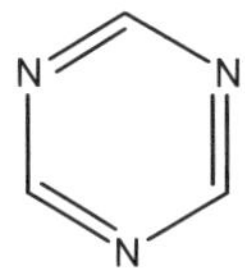
1,3,5-Triazine

(iii) Presence of different heteroatoms

When two or more different heteroatoms are present in the same ring, prefixes of heteroatoms are combined in the order of priority as given in Table (1) (Priority given in decreasing order). For example;

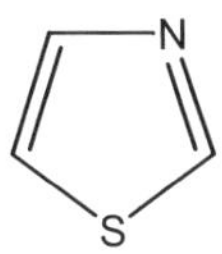
Thia + aza + ole = Thiazole
(1,3-Thiazole)

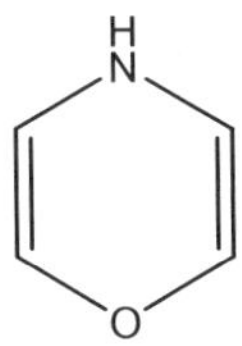
Oxa + aza + ine = Oxazine
(1,4-Oxazine)

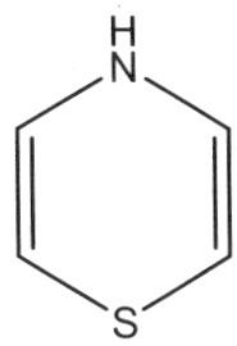
Thia + aza + ine = Thiazine
(1,4-Thiazine)

(iv) Numbering

(a) *With one heteroatom:* Heteroatom assigns the position-1 and proceeds in such a way as to give the lowest possible locant to the substituent if present. In Greek letters, position next to hetero atom is α and proceeded position is β.

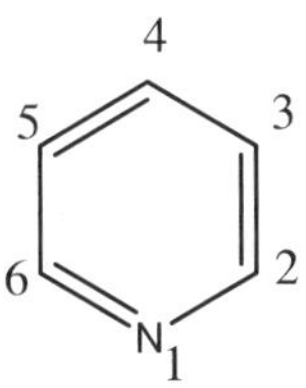
Pyridine

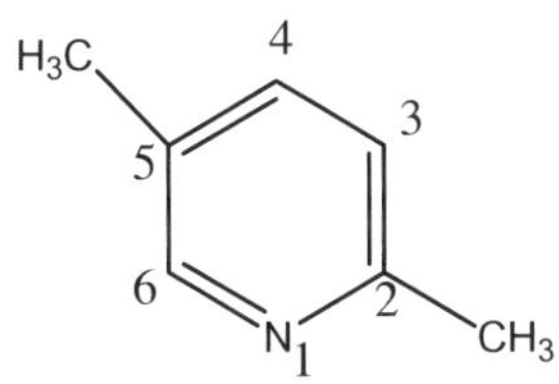
2,5-Dimethylpyridine

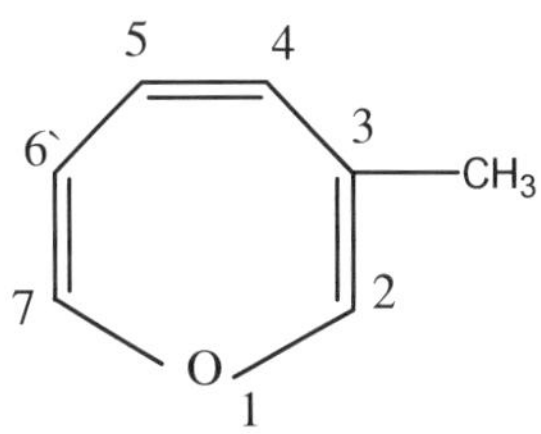
3-methyloxepin

(b) *With two or more identical heteroatoms:* In this case heteroatoms are assigned lowest set of number locants for example

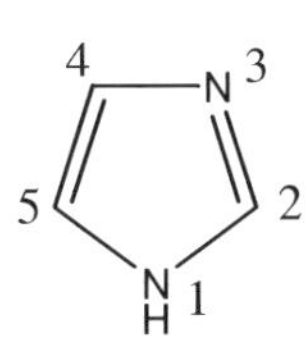
Correct one

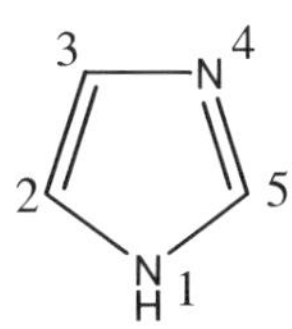
incorrect one

(c) *With multiple different heteroatoms*: In this case numbering starts at which heteroatom have highest priority remaining heteroatoms are given lowest number locants. for example

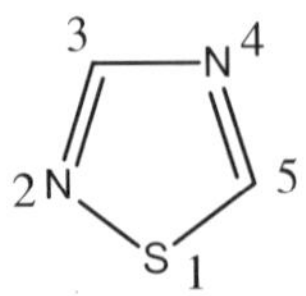

1,2,4 Thia diazole (correct one)

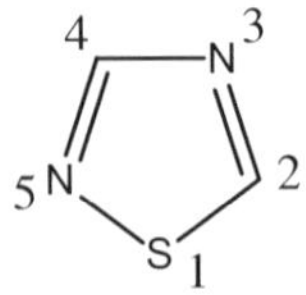

1,3,5 Thiadiazole (incorrectone)

Based on trivial system, names of important heterocyclic compounds are as follows;

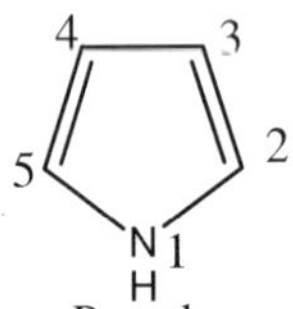

Pyrrole

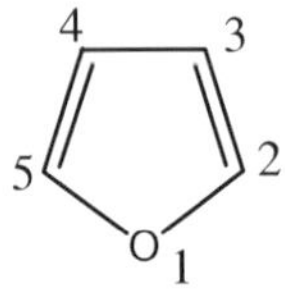

Furan

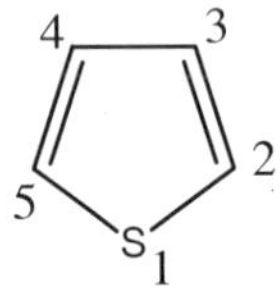

Thiophene

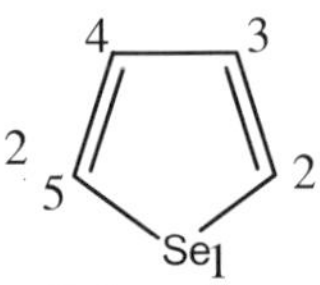

Selenophene

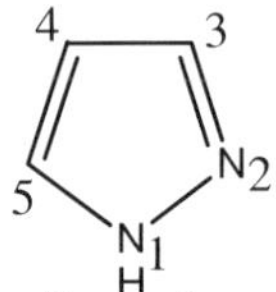

Pyrazole

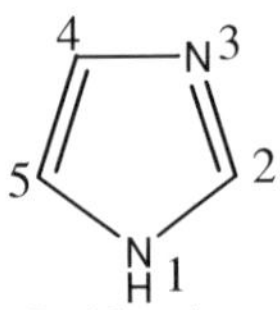

Imidazole

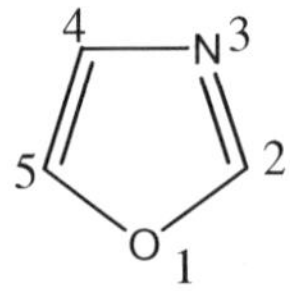

Oxazole

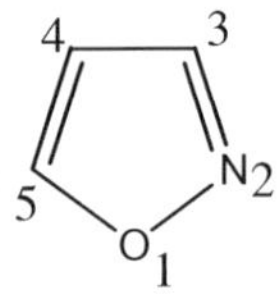

Isoxazole

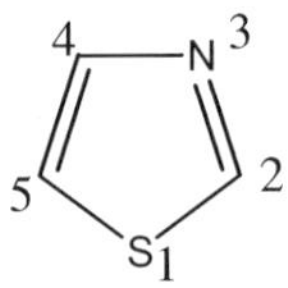

Thiazole

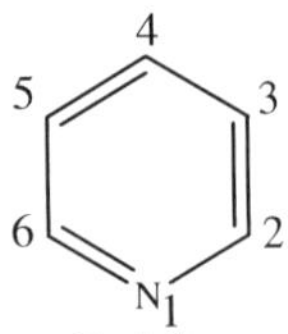

Pyridine

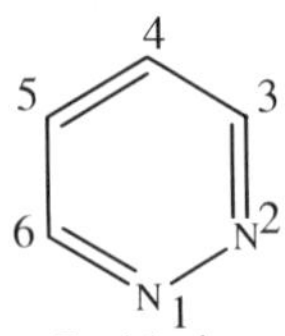

Pyridazine

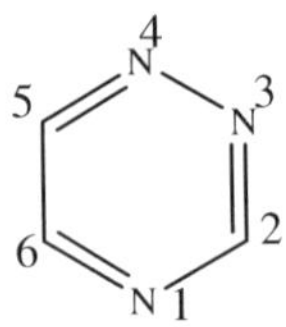

Pyrimidine

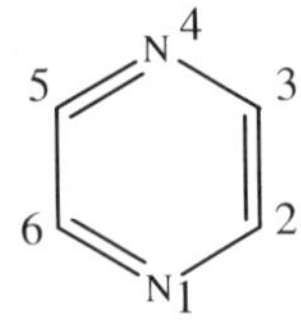

Pyrazine

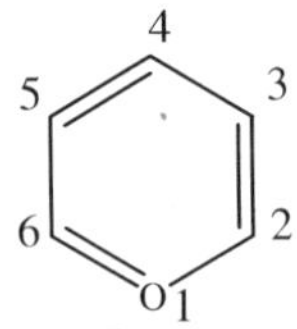

Pyran

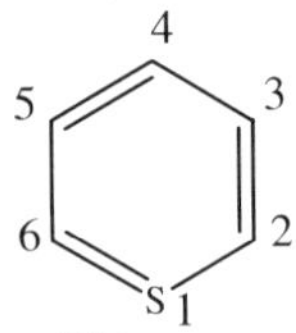

Thiopyran

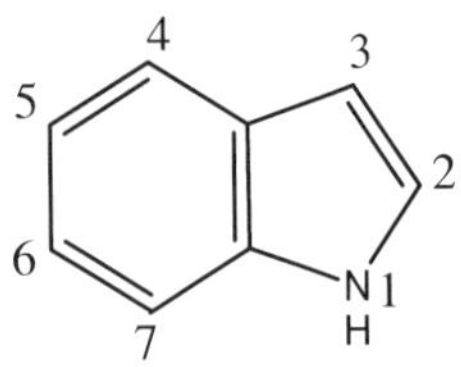

Indole

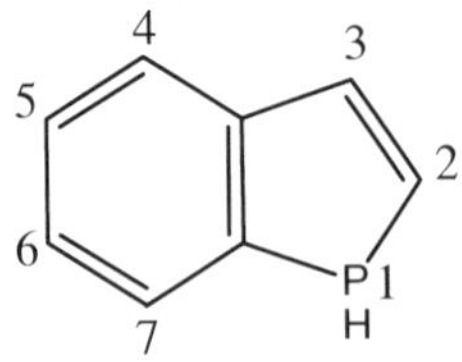

Phosphindole

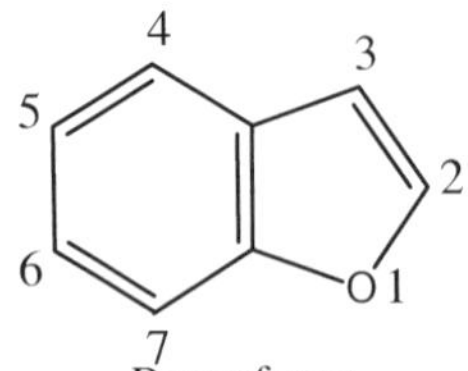

Benzofuran

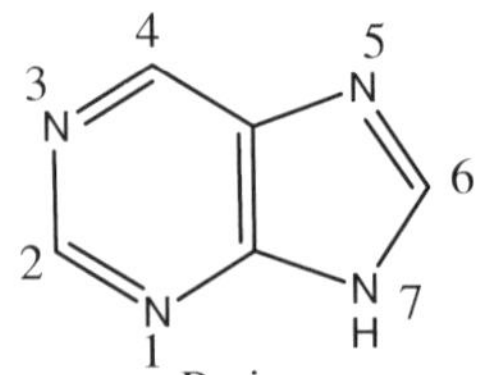

Purine

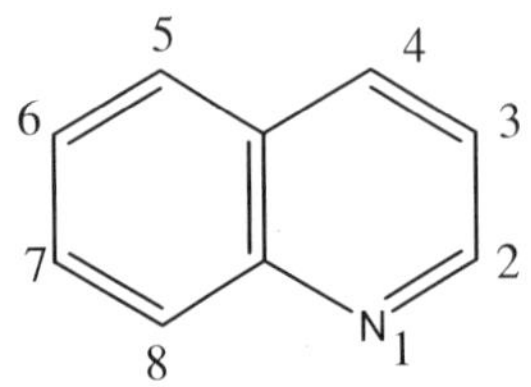

Quinoline

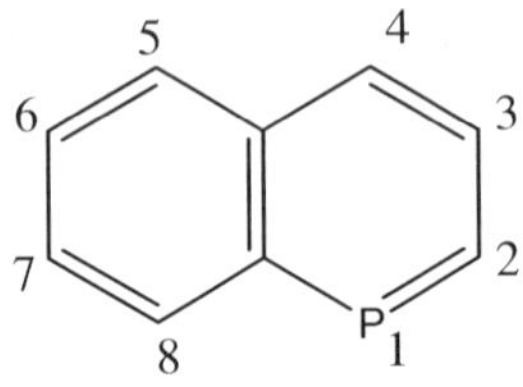

Phosphinoline

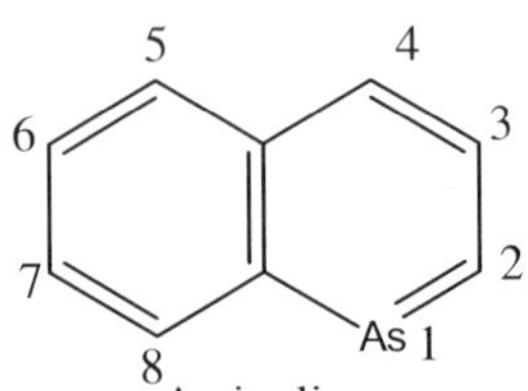

Arsinoline

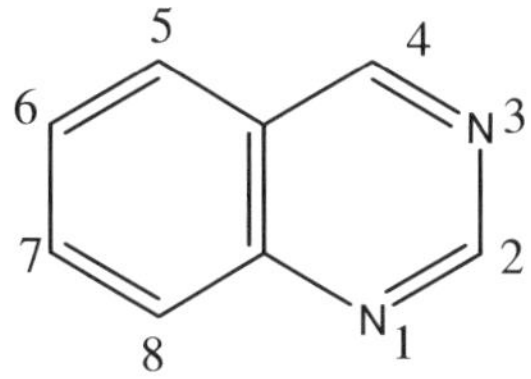
Quinazoline

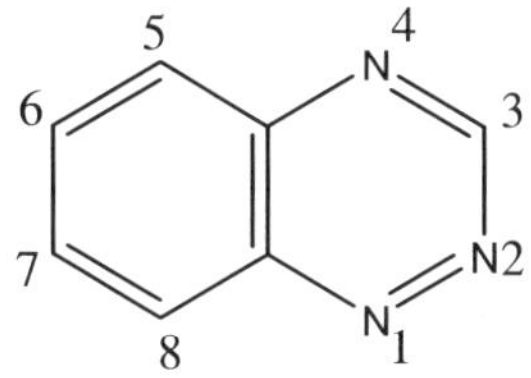
Cinnoline

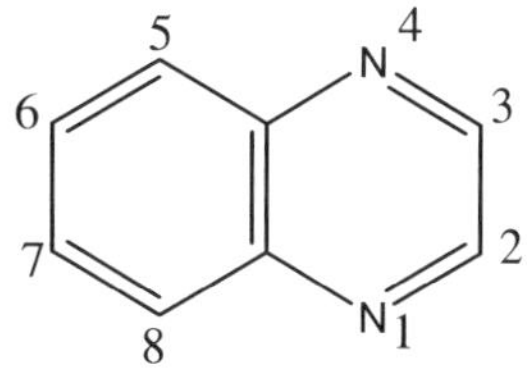
Quinoxaline

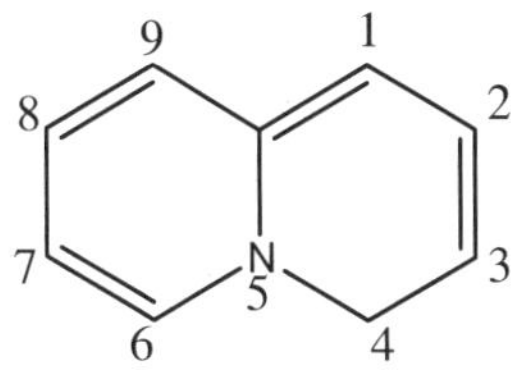
Quinolizine

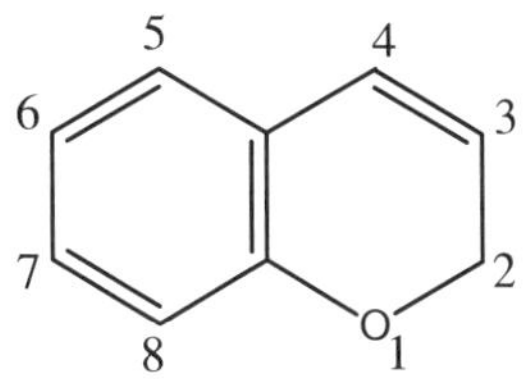
Chromene

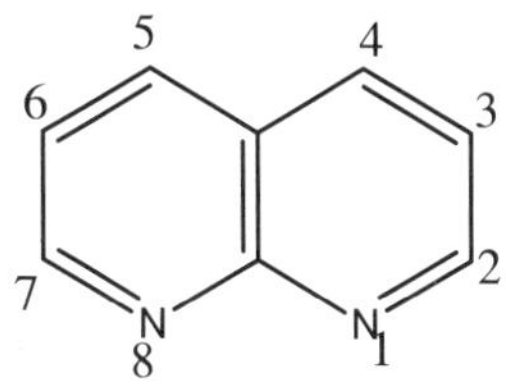
1,8-Naphthyridine

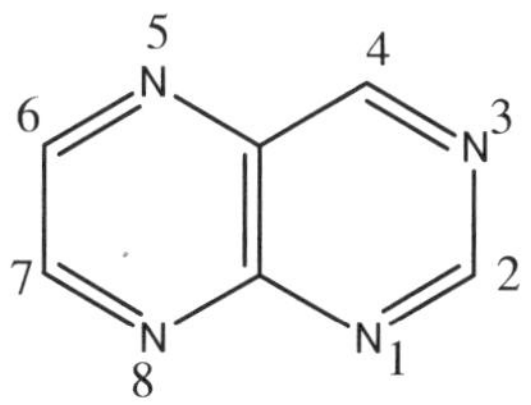
Pteridine

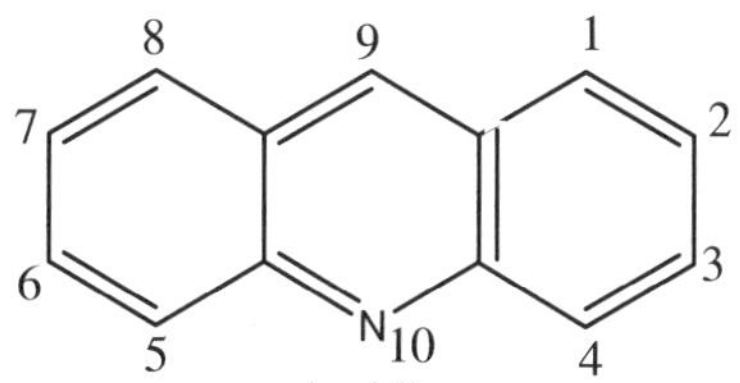
Acridine
(exception to systemic numbering)

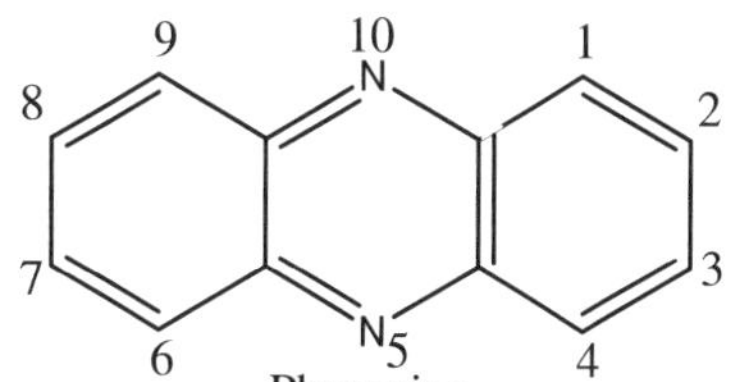
Phenazine

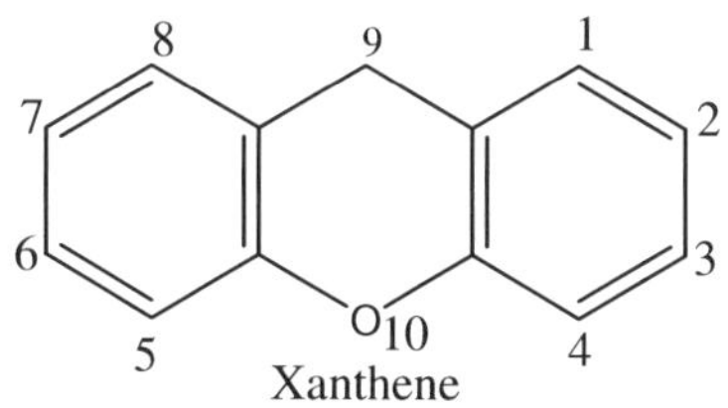
Xanthene

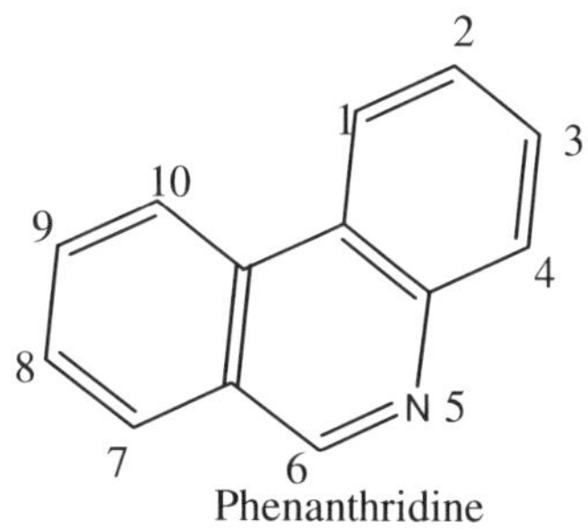
Phenanthridine

Spiro Heterocycles

These are compounds in which two rings are fused at a common point are known as Spiro compounds and the common atom which is quaternary in nature is designated as spiro atom. According to the number of spiro atoms, spiro compounds are classified into monospiro, dispiro and trispiro ring systems. For ex:

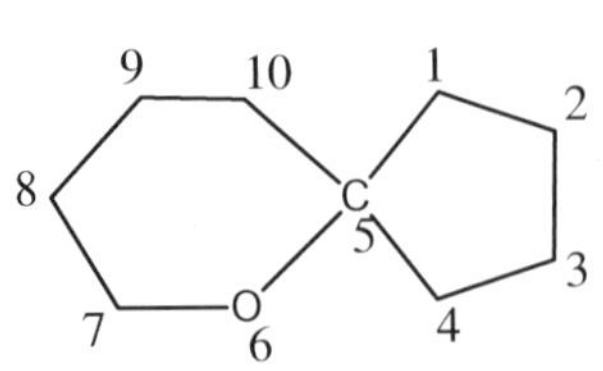

6-Oxaspirodecane

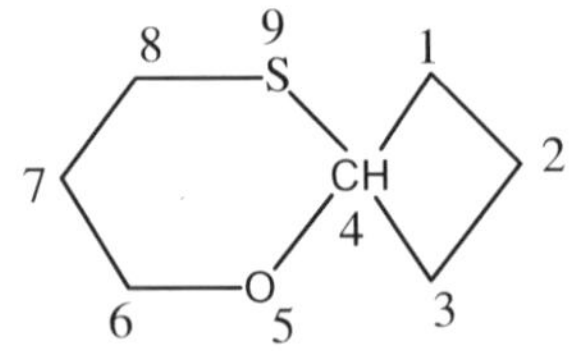

5-Oxa-9-thiaspiro nonane

Bridged Heterocycles

Heterocyclic systems in which two rings with two or more common atoms is known as Bridged heterocycles. for eg:

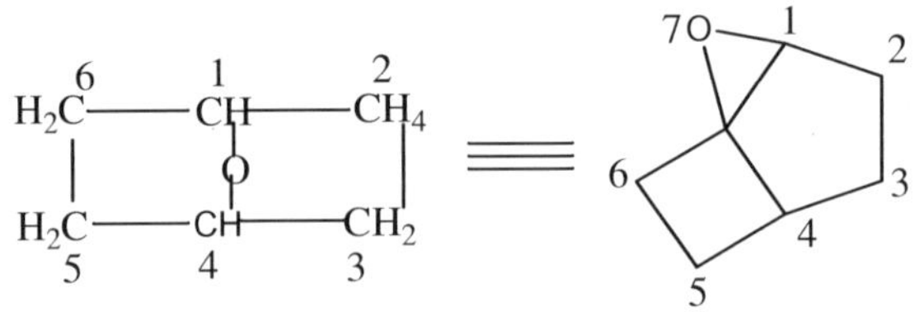

7-Oxabicyclo heptane

Chemical nature of Aromatic heterocycles

In the case of six membered aromatic heterocycles, the electronegative heteroatom causes withdrawl of electrons from the ring carbon atoms and thus affect localization of electrons with the result of electron deficiency on the ring carbon atoms. The six membered heterocycles are therefore known as π deficient aromatic heterocycles. Introduction of further heteroatom in the ring again decreases π electron density in the ring carbon atoms. But in the case of five membered aromatic heterocycles, lone pair of electron on the heteroatom delocalize six π electrons over five π atoms. So the electron density on each carbon atom is more and therefore five membered heterocycles are referred as excessive aromatic heterocycles. The order of aromaticity in five membered heterocycle is sulfur heterocycles > nitrogen heterocycles > oxygen heterocycles.

Reactivity in Aromatic heterocycles

Aromatic compounds are characterized by their extra stability due to delocalized π electron system, & substitution reactions rather than addition reactions with the retention of aromatic character. Nucleophilic attack and Electrophilic attack are the expected reactions can occur in aromatic heterocycles.

Nucleophilic attack

Heteroatom - Oxygen/Nitrogen/Sulfur bonded to carbon atom with multiple bond can accept shared pair of π electrons and permits the attack of Nucleophile. Diagramatically we can represent as;

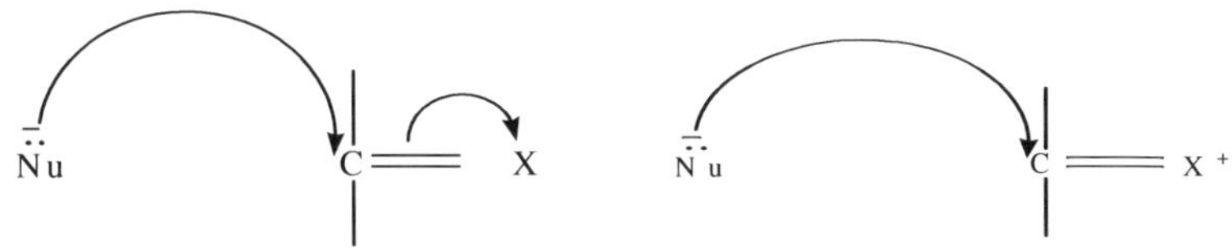

Nucleophilic attack takes place at the atom of low electron density.

Electrophilic attack

Lone pair of electrons on the heteroatom - Oxygen/Nitrogen/Sulfur can be made available for the electrophilic attack. Diagramatically we can represent as;

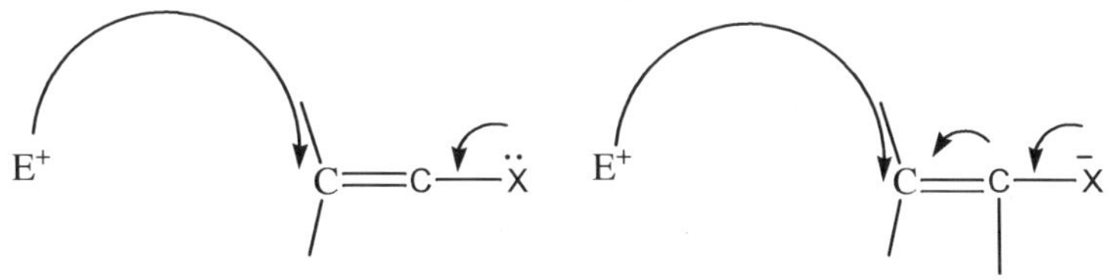

Electrophilic attack takesplace at the atom having high electron density Now we shall discuss some important heterocycles in detail.

PYRROLE

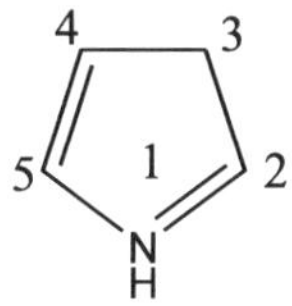

Pyrrole

Pyrrole is an important π excessive aromatic five membered heterocycle present in many natural substances like Alkaloids, Chlorophyll, Haematin, Vitamin B_{12} and Bile pigments.

Extraction

Pyrrole have been isolated in pure form from bone oil. Schematic representation for pyrrole extraction given below;

Bone oil $\xrightarrow{\text{washed } \bar{C} \text{ alkali}}$ Bone oil free from acidic substances $\xrightarrow[\text{dil.acid}]{\text{washed } \bar{C}}$ Bone oil from bases $\xrightarrow{\text{free fractionol distillation}}$ Fraction (`100-150°C) $\xrightarrow{\text{KOH fusion}}$ Potassio pyrrole $\xrightarrow[\text{distillation}]{\text{steam}}$ Pyrrole

Characterestic Chemical test for pyrrole. (Ehrlich test)

Pyrrole reacts with 4-dimethylaminobenzaldehyde in the presence of hydrochloric acid produces purple colour.

Now, will discuss some important synthetic routes for pyrrole;

Pyrrole can be synthesised by passing a mixture of acetylene and ammonia through a red hot tube

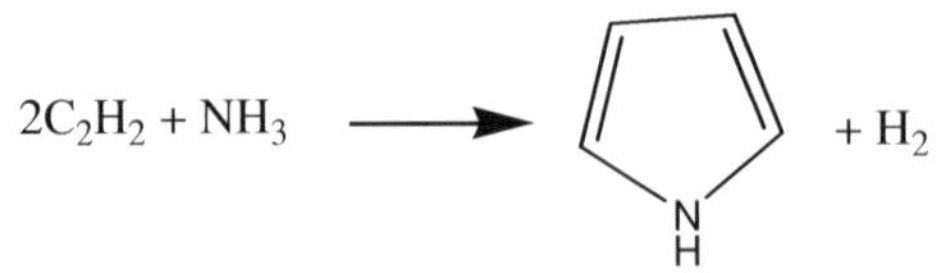

When succinimide distilled with zinc dust, pyrrole produced

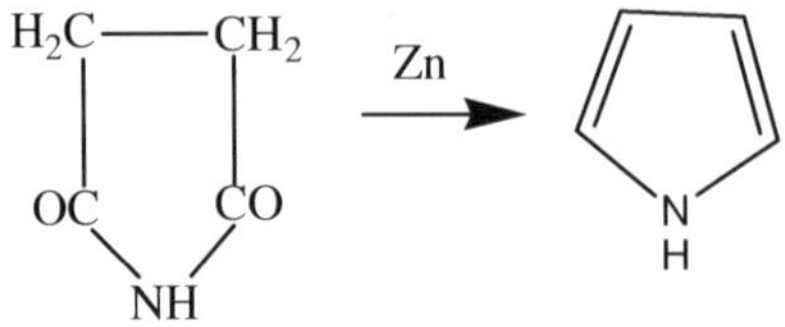

Pyrrole is manufactured by passing a mixture of furan, ammonia and steam over heated alumina.

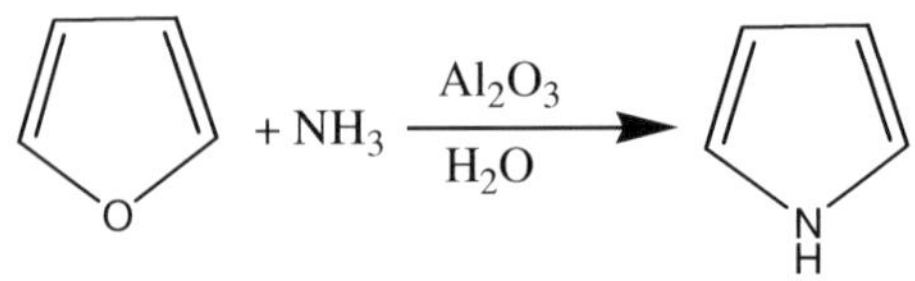

Knorr Pyrrole Synthesis

This synthesis involves Cyclic condensation of α amino ketones or α-amino β-keto esters with β-diketones or β keto esters.

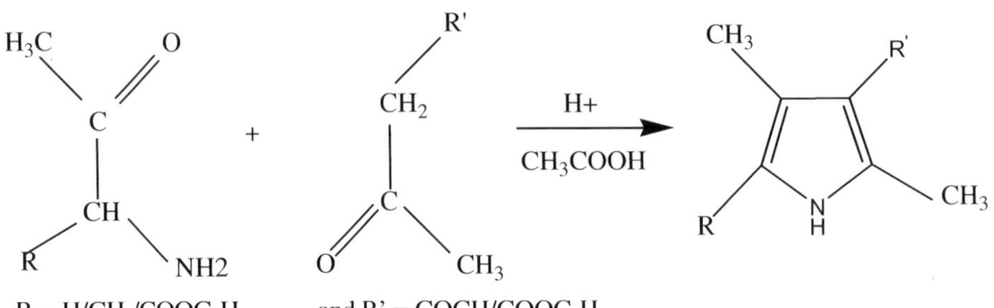

$R = H/CH_3/COOC_2H_5$ and $R' = COCH/COOC_2H_5$

Hantzsch Pyrrole Synthesis

It involves the reaction of β-diketones or β keto esters with β-halo ketones or aldehydes in the presence of ammonia or primary amine.

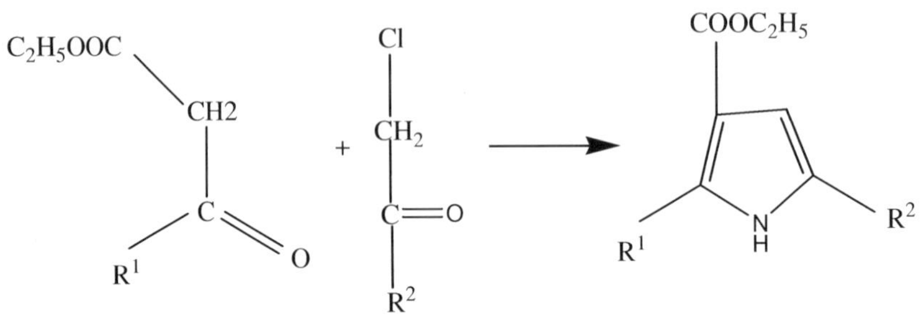

Paal - Knorr synthesis

This method involves cyclic condensation of 1,4-diketones with ammonia or its derivatives.

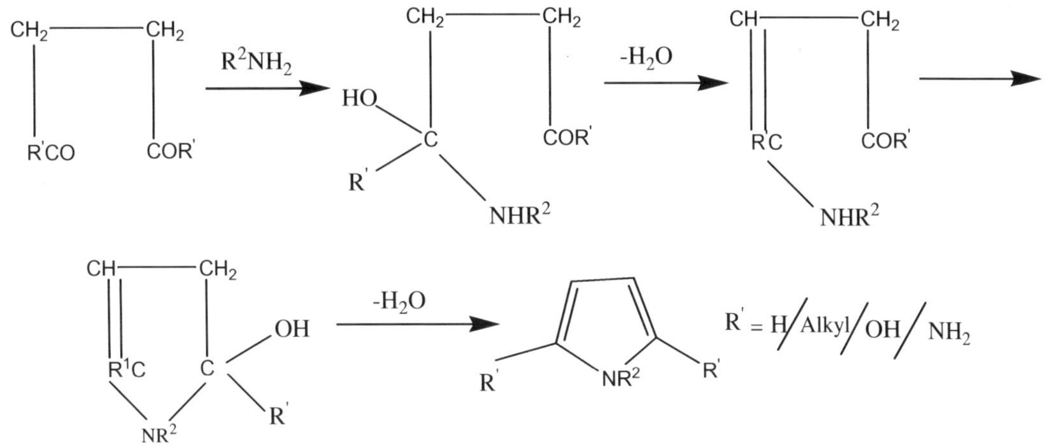

Substituted pyrroles by reaction of 1,4-dienes with Amines

Metal ion assisted amination of 1,4-dienes with primary amines followed by cyclization provides N-Substituted pyrroles.

eg: 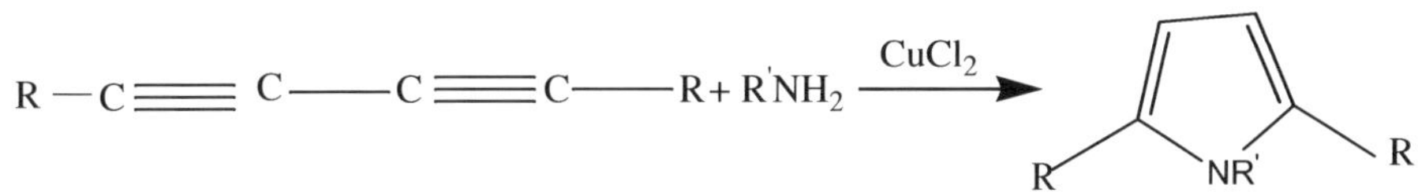

Basicity of pyrrole

Pyrrole is a weak base, since lone pair of electrons on the nitrogen atom is involved in cyclic delocalization [(4n + 2) π electron system] and is less available for protonation.

Chemical properties of Pyrrole

A. Electrophilic Substitution Reactions

Pyrrole is a π excessive aromatic heterocycle which undergoes electrophilic susbstitution preferentially at carbon-2.

A1. Nitration

Pyrrole undergoes nitration by nitric acid in acetic anhydride at low temperature gives 2-nitropyrrole as major product together with 3-nitropyrrole.

$$HNO_3 + (CH_3CO)_2O \longrightarrow \underset{\text{Nitrating agent}}{CH_3\text{-}\overset{\overset{\displaystyle O}{\|}}{C}\text{-}ONO_2} + CH_3COOH$$

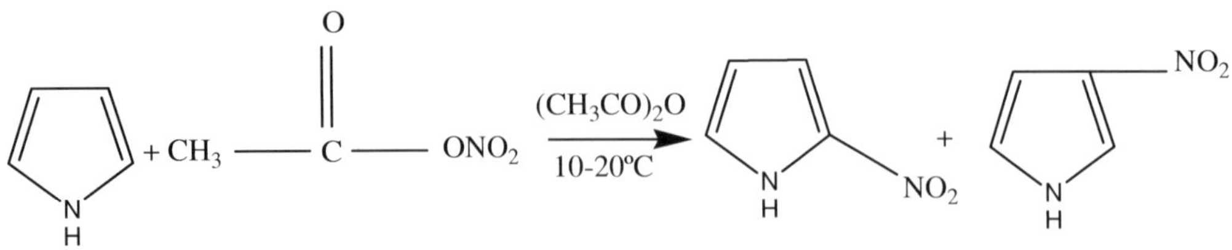

A2. Halogenation

Pyrrole undergoes halogenation at all strongly activating positions.

Chlorination

Sulfonyl Chloride in ether can be used to chlorinate pyrrole.

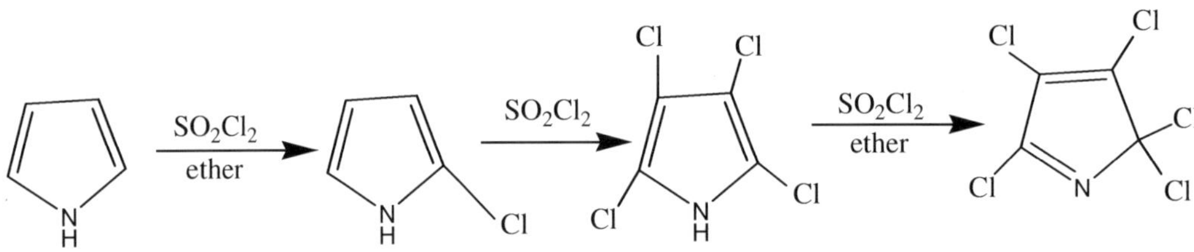

Bromination

Pyrrole on bromination with bromine in acetic acid gives 2,3,4,5-tetra-bromopyrrole.

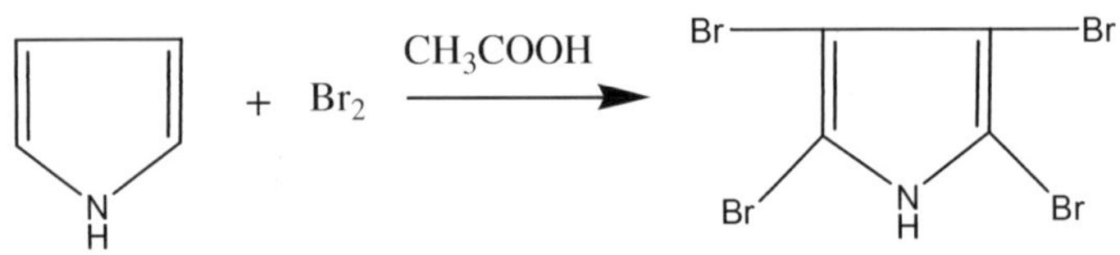

Iodination

Iodination of pyrrole with iodine in aqueous potassium iodide gives tetraiodopyrrole-which is used as a substitute for Iodoform

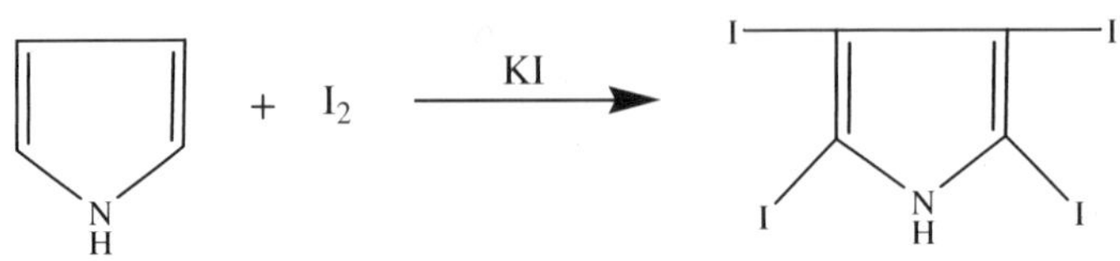

A3. Sulfonation

Pyrrole undergoes polymerization by concentrated sulfuric acid under ordinary conditions. Therefore sulfonation done by mild sulfonating agent like pyridine-sulfur trioxide.

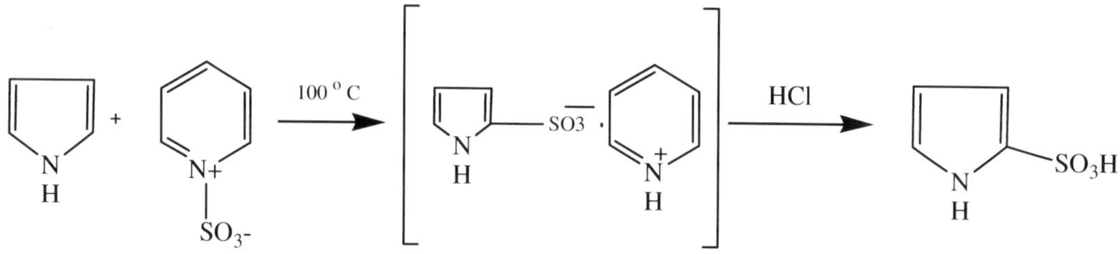

A4. Acylation

Pyrrole on acylation by acetic anhydride at 100-150°C give 2-acyl and 2,5-diacyl pyrroles.

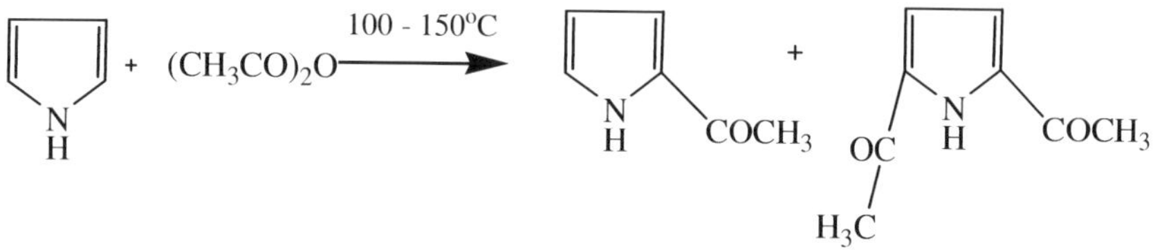

Pyrrole on acylation by acetic anhydride in the presence of sodium acetate gives N-acylpyrrole.

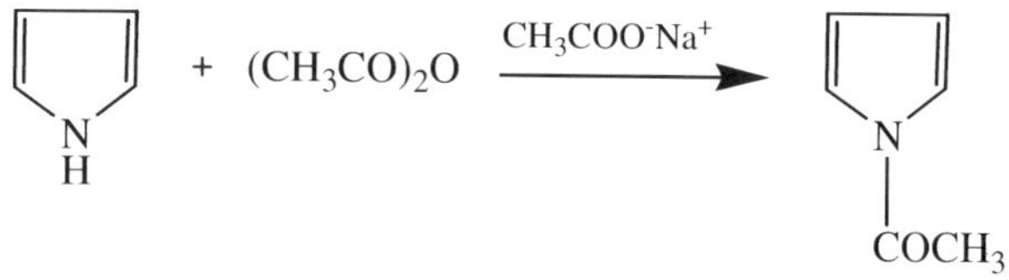

Houben - Hoesch Reaction

In this acylation reaction pyrrole reacts with aliphatic nitrile and hydrochloric acid in the presence of Lewis acid introduces an acyl group at α position.

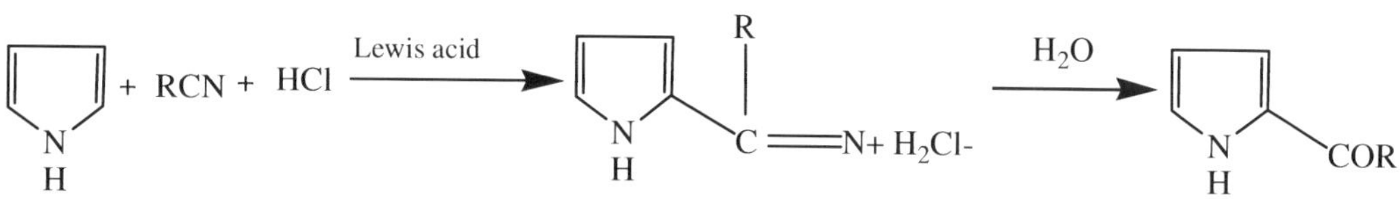

A5. Formylation

Formylation in pyrrole takesplace mainly at 2nd position.

Gatterman Formylation

Pyrrole when reacts with zinc cyanide and hydrochloric acid undergoes formylation.

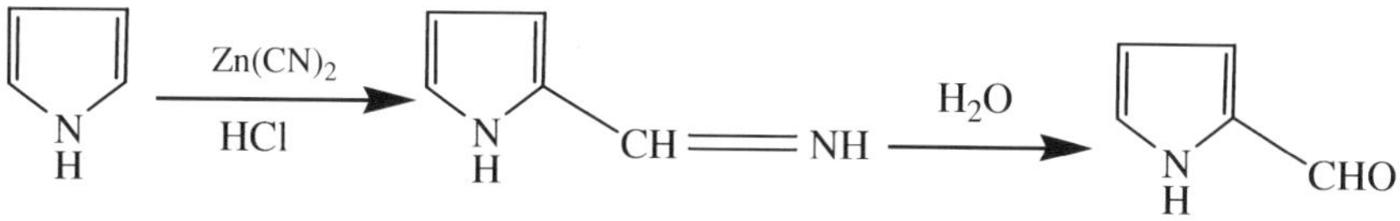

A6. Alkylation

Friedel - Crafts alkylation of pyrrole with Grignard reagent produces 2-alkylpyrrole via 1-alkyl pyrrole involving Hofmanmartius type rearrangement.

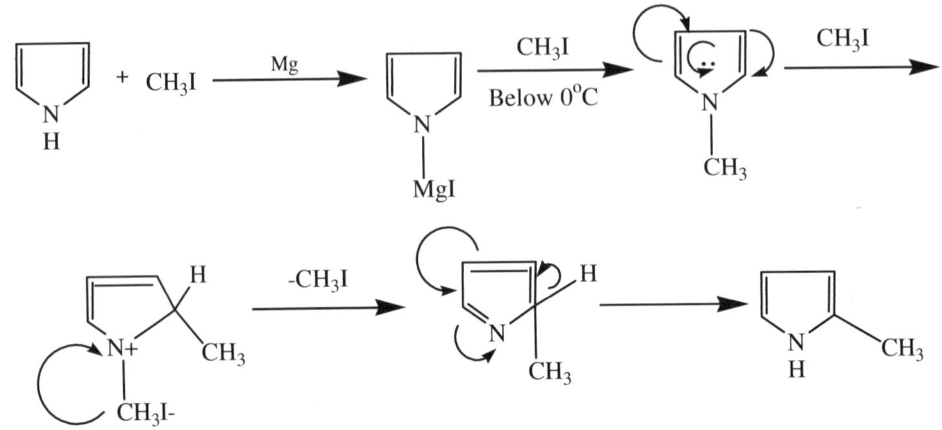

A7. Hydroxymethylation (Mannich Reaction)

Pyrrole undergoes Mannich reaction with formaldehyde and primary or secondary amine in the presence of an acid with the introduction of functionalized alkyl group at α-position.

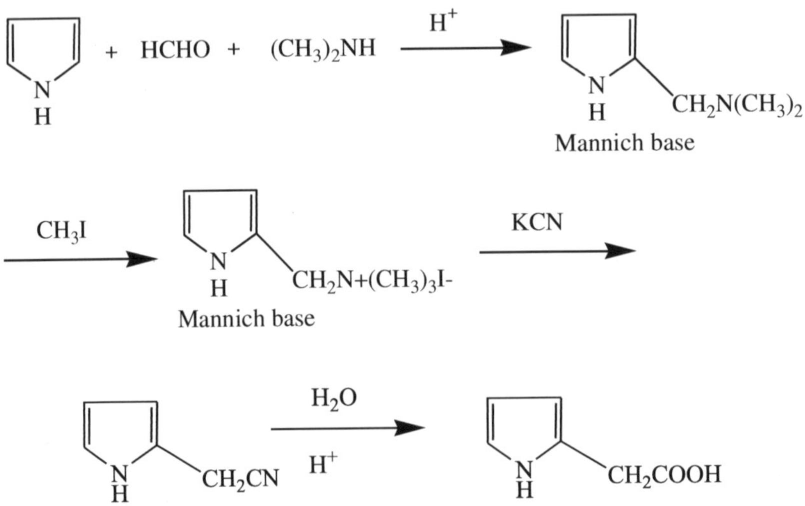

A8. Diazo coupling

Pyrrole undergoes diazo coupling reaction readily with benzene diazonium salts in the presence of alkali.

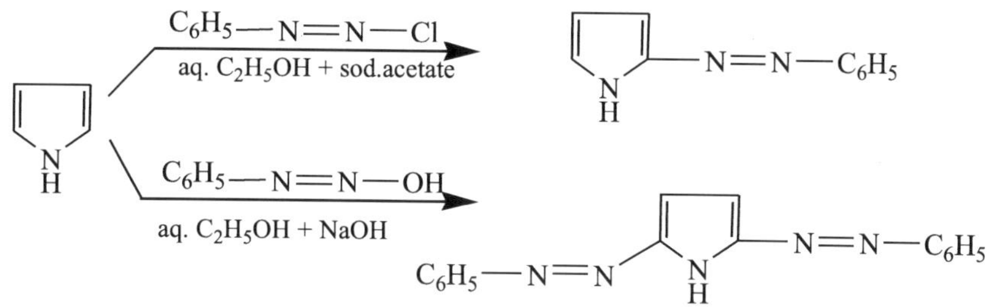

B. Nucleophilic substitution reactions

Nucleophilic substitution reactions are difficult in pyrrole due to its α-electron excessive character.

C. Oxidation

Pyrroles undergo oxidation very easily and forms polymeric products.

C1. Photo-Oxidation

Photosensitized oxidation of pyrrole produces 5-hydroxy 3-pyrrolin-2-one.

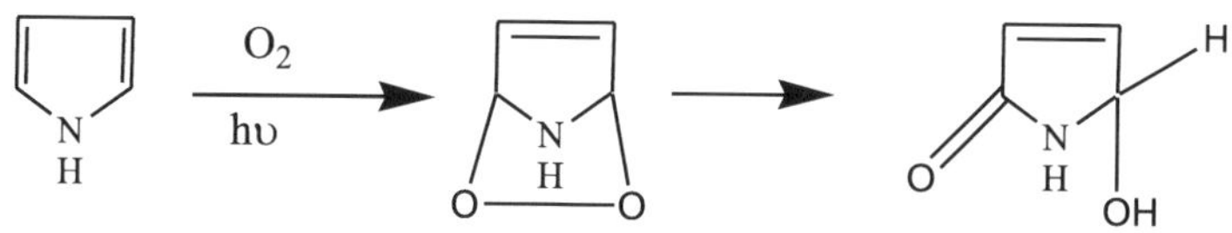

C2. Oxidation with Chromium Trioxide

Oxidation of pyrrole by strong oxidising agents like Chromium trioxide - Sulfuric acid produces maleinimide.

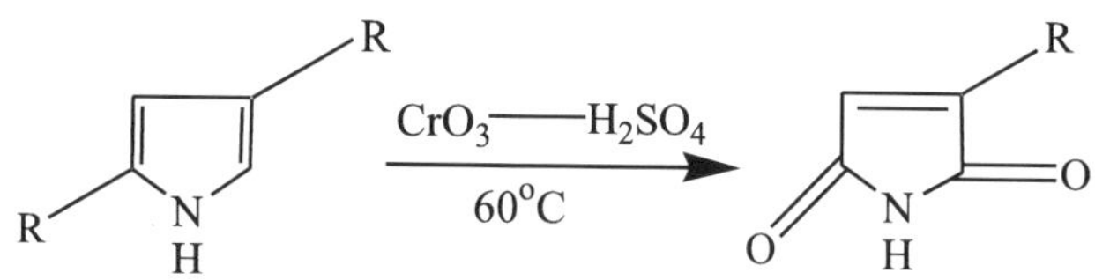

C3. Oxidation with Hydrogen Peroxide

Oxidation of pyrrole with warm hydrogen peroxide in pyridine over a pH range of 4-6 produces a mixture of tautomeric forms of pyrrolin-2-ones.

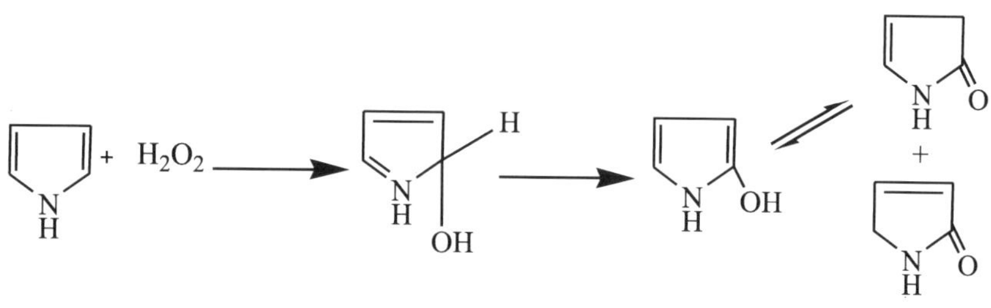

D. Reduction

Zinc and acetic acid reduces pyrrole to pyrroline which on heating with hydriodic acid and red phosphorous gives pyrrolidine.

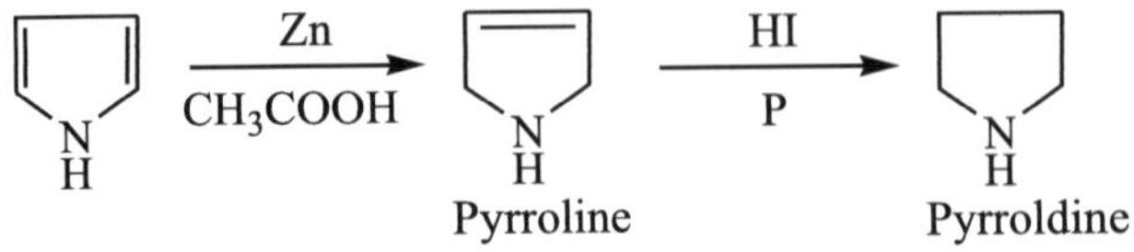

E. Ring expansion

Pyrrole reacts with sodium methoxide and methylene iodide gives pyridine.

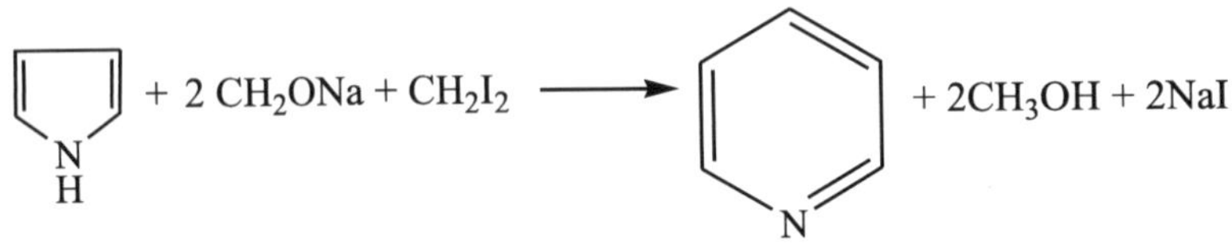

FURAN

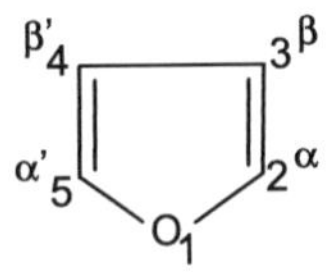

Furan can be isolated from pine wood by distillation commercially importance of furan is attributed to its role as a precursor for a widely used solvent tetrahydrofuran (THF).

Furan can be prepared in many ways; Dry distillation of mucic acid give furoic acid. which on heating undergoes decarboxylation to form furan.

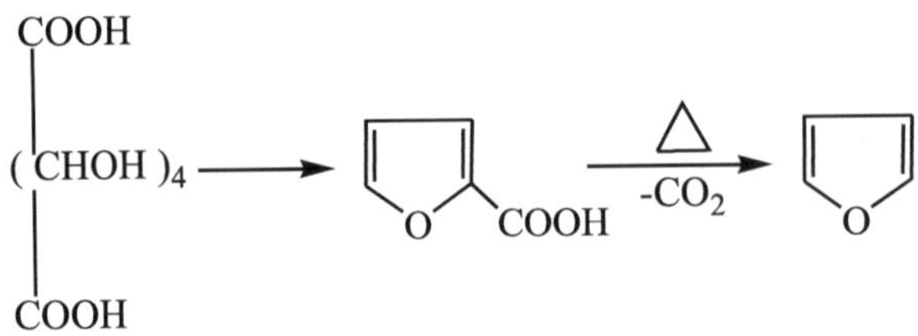

From Aldopentoses or Ketopentoses

Acid catalyzed consecutive dehydrations of aldoses or ketoses result in the formation of α ketoaldehydes which undergoes catalyzed cyclization forms furfural which on steam distillation at 400°C in the presence of oxide catalyst gives furan.

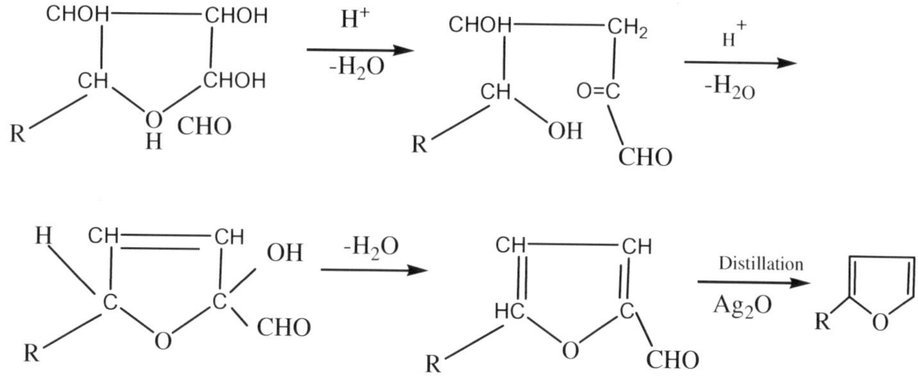

Furan by Photochemical Cyclization

Photochemical reaction of alkynic Ketones in alcohol produces an adduct as intermediate which undergoes dehydrative cyclization produces corresponding furans.

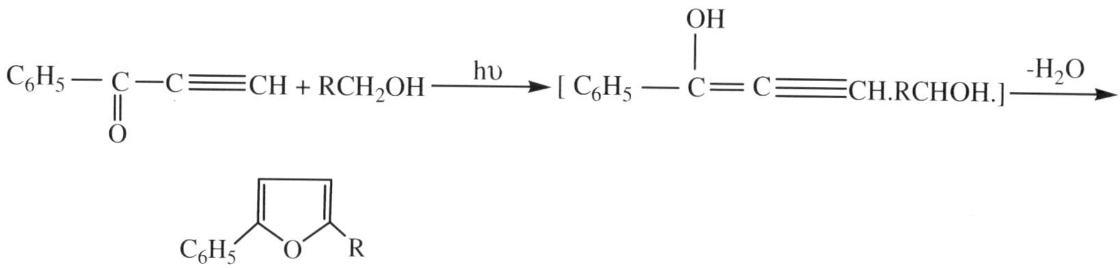

Furan from Alkynyl Sulfonium salts

Alkynyl bromide reacts with dimethyl sulfide in acetonitrile results in alkynyl sulfonium salt which reacts with β diketones give furans.

$$HC \equiv C - CH_2Br + (CH_3)_2S \xrightarrow{CH_3CN}$$

$$HC \equiv C - CH_2S^+(CH_3)_2Br^- \xrightarrow[\text{Prototropic rearrangement}]{C_2H_5OH}$$

$$\underset{\text{alkynyl sulfonium salt}}{H_2C = C = CHS^+(CH_3)_2Br^-} + CH_3COCH_2COCH_3 \xrightarrow{C_2H_5O^-Na^+}$$

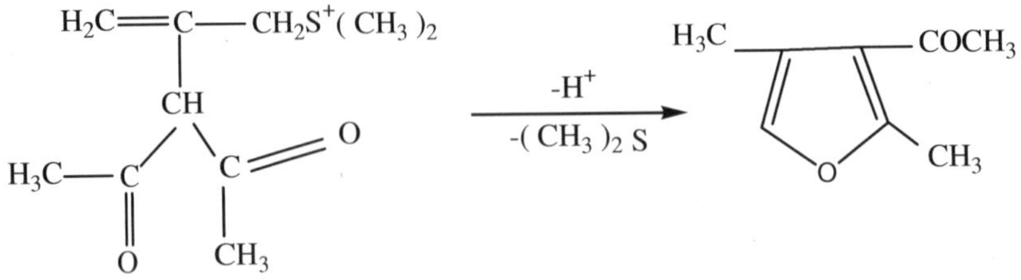

Furan from Sulfur ylides

Sulfur ylides reacts with β-diketones or β-Ketoesters produces furan.

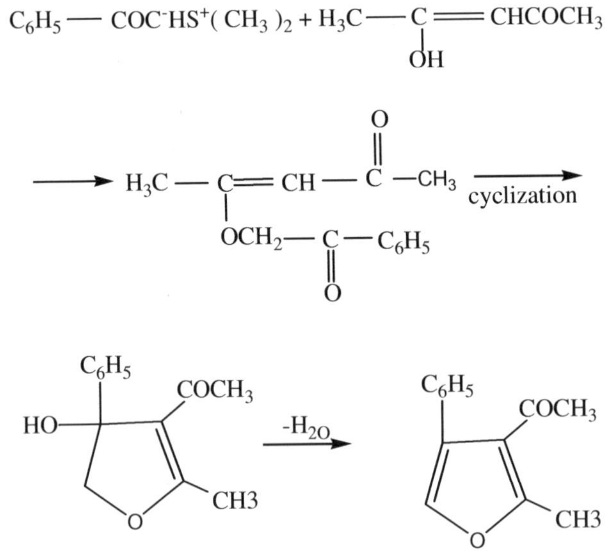

Furan from Phosphorous ylides

Sodium salt of α-hydroxy ketone reacts with β-ethoxyvinyltriphenyl phosphonium salt gives phosphorus ylide which undergoes intramolecular wittig reaction give dihydrofuran. From dihydrofuran one molecule of ethanol losses and forms furan.

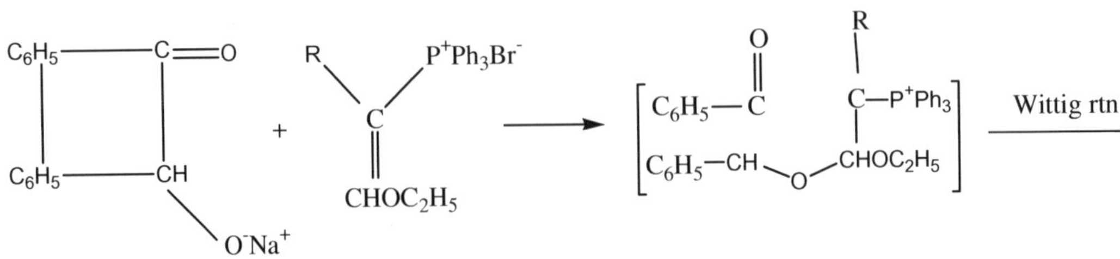

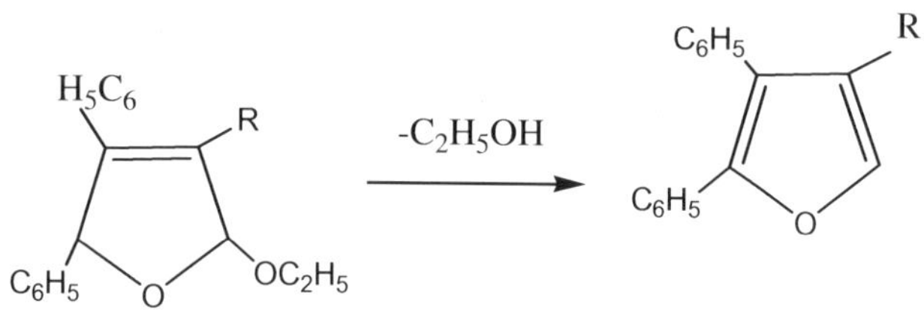

Furan by ring expansion of three membered heterocycle

Alkynic oxiranes in the presence of sulfuric acid and mercuric sulfate gives alkynic diols which rearrange to give Furan.

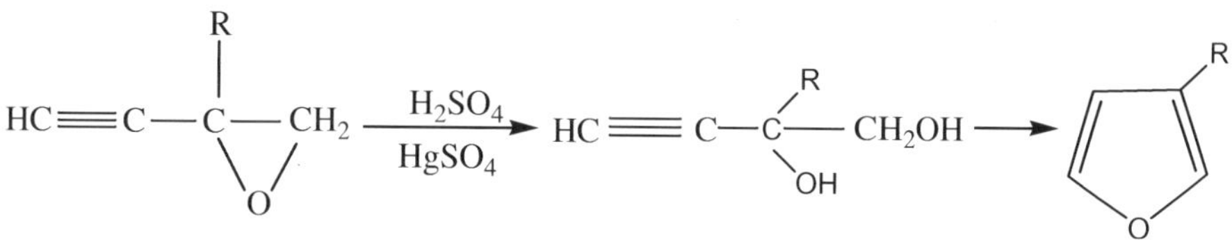

Furan by ring contraction of six membered heterocycle

1,2-dioxins in the presence of alcoholic alkali gives Furan.

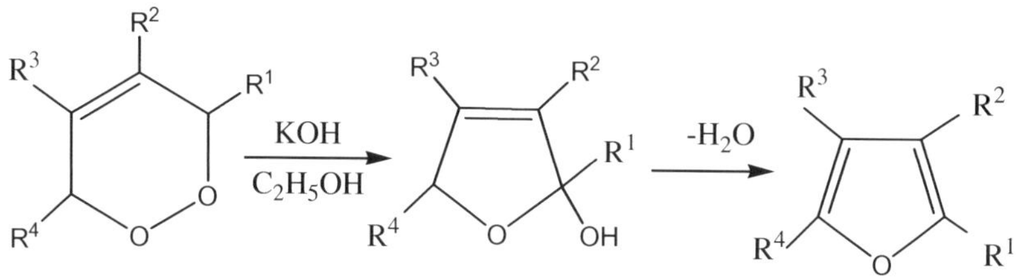

Chemical properties of Furan

Furan is a π-excessive heterocycle and mainly undergoes electrophilic substitution reactions. Electrophilic substitution preferentially takesplace at C-2 and C-5 (α positions).

A1. Nitration

Furan can be nitrated with mild nitrating agent, acetyl nitrate, at low temperature give 2,5-addition product. Pyridine acted upon it to eliminate acetic acid.

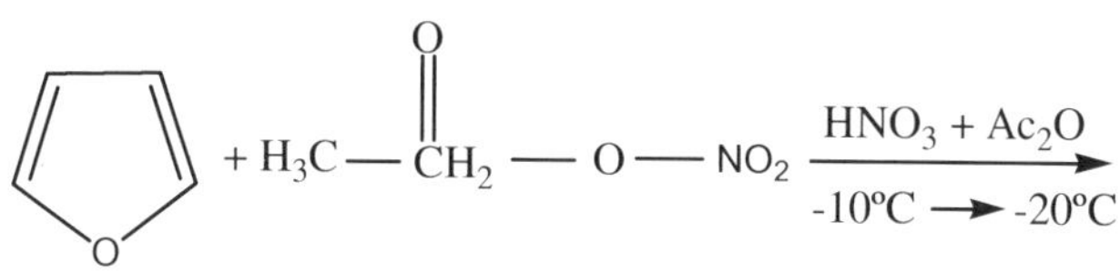

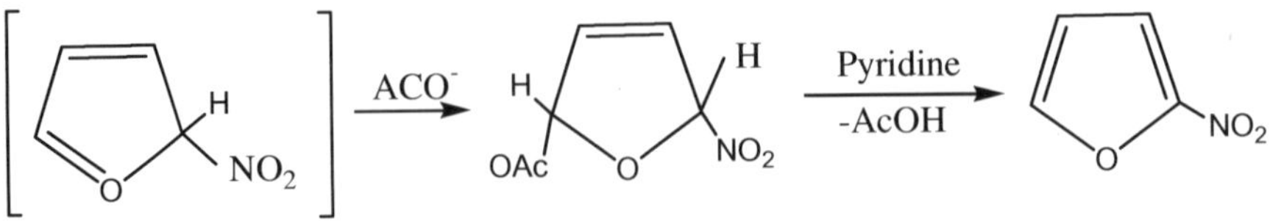

A2. Sulfonation

Furan can be sulfonated with the complex of sulfur trioxide with pyridine.

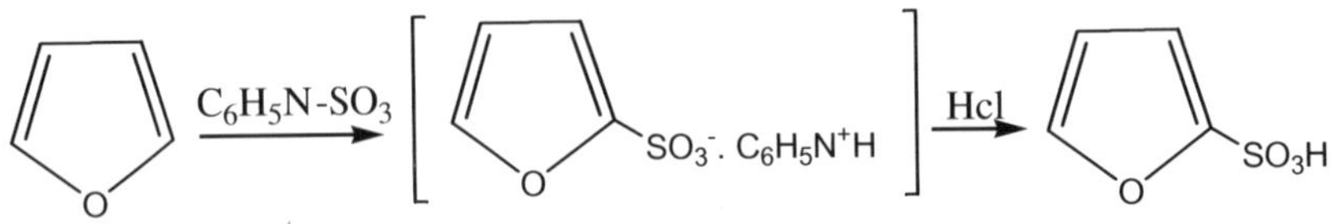

A3. Halogenation

Bromination of furan with dioxane - dibromide at -5°C gives 2-bromofuran

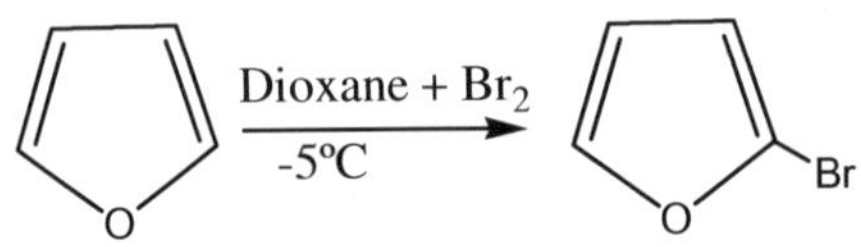

Chlorination of furan with Chlorine in the presence of dichloromethane at - 40°C gives 2-chlorofuran.

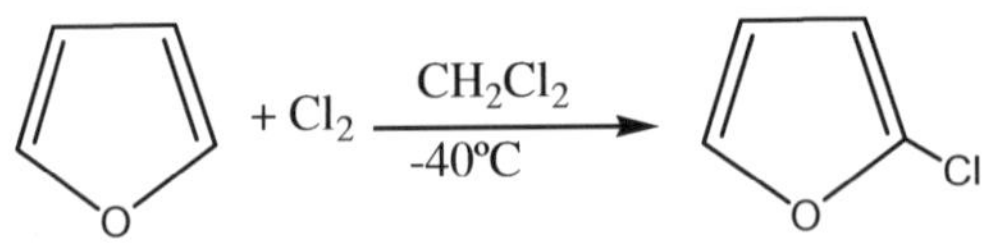

A4. Alkylation

Furan undergoes alkylation by alkenes at 2nd position in the presence of mild catalysts.

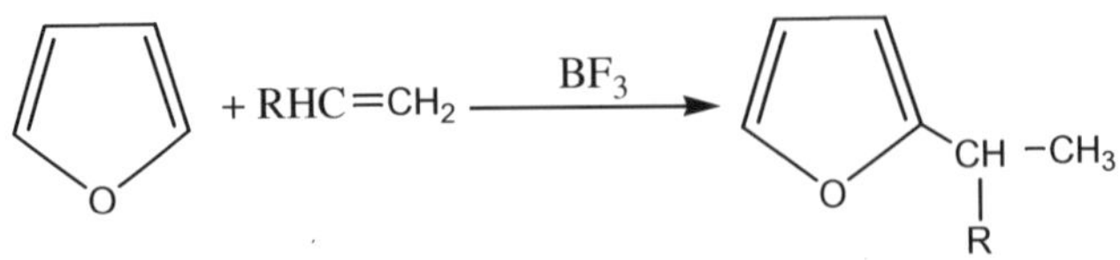

A5. Acylation

Acylation of furan to 2-acylfuran can be done with acid anhydrides in the presence of mild catalysts such as phosphoric acid or boron trifluride.

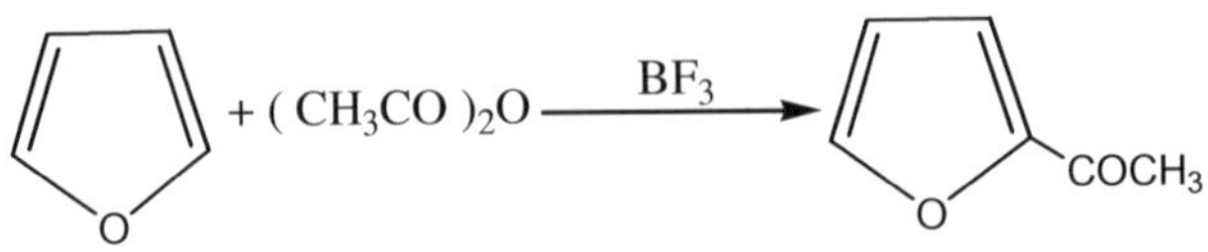

A6. Reaction with diazonium salts

Furan undergoes phenylation instead of diazocoupling with benzenediazonium salts. (Gomberg reaction)

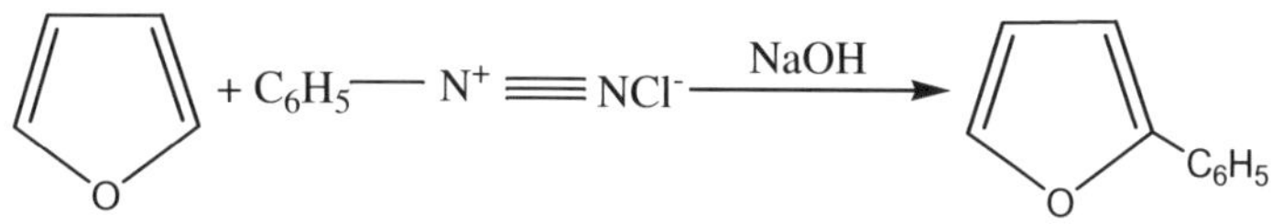

B. Nucleophilic reactions

Nucleophilic substitution mainly takesplace in halogenated Furans - which involves substitution of the halogen atom.

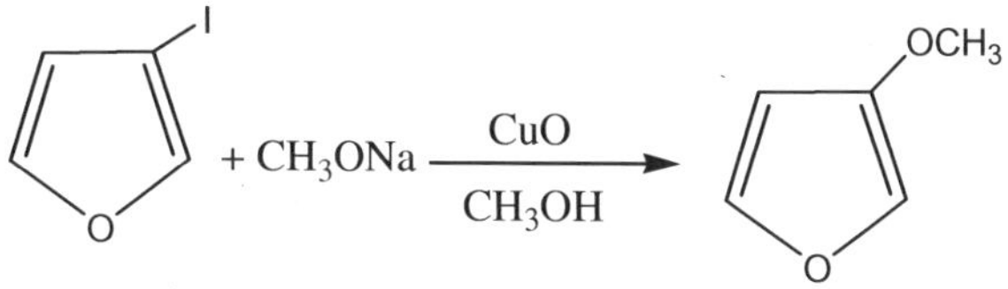

C. Reduction

Furan catalytically reduced by Raney nickel to Tetrahydrofuran.

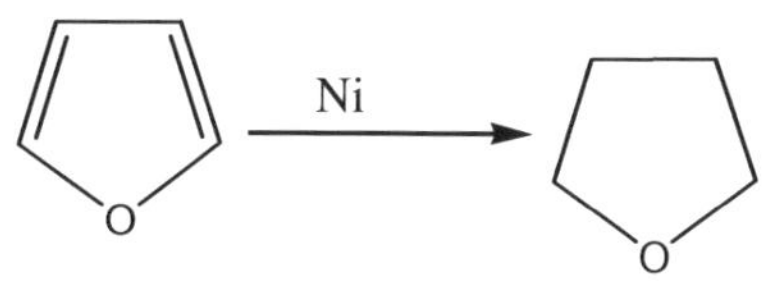

D. Cyclo addition reactions

Furan can acts as diene and react with dienophile to form adduct. Furan reacts with maleic anhydride in acetonitrile at 40°C gives an endo adduct which converts into an exo adduct.

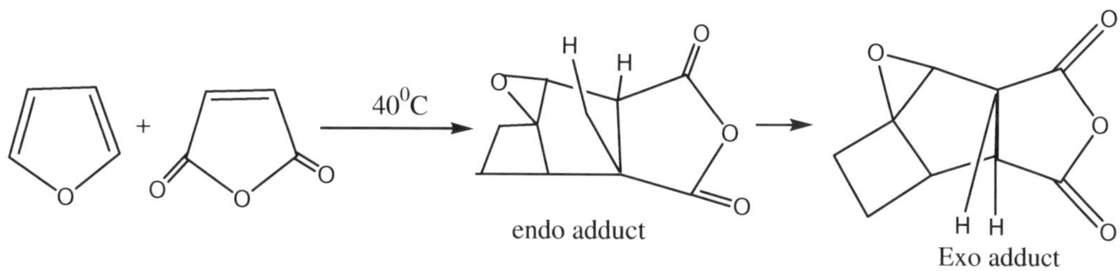

E. Photo Chemical Cyclo addition reaction

Furan undergoes photo chemical Cycloaddition reactions when irradiated with carbonyl compounds produce oxetanes.

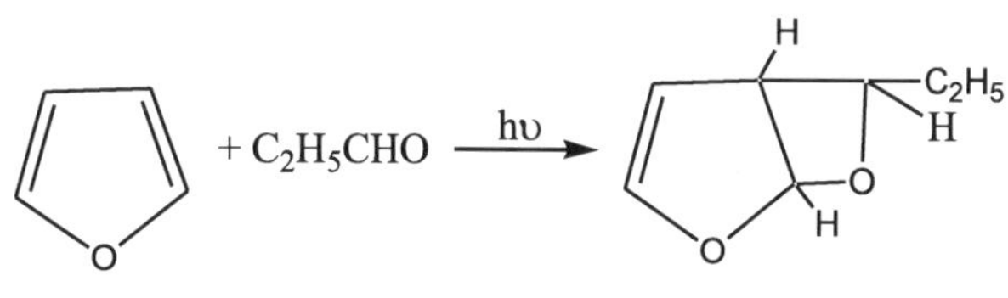

THIOPHENE

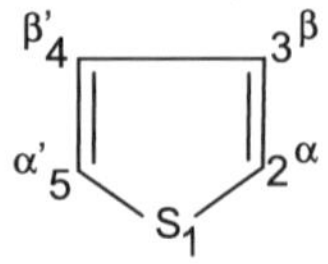

Thiophene present as an important component in the synthetic pharmaceuticals and dyes. Tetrahydrothiophen occur in Biotin-(Vitamin-H). Thiophene occurs in benzene fraction of coal tar which is converted to thiophene-2-sulfonic acid with cold concentrated sulphuric acid, which is soluble in water seperated from water insoluble benzene. Now will discuss some synthetic methods for preparing Thiophene.

From Hydrocarbons by Cyclization reactions

Cyclization of hydrocarbons like butanes, butenes or butadienes react with sulfur at high temperature gives thiophene.

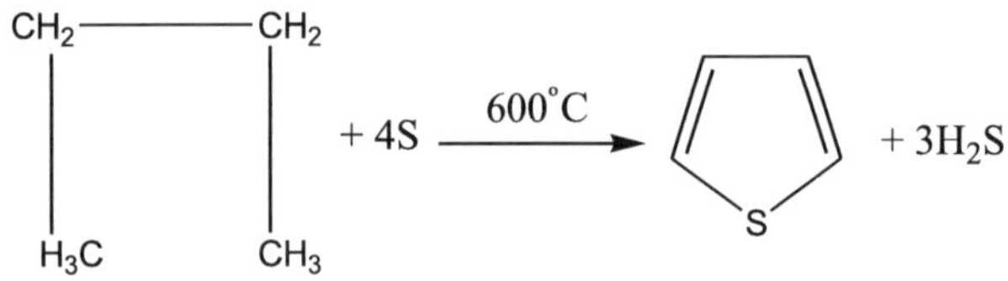

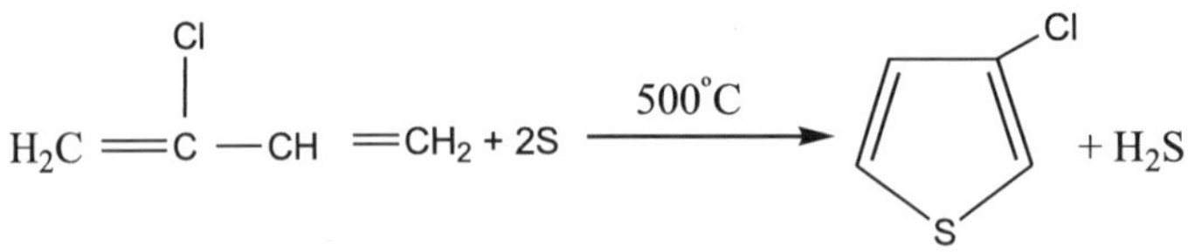

Alkenes & alkadienes substituted with acyl groups are cyclized readily with sulfur at low temperature give Thiophene.

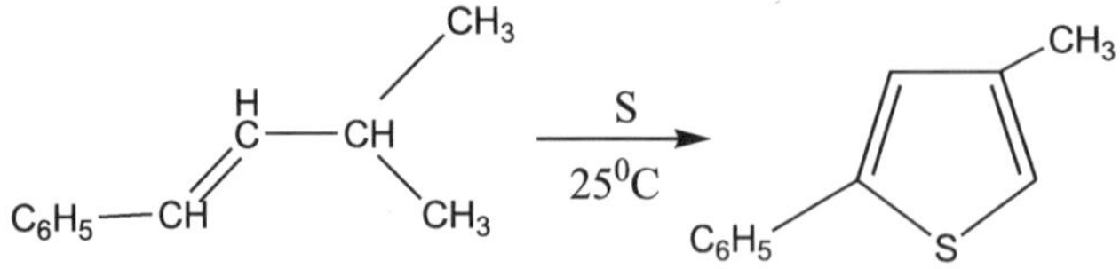

Thiophene from 1,4-diketones by paal synthesis

Diketones react with phosphorous pentasulfide forms Thiophene.

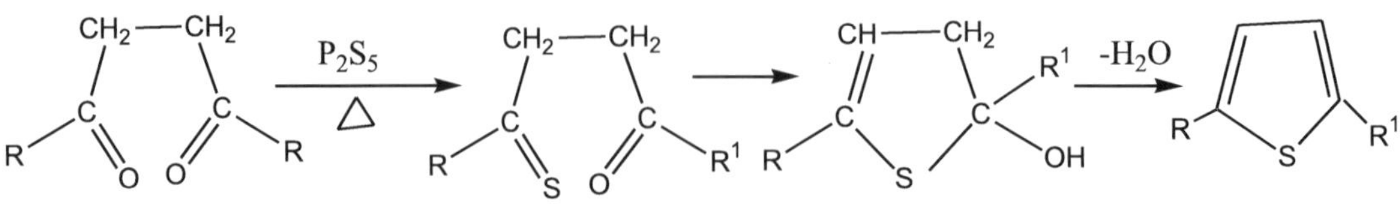

Thiophene by the reaction of activated alkynes with α mercpto ketones

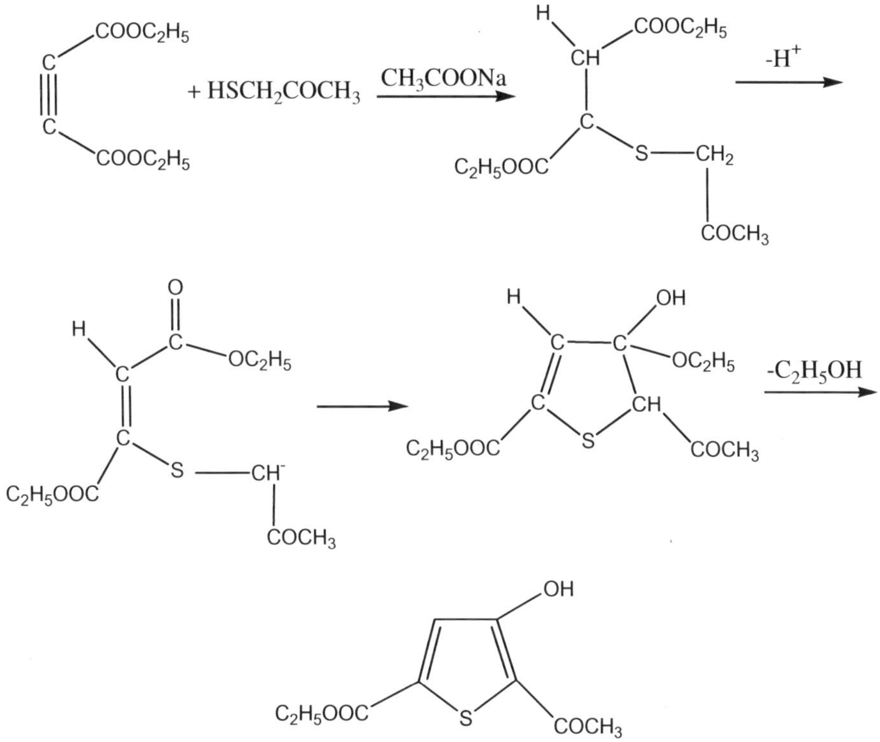

Thiophene by Gewald Synthesis

Condensation of α-mercapto ketones with activated methylene nitriles in the presence of a base gives 2-aminothiophene.

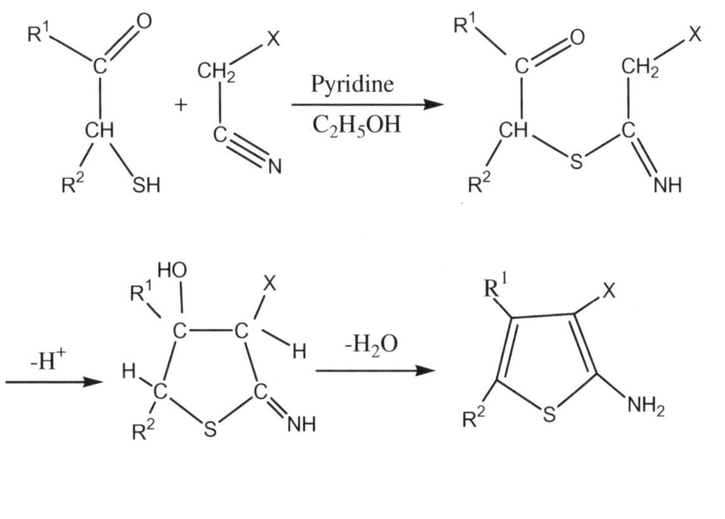

Thiophene by Hinsberg Synthesis

Condensation of α-diketones with dimethylene sulfides in the presence of alcoholic sodium ethoxide give Thiophene.

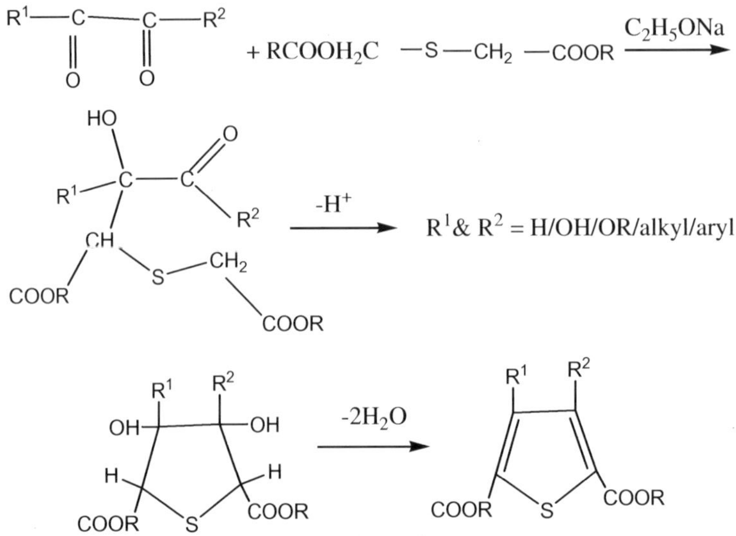

Thiophene by Cyclization reactions

Stilbene react with sulfur give tetraphenylthiophene.

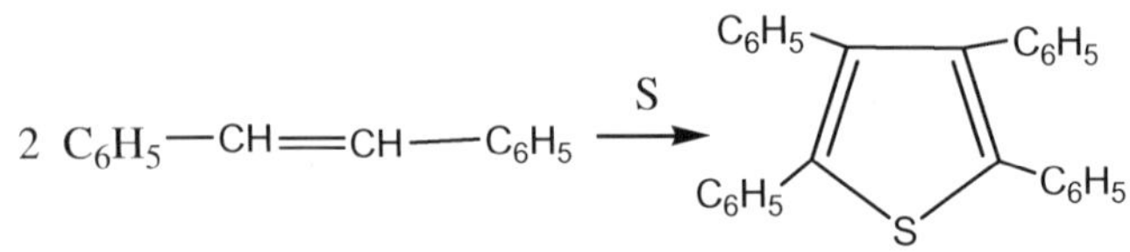

Chemical Characterestics of Thiophene

Thiophene is a π-excessive aromatic heterocycle. Electrophilic attack mainly at α-position to sulfur.

A1. Nitration

Thiophene undergoes nitration by acetyl nitrate at 10°C.

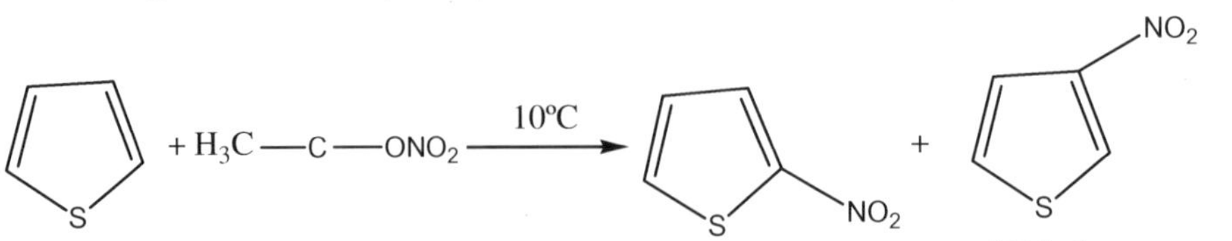

95%   5% in less amount

α-selectivity in nitration decreases with strong nitrating agents.

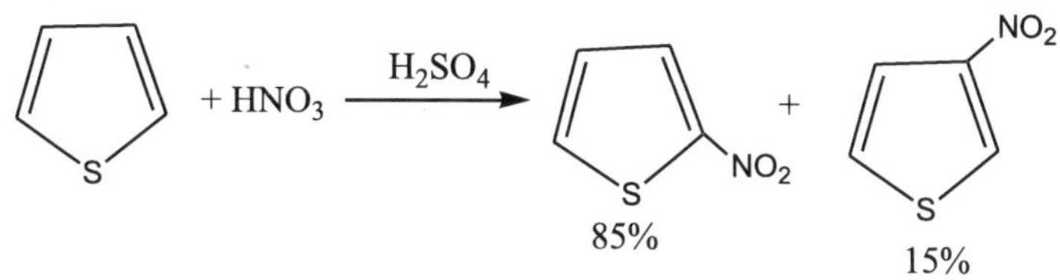

A2. Sulfonation

Thiophene readily sulfonated with 85% H_2SO_4 at room temp.

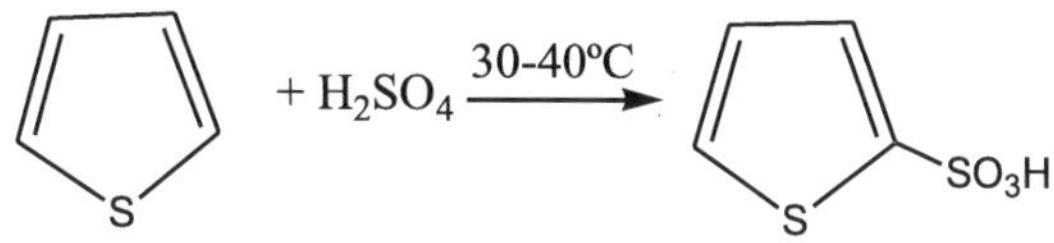

But, Thiophene react with Chlorosulfonic acid give Thiophene-2-Sulfonyl Chloride.

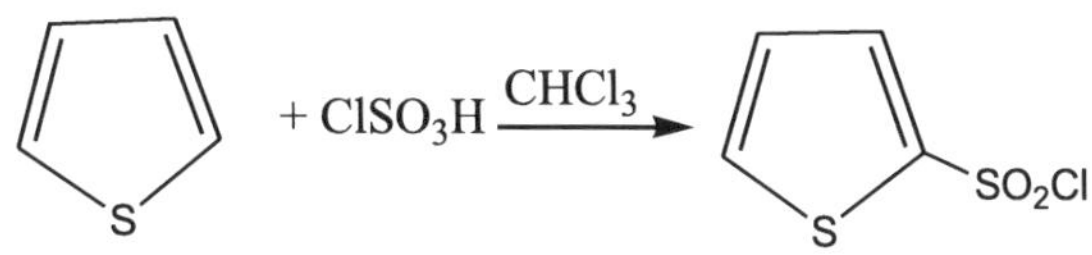

A3. Halogenation

Chlorination

Thiophene readily reacts with chlorine give a mixture of chlorinated thiophenes.

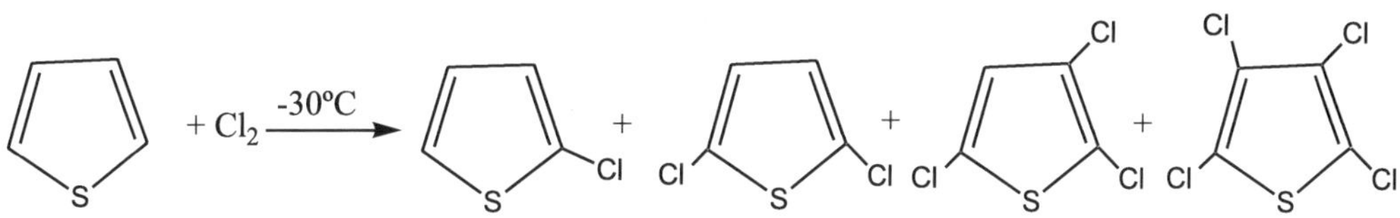

Bromination

Thiophene can be brominated by molecular bromine in acetic acid in the presence of ether or carbon tetra chloride give 2-bromothiophene.

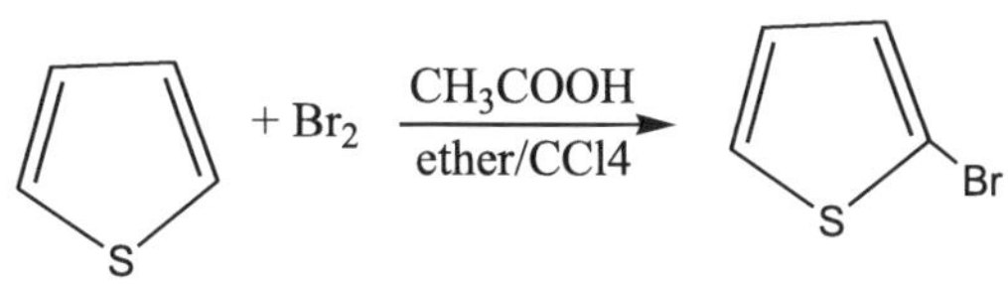

Bromination of thiophene in the presence of base give dibromothiophene.

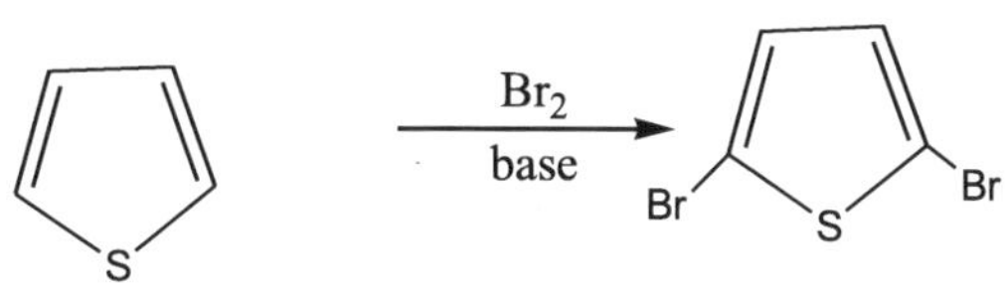

Iodination

Iodination of thiophene with iodine in the presence of mercury oxide gives 2-iodothiophene & 2,5-iodothiophene.

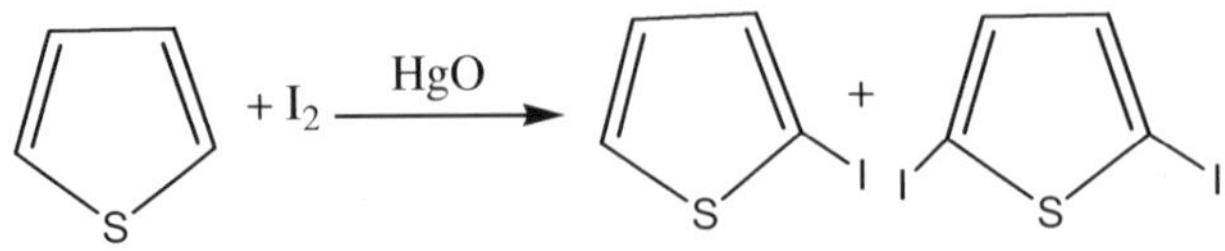

A4. Alkylation

Alkylation of thiophene with alkenes in the presence phosphoric acid or boron trifiuoride gives a mixturc of α and β-isomers.

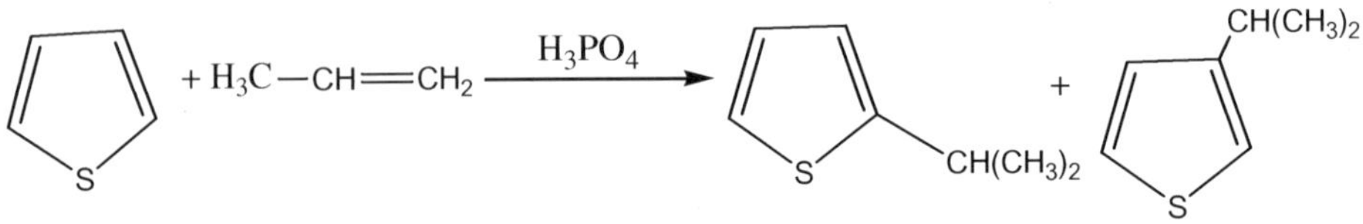

A5. Acylation

Thiophene can be acylated by acid anhydrides in the presence of phosphoric acid or by acid chlorides in the presence of stannic chloride.

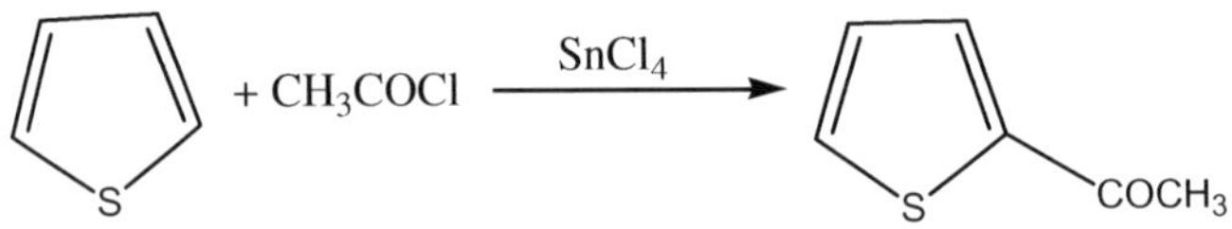

A6. Mercuration

Thiophene reacts with mercury acetate resulting in acetoxymercuration at all free nuclear positions.

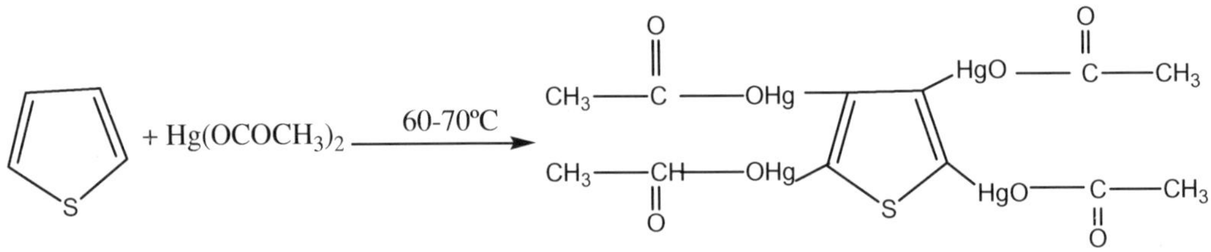

B. Nucleophilic reactions

Nucleophilic substitution is rare in Thiophene.

C. Reactions of Thiophene with Reducing agents

C1. Catalytic reduction

Thiophene can be catalytically reduced to Tetrahydrothiophene (Thiophane)

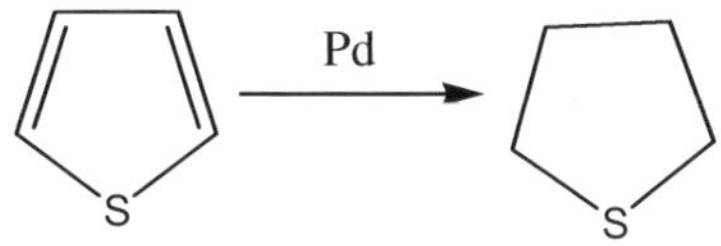

C2. Birch reduction

Reduction of thiophene with lithium - ammonia or sodium-ammonia in the presence of alcohol give mixture of 2,3-dihydro & 2,5-dihydrothiophene.

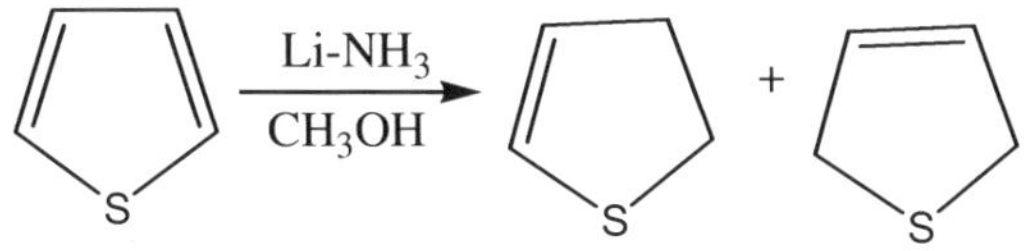

C3. Reductive Desulfurization

Thiophenes reductively desulfurized by Raney nickel in alcohol at 60-70°C.

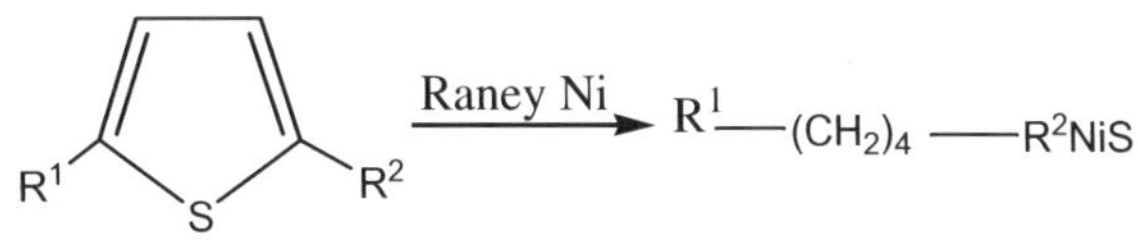

D. Thiophene with electron deficient species

D1. Reaction with Carbenes

Thiophene undergoes cycloaddition reaction with carbenes forms cyclopropane derivative.

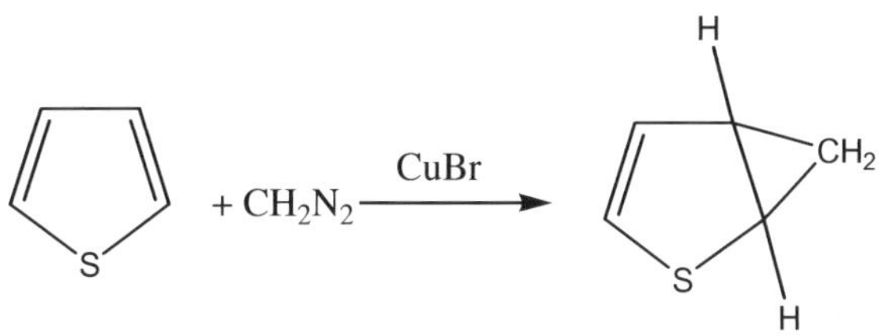

D2. Reaction with Nitrenes

Thiophene reacts with ethoxycarbonylnitrene forms N-ethoxycarbonylpyrrole.

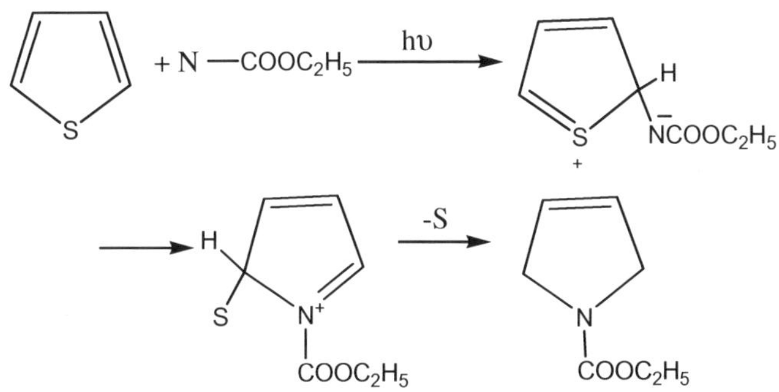

E. Cycloaddition reactions of Thiophene

Tetramethylthiophene undergoes cycloaddition reaction with dicyanoacetylene in the presence of aluminium chloride gives cycloadduct.

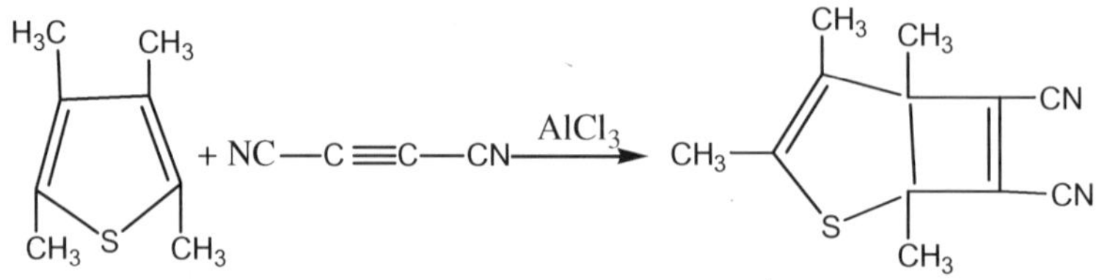

IMIDAZOLE

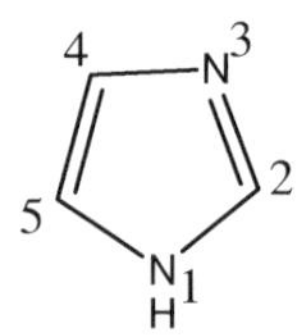

Imidazole is a five membered heterocycle and is also known as 1,3-diazole. Nitrogen in the first position is pyrrole type nitrogen. Nitrogen in third position is pyridine type. Imidazole occur in many natural compounds like histidine, Purine, biotine ...etc. Imidazole can be prepared in many ways. We shall discuss them one by one.

Imidazole by Marckwald synthesis

α-amino ketones reacts with Cyanates, thiocyanates or isothiocyanates give 3H-imidazoline-2-thiones (2-mercaptoimidazoles) which oxidised or dehydrogenated to give corresponding imidazoles.

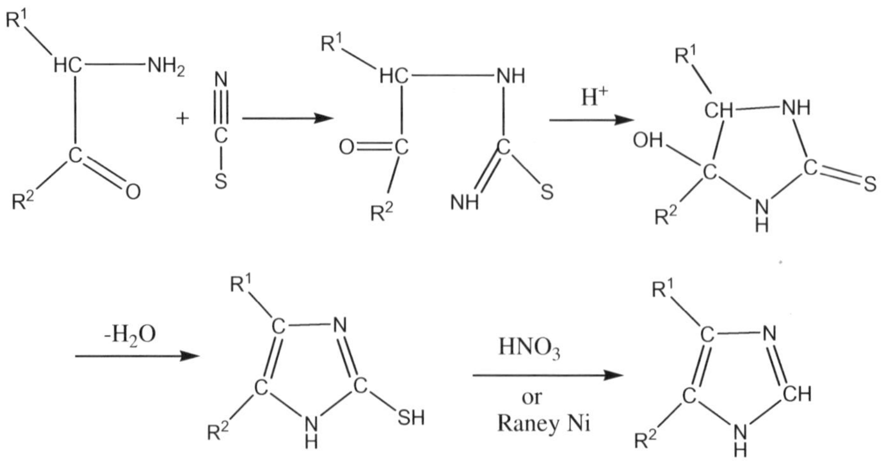

Imidazole by Formamide synthesis

It involves reaction of α-diketones, α-hydroxy, α-halo or α amino Ketones with formaldehyde and ammonia.

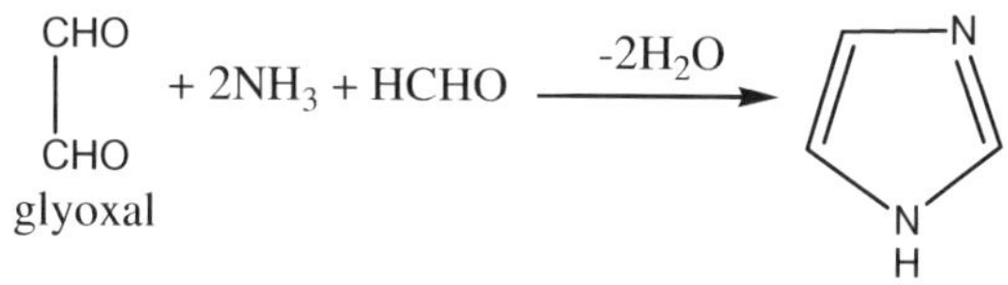

Imidazole by Wallach synthesis

N, N1-disubstituted oxamide react with phosphorous oxychloride give a chlorinated derivative which on reduction by hydroiodic acid give 1-substituted imidazole.

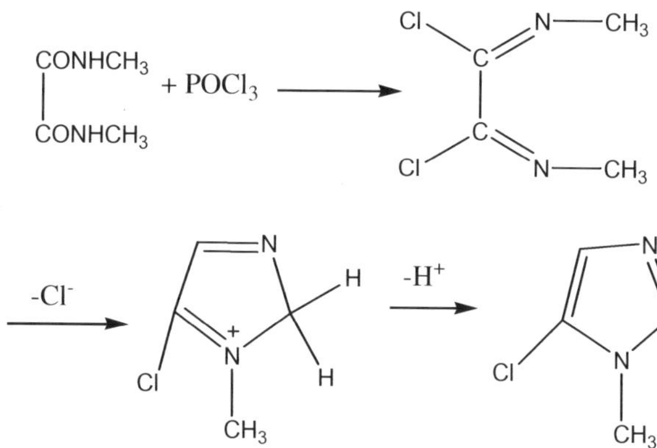

Imidazole by reaction of Arylaldoximes with propiolate ester

Cyclization of arylaldoximes with propiolate ester gives an amidine intermediate which on dehydration gives substituted imidazole.

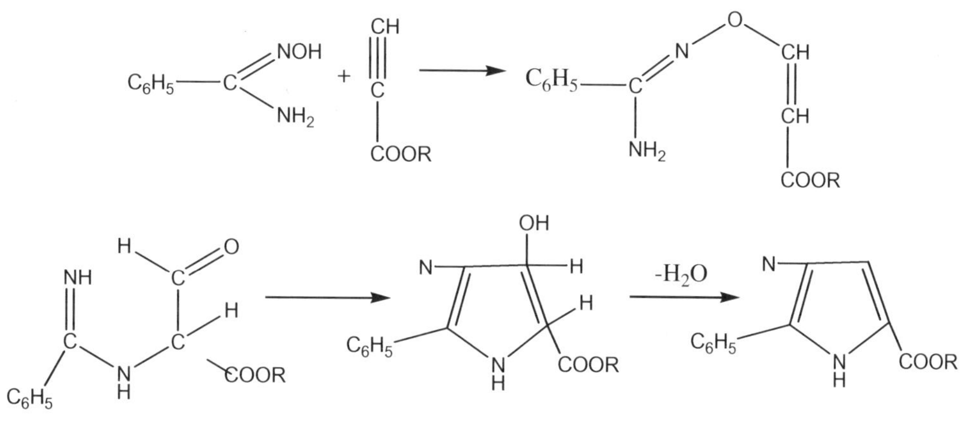

Imidazole by reaction of carboxylic acid & aldehyde or Ketone

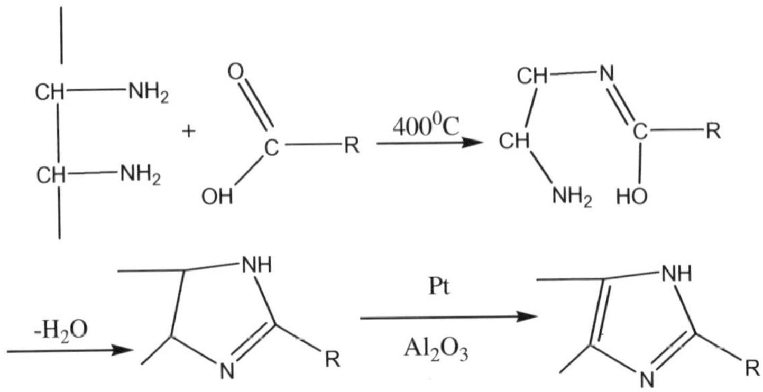

Imidazole by ring contraction

2-Chloropyrazine reacts with potassium amide in liquid ammonia gives imidazole.

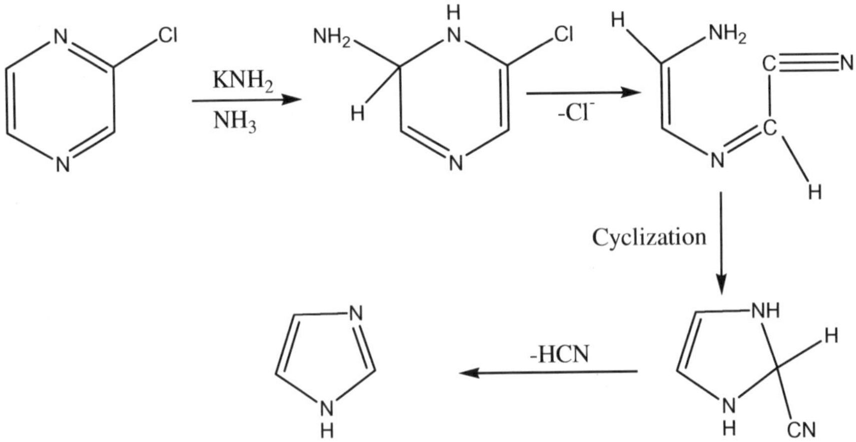

Imidazole from tartaric acid by nitration

Tartaric acid on nitration by concentrated nitric acid and concentrated sulphuric acid gives tartaric acid dinitrate. Which on treatment with formalin and ammonia solution get imidazole 4,5 dicarboxylic acid which on decarboxylation yield Imidazole.

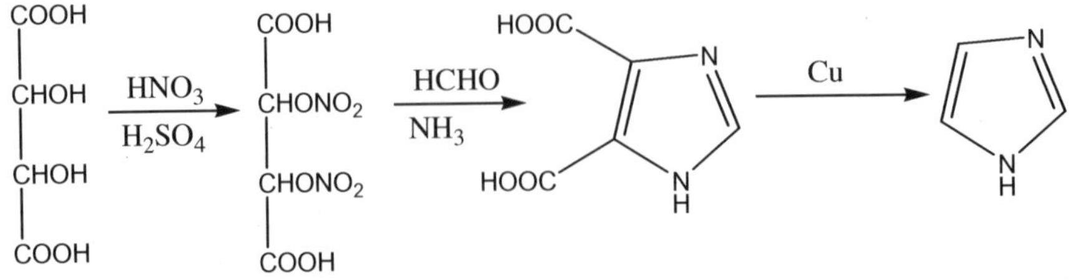

Chemical characterestics of Imidazole

Imidazole exerts tautomerism. It exhibits amphoteric nature since one nitrogen is pyrrole type and other one is pyridine type.

A. Etectrophilic Substitution

Electrophilic attack occurs at N-3 (pyridine type) but not at N-1 (pyrrole type) because lone pair of pyrrole type nitrogen is involved in aromatic sextet. Electrophilic attack occur at C_4 and C_5 also.

A1. Nitration

Imidazole nitrated by a mixture of concentrated nitric acid and sulfuric acid at 160°C to give 4-nitroimidazole.

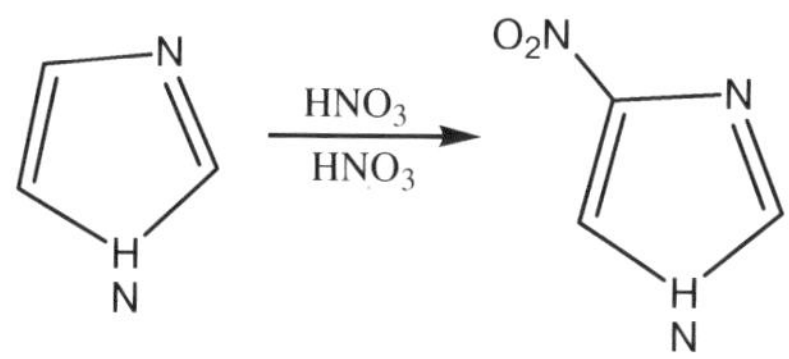

A2. Sulphonation

When imidazole treated with oleum (H_2SO_4 – SO_3) at 160ºC, sulphonation takesplace at 4th position.

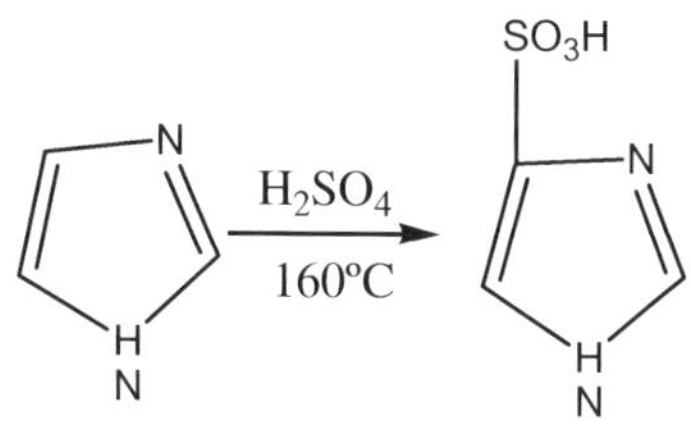

A3. Halogenation

Imidazole undergo bromination at all vacant nuclear positions by bromine in aqueous solution or organic solvent.

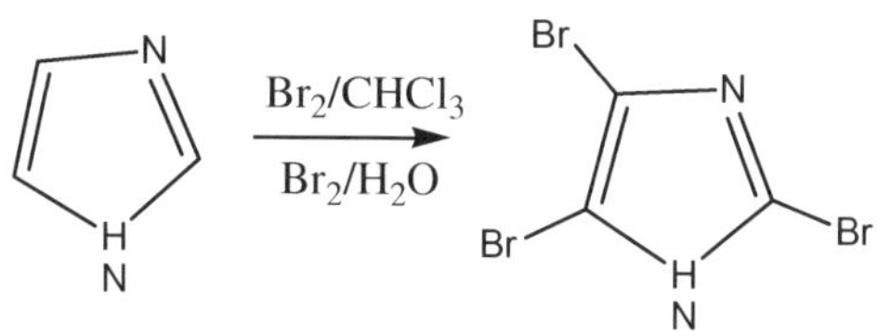

A4. Acylation

Imidazole does not undergo Friedel - Crafts reactions as imidazole markedly deactivated in the presence of Lewis acids. 1-substituted imidazole when treated with acyl or aroyl halide in the presence of triethylamine undergo C-acylation or C-aroylation.

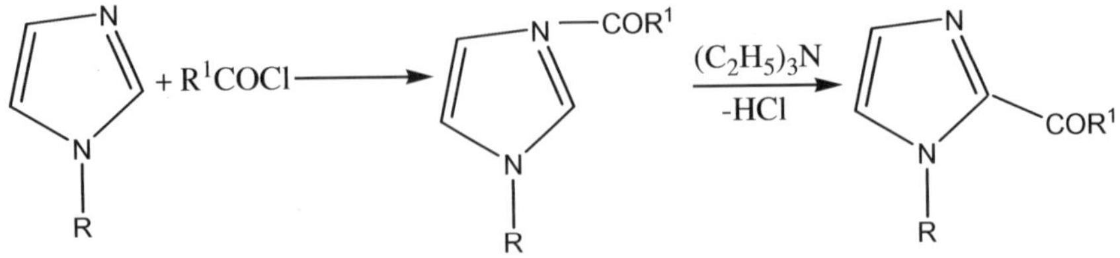

A5. Diazo coupling

When imidazoles are activated by electron releasing group, undergo diazocoupling in alkaline medium. preferentially at 2nd position.

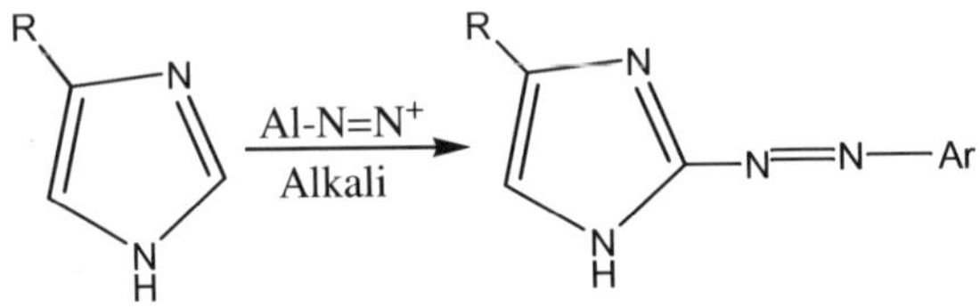

A6. Oxidation

Imidazole is inert to oxidation, but degraded by hydrogen peroxide as well as by per benzoic acid.

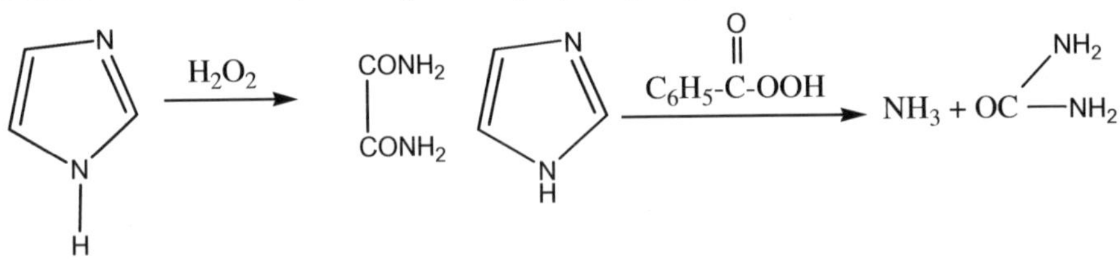

B. Nucleophilic substitution

Imidazole undergo nucleophilic substitution preferentially at second position. Nucleophile replaces halogen in 2-Halo-imidazole.

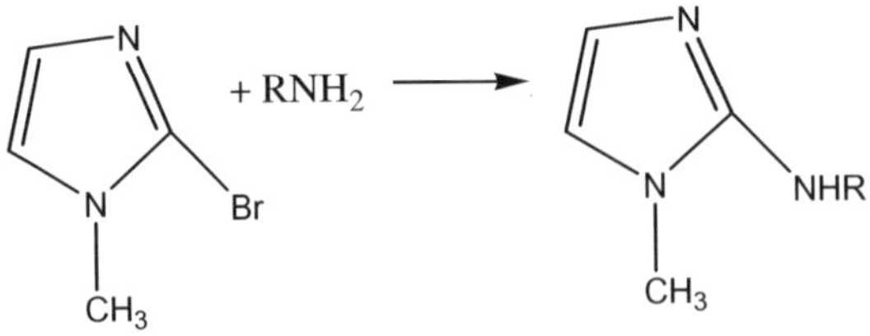

Sometimes nucleophile open the imidazole ring.

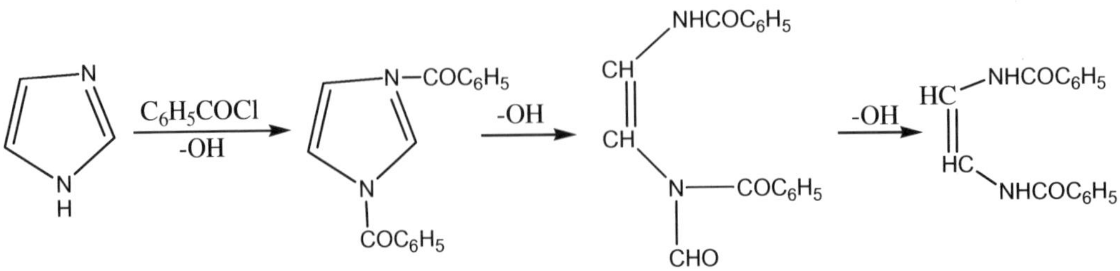

C. Ring expansion of Imidazole by electron deficient species

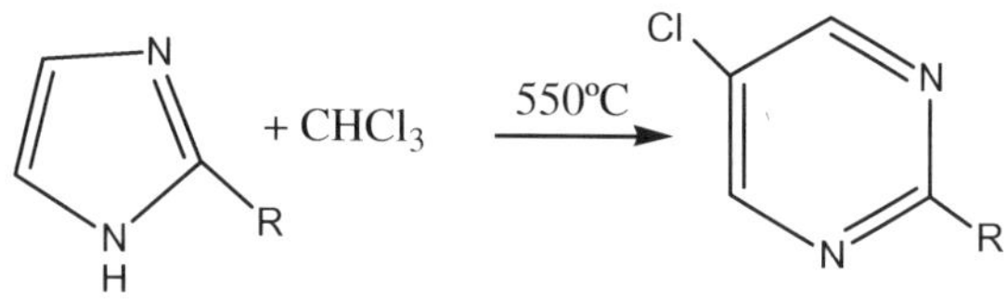

D. Cyclo addition reaction of Imidazole

Imidazole undergo addition accross the carbon-carbon double bond under photochemical conditions.

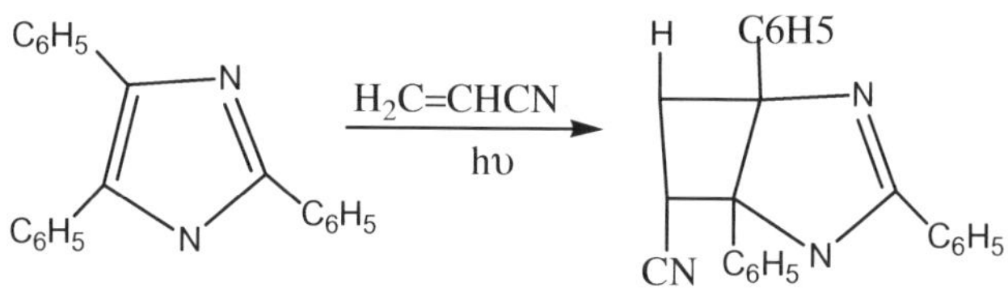

OXAZOLE

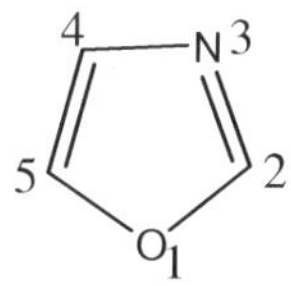

Oxazole is a 1,3-azole having an oxygen atom and a pyridine type nitrogen atom at 3rd position. Now will see different synthetic methods for oxazole one by one.

Oxazole by Robinson Gabriel Synthesis

It involves cyclodehydration of α-acylamino ketones in the presence of dehydrating agents like H_2SO_4, PCl_5, $POCl_3$ & $SOCl_2$.

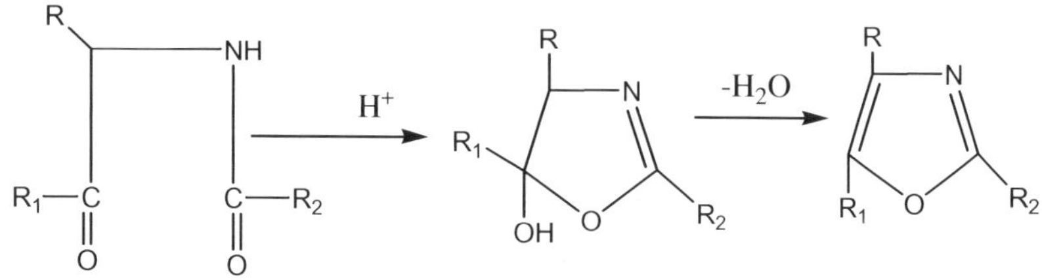

Oxazole by Blumlein Lewy Synthesis

α-halo Ketones undergo condensation with primary amides leads to the formation of Oxazoles.

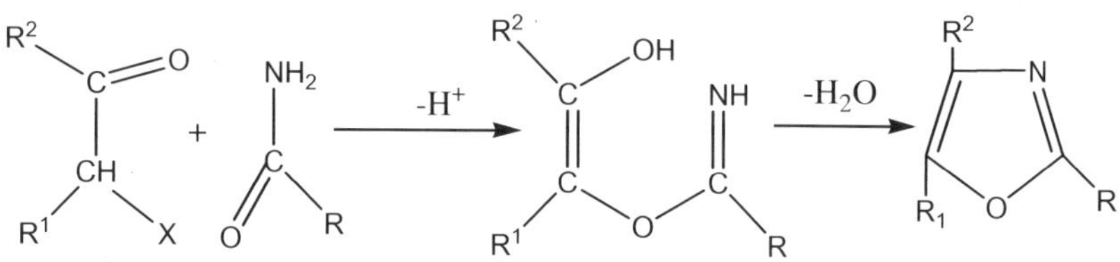

Oxazole by α-Hydroxyamino Ketones with Aldehydes

α-hydroxy amino ketones react with aldehydes in the presence of sulfuric acid and acetic anhydride give oxazoles

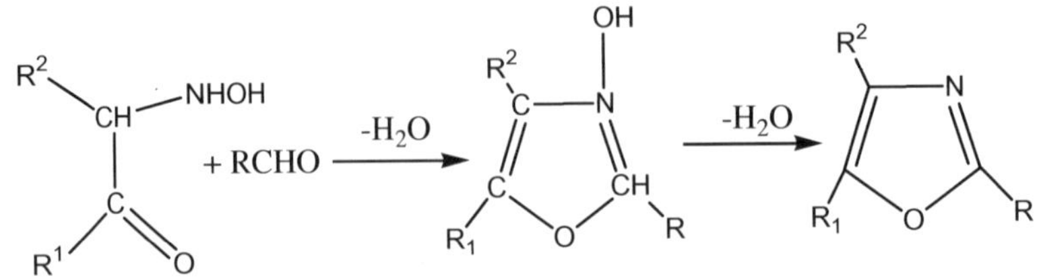

Oxazole from Isocyanide

Reaction of α-metallated isocyanides with carbylamine derivatives yield substituted oxazoles.

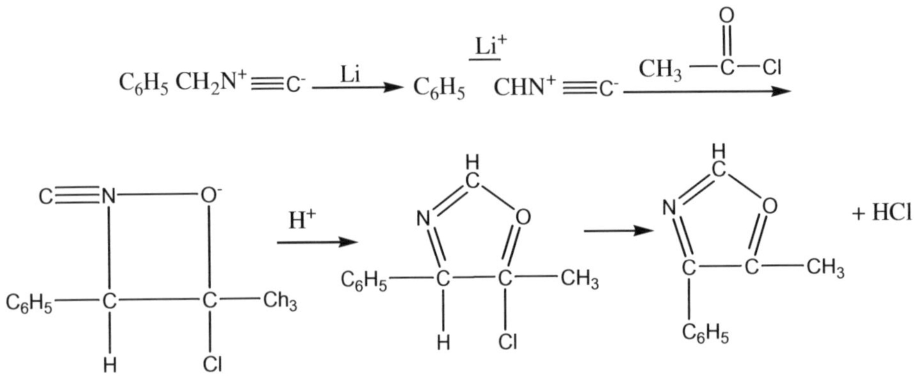

Oxazole from ethyl &-hydroxy keto succinate

Ethyl α-hydroxy keto succinate react with formamide give diethyl oxazole-4,5 dicarboxylate which is subsequently hydrolysed and decarboxylated give isoxazole.

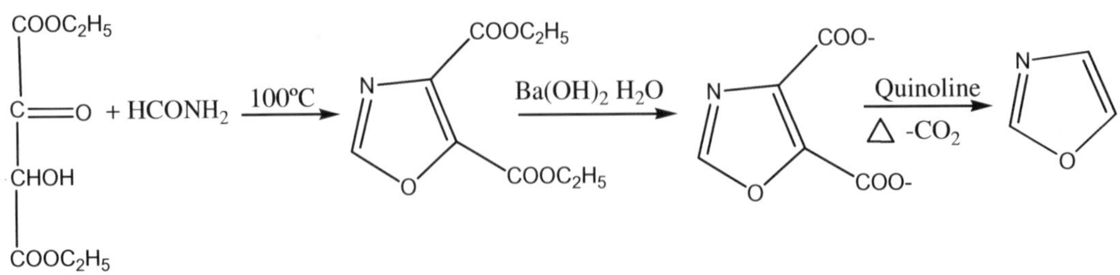

Oxazole from Acylaziridines

Thermolysis of 1-substituted-2-aroyl-3-phenyl aziridine give azomethine which cyclizes and oxidised to give oxazole derivative.

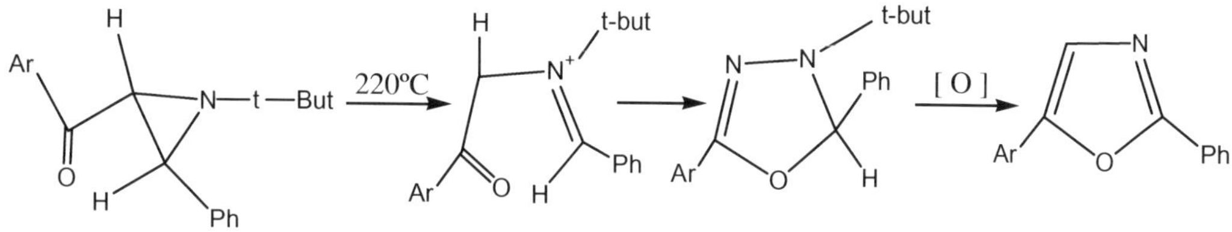

Chemical characterestics of Oxazole

Electrophilic reactions

Electrophilic attack takesplace when the ring is activated by electron donating substitutents. The order of susceptibility of the carbon atoms of the oxazole ring towards electrophilic attack is as C-4>C-5>C-2. Electrophilic substution reactions like nitration, sulfonation and chlorosulfonation do not occur in oxazole.

Bromination

2-methyl-4-phenyl isoxazole undergo bromination at 5th position.

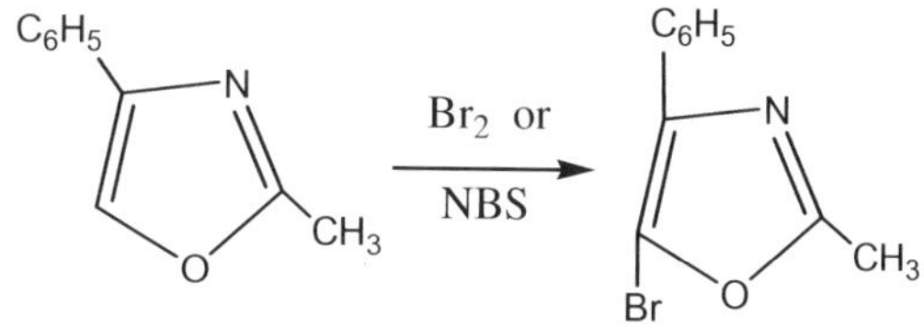

Mercuration

Mercuration in oxazole takesplace at C-4 or C-5, if both positions are occupied, mercuration occurs at 2nd position.

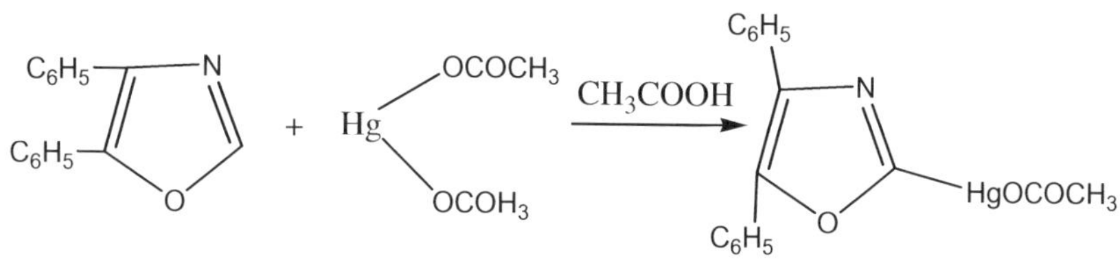

Vilsmeier-Haack formylation

Formylation in 5-methyl-2-phenyloxazole takesplace at 4th position in the presence of Dimethyl formamide and phosporous oxychloride.

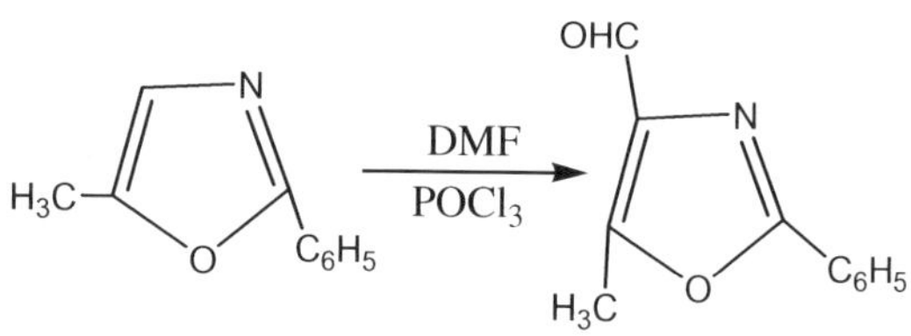

Nucleophilic reactions of Oxazole

Oxazoles when treated with ammonia or formamide at 200°C, nucleophile attacks at second position and converted into imidazole.

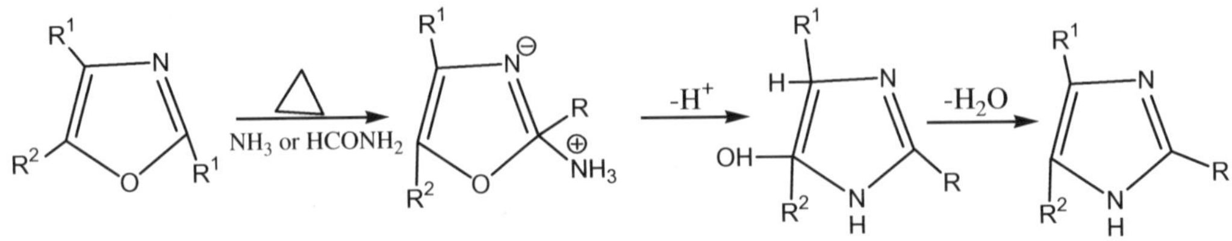

Thermal reaction of Oxazole

Oxazoles containing a carbonyl substitutent (aldehyde, ester, amide or acyl Chloride) at 4th position are rearranged on heating at 90-120°C to isomeric oxazoles in which the cabonyl substituent becomes a part of the oxazole ring. The reaction is called as cornforth rearrangement.

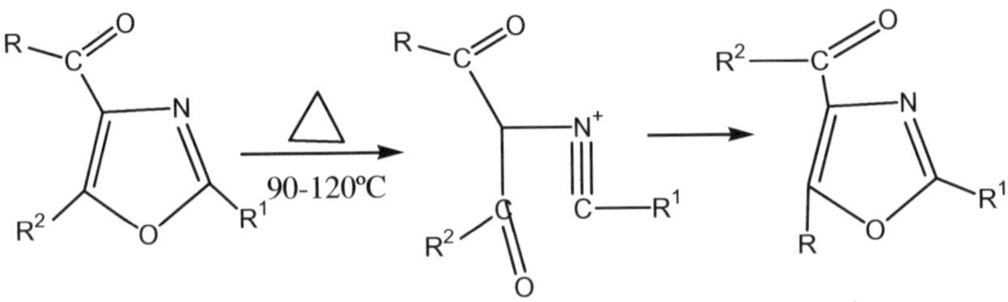

Cycloaddition Reactions

Oxazole acts as diene and undergo Diels-Alder reaction with alkenic and alkynic dienophiles.

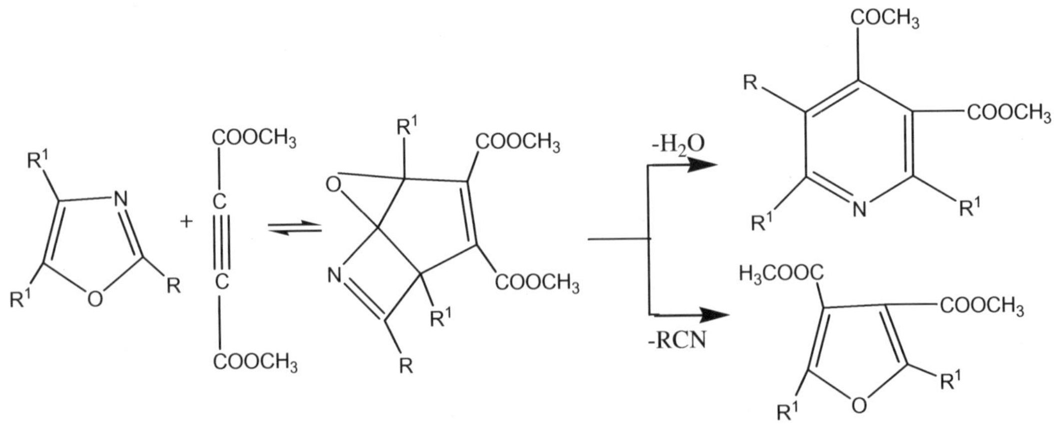

Thus the adducts become important precursors for the preparation of pyridine or furan derivatives by the loss of appropriate fragments.

Oxazole with reducing agents

Oxazolcs can be reduced to oxazolidines by sodium in ethanol. Oxazoles on catalytic hydrogenation with platinum oxide or platinum in acetic acid yield acyclic products. 2,5 diphenyl oxazole reduced to 2-benzylamino-1-phenyl ethanol by LAH.

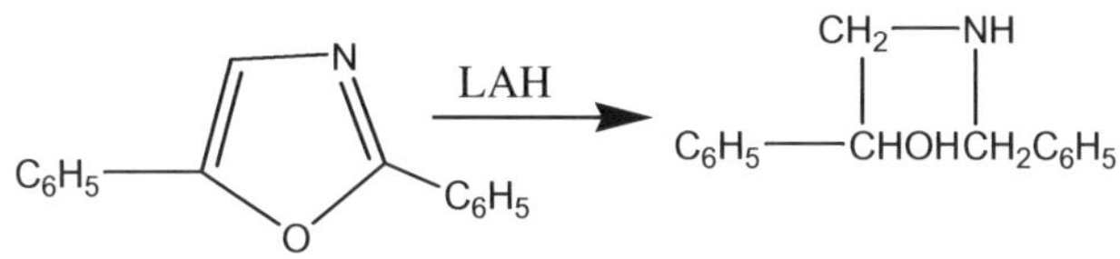

THIAZOLE

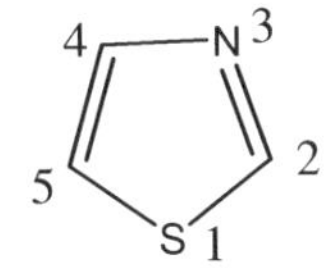

Thiazole contain sulphur in 1st position and nitrogen in 3rd position. Thiazole occur in many natural compounds like Thiamine, Penicillins....etc.

Hantzschis synthesis for Thiazoles

An α-haloketone reacts with thioamide or thio urea thiazoles are formed.

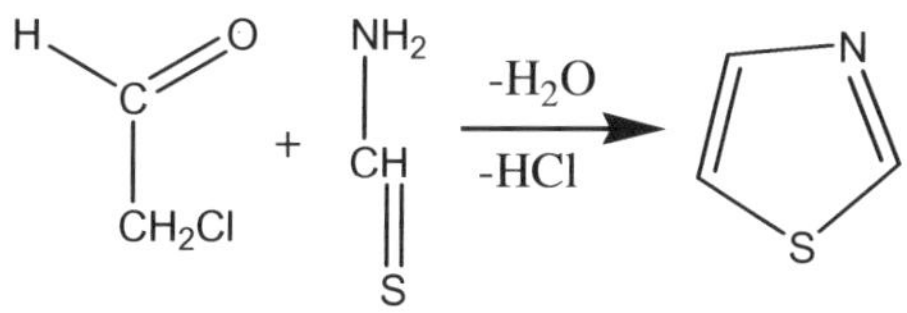

Thiazole by Gabriel Synthesis

It involves heating acylamino compounds with phosphorous pentasulphide to give thiazole derivatives.

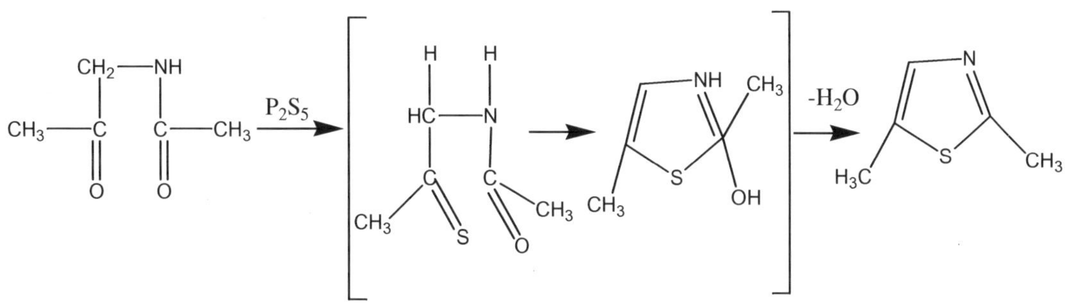

Thiazole by Cook - Heilborns synthesis

α-aminonitriles reacts with dithioacids or esters, carbon disulfide, carbon Oxysulfide and isothiocyanates under mild conditions give 5-aminothiazoles

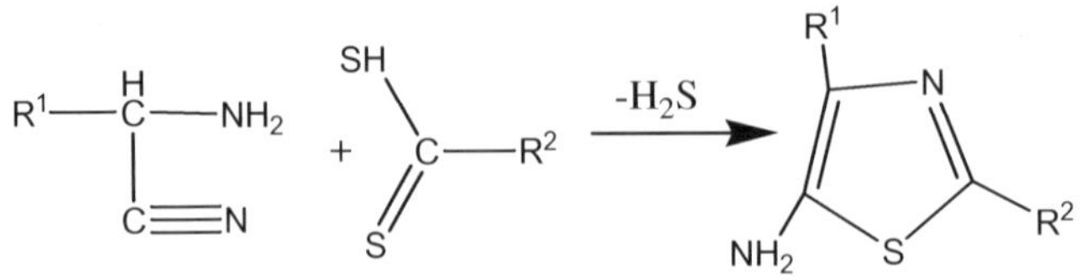

Thiazole by Tcherniacs synthesis

2-substituted thiazoles are obtained by acid hydrolysis of α thiocyano ketones or treatment with amines or sulfur compounds.

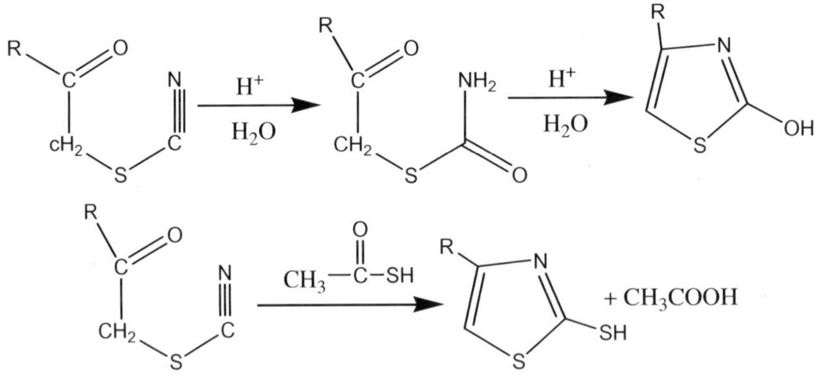

Thiazole by α-Mercapto Ketones with Nitriles

α-Mercapto ketones react with nitriles, cyclizes to give thiazoles

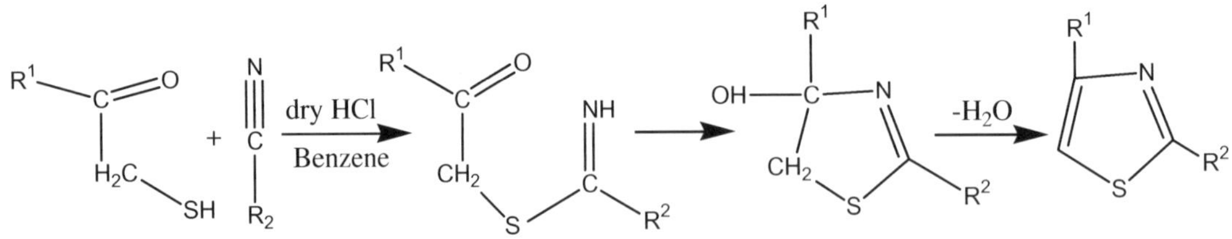

Chemical characterestics of Thiazole

Nitrogen present in thiazole is pyridine-type and sulfur is that of thiophene type. Thiazole is a π excessive heterocycle.

A. Electrophilic reactions of Thiazole

Presence of pyridine type nitrogen deactivates thiazole ring towards electrophilic attack.Thiazole undergo electrophilic substitution readily, if thiazole ring is substituted with electron releasing substitutents (–OH and –NH_2). Electrophilic attack occur at mainly on 5th position.

A1. Nitration

Thiazole itself does not undergo nitration. But methyl thiazole can be nitrated under mild conditions.

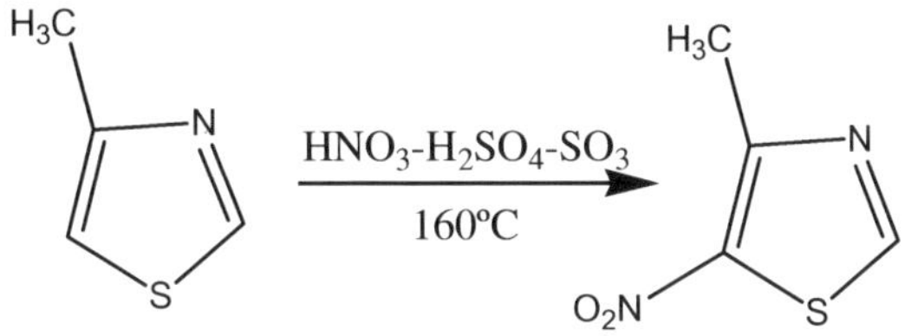

A2. Sulfonation

Sulfonation of thiazole occurs at drastic conditions with oleum but, 2-aminothiazole can be sulfonated at low temperature.

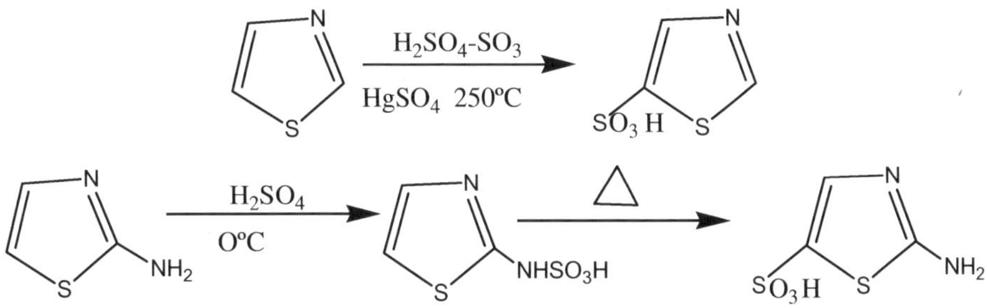

A3. Halogenation

Thiazole itself doesnot undergo halogenation but 2- methyl thiazole undergo bromination. Similarly 2-amino thiazole also undergo bromination.

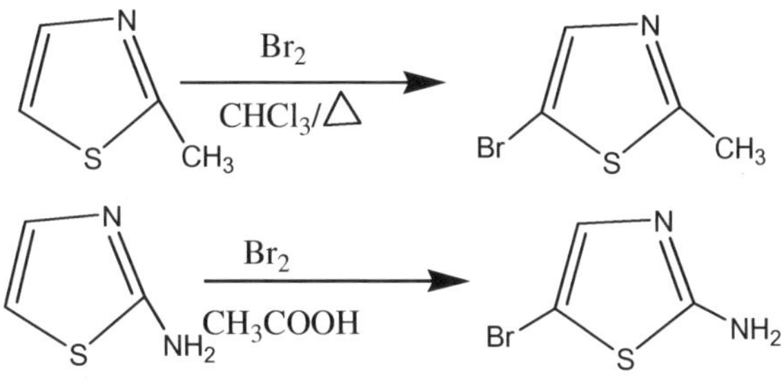

A4. Alkylation

If thiazole is activated at 2nd & 4th position, then alkylation takesplace at 5th postion.

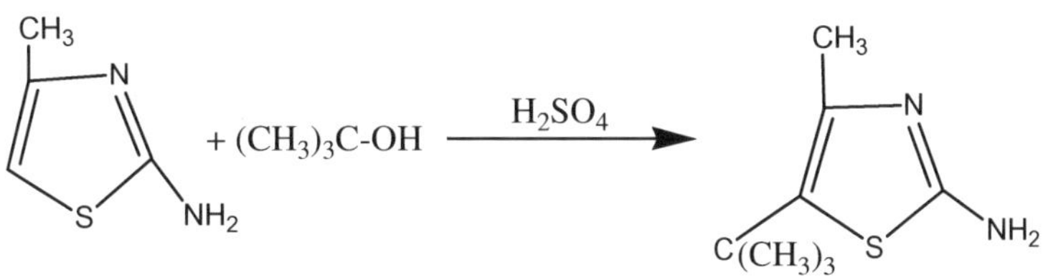

A5. Mercuration

Thiazole is mercurated by mercuric acetate in the presence of aqueous acetic acid to give 2,4,5-tri acetoxymercury thiazole.

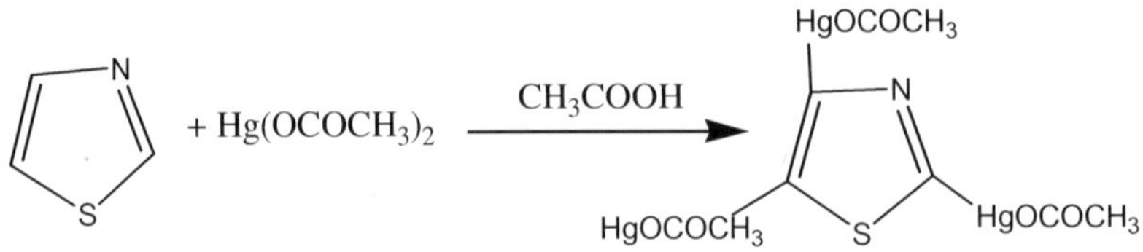

A6. Diazo coupling

2-Aminothiazole undergo diazocoupling and diazo group get substituent at 5th position.

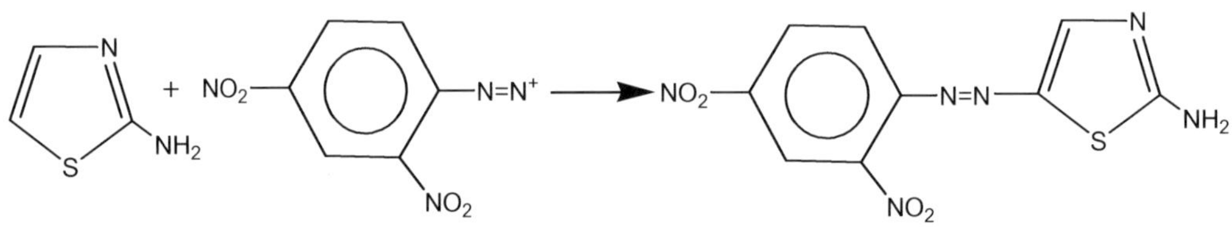

B. Condensation reactions

2-aminothiazoles undergo condensation reaction with aromatic aldehydes and ketones under mild conditions.

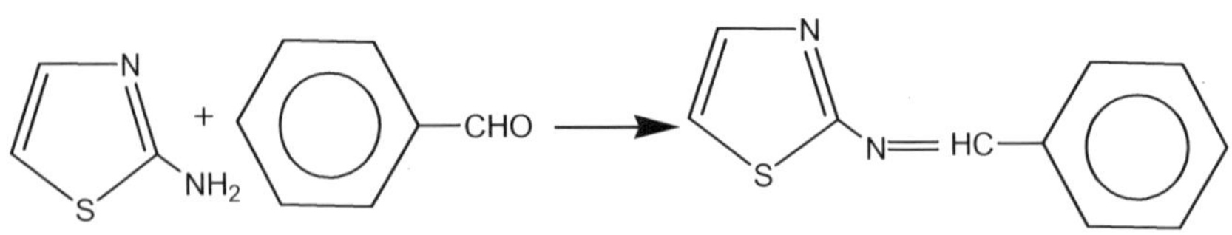

This condensation reaction can be used to synthesize a number of biheterocycles. eg.

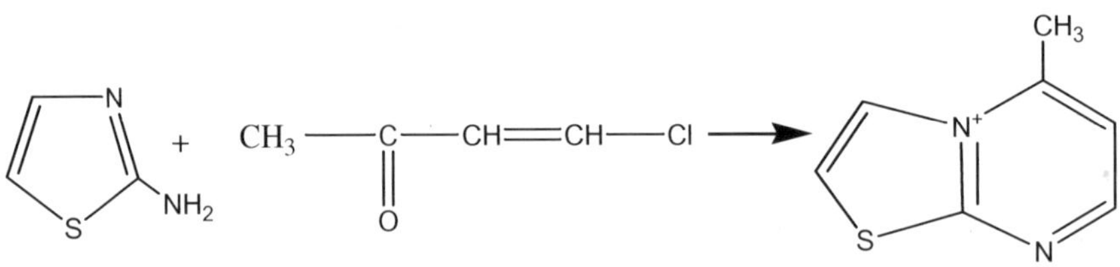

C. Oxidation

Thiazole is inert to oxidation, but if the ring activated, then oxidized to give N-oxides, by hydrogen peroxide or peracetic acid.

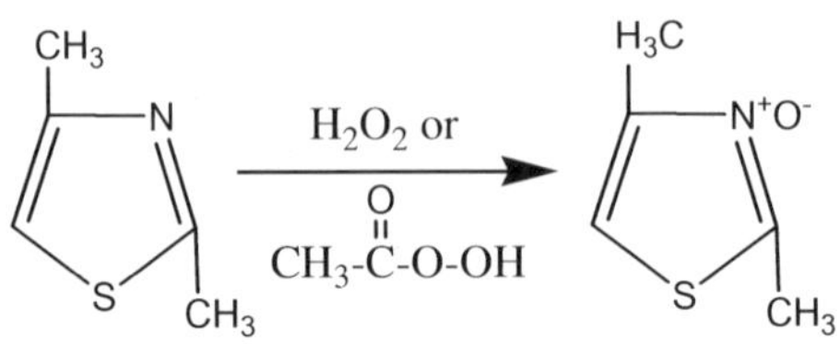

D. Desulfurization

Substituted thiazoles undergo desulfurization to give different products in different conditions.

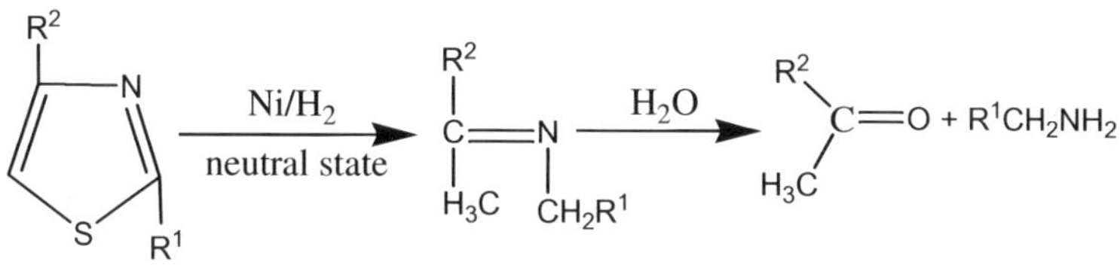

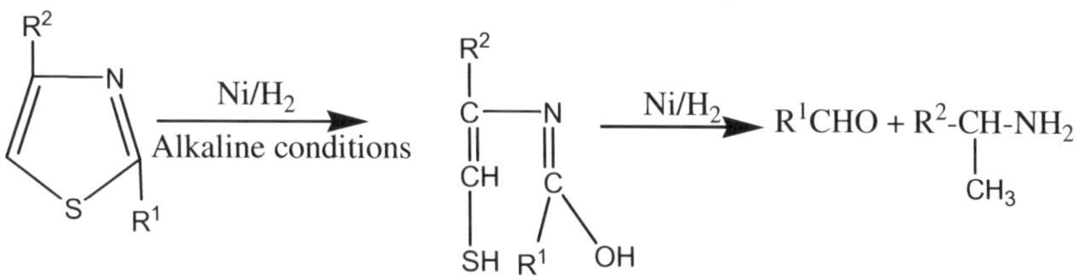

E. Nucleophilic reactions

Nucleophilic reactions occurs mainly on activated thiazole ring. For example amination does not takes place in thiazole, but methylated thiazole get aminated by sodamide.

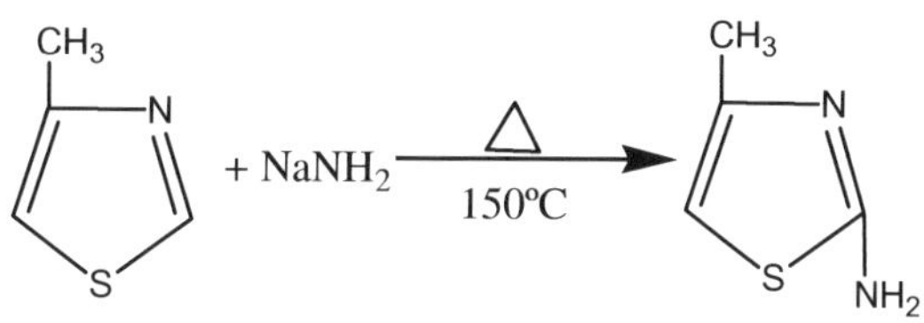

E1. Metallation

Thiazoles are deprotonated preferentially at C-2 by a strong base Thus thiazole is metallated with the abstraction of acidic hydrogen at C-2 when treated with n-butyl - lithium or ethyl magnesium bromide.

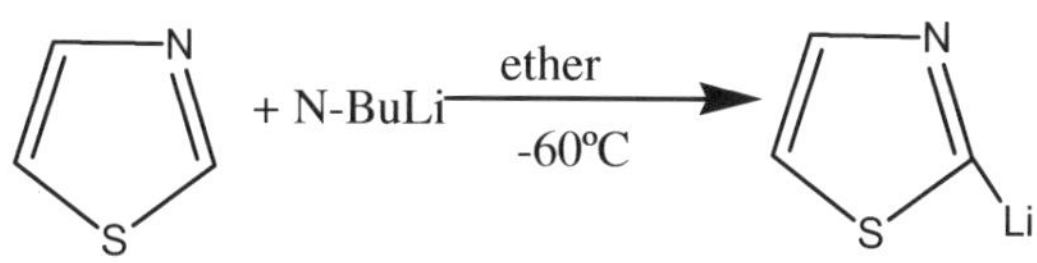

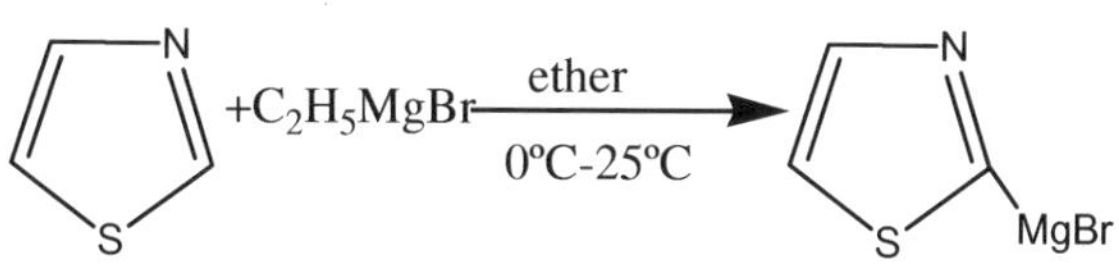

PYRAZOLE

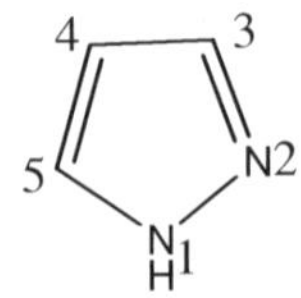

Pyrazole ring is incorporated in many pharmaceuticals. Nitrogen present in the first position is pyrrole type and that of 2nd position is pyridine type. Pyrazole exhibits tautomerism.

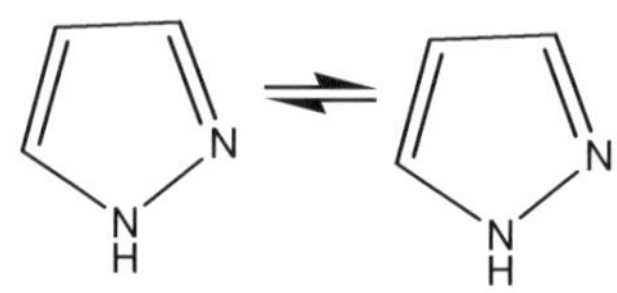

Now will see some synthetic pathways for preparing pyrazole.

Pyrazole by the reaction of β-Diketones with Hydrazines

It involves reaction of β-diketones with hydrazine in the presence of acid.

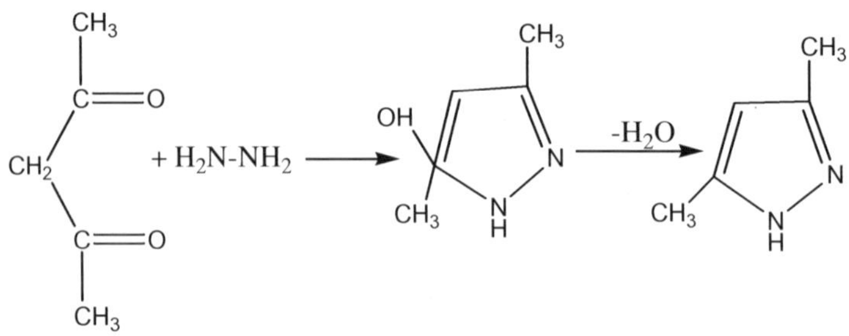

Pyrazole by reaction of α, β-unsaturated carbonyl compounds with Hydrazines

α, β-ethylenic carbonyl compounds reacts with hydrazines form pyrazoles.

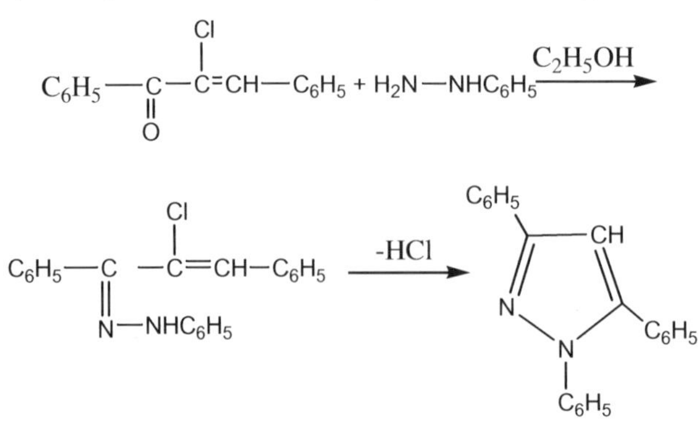

Pyrazole by 1,3-dipolar Cydoadditions

1,3-Dipolar Cycloaddition of diazoalkanes with functionalized alkynes give pyrazoles.

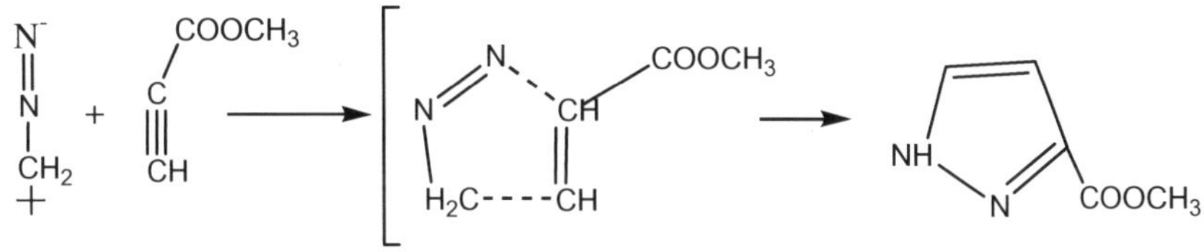

Chemical Characterestics of Pyrazole

Pyrazole have pyrrole type nitrogen at 1st position and pyridine type nitrogen in 2nd position.

Electrophilic reactions

Electrophilic attack in pyrazole takesplace at C-4.

A1. N-Alkylation

This is due to electrophilic attack at Nitrogen atom. Pyrazoles with free NH group are readily alkylated by methyl iodide or dimethyl sulfate forms N-alkylpyrazoles.

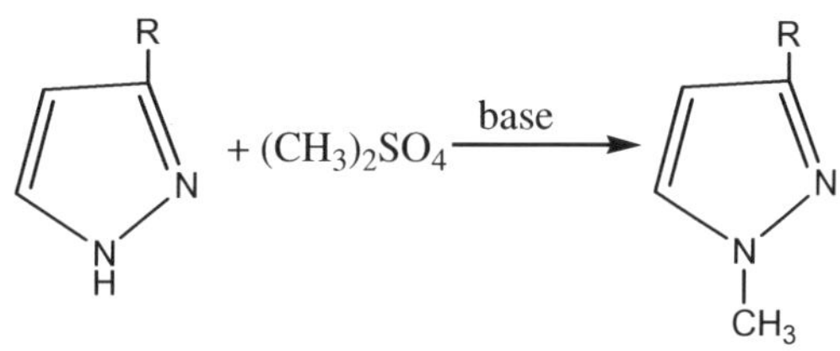

A2. N-acylation

Pyrazoles with free NH group undergo acylation when treated with acetyl chloride or acetic anhydride.

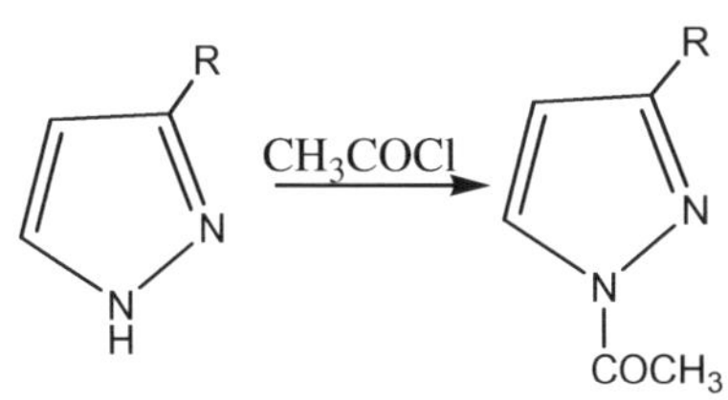

A3. Michael Addition

Pyrazoles undergo Michael addition with activated alkenes and alkynes.

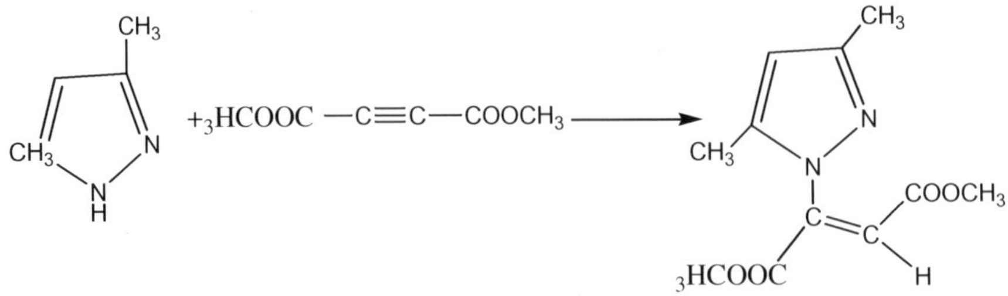

But, when pyrazole reacts with methyl ethyl Ketone, two successive additions occur at same catrbon atom.

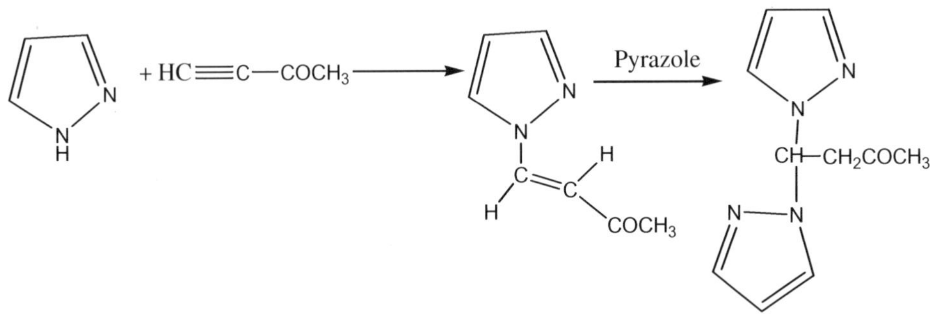

A4. Nitration

Nitration of pyrazole with nitrating mixture takesplace at 4th position.

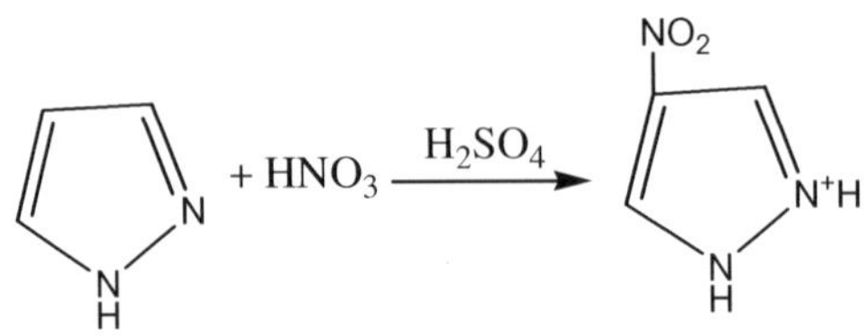

If pyrazole is substituted with phenyl group at 1st position, it competes with pyrazole ring and nitration occurs at para position.

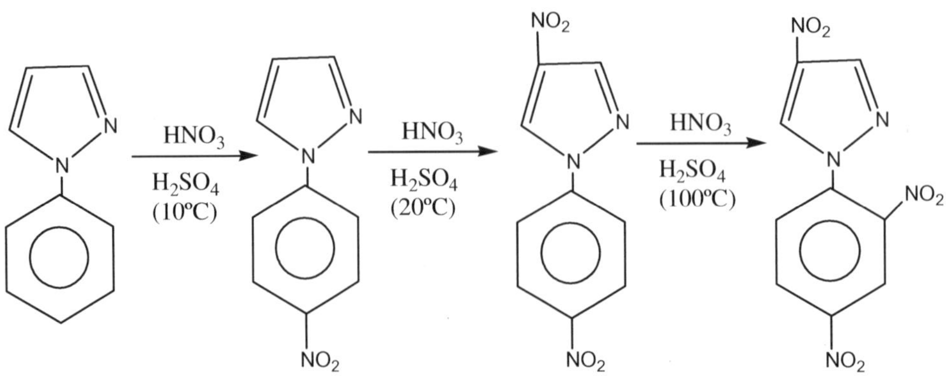

A5. Sulfonation

Pyrazole undergo sulfonation at vigorous condition with oleum.

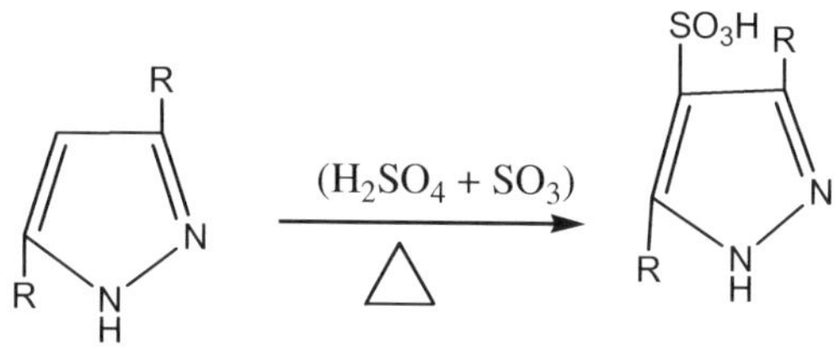

A6. Halogenation

Pyrazole can be halogenated at 4th position.

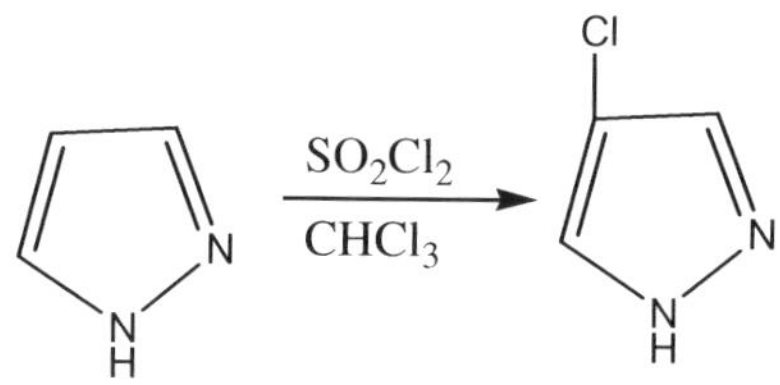

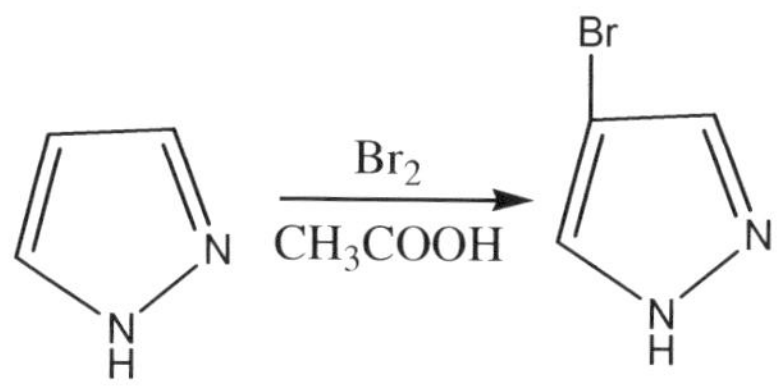

A7. Mercuration

Pyrazoles are chloromercurated at 4th position by reacting with mercury chloride.

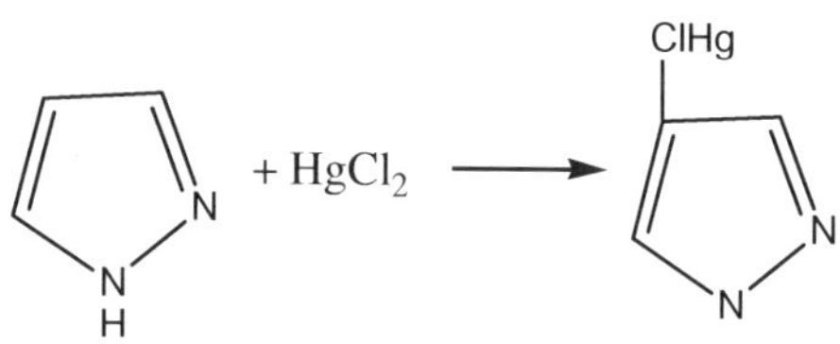

A8. Oxidation

Pyrazole react with hydrogenperoxide to form 2-oxide-

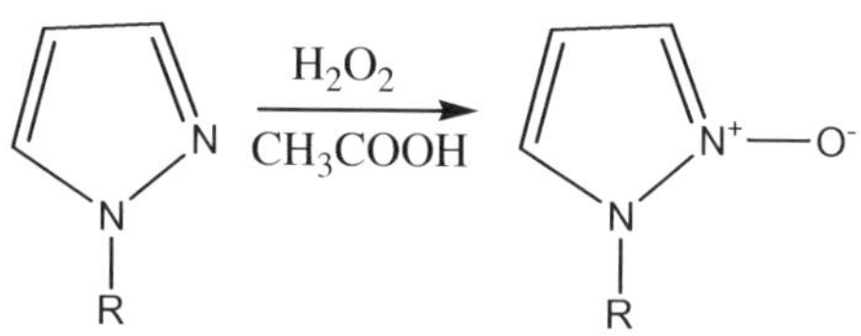

When alkyl pyrazoles are treated with alkaline $KMnO_4$, alkyl group converted into carboxylic group.

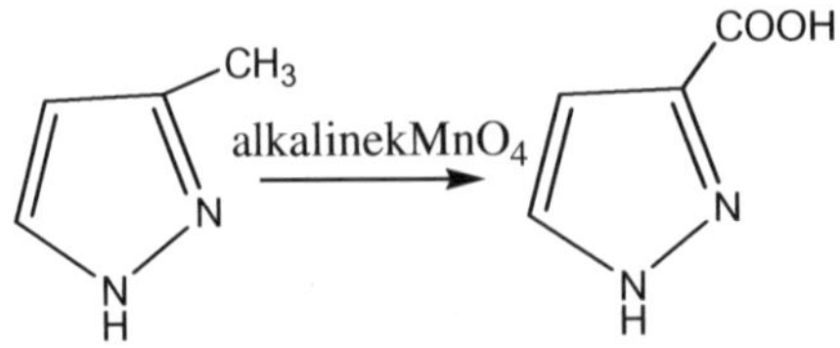

C. Reduction

Pyrazole can be reduced to 2-pyrazolines again to pyrazolidines.

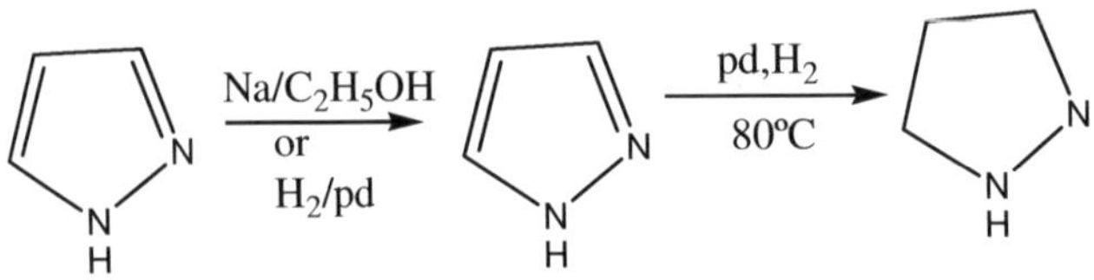

D1. Nucleophilic reactions

When pyrazoles have electron - withdrawing substituent attached at α -to halogen atom, undergo nucleophilic substitution.

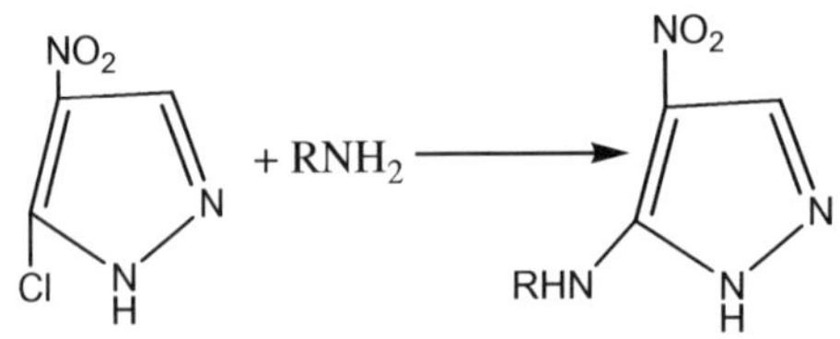

D2. Metallation

N-substituted pyrazoles are lithiated at 5th position, when treated with n-butyl-lithium.

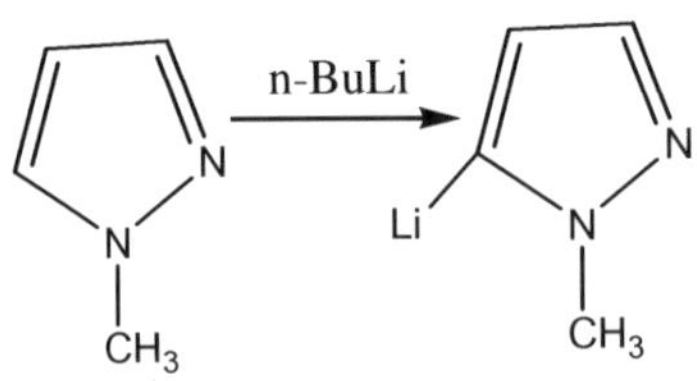

E. Ring clevage in pyrazole ring

If 3rd position in pyrazole is free, then ring can be open by strong base like sodamide.

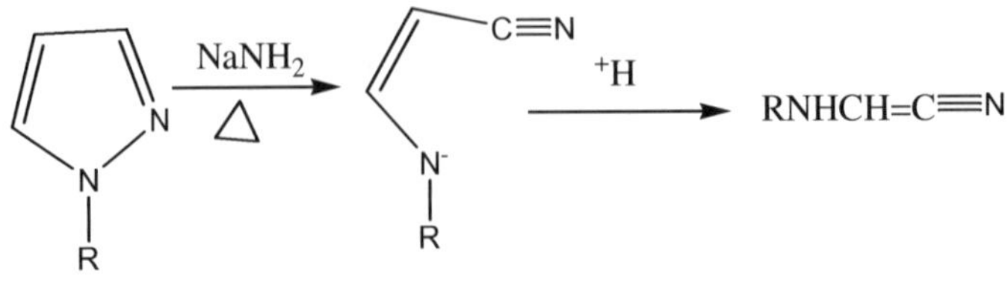

ISOXAZOLE

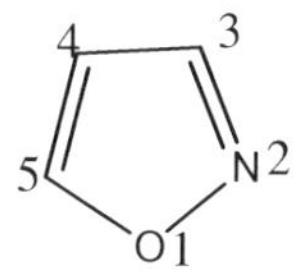

Isoxazole is a π-excessive heterocycle with furan type oxygen and pyridine type nitrogen.

Now we shall discuss some synthetic methods for Isoxazole.

Isoxazoles from Diketones

An, α-β-diketone reacts with hydroxylamine forms a mixture of isomeric isoxazoles.

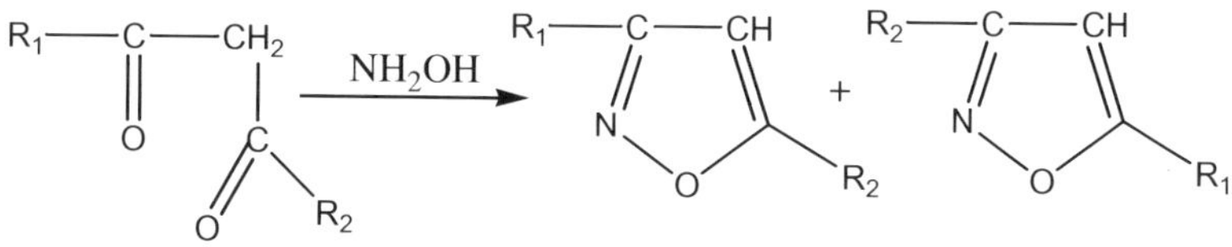

Isoxazoles from tetra-alkoxy alkanes

1,1,3,3-tetraethoxypropane on reaction with hydroxylamine yields isoxazole.

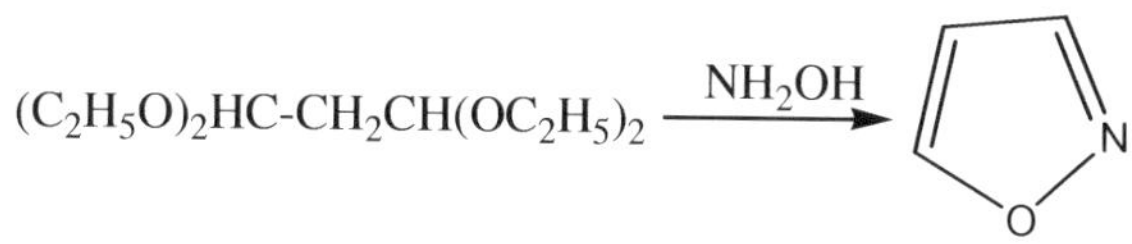

Isoxazoles from Nitrile oxides

Isoxazoles are generally prepared by cycloaddition of olefins or acetylenes to nitrile oxides. The treatment of chloroximes with bases like triethylamine forms nitrile oxides.

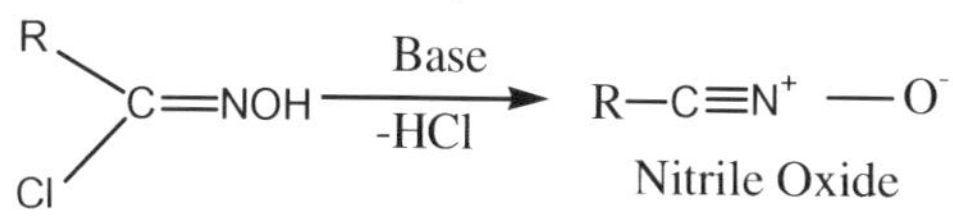

The nitrile oxides react with a monosubstituted alkyl or aryl-alkyne regioselectively via 1,3 cycloaddition to yield 5-substituted isoxazole.

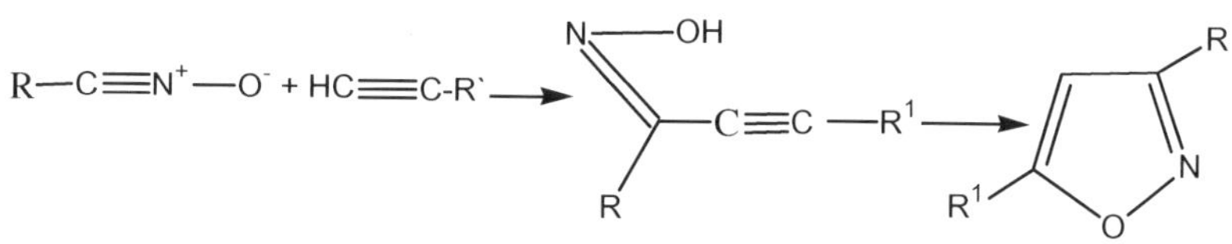

Isoxazole from fulminic acid

Fulminic acid react with vinyl acetate gives isoxazole.

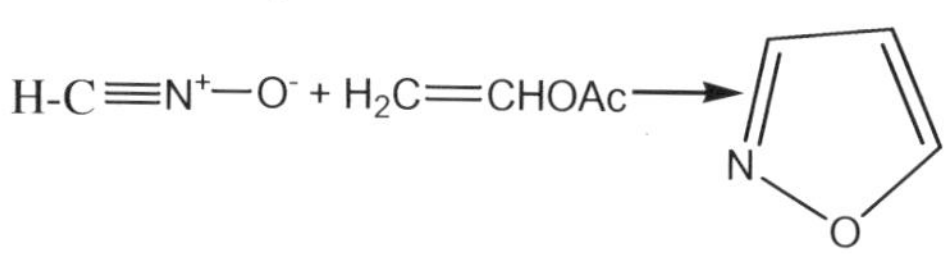

Chemical Characterestics of Isoxazole

A. Electrophilic reactions

Electrophilic attack at nitrogen are rare.

A1. Nitration

Under controlled conditions isoxazole is nitrated at 4th position.

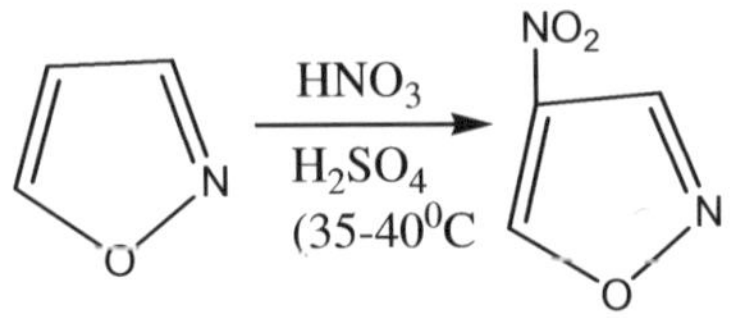

Nitration of 5-methyl isoxazole gives 5-methyl 4-nitro isoxazole.

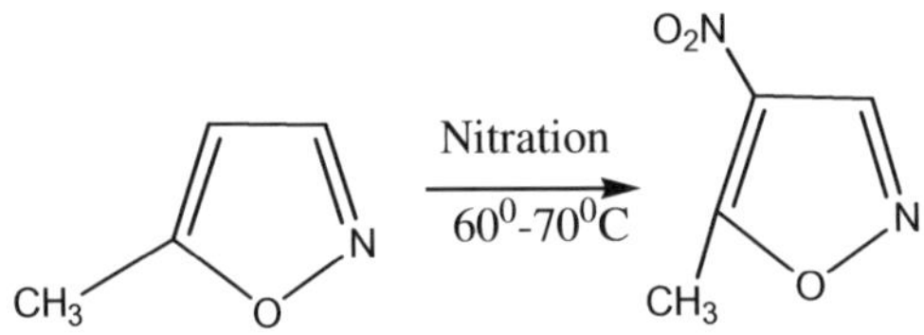

A2. Sulfonation in Isoxazole

Sulfonation of Isoxazole takesplace in drastic conditions with oleum.

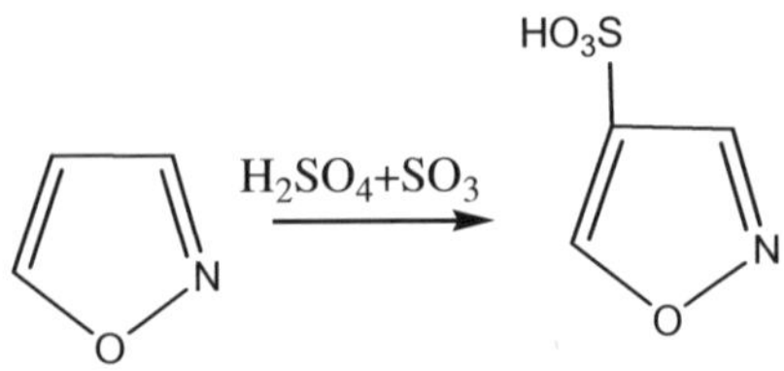

A3. Halogenation in Isoxazole

Isoxazole undergo halogenation at 4th postion.

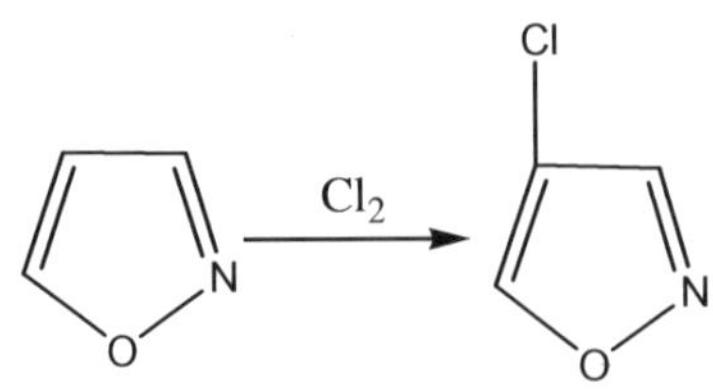

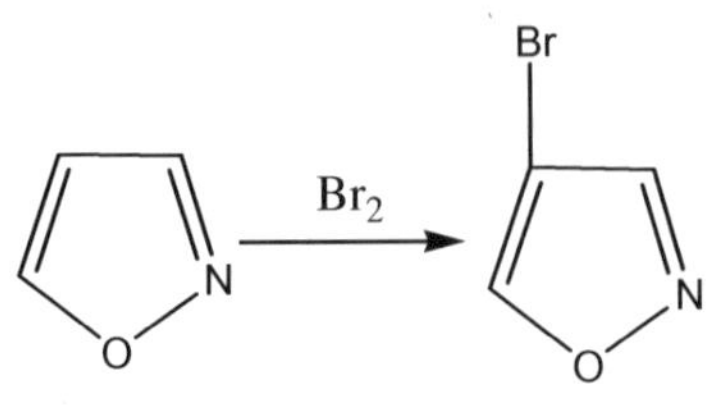

Dimethyl isoxazoles are iodinated with iodine in the presence of concentrated nitric acid.

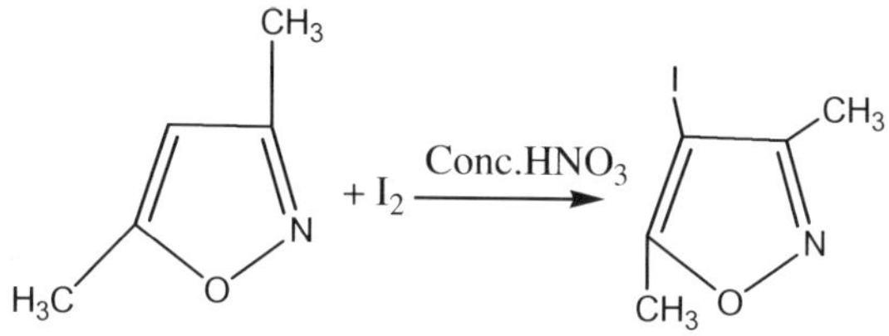

A4. Chloromethylation

Dimethyl isoxazole react with formaldehyde and hydrochloric acid in the presence of zinc chloride give chloromethylated product.

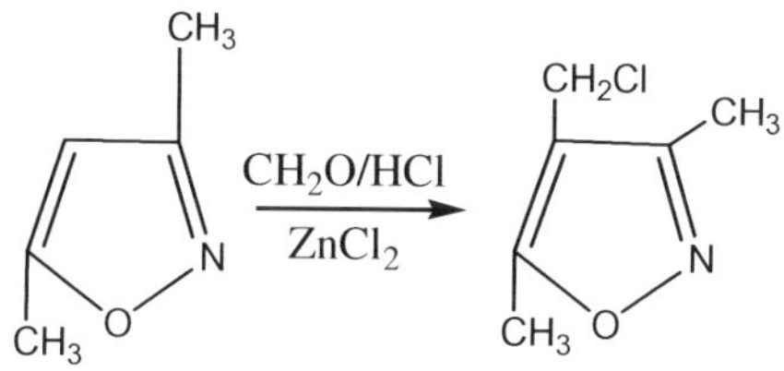

A5 Hydroxy methylation

When Dimethyl isoxazole react with formaldehyde in the presence of sulfuric acid, 4th position of isoxazole ring get hydroxymethylated.

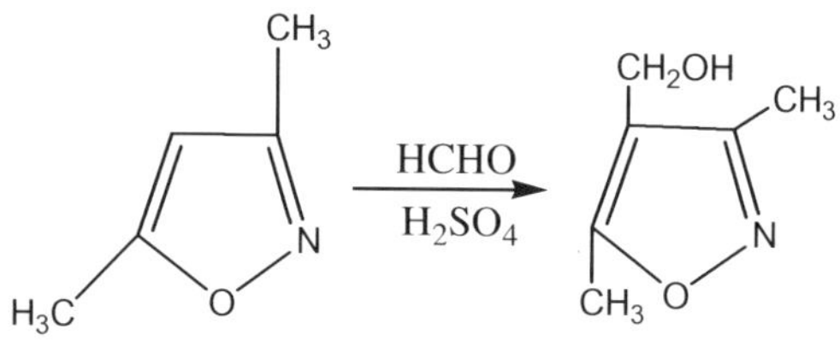

A6. Mercuration

Phenyl isoxazole is mercurated at 4th position, when treated with mercury acetate.

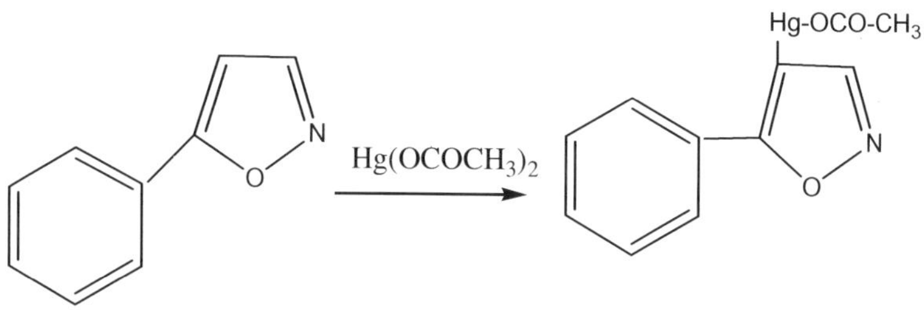

B. Oxidation

Isoxazole ring is inert to oxidation reactions. but, when unsaturated side chains or oxo functional groups are there, they will oxidise to corresponding acids.

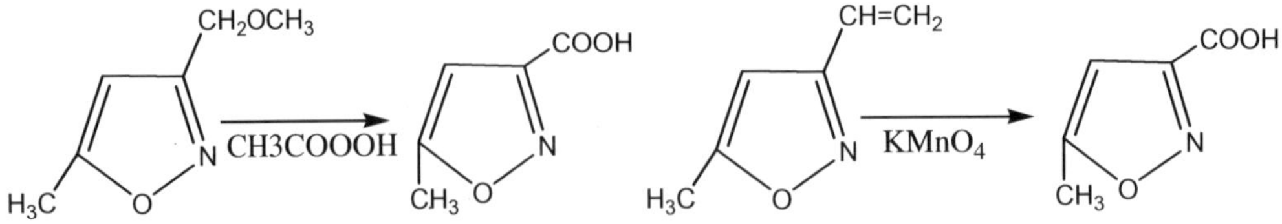

C. Nucleophilic reactions

If isoxazole ring activated then halogens at 3rd and 5th position can be replaced by nucleophiles.

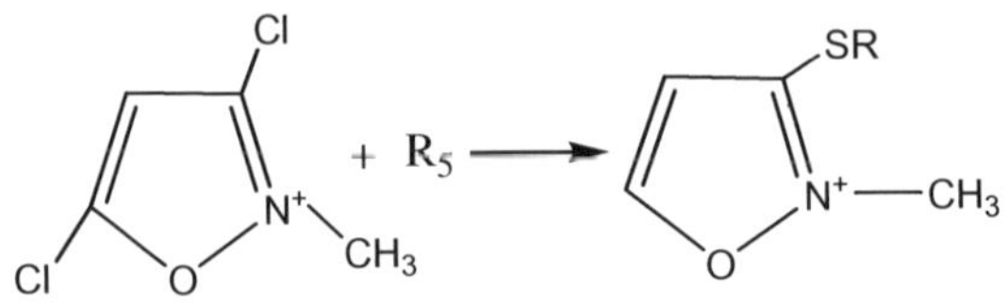

D. Reduction

Catalytic hydrogenation of isoxazole open the ring and form enaminone which on hydrolysis give diketones.

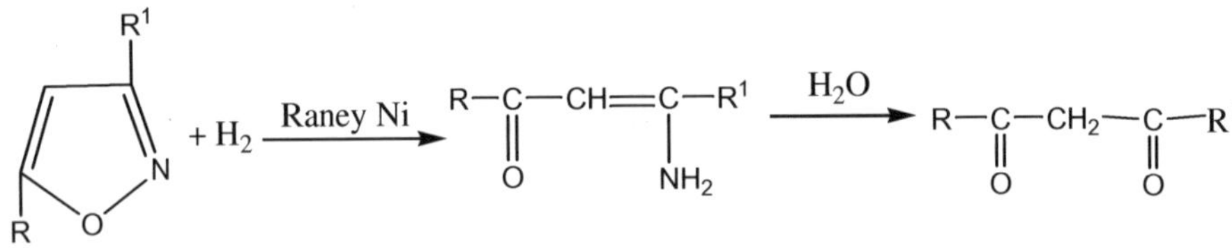

Reduction of isoxazole by LAH give amino ketones.

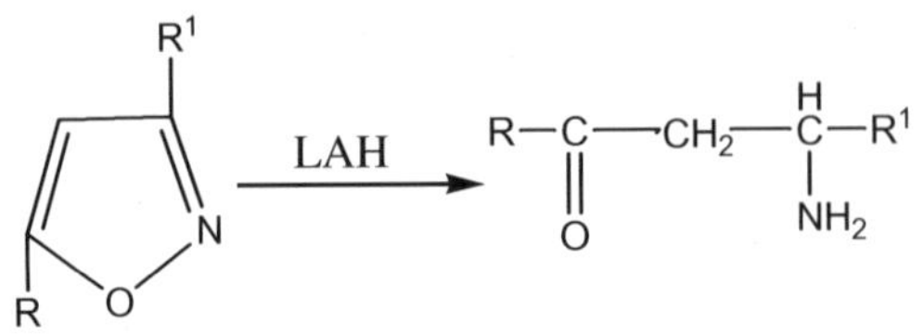

E. Condensation reactions

If 4th position is substituted with electron withdrawing group like, NO_2, then methyl group at 5th position will be more reactive than 3rd position, thus it can be condensed with aromatic aldehydes in the presence of diethylamine.

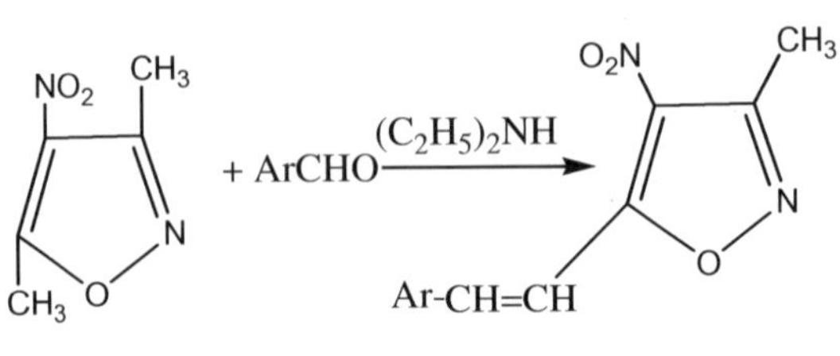

INDOLE

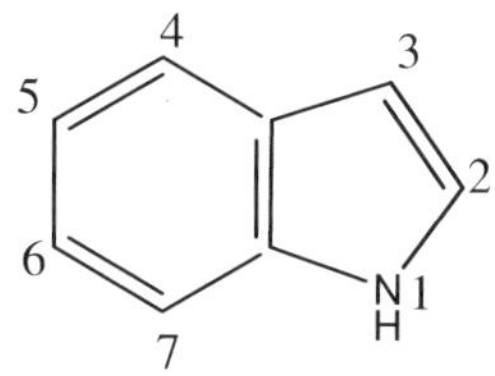

Indole occurs in many natural compounds like alkaloids.

Indole can be prepared in many ways.

Reissert Indole Synthesis

O-Nitrotoluene react with diethyl oxalate in the presence of a base (Claisen condensation) gives o-nitrophenylpyruvate, which on reductive cyclization followed by dehydration leads to the formation of indole-2-carboxylate which undergo decarboxylation to give Indole.

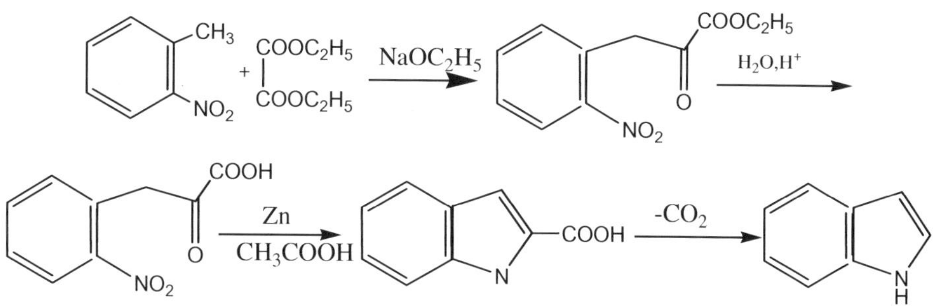

Indole from o-nitrophenylnitroethylene

O-nitrophenylnitroethylene undergo reductive cyclization followed by subsequent aromatization with the elimination of ammonia results in indole formation.

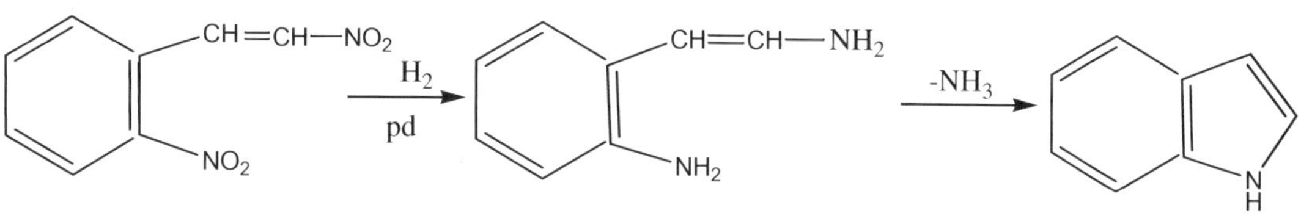

Madelung Synthesis

It involves cyclic dehydration of acyl o-toludine in the presence of a strong base like sodamide or tertiary butoxide at a high temperature.

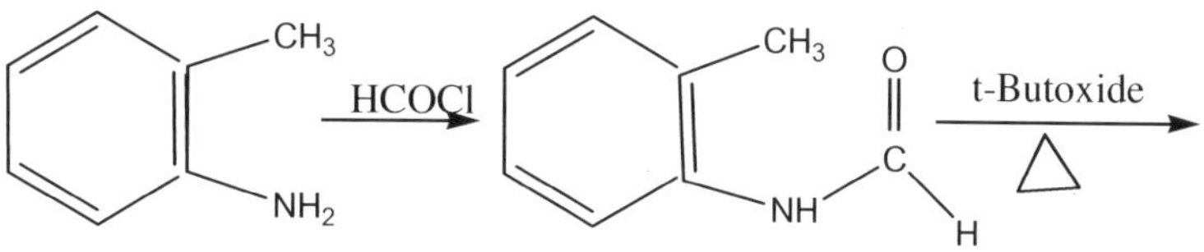

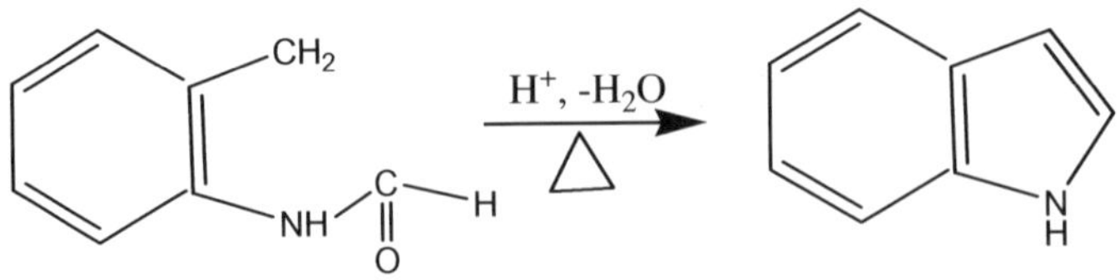

Indole by Isonitrile cyclization

O-tolyl isocyanide react with lithium dialkylamide at -78°C undergo lithiation of methyl group which undergo cyclization to form lithiated indole, which on hydrolysis give indole.

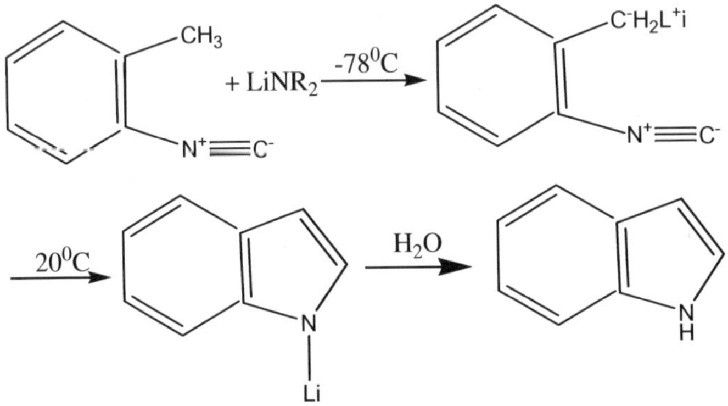

Bischler Indole Synthesis

The reaction of α-hydroxy or α-halo ketones with acylamine in the presence of acid give indole. The reaction involves N-alkylation, electrophilic intramolecular cyclization and aromatization.

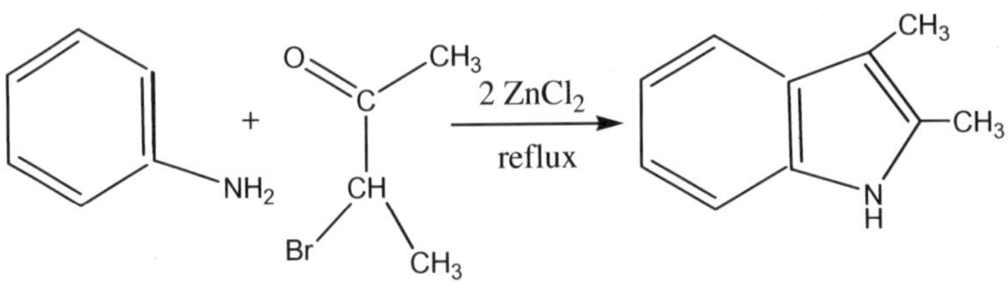

Fischer Indole Synthesis

It involves acid catalyzed cyclization of arylhydrazenes of appropriate aldehydes and ketones with the elimination of ammonia. The conventional catalysts employed are zinc chloride, polyphosphoric acid or Lewis acid.

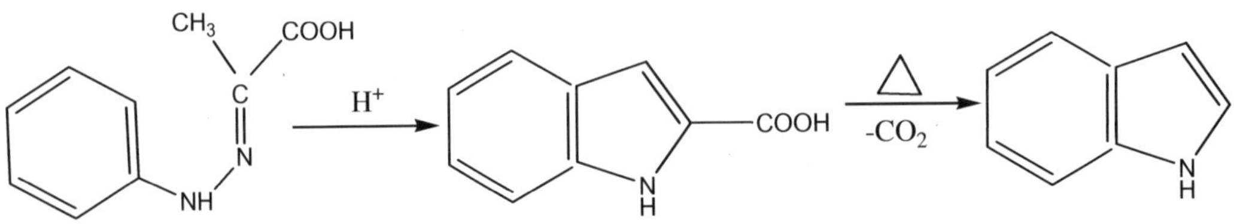

Gassman Indole Synthesis

In this reaction aniline react with tert-butyl hypochlorite gives N-chloroaniline which on treatment with β-keto-sulfide give azasulfonium salt, which deprotonated to give sulfur ylide which undergo sigmatropic reararrangement and give α-amino ketone. It cyclizes to give 3-methyl thio indole. From which methylthio group removed by its reaction with Raney nickel.

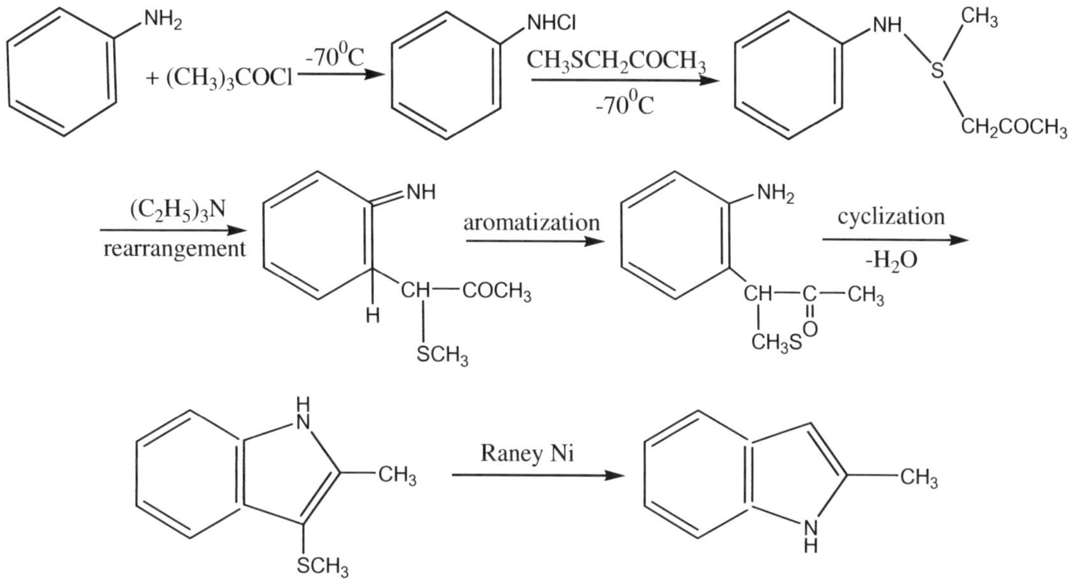

Indole from Pyrrole

Vinyl pyrrole reacts with π-electron deficient alkynes undergo cyclicaddition reaction form dihydroindoles which undergo aromatization.

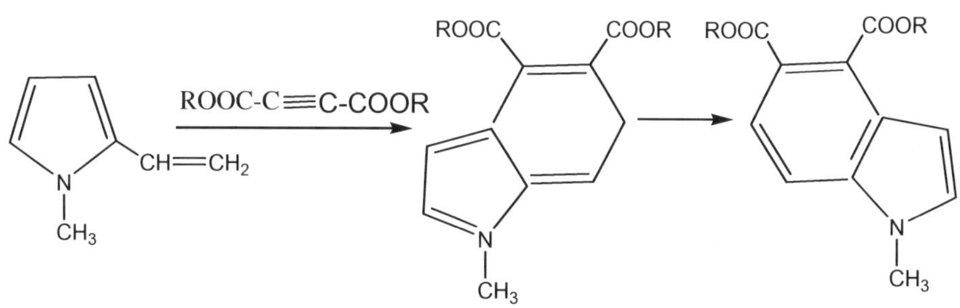

Chemical Characterestics of Indole

Indole is the fusion of benzene ring to face b or α,β-positions of pyrrole ring.

A. Electrophilic reactions of Indole

Indole is π excessive heterocycle. Electrophilic substitution takesplace mainly at 3rd position.

A1. Nitration

Nitration of Indole with benzoyl nitrate in acetonitrile at low temperature gives 3-nitroindole.

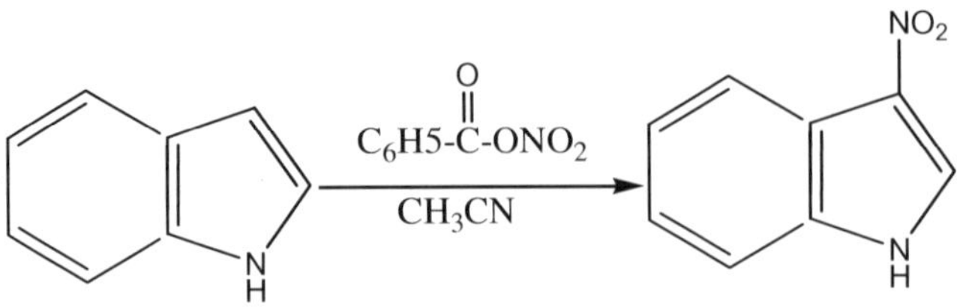

A2. Nitrosation

Indole reacts with nitrous acid give mixture of dimeric products and 3-nitrosoindole.

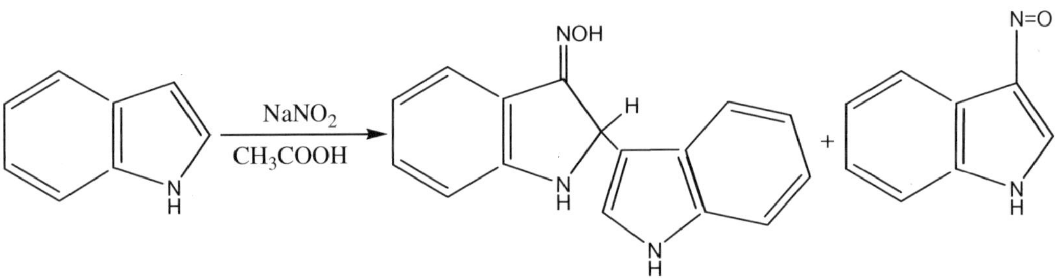

A3. Halogenation

Chlorination

Chlorination of Indole with sulfonyl chloride give 3-chloroindole.

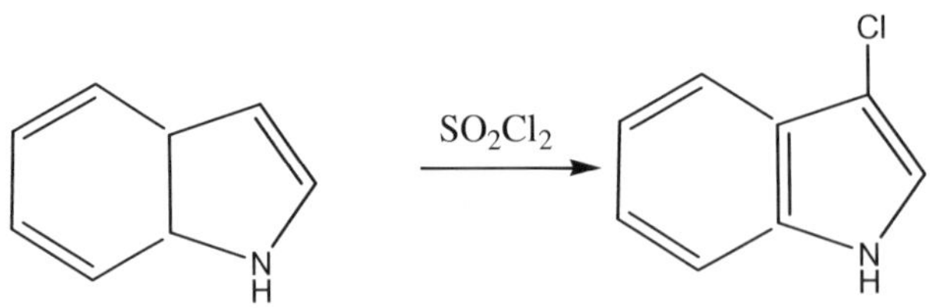

Bromination

Bromination of Indole takesplace at 3rd position.

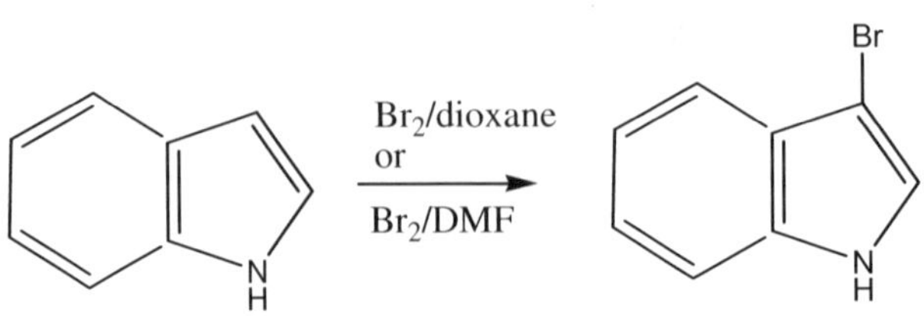

Iodination

Indole react with iodine in the presence of Choloroform at low temperature give 3-iodoindole.

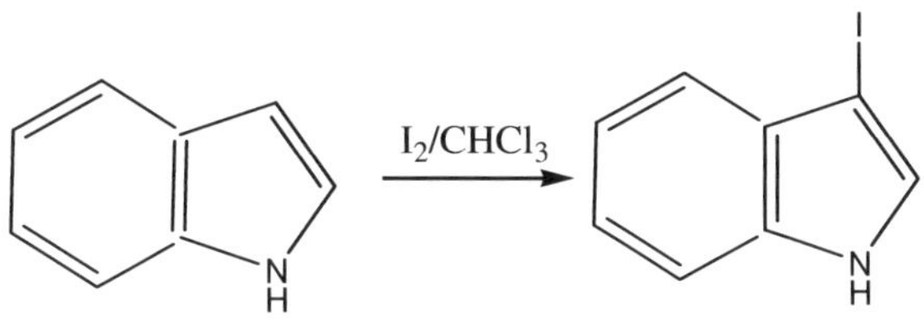

A4. Sulfonation

Indole sulfonated by pyridine-sulfurtrioxide complex give indole-3-sulfonic acid.

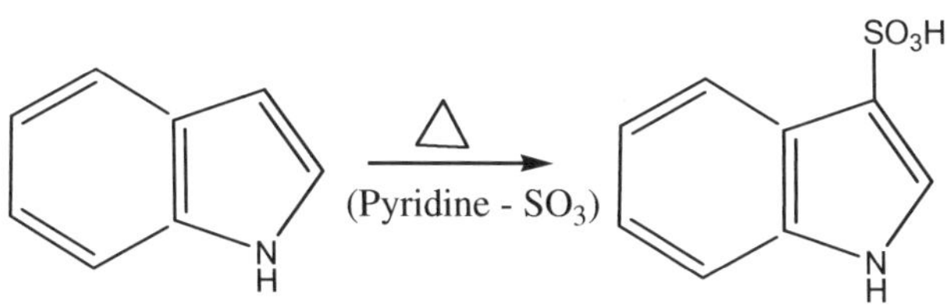

A5. Acylation

Indole with acetic anhydride in the presence of acetic acid give 1-acetyl and 1,3-diacetyl indoles.

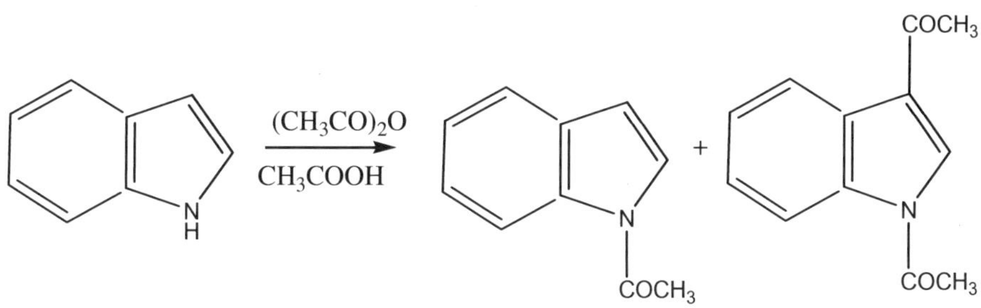

A6. Formylation

Indole react with N,N-dimethyl formamide in the presence of phosphorous oxychloride gives 3-Formyl indole.

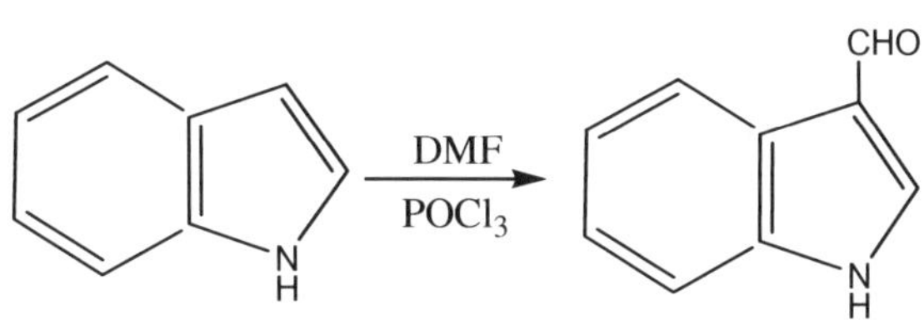

A7. Alkylation

Indole react with excess of methyl iodide in the presence of DMF at 80-90°C produces 3-methyl indole.

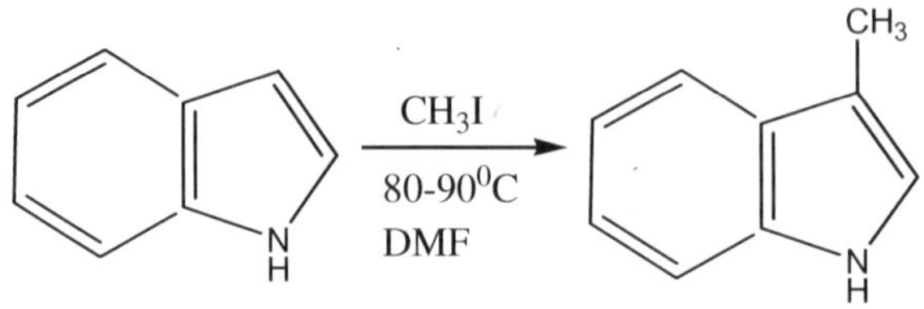

A8. Indole with aromatic aldehydes and ketones

Indole react with aromatic adehyde in the presence of acid give a cation, which again reacts with indole give a colourless bisindolylmethane which oxidised to give a coloured cation.

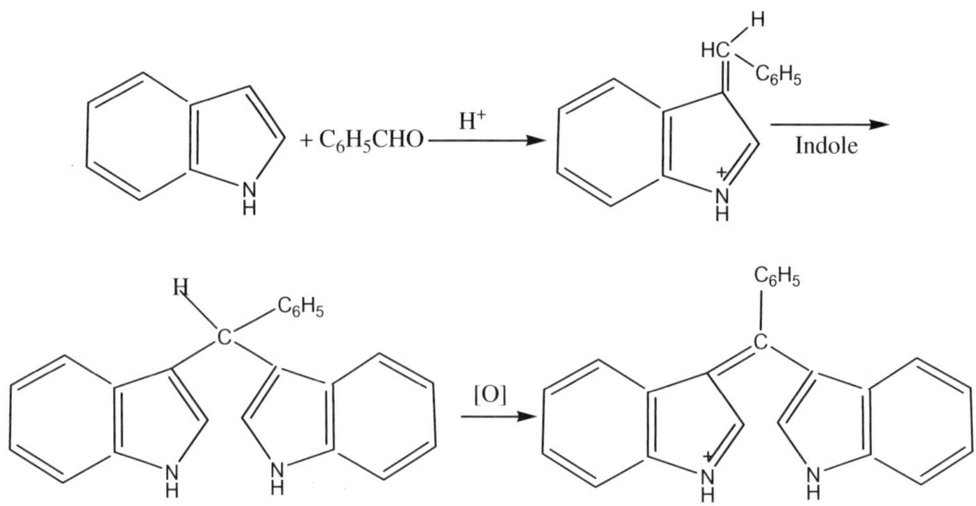

A9. Indole with α-β-unsaturated ketones

Indole undergo Michael type addition with α,β-unsaturated ketone to give α,β-alkylated product.

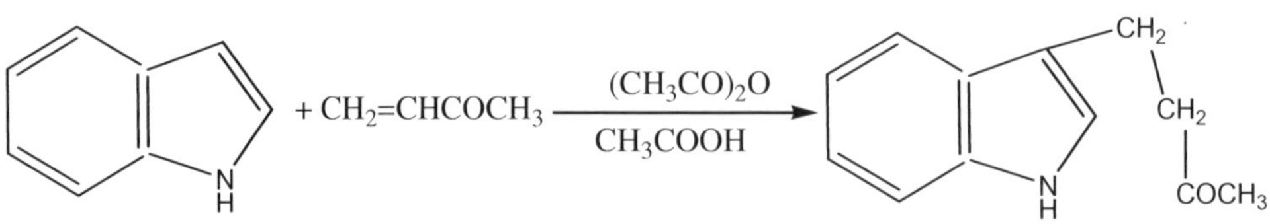

A10. Mannich reaction

Indole reacts with formaldehyde and N,N-dimethylamine in the presence of a weak acid results in aminomethylation with the formation of 3-N,N-dimethylamino methyl indole (gramine).

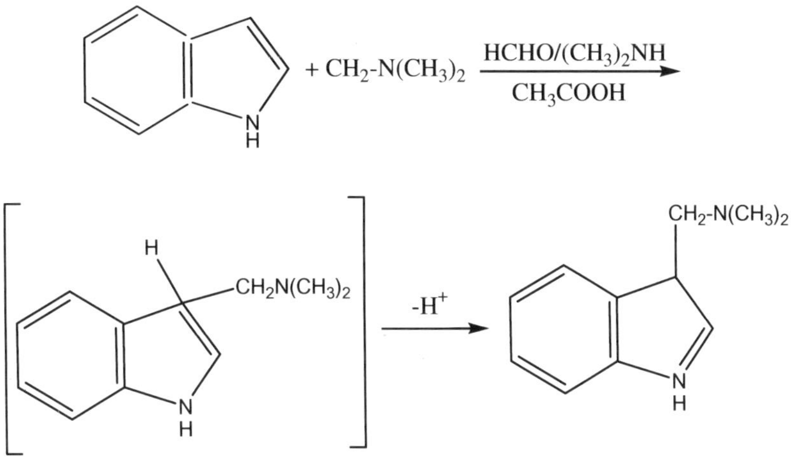

B. Reaction with Nucleophiles

Indole is π electron excessive, so inert towards nucleophilic attack.

C. Oxidation

Indole is Oxidised by air with the formation of indolin-3-one (indoxyl).

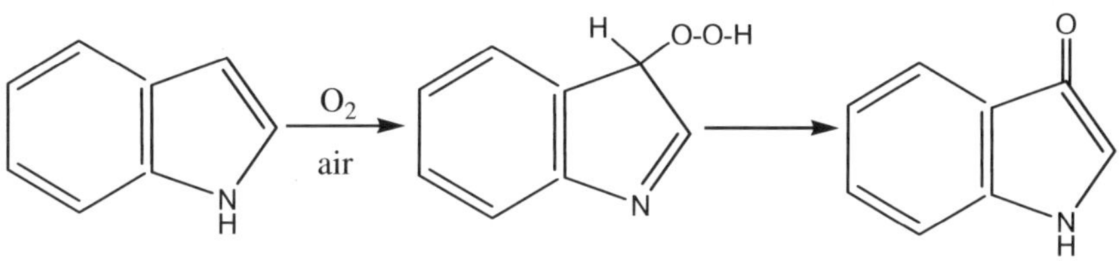

Indole undergo Oxidation by ozone to give 2-acylamino phenyl ketones.

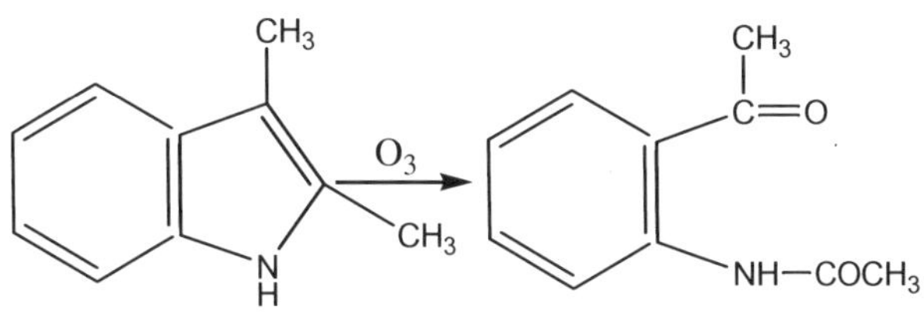

D. Reduction

Indole is Catalytically hydrogenated to Indoline by Raney nickel in ethanol.

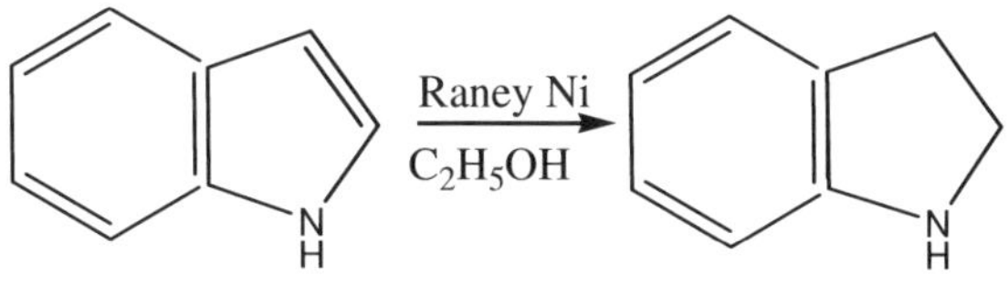

PYRIDINE

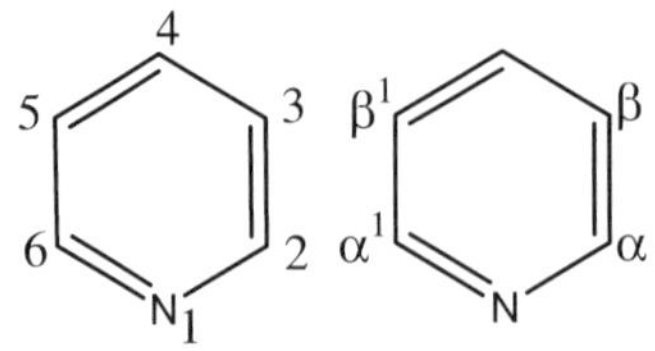

Nitrogen have a lone pair of electrons, which is available for protonation. Thus pyridine behaves as a tertiary base. Many synthetic methods are there to prepare pyridine.

Hantzsch Synthesis

It involves condensation of an aldehyde with two moles of a β dicarbonyl compound and ammonia.

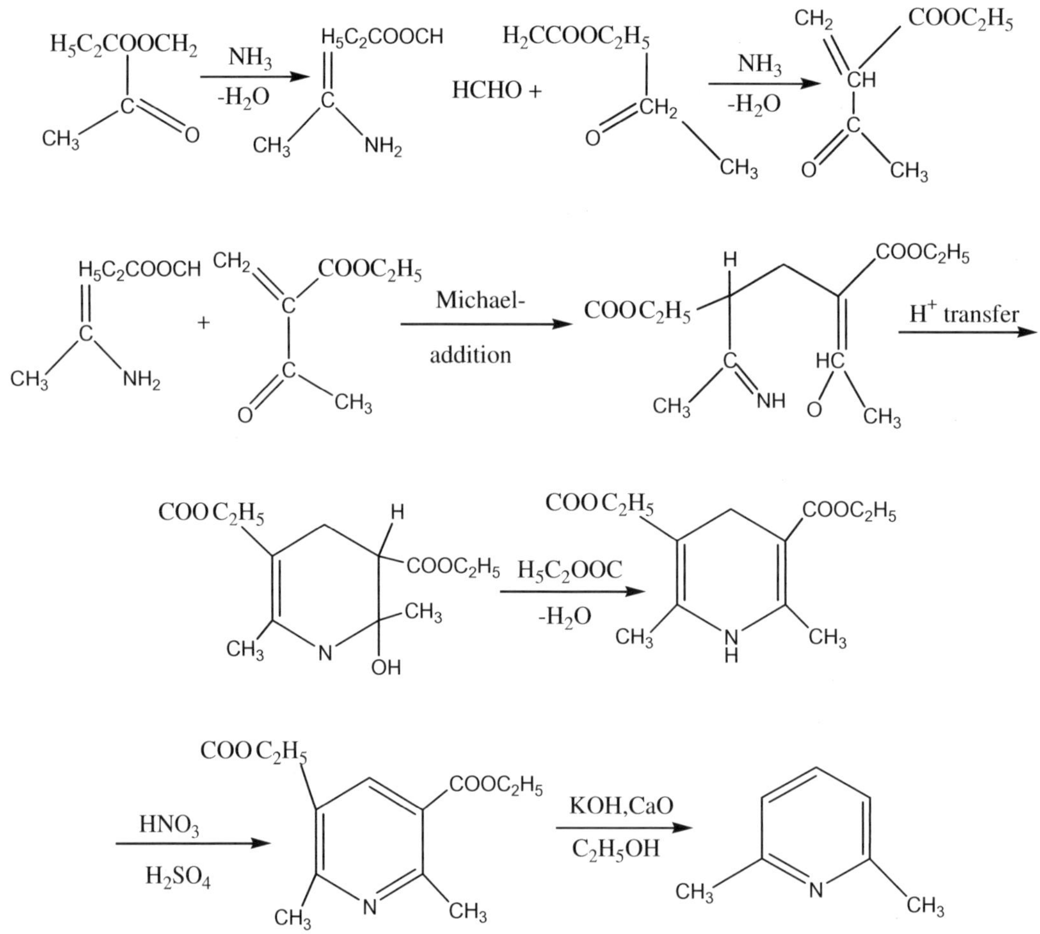

Guareschi Synthesis

It involves treating a cyanoacetamide with a diketone yield pyridone which converted to pyridine.

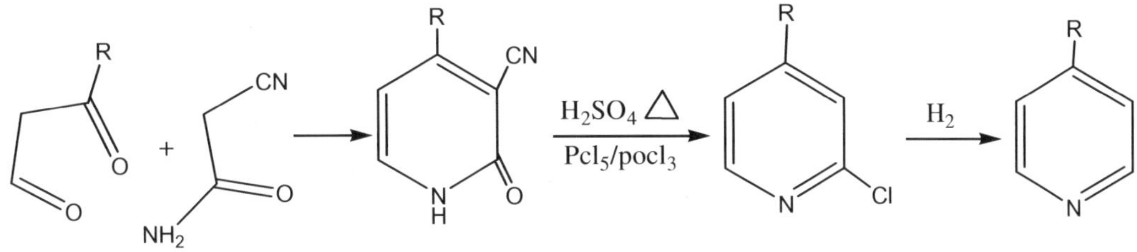

From aldehydes or ketones and ammonia

Aldehydes or ketones react with ammonia at high temperature give pyridines.

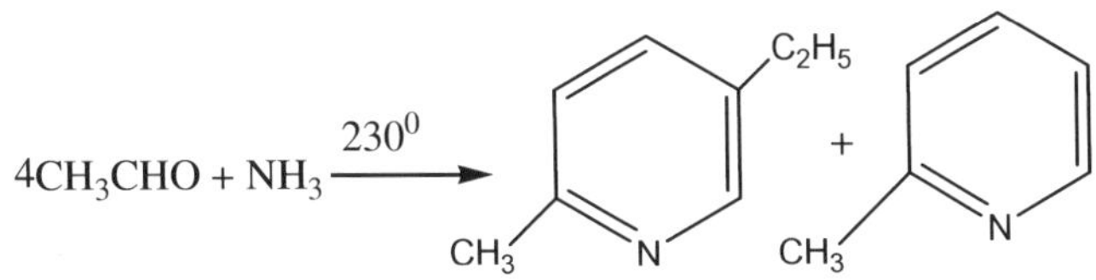

From pentamethylene diaminehydrochloride

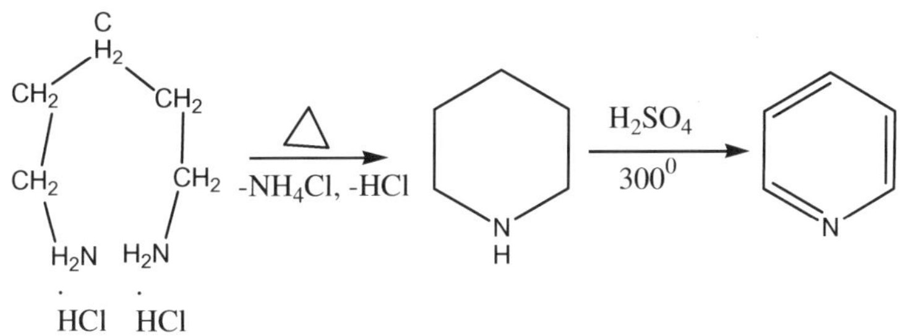

From furans

2-Furyl ketones give 3-hydroxy - 2 alkyl pyridines when heated with ammonia.

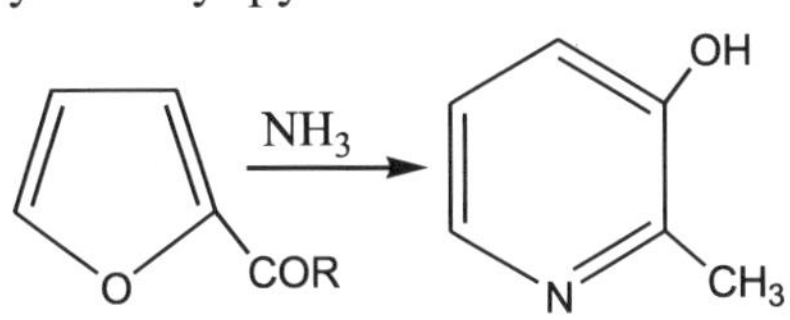

From Azawitting reaction

The Azawitting reaction of iminophosphorane prepared by the reaction of triphenylphosphorous on ethyl-2-azido-5-phenyl-2-4-butadiene carboxylate followed by its reaction with isocyanate yields a carbodiimide. It undergoes thermal electrocyclic ring closure and aromatized to give 2-aminopyridine derivative.

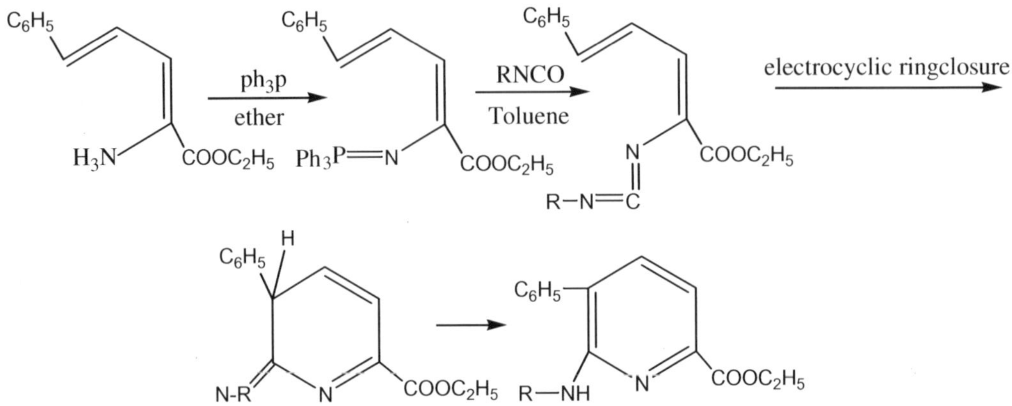

Chemical Properties of Pyridine

Pyridine is a π deficient heterocycle. Pyridine contains a doubly bonded nitrogen atom which attracts electrons from the ring, while the nitrogen atom of pyrrole donates electrons to the ring. Therefore electrophilic substitution takesplace only in drastic conditions.

Electrophilic substitution

A1. Nitration

3-nitro Pyridine formed in vigorous conditions.

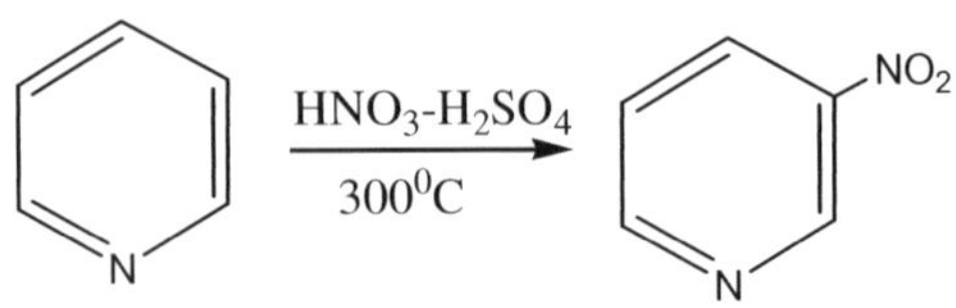

A2. Sulfonation

Pyridine is resistant to sulfonation by conc.sulfuric acid or oleum but presence of catalytic amount of mercuric sulfate facilitates sulfonation after prolonged heating at 230°C to form pyridine 3-sulfonic acid.

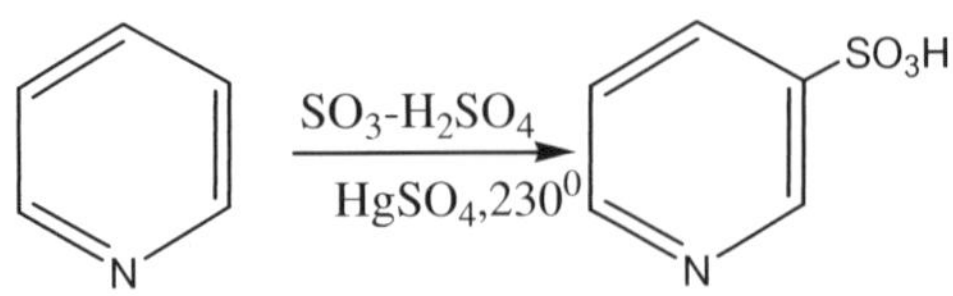

A3. Bromination

Pyridine reacts with Bromine in the presence of oleum at 300°C give Bromopyridine.

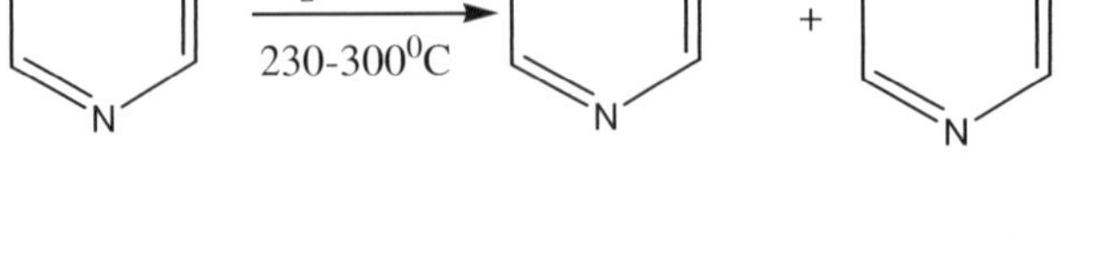

A4. Mercuration

Mercuration of Pyridine carried out by heating pyridine with mercuric acetate at 170-180°C. The initial salt formed will rearranges to give 3-pyridylmercuric acetate which is converted to pyridine mercuric chloride.

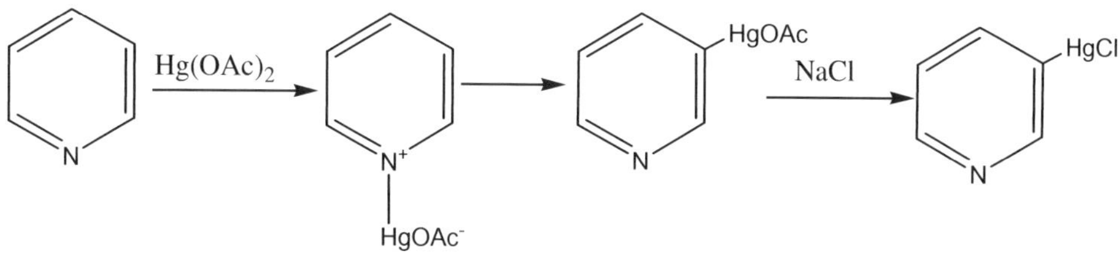

B. Diels-Alder reaction

Pyridine does not afford the normal Diels-Alder adduct but may react with powerful dienophiles like dimethyl acety lenedicarboxylate (DMAD) to form adduct. Initially a zwitterion is formed, which cyclizes and rearranged to give the adduct.

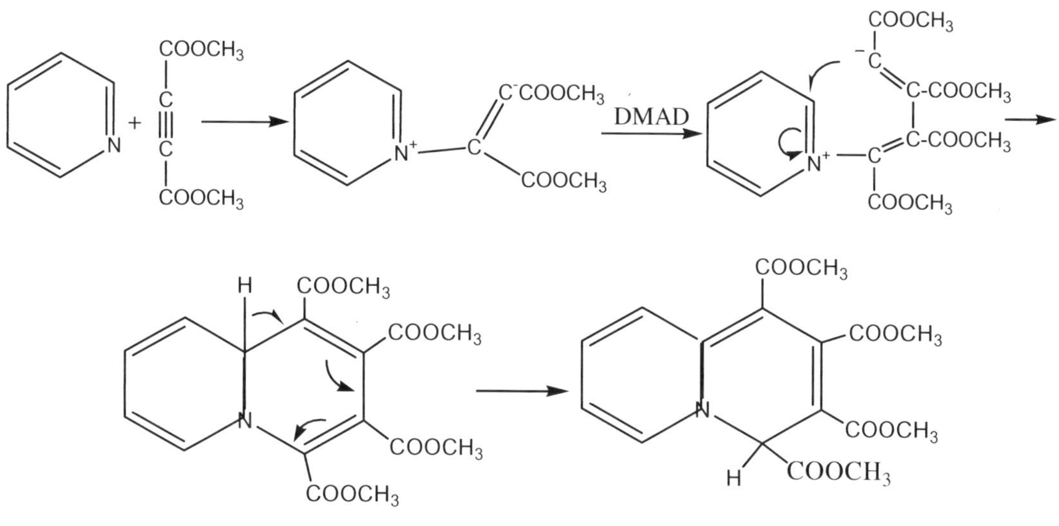

C. Reduction

Due to lower electron density about the carbon atoms the pyridine ring is more easily reduced.

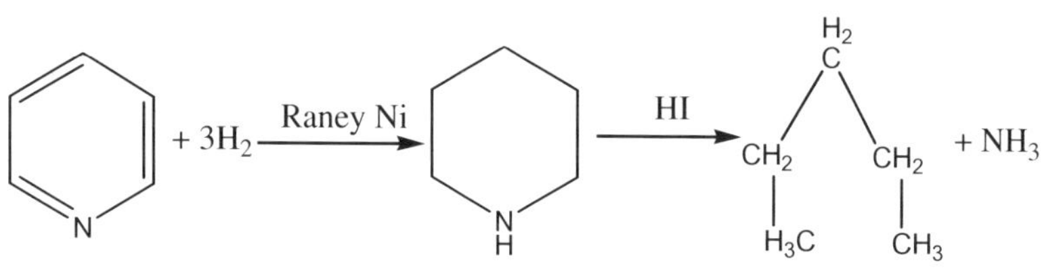

D. Reaction with oxidizing agents

Due to low electron density about its carbon atoms pyridine is resistant to most of the oxidising agents which are electron acceptors. However pyridine is oxidized by perbenzoic acid, peracetic acid or hydrogenperoxide in acetic acid to give pyridine-1-oxide.

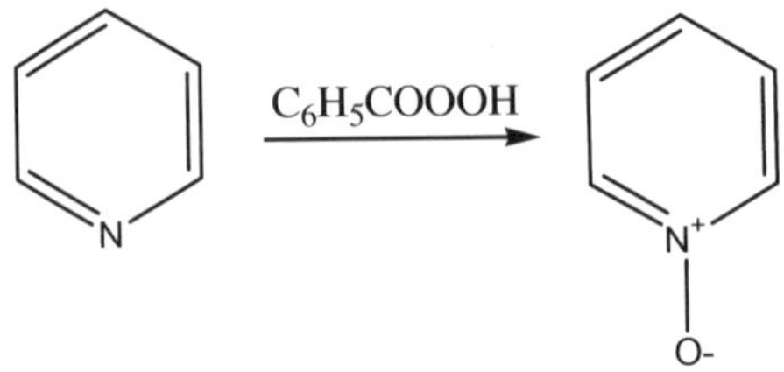

E. Nucleophilic Substitution

The electron deficient nature of 2nd 4th positions of pyridine makes these positions very reactive towards nucleophiles 2-amino pyridine can be prepared from pyridine by the reaction of sodamide (chichibabin reaction)

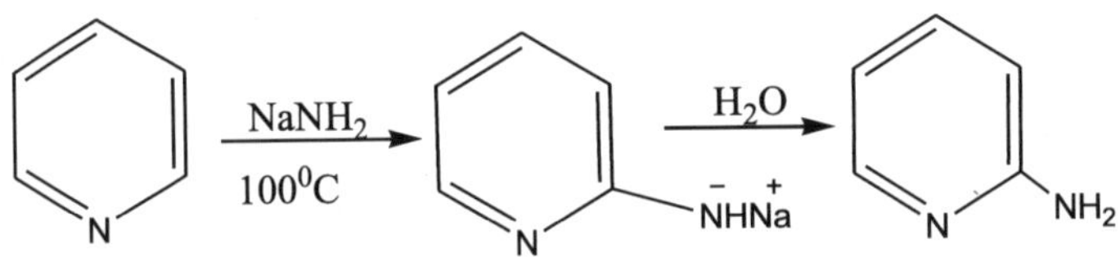

Same electronegativity of nitrogen that makes pyridine unreactive towards electrophilic substitution makes pyridine highly reactive towards nucleophilic substitution. Other important nucleophilic substitutions can be sketched as follows;

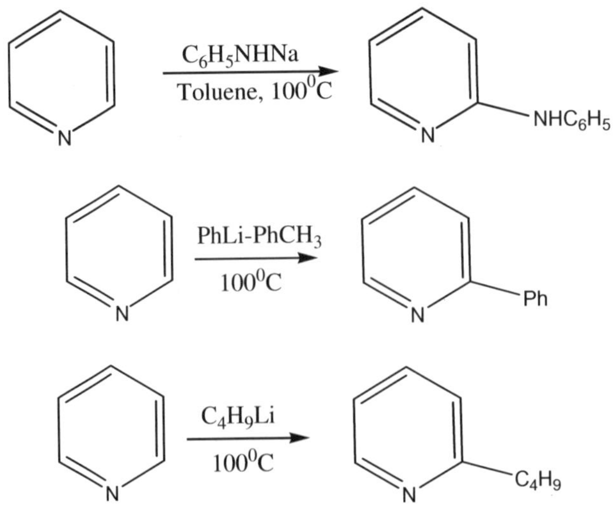

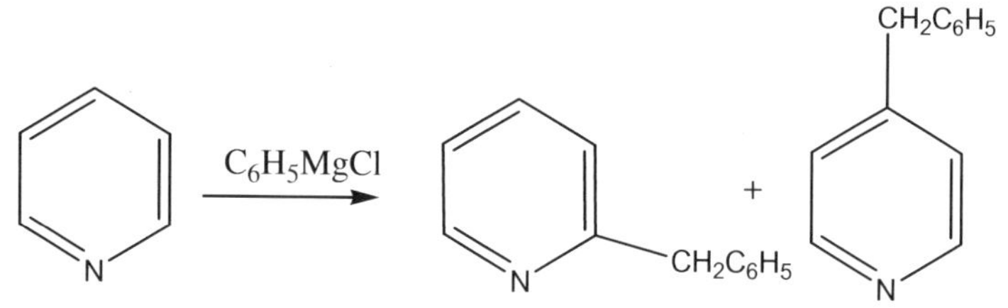

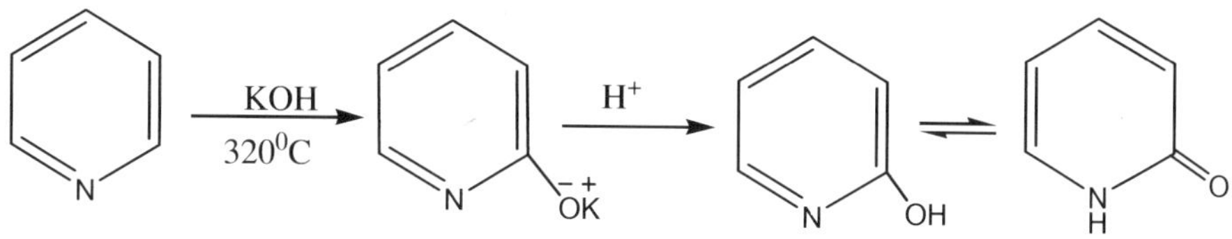

F. Ring Opening Reactions

Pyridine is not cleaved by acids and is stable in aqueous acids upto 300°C. But pyridine when reduced with sodium in 95% ethanol resulting in cleavage of ring to produce small amount of glutaconic dialdehyde OHC $(CH_2)_4$CHO. Pyridinium salts readily reacts with nucleophiles and ring cleaved to give gluconaldehyde derivative.

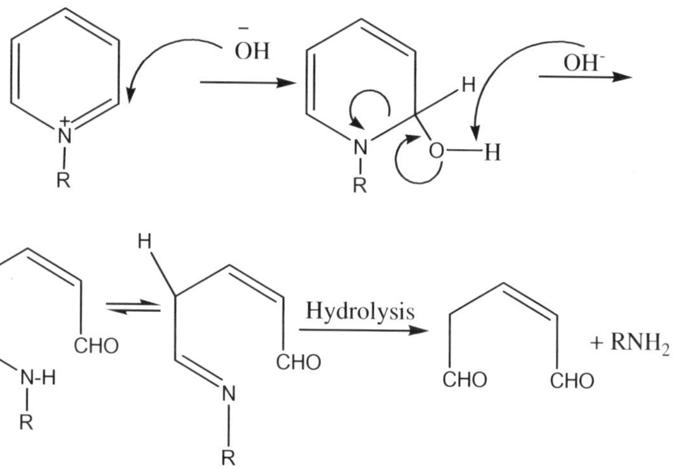

G. Photochemical Reaction

Irradiation (2537Å) of pyridine in butane converted to unstable Dewar pyridine, which have the half life of about 2mts, converted back to pyridine.

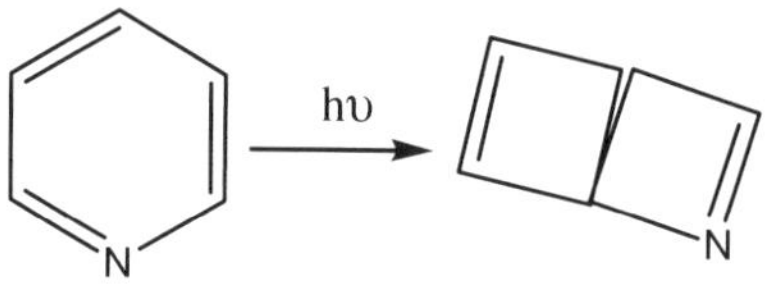

PYRIMIDINE

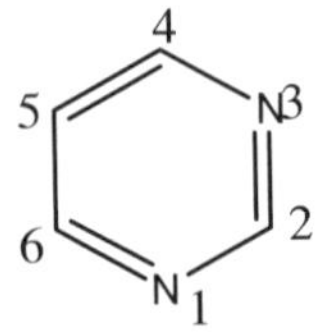

Pyrimidine widely distributed in nucleic acids. Pyrimidine is symmetrical about the line passing C-2 and C-5, the positions C-4 and C-6 are equivalent and so are N-1 and N-3. Now we will see some synthetic methods for pyrimidines

Gabriel's synthesis

Malonic acid react with urea gives Barbituric acid, which chlorinated to give trichloro derivative which dehalogenated by zinc dust give pyrimidine.

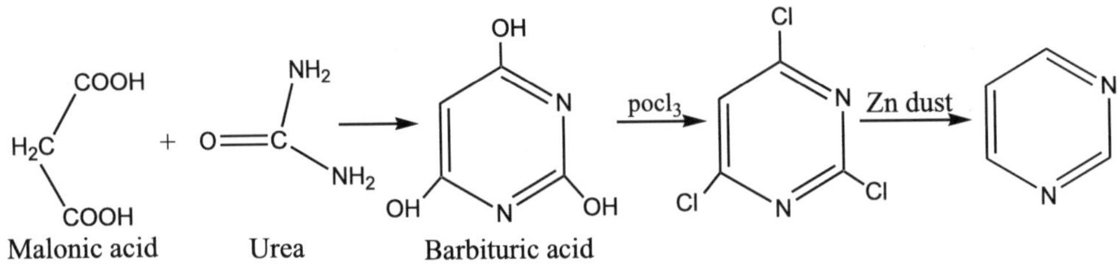

Pyrimidine from α,β-unsaturated ketones

α,β-unsaturated ketones react with amidines gives dihydropyrimidine, which is readily oxidized by a stream of air to give corresponding pyrimidine.

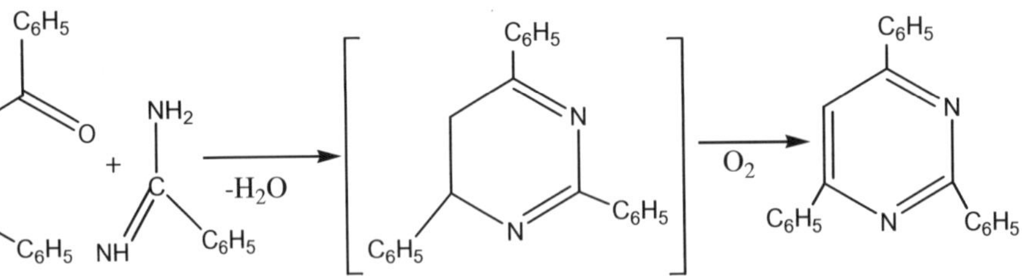

Pyrimidine from Aliphatic compounds

Pyrimidine can be prepared by the reaction in between 1,1,3,3-tetraethoxypropane and formamide.

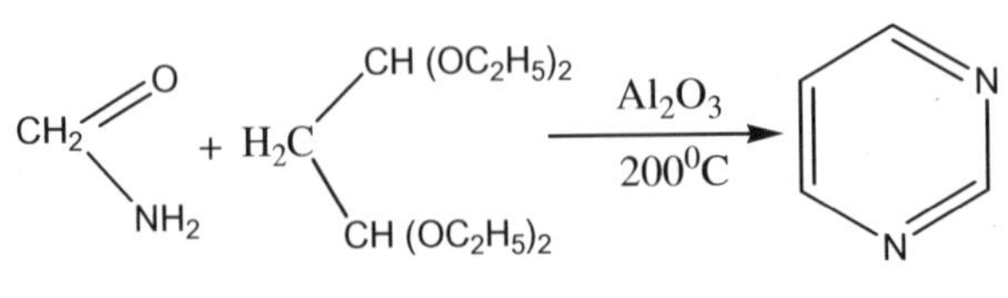

Pyrimidine by Whittaker's method

Catalytic reductive dechlorination of 2,4-dichloropyrimidine gives pyrimidine.

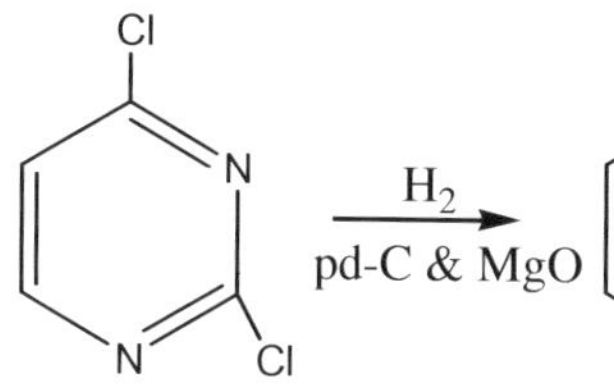

Chemical Properties of Pyrimidine

Reaction with acids

Pyrimidine can be protonated in the presence of acids.

Electrophilic Substitution

Pyrimidine is resistant to electrophilic substitution. The electrophilic attack at positions 2,4 and 6 is particularly retarded because of the electron deficiency at these positions. If one or more electron-releasing groups are present on the ring, then electrophilic substitution at 5th position is possible. Bromination of pyrimidine can be proceeded via perbromide intermediate.

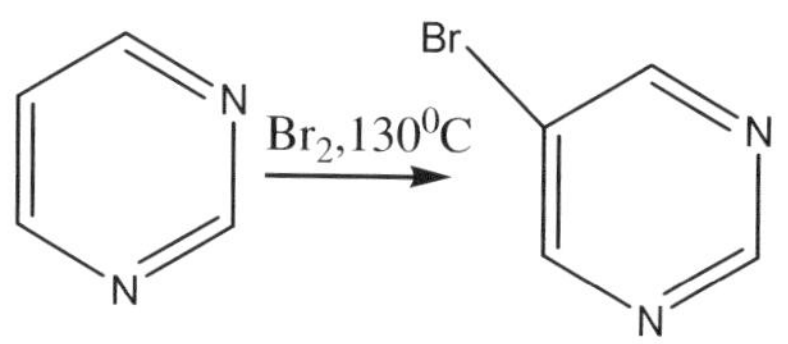

Pyrimidine does not undergo nitration. But 2,4-dihydroxy pyrimidine undergoes nitration in boiling fuming nitric acid give 2,4-dihydroxy-5-nitropyrimidine. Pyrimidines with two or more electron donating groups undergo diazocoupling at 5th position.

Nucleophilic Substitution

2nd, 4th, and 6th positions in Pyrimidine is easily suceptible to nucleophilic attack. Grignard and organolithium reagents readily add to 3,4-bond of pyrimidines at room temperature.

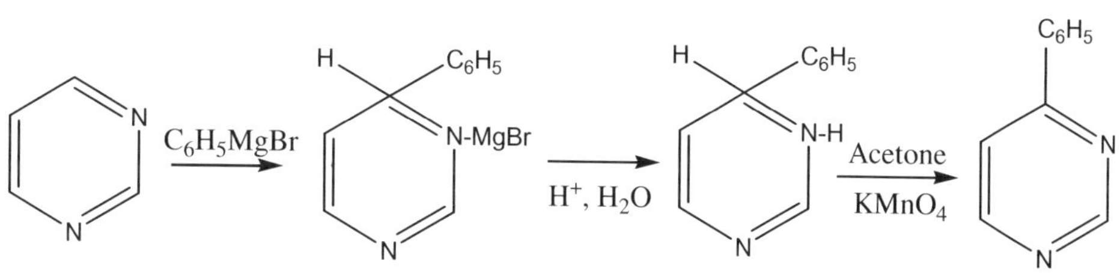

Reaction with oxidizing agents

With per acids Pyrimidine gives a low yield of N-oxide, but the ring is largely destroyed. But alkyl pyrimidines give a satisfactory yield of N-oxides.

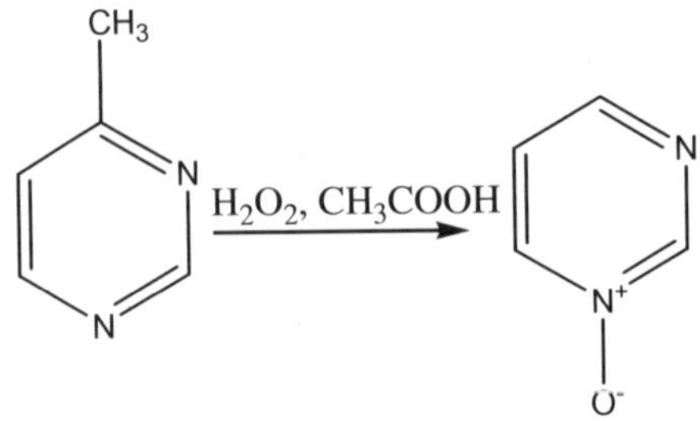

Thio-Claisen Rearrangement

Substituted thiopyrimidines undergo thio-claisen rearragement. 3-methyl- 4-allylthio-Pyrimidine-2-one on heating yields 5-allyl-4-thiouracil.

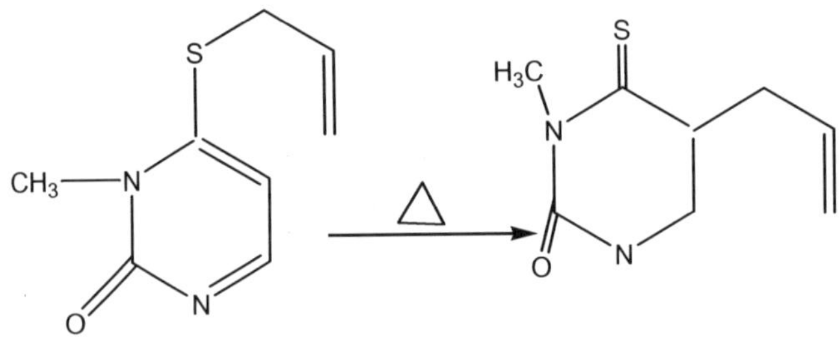

QUINOLINE

Quinoline occurs in coal-tar and bone oil from which it can be extracted with acids.

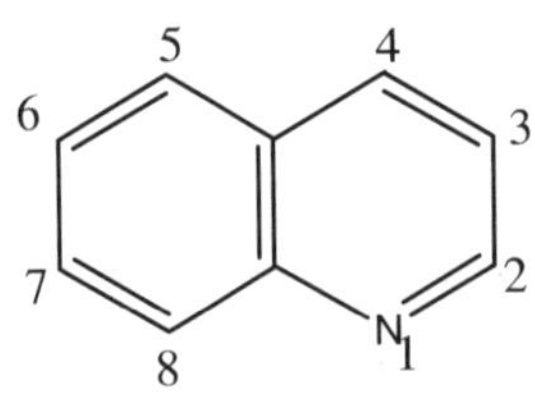

Quinoline ring structure is obtained by ortho-condensation of benzene ring with pyridine. It can also called 1-azanaphthalene or benzo pyridine. Many methods are there to synthesise quinoline. Important among them are as follows;

Skraups Synthesis

In this method an aniline derivative having a vacant ortho position is heated with glycerol, conc.sulfuric acid and an oxidizing agent.

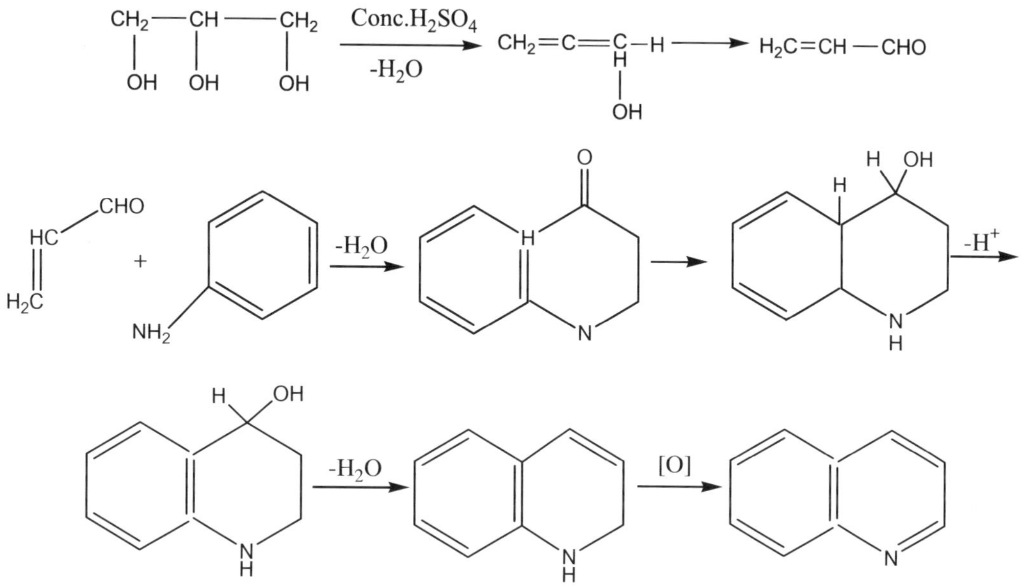

Doebner-Miller Synthesis

In this method, an aromatic amine and two molecules of an aldehyde are heated in the presence of hydrochloric acid.

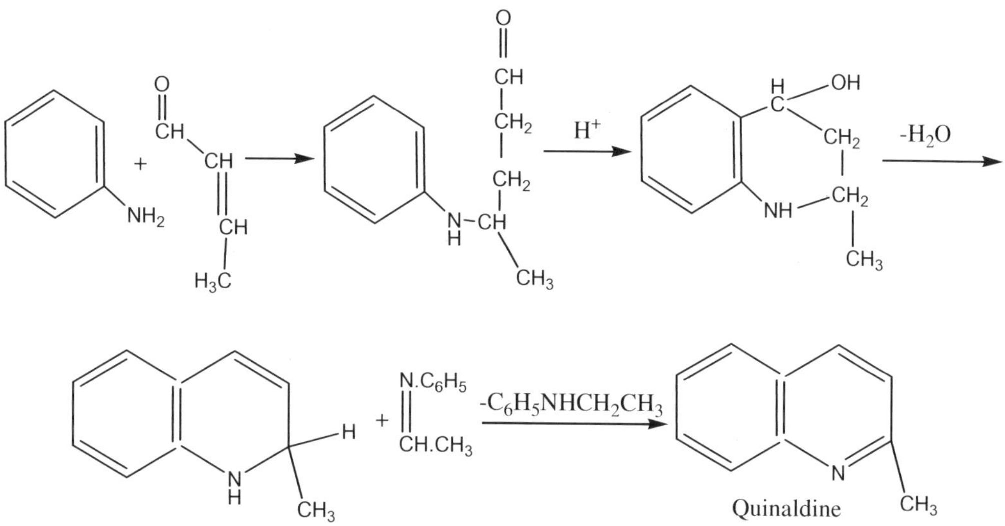

Friedlanders Synthesis

This method consists of condensing the o.amino benzaldehyde with aldehyde or ketone containing a reactive methylene group adjacent to the carbonyl group in aqueous sodium hydroxide.

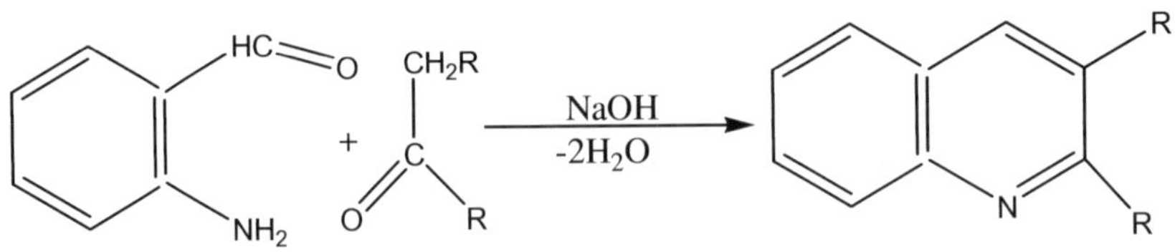

Pfitzinger synthesis

It employs isatin instead of o-amino benzaldehyde in Friedla nders synthesis.

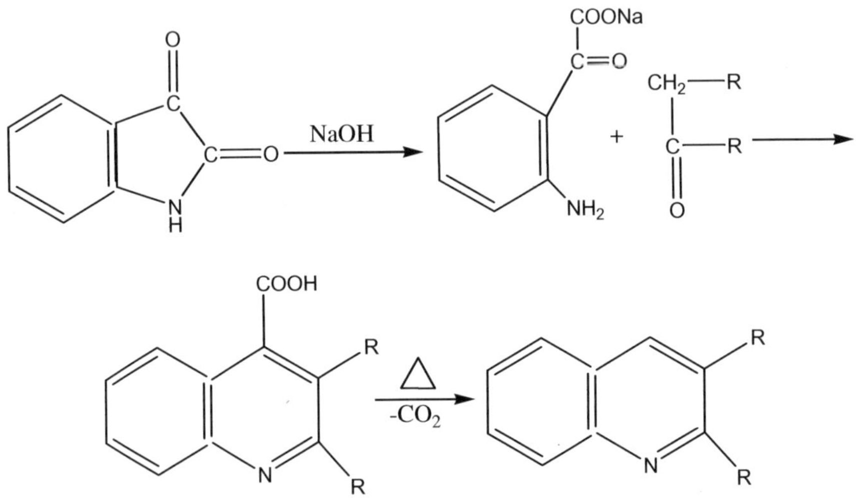

Conardt-Limpach synthesis

It involves condensation of β-ketoester and aniline. The reaction takesplace at low temperature and ketonic group of β-ketoester form schiff base.

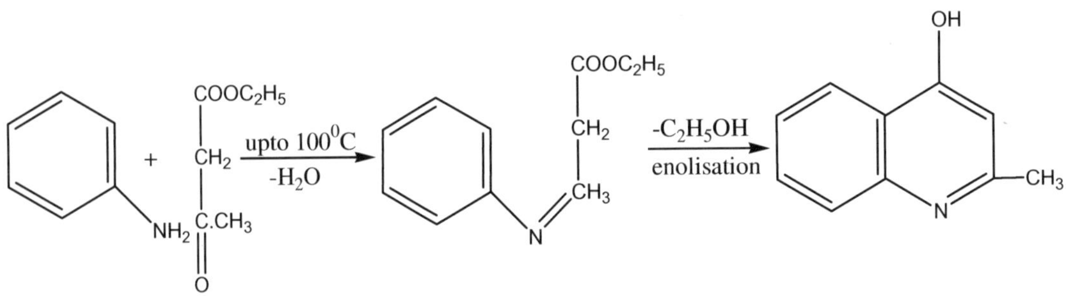

Knorr Synthesis

It also involves condensation of β-ketoester with aniline. Here the reaction takesplace at high temperature and involves ester group of β-ketoester to form amide.

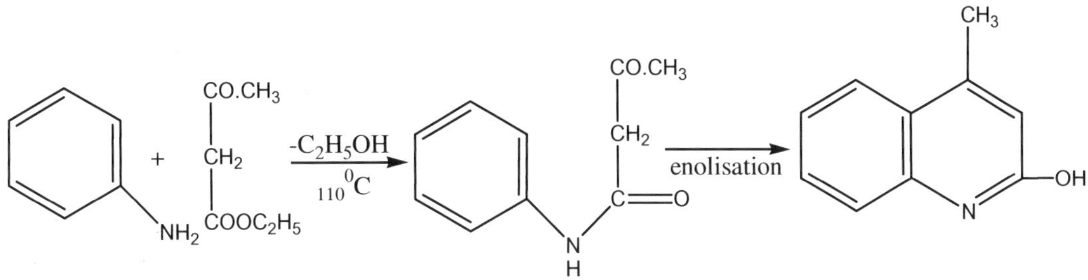

Camps method

This method employed to prepare hydroxy quinolines and involves intramolecular cyclization of o-acylamino acetophenone in the presence of sulphuric acid.

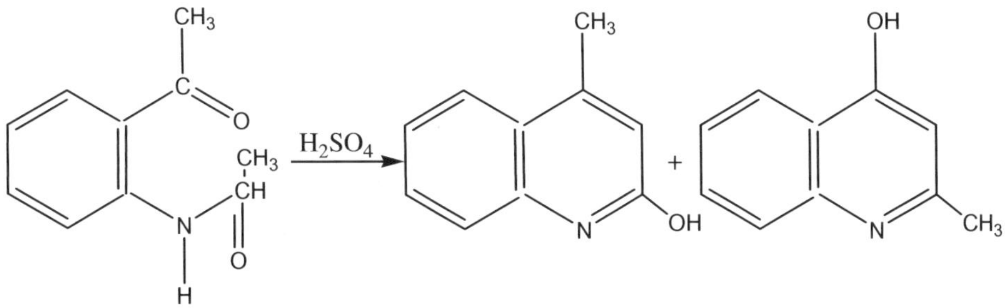

Properties of Quinoline

Quinoline displays chemical properties associated with a tertiary amine.

Electrophilic substitution

Electrophilic substitution preferentially takesplace at 5th, 6th, and 8th position

Sulphonation

In strong acidic medium Quinolinium ion get sulphonated.

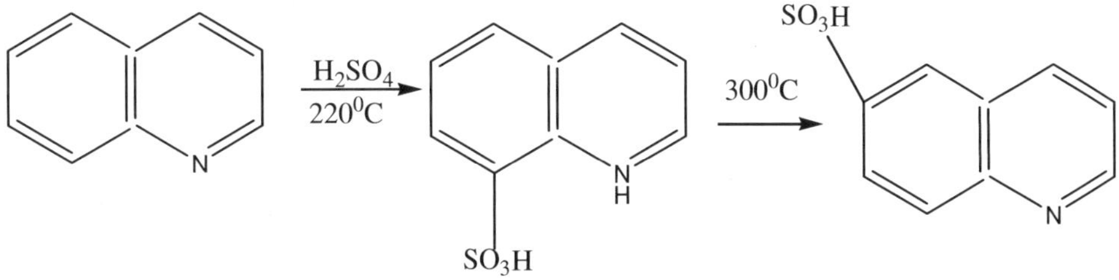

8-sulphoquinoline 6-sulphoquinoline

Nitration

Quinolinium ion get nitrated in strong acidic medium.

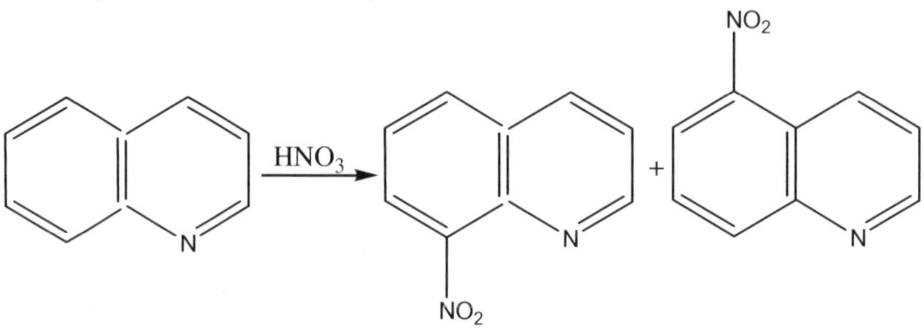

Halogenation

Halogenation occurs contrary to prediction. Bromination takesplace in Benzene ring.

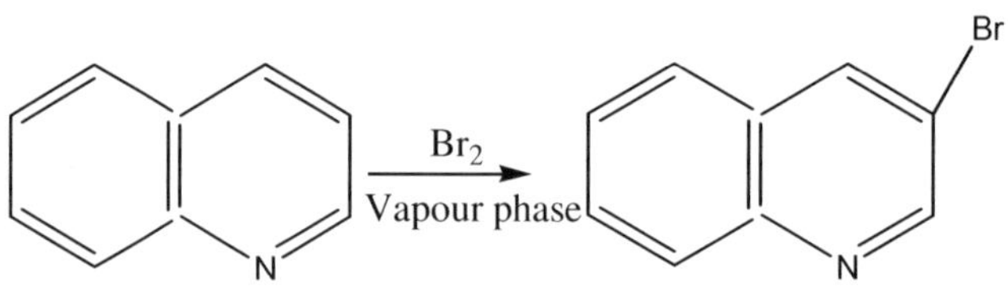

3-bromoquinoline

Mercuration

With mercuric acetate quinoline forms quaternary N-mercuricacetate at room temperature. On treatement with sodium chloride, gives a mixture of 3 and 5 mercuric chlorides.

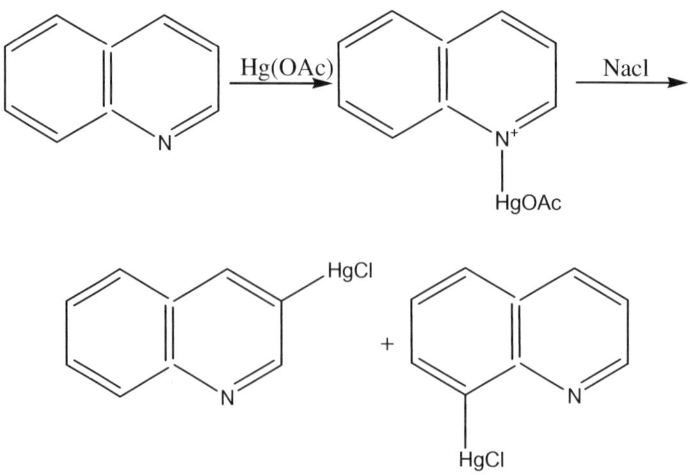

Nucleophilic Substitution

In Chichibabin reaction nucleophile attack at C-2.

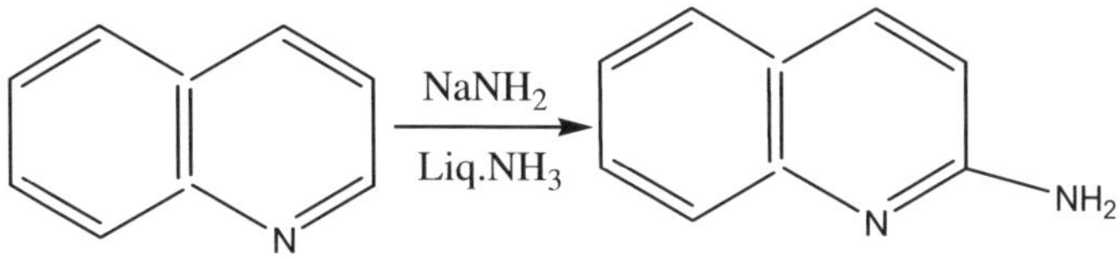

Oxidation

Since Oxidation is dependent on electron availability, permanganate oxidation will destroy the benzene ring, & leave the π deficient pyridine ring intact. Thus vigorous oxidation of quinoline oxidises the benzene ring to form quinolinic acid.

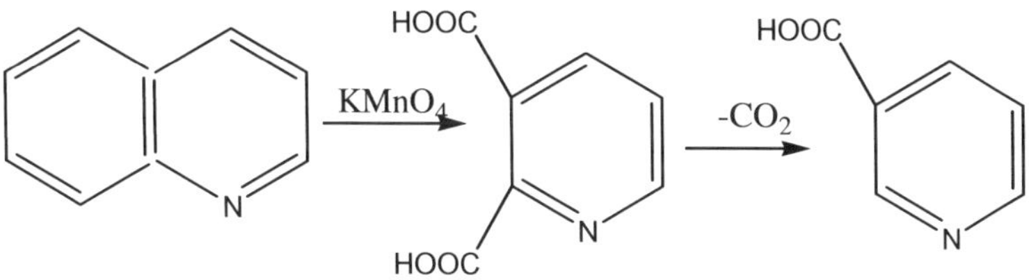

Reduction

Catalytic reduction attacks preferentially at more electron deficient pyridine ring of quinoline.

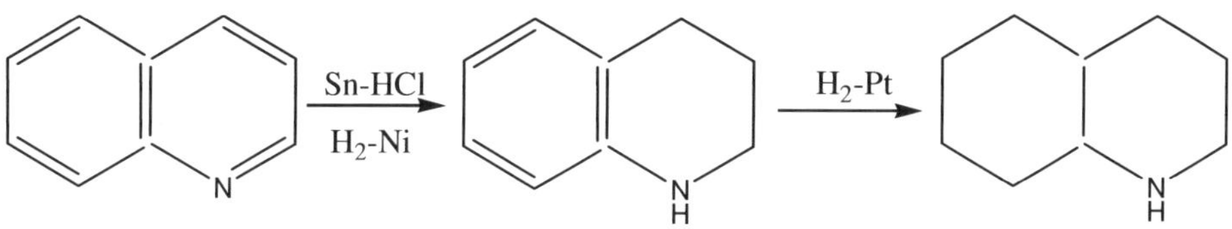

1,2,3,4 Tetrahydroquinoline

Decahydroquinoline

ISOQUINOLINES

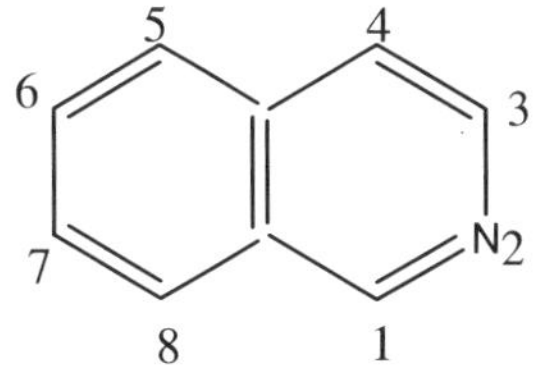

Isoquinoline can be prepared in many ways, some of them are as follows;

Bischler-Napieralski Synthesis

This method involves a cyclodehydration, of an acyl derivative of β phenylethylamine to lead to 3,4-dihydroiso quinoline in the presence of polyphosphoric acid, zinc chloride or phosphorous pentoxide. This is dehydrogenated to isoquinoline.

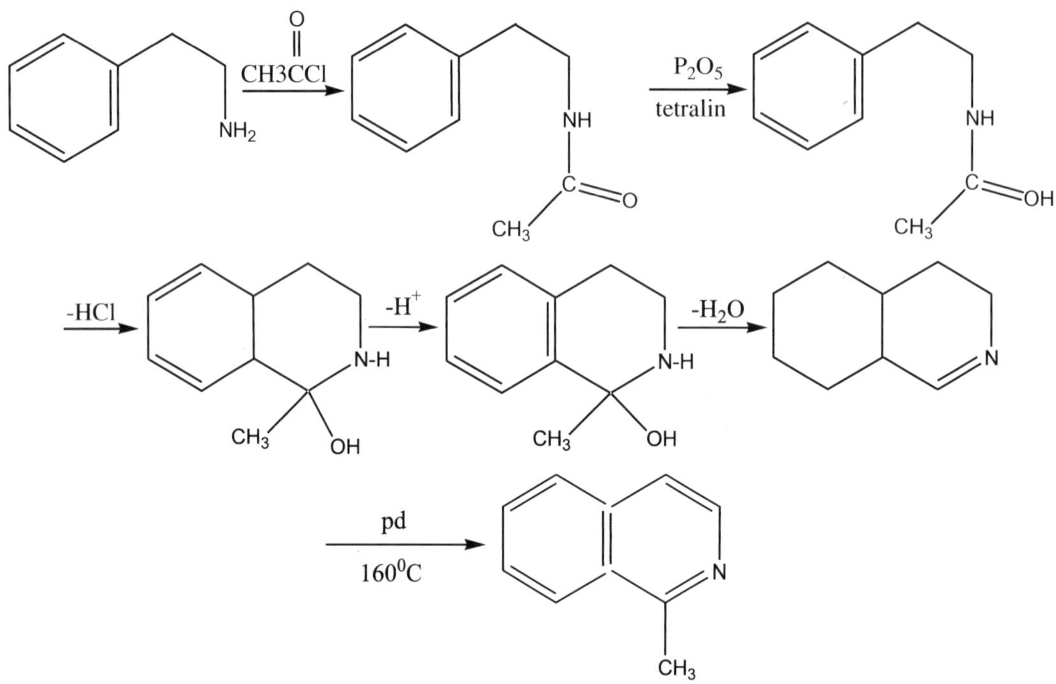

Gabriel synthesis

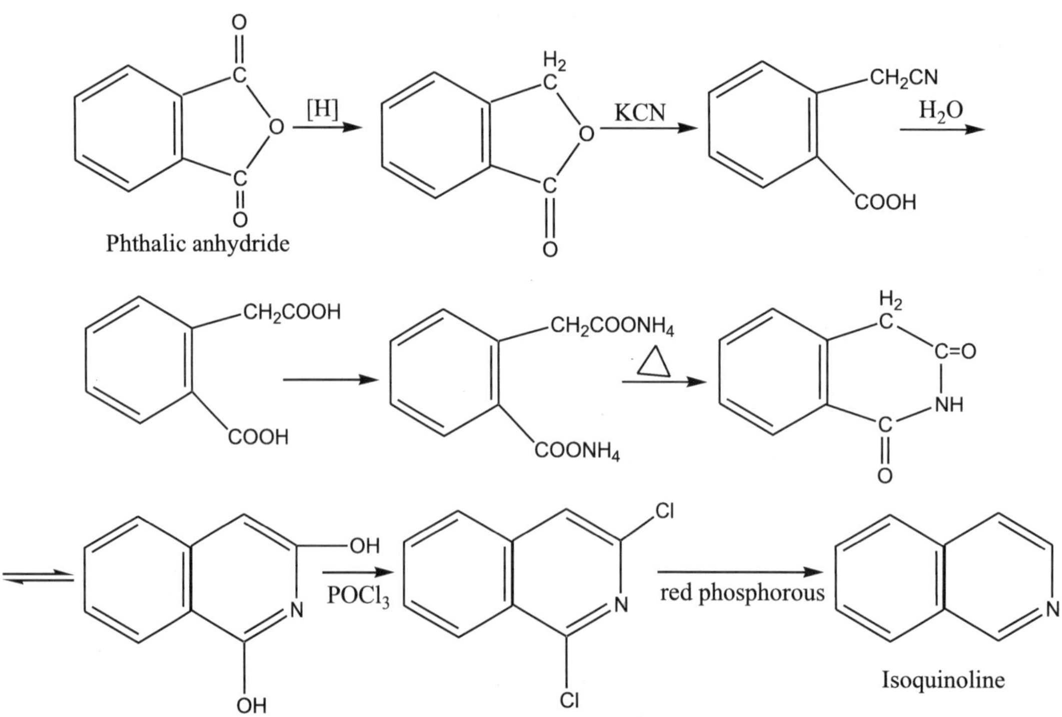

Isoquinoline from benzylidenes

Isoquinoline can be prepared by passing benzylidene ethy lamine vapours through red hot tube.

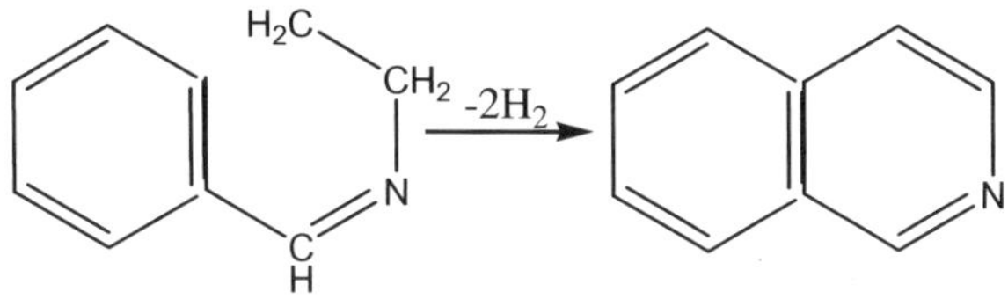

Pictet-spengler method

It consists of condensation of β-arylethylamine with an aldehyde in the presence of dilute hydrochloric acid to form techahydroisoquinoline which is dehydrogenated by palladium.

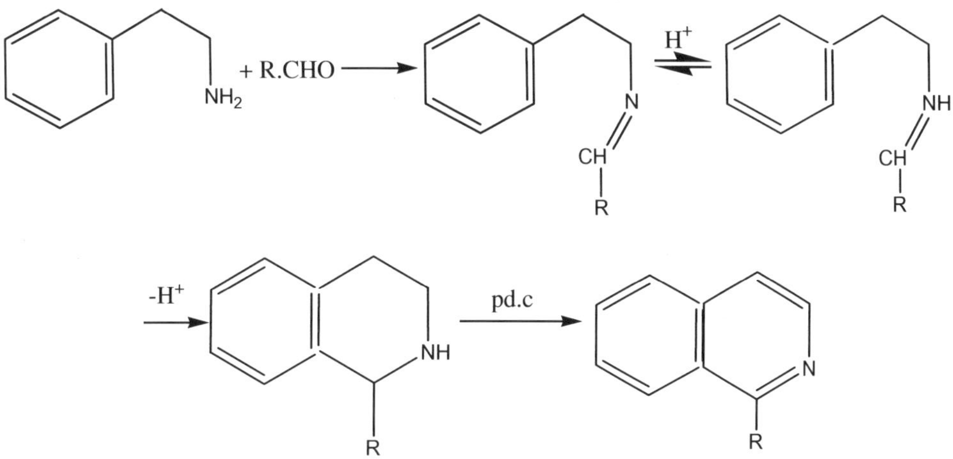

Isoquinoline from Indene

Here indene is treated with ozone at -70°C followed by reduction with dimethylsulfide in the presence of NH_4OH.

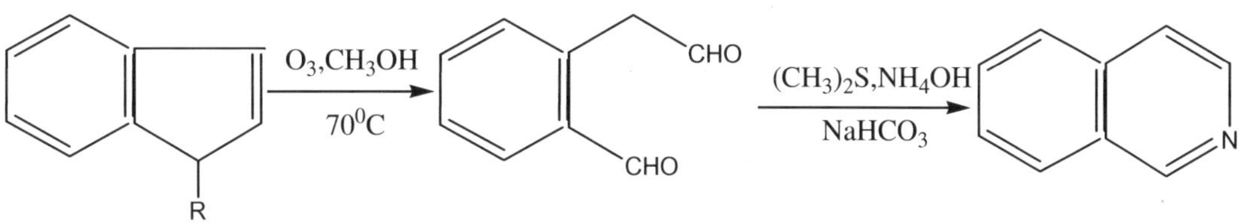

Pomeranz-Fritsch Synthesis

It consists of condensation of an aromatic aldehyde with amino acetal, the intermediate formed is then cyclized in the presence of sulfuric acid or phosphorous pentoxide.

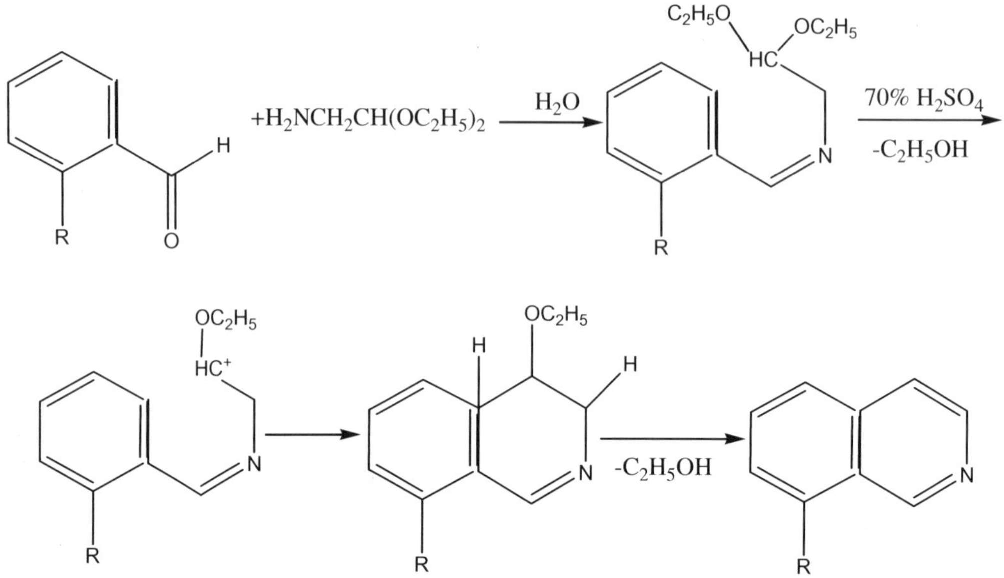

Properties of Isoquinoline

Electrophilic substitution

Isoquinoline and quinoline are similar in their chemical behaviour. Isoquinoline undergo nitration and sulphonation at 5th & 8th positions. But bromination and mercuration occurs at 4th position. (refer electrophilic reactions of Quinoline)

Reaction with Oxirane

Isoquinoline reacts with oxirane in acetic acid to form oxazolidine.

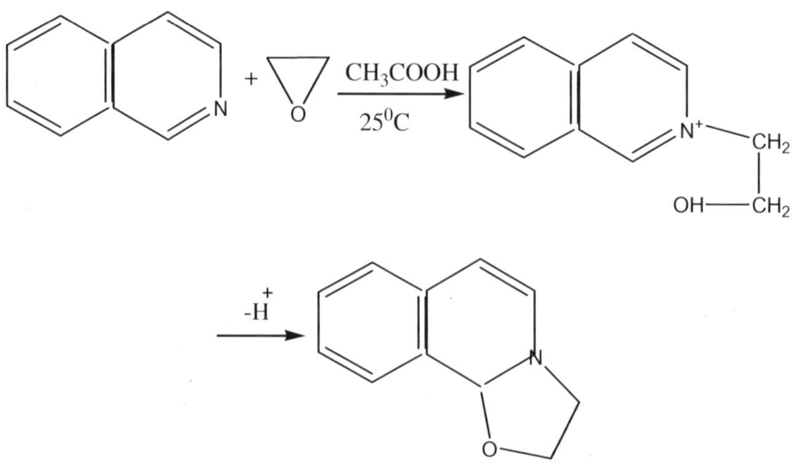

Nucleophilic Substitution

Nucleophilic attack takesplace at 1st position, if 1st position occupied, 3rd position is attacked. Chichibabin reaction takesplace as usual.

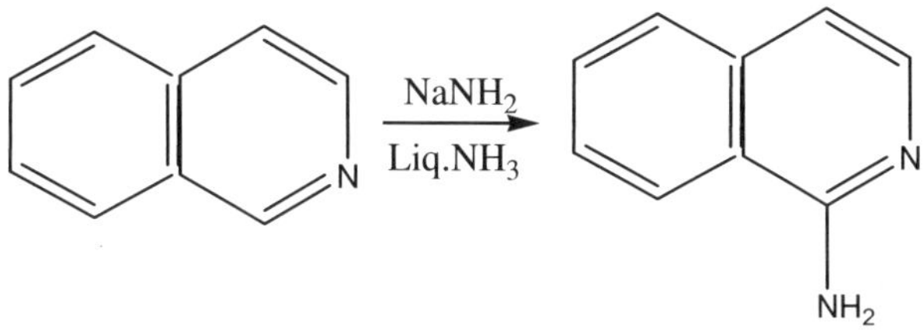

Reduction

Isoquinoline is reduced to different products by different reducing agents.

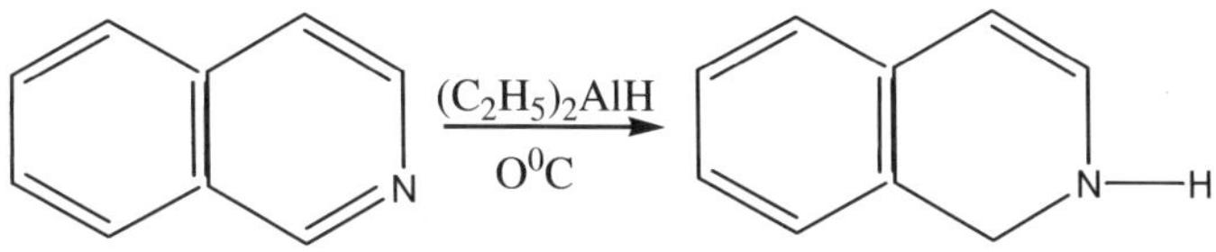

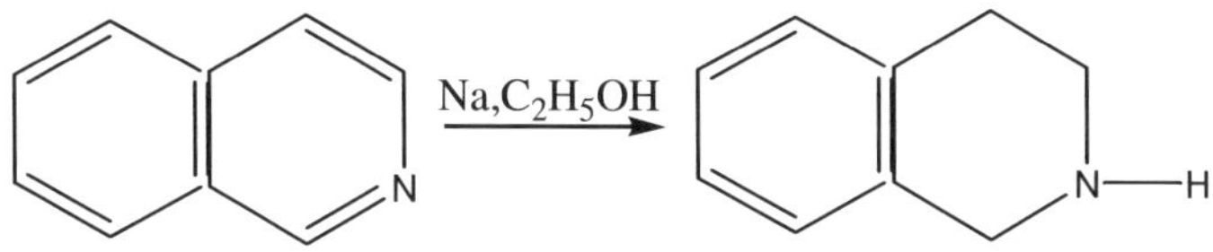

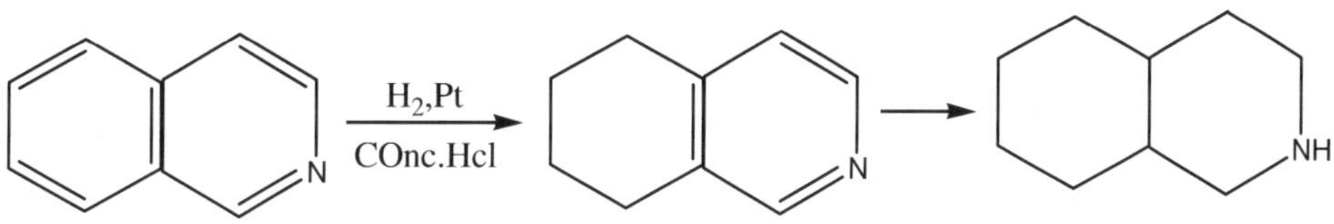

Reaction with Oxidizing agents

Isoquinoline is resistant to most of the oxidizing agents but is attacked by alkaline potassium permanaganate to give pyridine 3,4 dicarboxy.

lic acid (cinhomercuric acid) and phthalic acid.

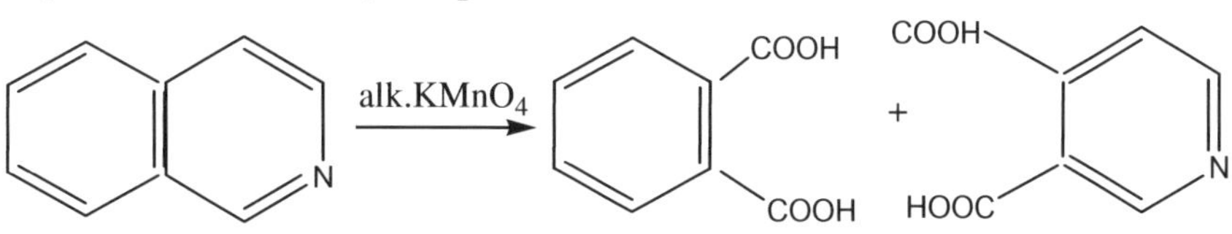

Neutral potassium permanganate convert isoquinoline into phthalimide.

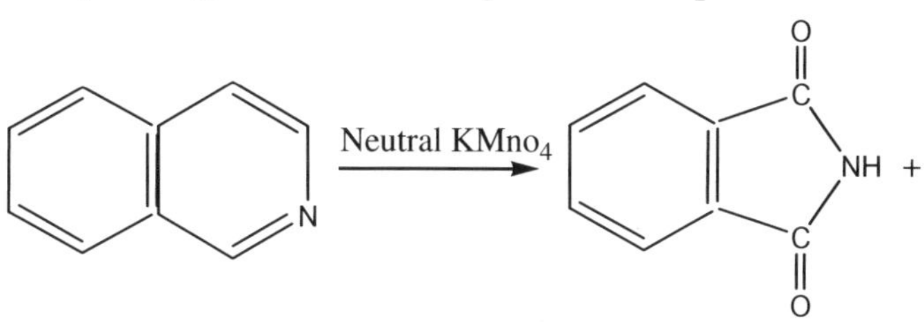

ACRIDINE

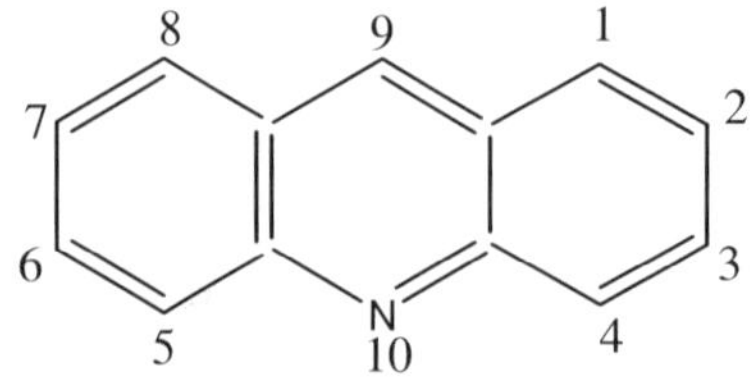

Acridine is the aza derivative of anthracene. It can be also called as benzoquinoline or dibenzpyridine. It can be synthesised in many ways.

Acridine from Diphenylamine

Acridine can be prepared by oxidation of diphenylamine using lead oxide as oxidising agent.

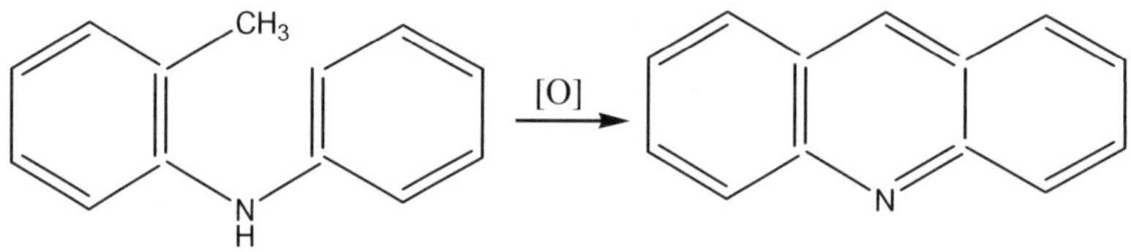

Acridine from o-aminodiphenylmethane

Acridine can be prepared by passing o-amino diphenylmethane through red hot tube.

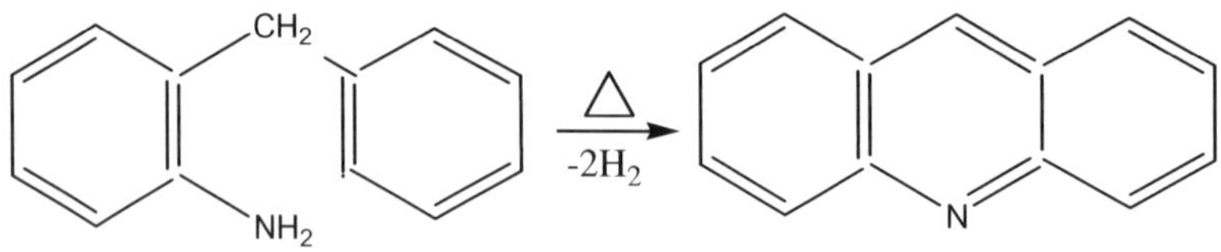

Acridine from benzylaniline

Acridine can be prepared by passing benzylaniline through a red hot tube.

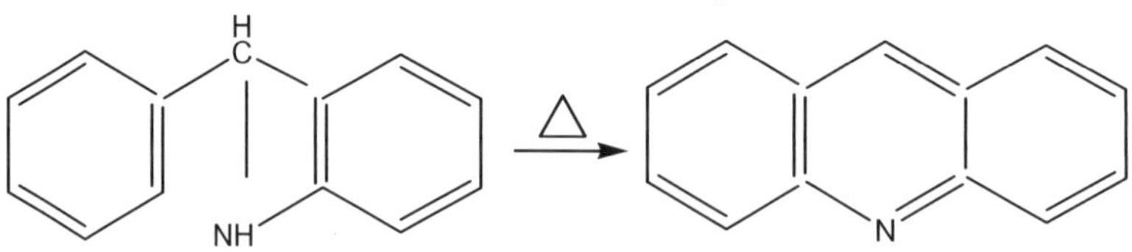

Acridine by Ullmann method

It consists of heating o-halogenobenzoic acid with an arylamine in presence of copper powder to form acridone which can be reduced into acridine by zn dust distillation.

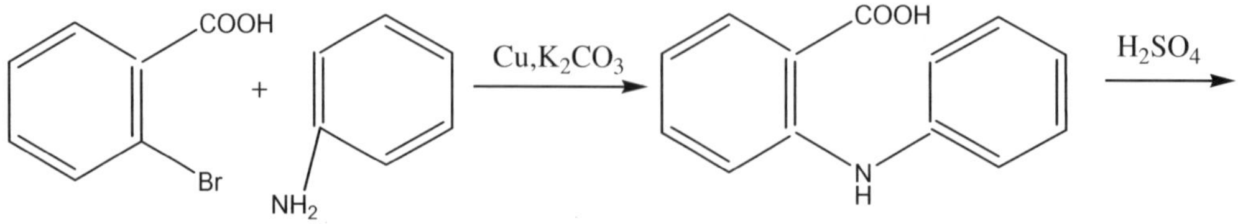

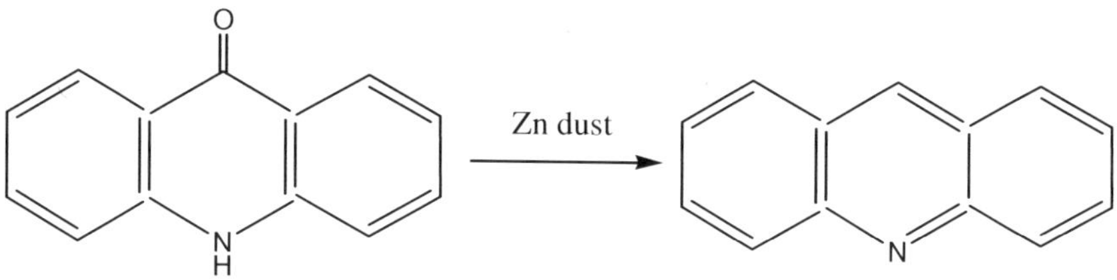

Acridine by Goldberg method

It is an analogous method to Ullmann method. It involves heating of o-aminobenzoic acid with Bromobenzene.

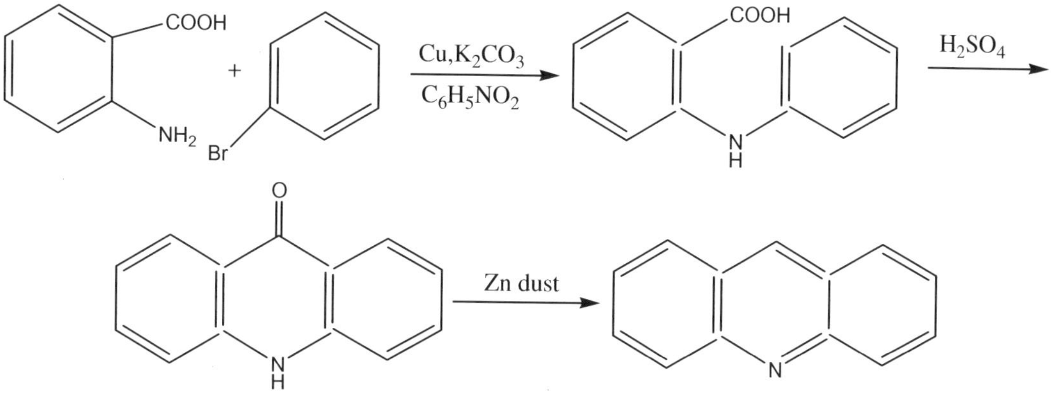

Properties of Acridine

Properties of acridine can be derived by extrapolation from the chemistry of pyridine and Quinoline.

Electrophilic substitution

Electrophilic reactions mainly takesplace in benzenoid rings.

Halogenation

Bromination of acridine gives 2 and 2,7-dibromo products.

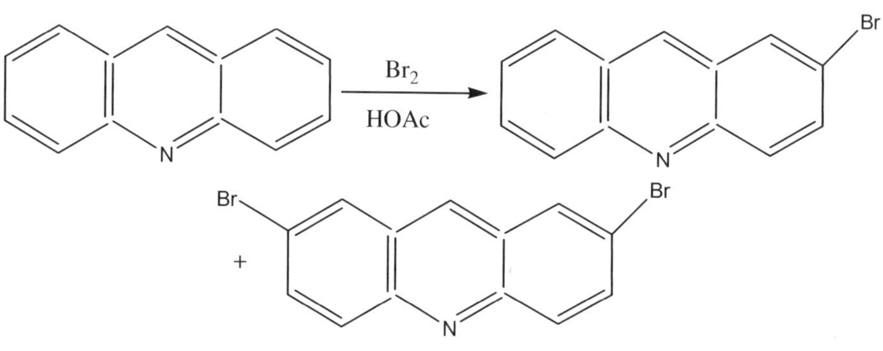

Nucleophilic Substitution

Acridine undergoes nucleophilic attack at 9th position due to its less electron density at 9th position compared to other positions. Acridine reacts with sodamide in liquid ammonia gives 9-aminoacridine.

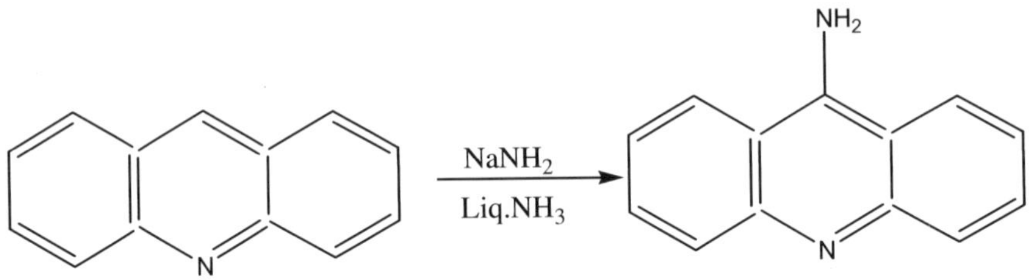

Reaction with Oxidizing agents

Acridine is a stable ring towards oxidation but is converted to N-oxide with peracids.

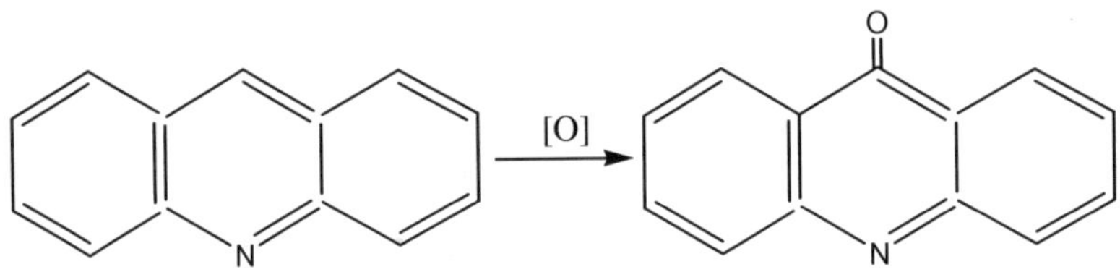

Reaction with Reducing agents

Benzene ring of acridine can be selectively reduced by pd or Rh/C in hydrochloric acid, platinium oxide in trifluoroacetic acid to produce octahydroacridine.

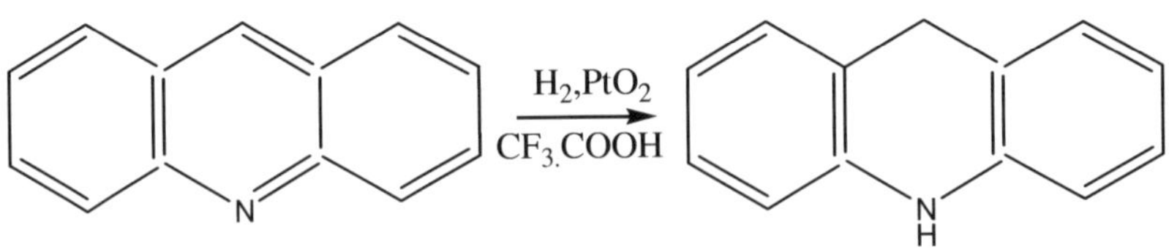

Acridine on reduction by lithium in liquid ammonia gives 1,4,5,8-Tetra hydroacridine.

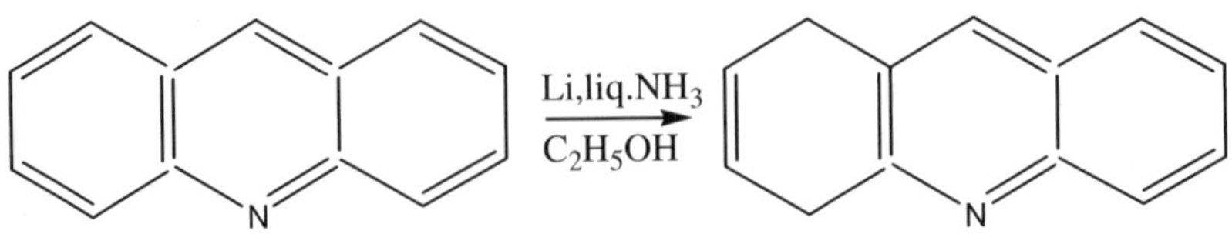

AZEPINES

Azepines are 7-membered heterocycle and can be called as azacyclo heptatriene. Several methods are there to prepare Azepines.

Azepines by Valence Bond Isomerization

In valence bond migration, the atoms involved in bond reorganization be apparently in a parallel plane so that small adjustments in bond distances, angles and electron distribution can be achieved. so it is a reorganisation in which σ & π electrons are reorganized.

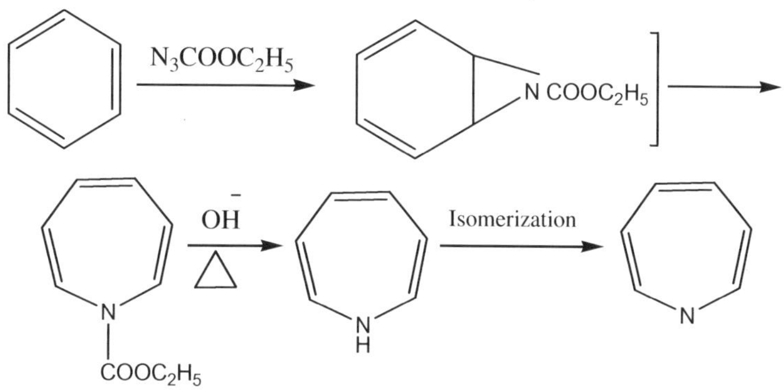

Azepine from Phenylazide

A phenylazide on decomposition in boiling primary or secondary amine undergoes ring expansion to yield 3H azepine.

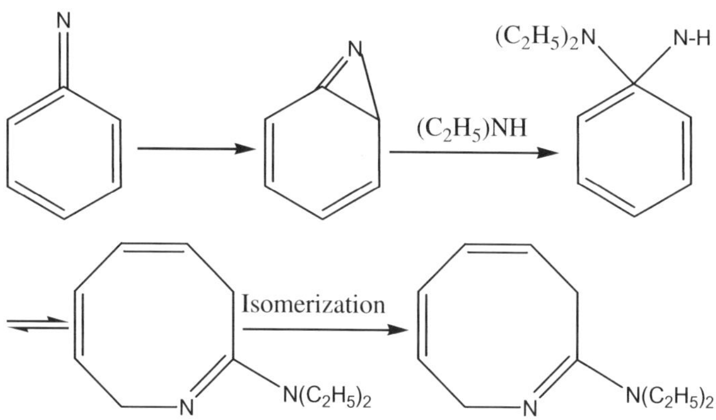

Azepine from Nitrobenzene

2-alkoxy - 3H - azepine can be prepared from nitrobenzene by its deoxygenation with tributylphosphine.

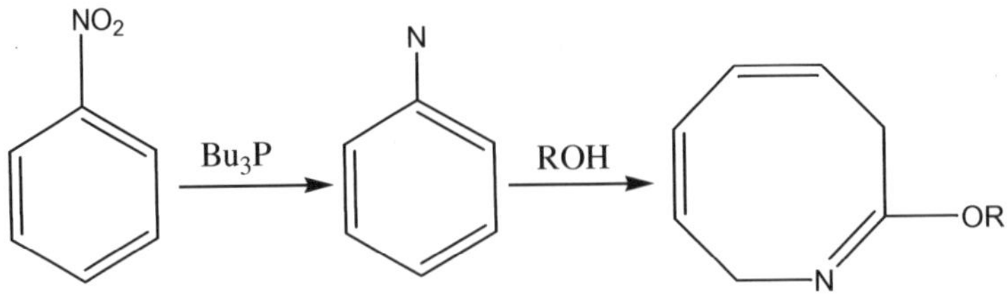

Chemical reactions of Azepines

Ring contractions

Azepines underogo photo-ring contraction to bicyclic valence tautomers. 2-methyl-N-carbomethoxyazepine on photolysis yield 2-carbomethoxy-3-methyl-2-azabicyclo hepta-3,6-diene.

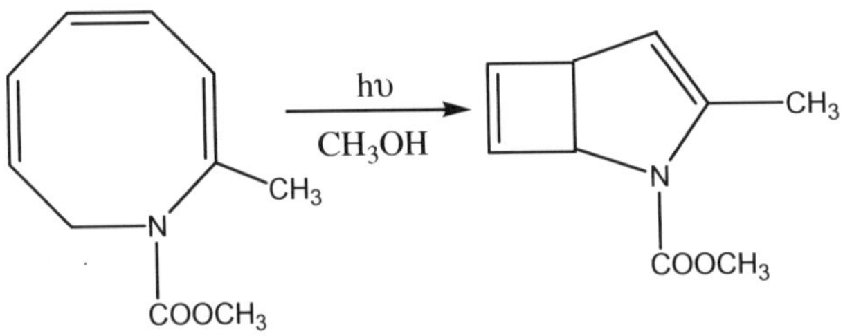

Diels-Alder reaction

N-carbo-ethoxyazepine cycloadds to 1,5-dicarbomethoxy-3,4-diphenyl cyclopentadienone to yield cycloadduct.

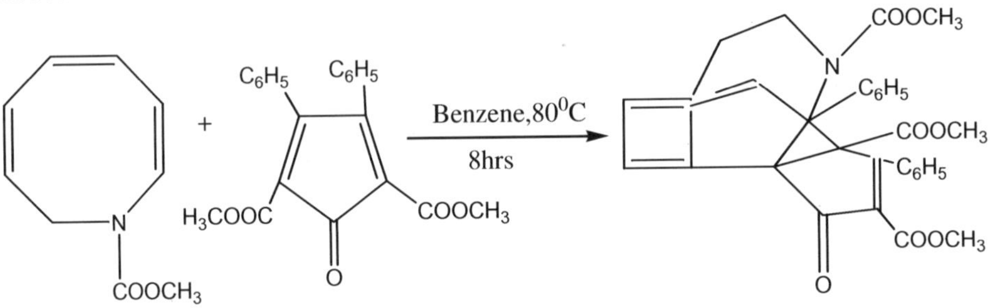

PHENOTHIAZINE

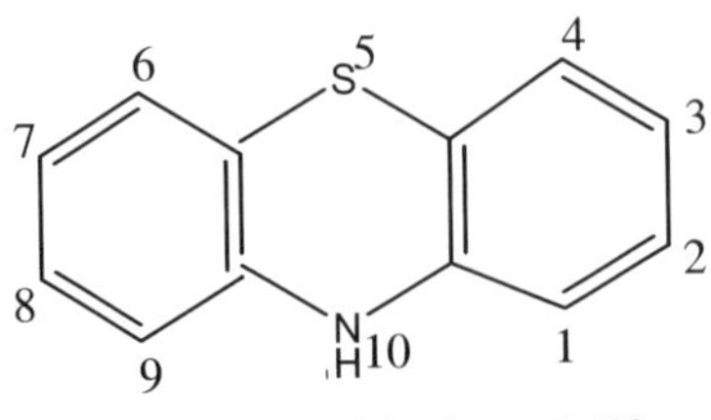

Phenothiazine can be called as Dibenzo 1,4 thiazine. Different synthetic routes are there to prepare phenothiazine

Phenothiazine from o-aminothiophenol

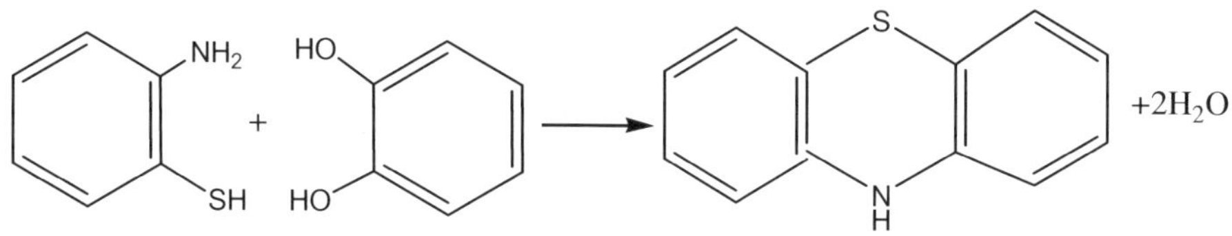

O-aminothiophenol Catechol

Phenothiazine from Diphenyl amine

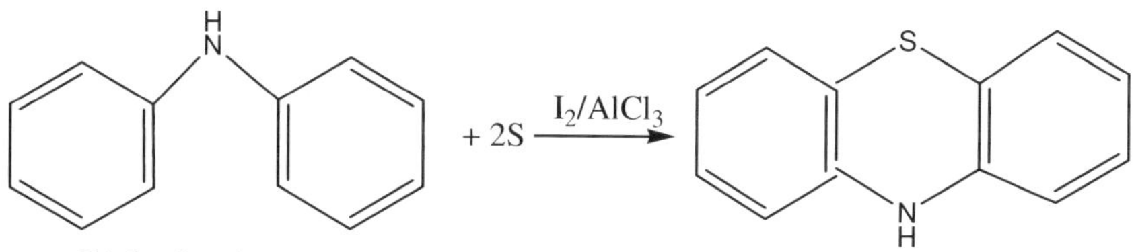

Dipheyl amine

Prpperties of Phenothiazine

Oxidation

Phenothiazine on Oxidation gives a ketone

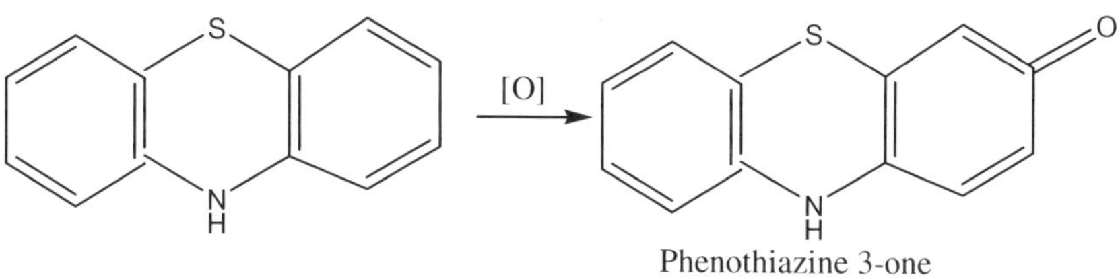

Phenothiazine 3-one

Sulphonation

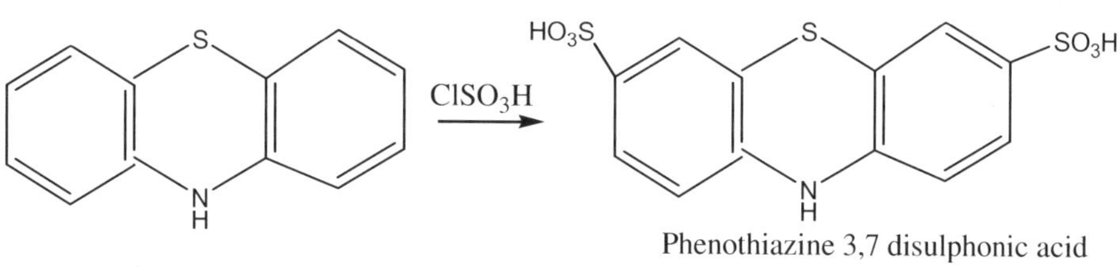

Phenothiazine 3,7 disulphonic acid

Chlorination

Chlorination of phenothiazine by different chlorinating agents give different products.

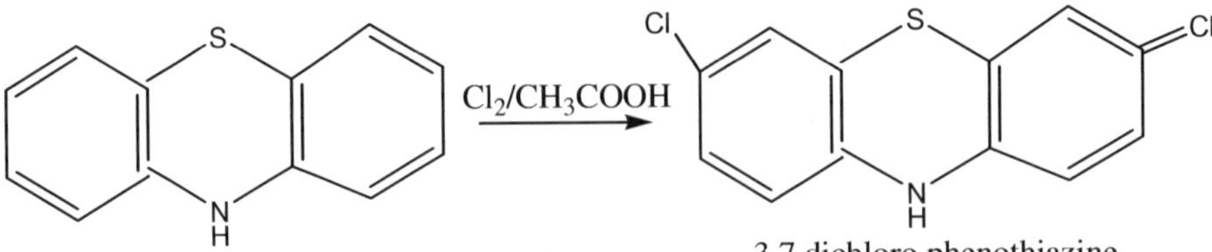

3,7 dichloro phenothiazine

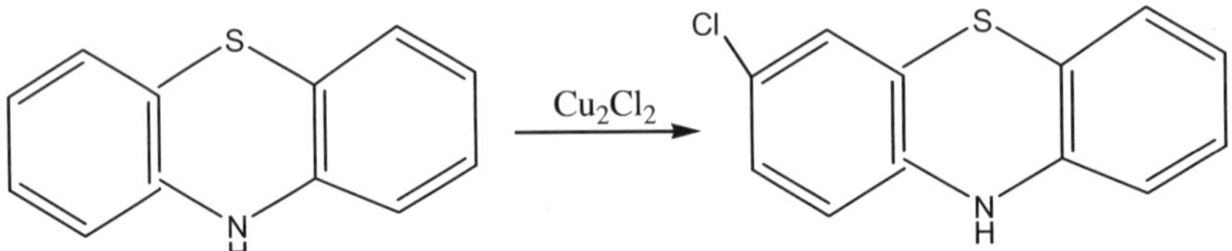

1,7 dichloro phenothiazine

Acetylation

Phenothiazine by actylation gives 10-acetyl phenothiazine

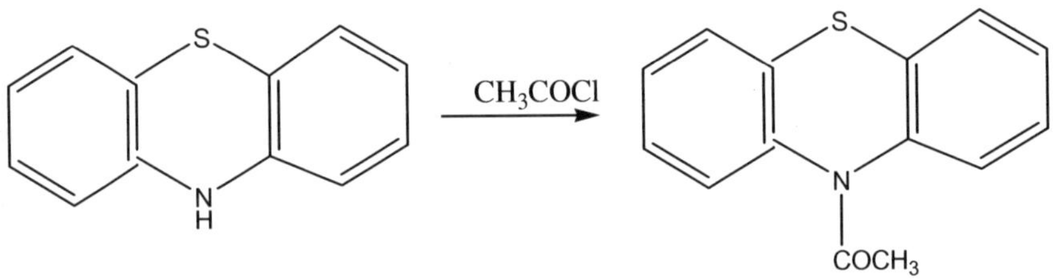

Alkylation

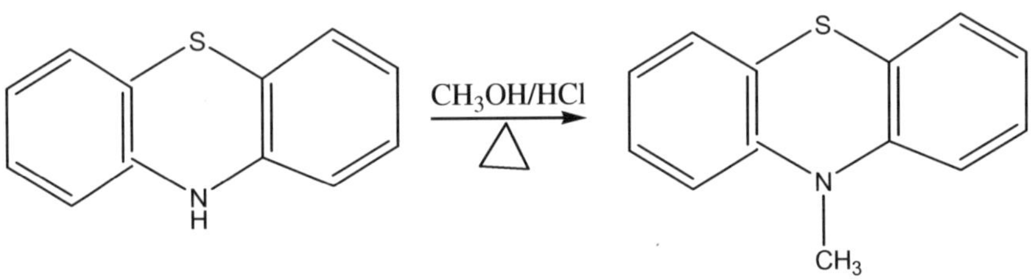

Phenothiazine on alkylation gives 10-methyl phenothiazine.

2

Polynuclear Hydrocarbons

INTRODUCTION

Compounds having more than one aromatic nucleus are known as polynuclear aromatic hydrocarbons.

Diphenylmethane

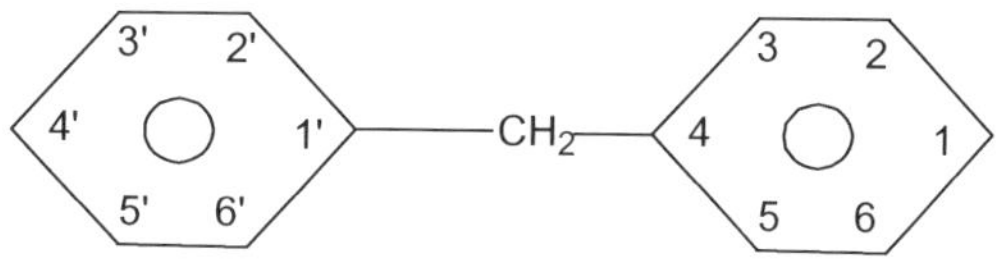

Preparation

1. By the friedel - craft's condensation between benzyl chloride and benzene.

$$C_6H_5CH_2Cl + C_6H_6 \xrightarrow{AlCl_3} C_6H_5CH_2C_6H_5 + HCl$$

2. Diphenyl methane can be prepared by condensation between one molecule of formaldehyde and two molecules of benzene in the presence of concentrated sulphuric acid.

$$2C_6H_6 + HCHO \xrightarrow{Conc.\ H_2SO_4} C_6H_5CH_2C_6H_5 + H_2O$$

3. Diphenyl methane can be prepared by heating benzophenone with hydriodic acid and red phosphorous at 160°C under pressure, by wolf - kishner reduction or by Lithium Aluminium Hydride - Aluminium trichloride.

$$C_6H_5COC_6H_5 + \xrightarrow{HI / P} C_6H_5CH_2C_6H_5$$

4. By Grignard reaction also Diphenyl methane can be prepared.

$$C_6H_5MgBr + C_6H_5CH_2Cl \longrightarrow C_6H_5 . CH_2 . C_6H_5 + MgBrCl$$

IMPORTANT REACTIONS OF DIPHENYL METHANE

Nitration

On nitration, a nitro group is introduced at 4th nuclear position; while further nitration gives 4,4'-dinitro product.

Oxidation

Diphenyl methane on oxidation by chromic acid in glacial acetic acid gives benzophenone.

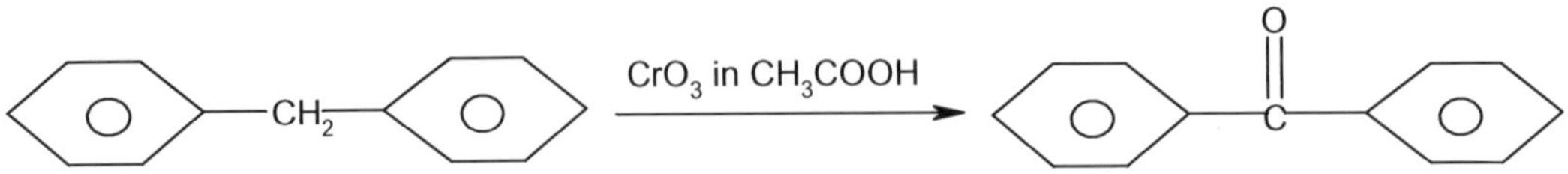

Formation of Fluorene

When Diphenyl methane vapours passes through red hot iron tube fluorene is formed.

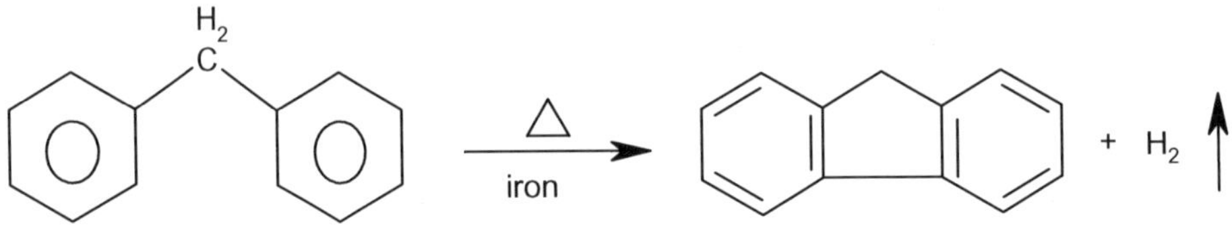

Triphenyl methane (Tritane)

Triphenyl methane is a colourless, Crystalline solid. It can be prepared by Friedel crafts reaction. Benzene is condensed either with chloroform or benzyl chloride in presence of anhydrous aluminium chloride

$$3C_6H_6 + CHCl_3 \xrightarrow{AlCl_3} (C_6H_5)_3CH + 3HCl$$

$$2C_6H_6 + C_6H_5CHCl_2 \xrightarrow{AlCl_3} (C_6H_5)_3CH + 2HCl$$

Triphenyl methane can also prepared from Benzaldehyde

$$2C_6H_6 + C_6H_5CHO \xrightarrow[\triangle]{ZnCl_2} (C_6H_5)_3CH + H_2O$$

IMPORTANT REACTIONS OF TRIPHENYL METHANE

Bromination

Triphenyl methane on bromination gives, triphenyl methyl bromide.

$$(C_6H_5)_3CH \xrightarrow{Br_2} (C_6H_5)_3CBr + HBr$$

Oxidation

Triphenyl methane on oxidation by lead oxide or chromic acid gives Triphenyl carbinol

$$(C_6H_5)_3CH \xrightarrow{CrO_3} (C_6H_5)_3COH$$

Reaction with sodium

Triphenyl methane on reaction with sodium in ether or liquid ammonia gives triphenyl methyl sodium

$$(C_6H_5)_3\,CH \xrightarrow{Na} (C_6H_5)_3\overset{-}{C}\text{-}\overset{+}{Na} + H_2\uparrow$$

Naphthalene

Naphthalene is the largest single constituent of coal-tar

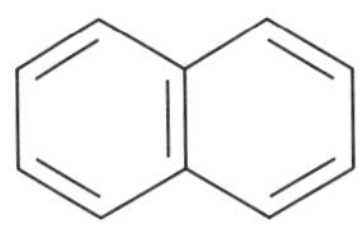

It is a white solid, insoluble in water. It can be isolated from coal-tar as well as petroleum. Naphthalene can be synthesised in many ways;

1. When 4-phenyl but -1-ene is passed over red hot calcium oxide naphthalene is formed.

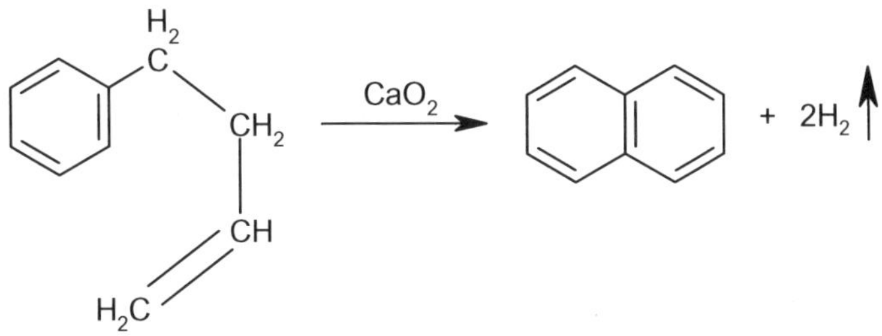

2. When 4-phenyl but -3 enoic acid is warmed with sulphuric acid,1-naphthol is formed, which on distillation with zinc dust gives naphthalene.

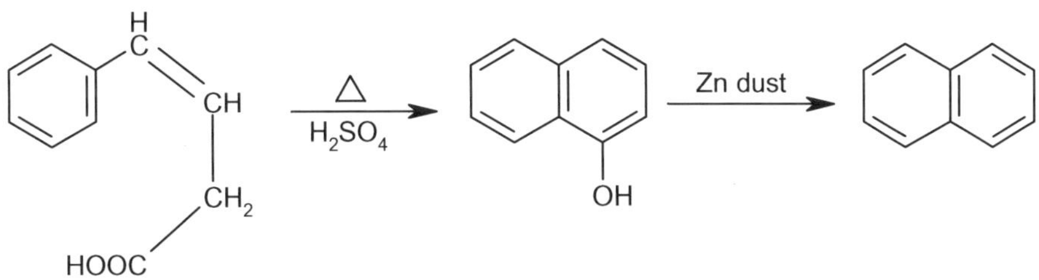

3. **Haworth synthesis:** Three important synthetic tools are applied here like Friedel craft's reaction, Clemmensen reduction, & Catalytic dehydrogenation. Benzene is condensed with succinic anhydride in the presence of anhydrous alumimiun chloride (Friedel crafts reactiom), a ketonic acid is formed, which is reduced by clemmensen method. The ring is closed by heating with concentrated sulphuric acid. Product formed α-tetralone again reduced by clemmensen method. This compound dehydrogenated to naphthalene by heating with selenium or palladised charcoal.

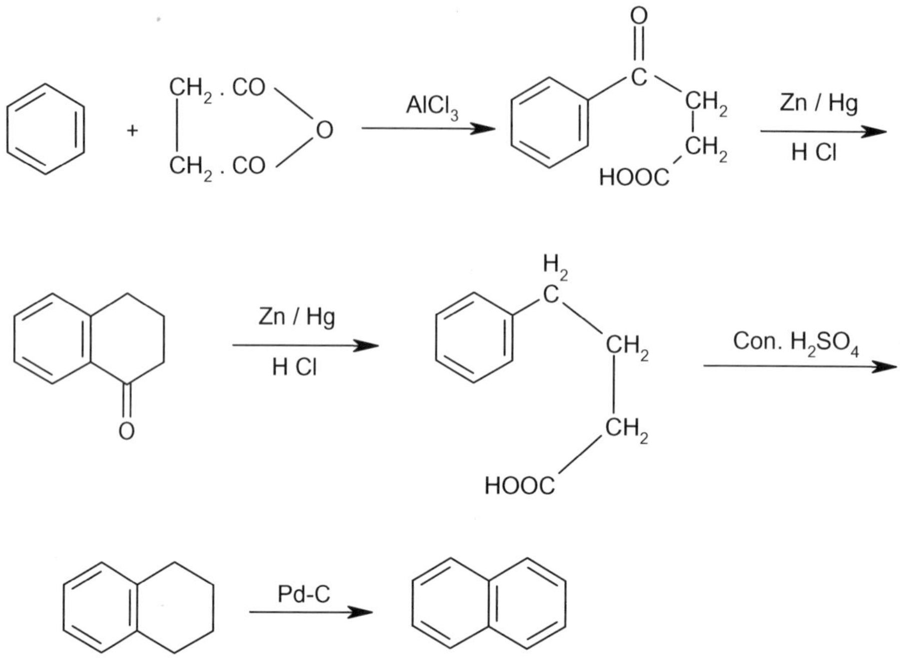

IMPORTANT REACTIONS OF NAPHTHALENE

Reduction

Hydrogen is added (reduction) in different conditions yield different products.

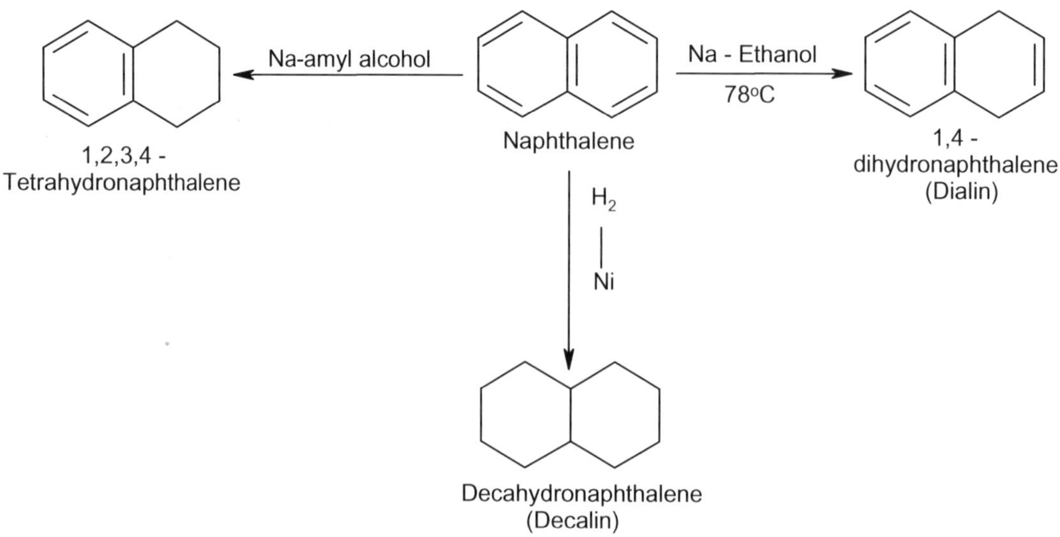

Oxidation

Naphthalene oxidised in different conditions give different products.

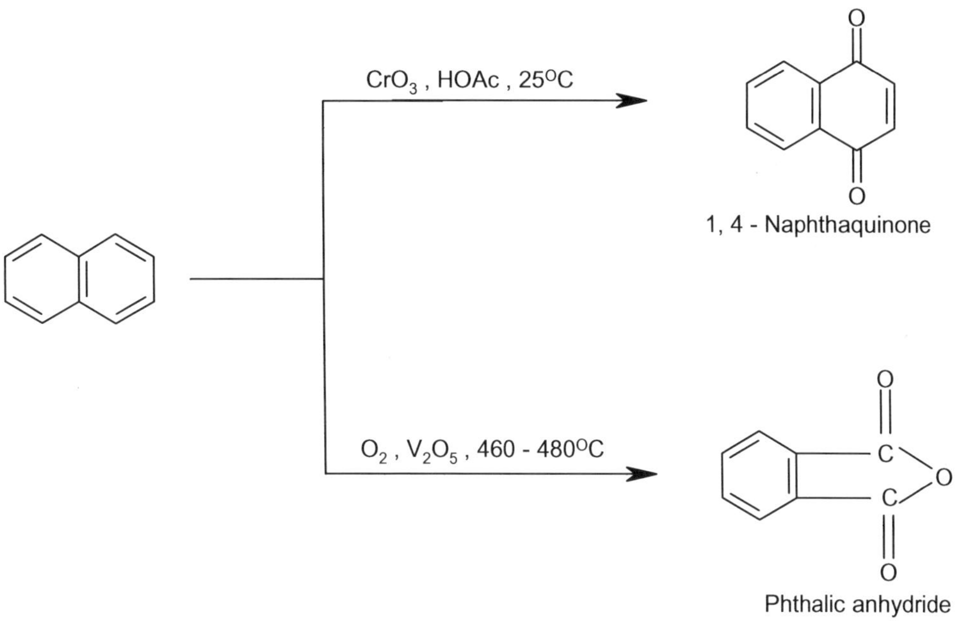

Nitration

Naphthalene on nitration gives 1-nitro naphthalene.

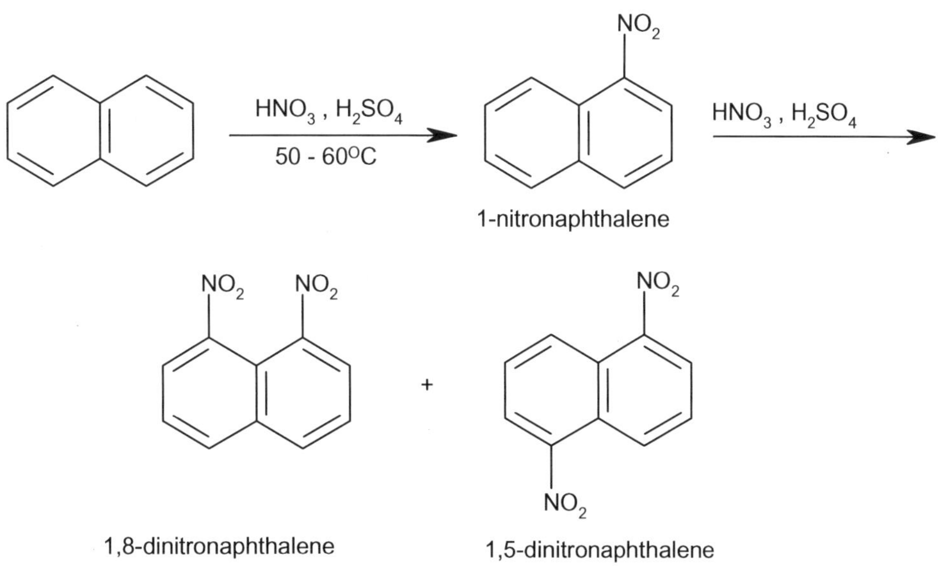

Halogenation

Naphthalene on bromination gives 1-bromonaphthalene.

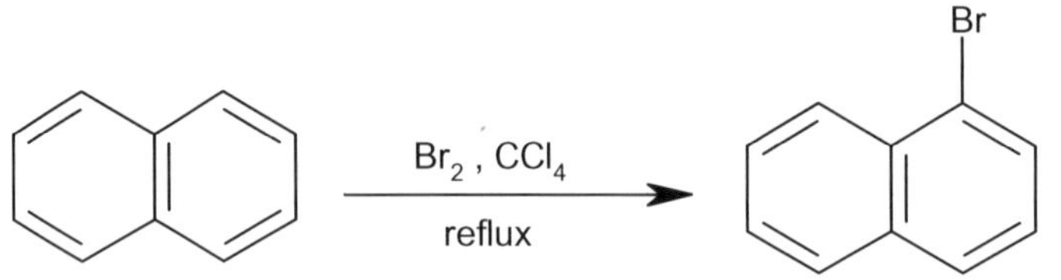

1-bromonaphthalene

Sulphonation

Sulphonation of Naphthalene at varied temperatuses give different products

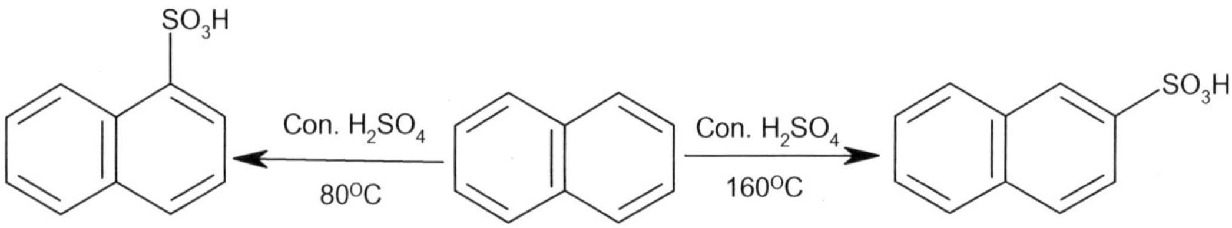

1-Naphthalene Sulphonic Acid

Naphthalene

2-Naphthalene Sulphonic Acid

Frieded-Crafts acylation

In the presence of different solvents give different products.

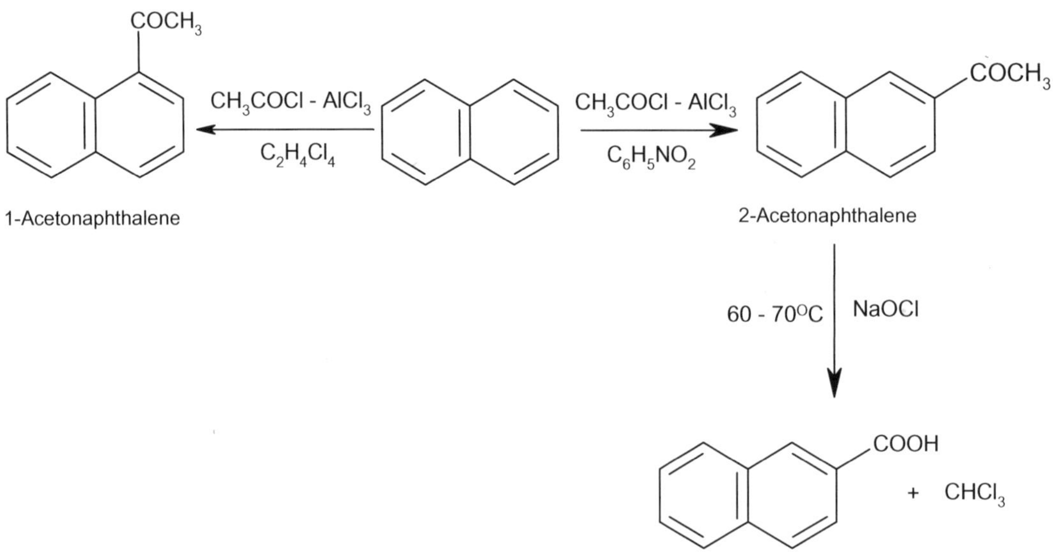

Addition of ozone

Ozone adds to naphthalene to form di-ozonide which on hydrolysis gives phthalaldehyde.

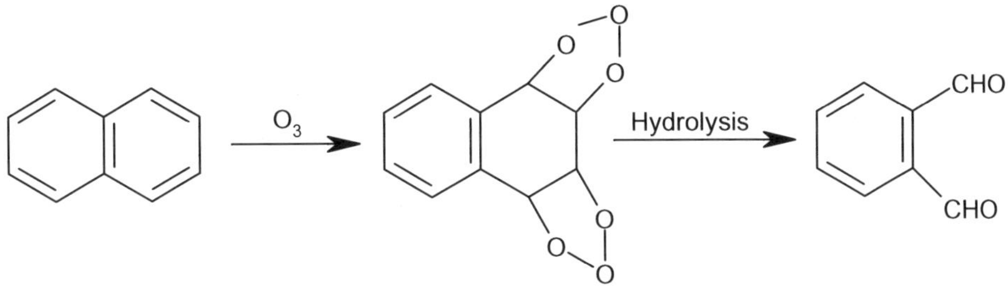

Chloromethylation

Naphthalene can be chloromethylated by heating with a mixture of fomaldehyde, glacial acetic acid, 5% H_3PO_4 & conc. HCl.

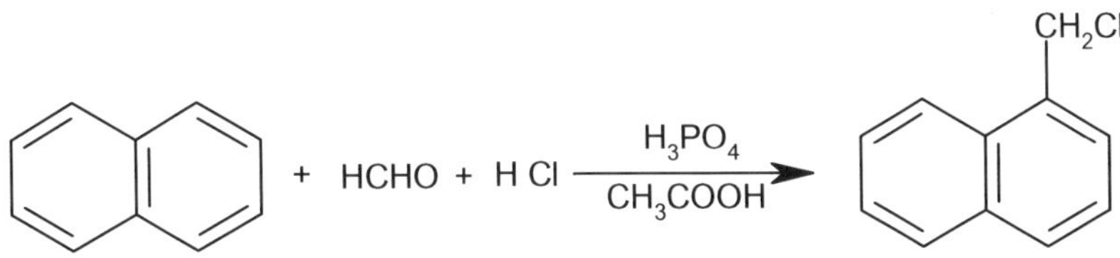

1-Chloromethyl naphthalene

STRUCTURE OF NAPHTHALENE

Naphthalene classified as aromatic. Naphthalene undergoes addition reactions, which is characterestic of unsaturated compounds During electroplilic substitution reactions, hydrogen is displaced as hydrogen ion and naphthalene ring is preserved.

Naphthalene contains two flat six membered rings and consideration of atomic orbitals shows that the structure can provide π clouds containing six-electrons-the aromatic sextet. Ten carbons lie at the corners of two fused hexagons. Each carbon is attached to three other atoms by σ bonds. Since these bonds result from the overlap of trigonal SP^2 orbitals, all carbon and hydrogen atoms lie in a single plane. Above and below this plane, there is a cloud of electrons formed by overlap of 'p'orbitals. We can consider this cloud as two partially overlapping sextets that have a pair of π electrons in common.

X-ray analysis showed that in contrast to benzene, all carbon-carbon bonds in naphthalene are not same, especially C_1-C_2 bond is cosiderably shorter than C_2-C_3 bond.

Elemental analysis and molecular weight determination showed, molecular formula of naphthalene is $C_{10}H_8$. Naphthalene on oxidation gives phthalic acid suggests presence of benzene rings with two ortho side chains.

Presence of two fused benzene rings have been confirmed from the following reactions. Nitration of naphthalene produced nitronaphthalene which on oxidation gave o-nitrophthalic acid. Reduction of nitronaphthalene gave amino naphthalene which on oxidation yielded phthalic acid.

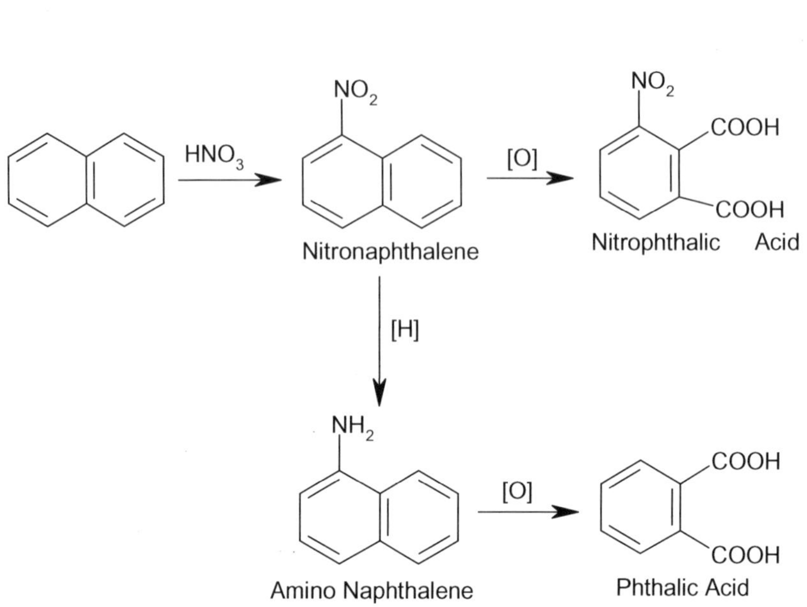

From these reactions, it is clear that naphthalene is made up of two benzene rings joined in ortho positions.

Naphthalene exists in three resonating structures, as follows;

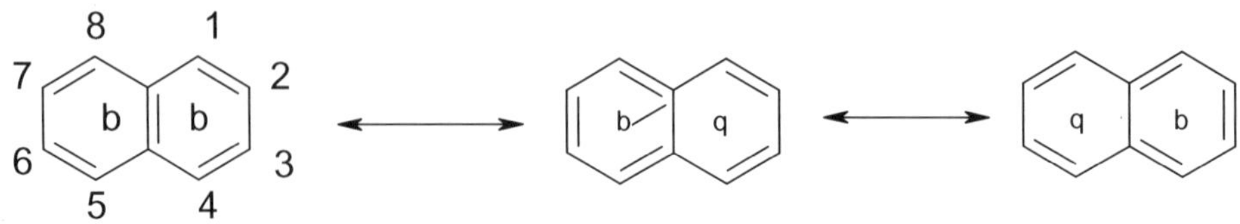

I II III

b = benzenoid ring; q = quinonoid ring.

Among these resonating structures, I have both rings benzenoid while in II & III one of the ring is benzenoid and other is quinonoid. According to fries rule, among the different resonating structures of a polynuclear hydrocarbon, the one having maximum number of benzenoid rings is most stable structure.

ANTHRACENE

Anthracene is otherwise known as green oil. Anthracene can be synthesised in many ways.

1. Anthracene by Friedel-craft's reaction

Here two specific reactants are condensed in presence of anhydrous Aluminium chloride.

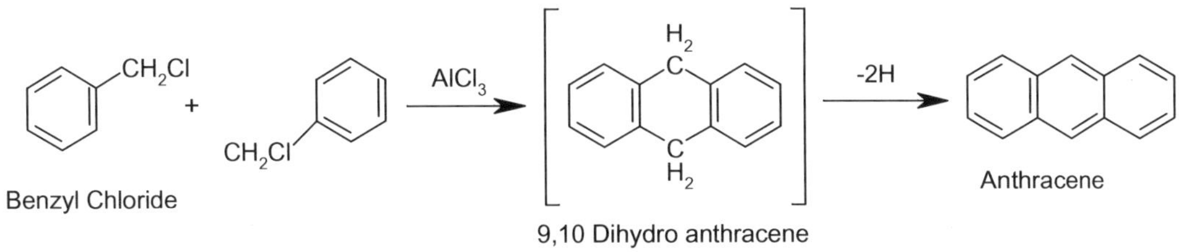

B)

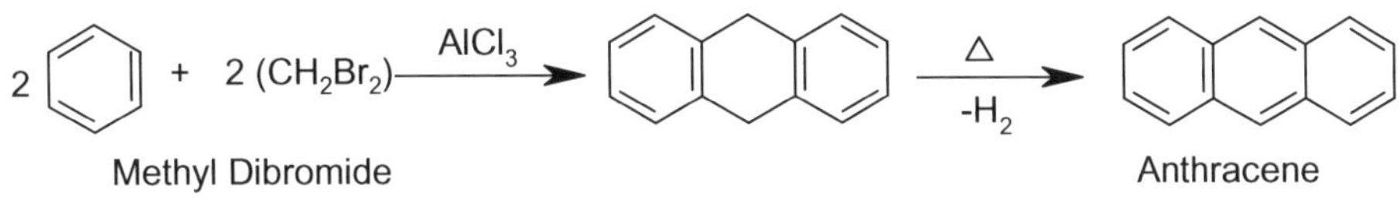

C)

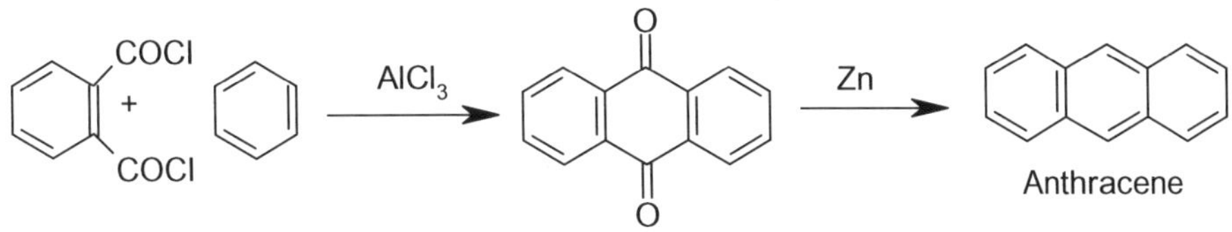

D)

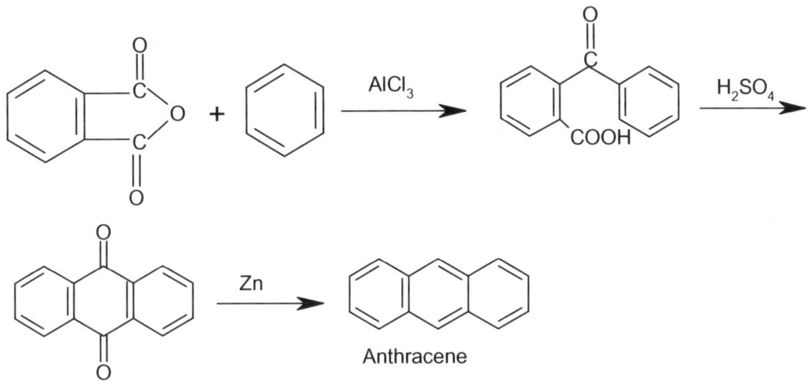

2. **Anthracene by Elbs reaction:** Pyrolysis of diaryl ketone containing a methyl or methylene group ortho to carbonyl group gives polyhydrocarbon.

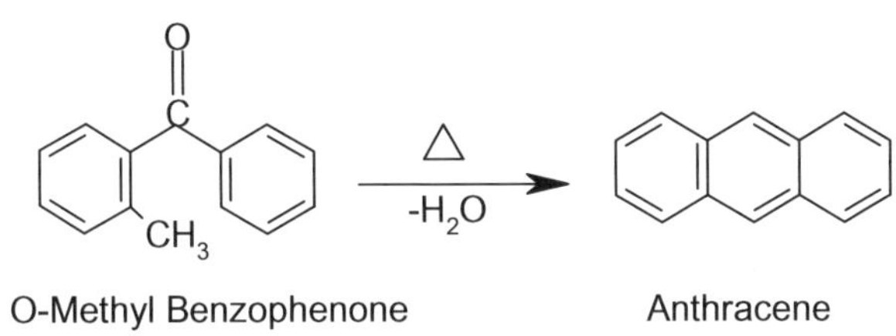

3. **Anthracene by fittig reaction:** O-bromobenzyl bromide is heated with sodium in presence of ether give dihydro anthracene which on mild oxidation gives anthracene.

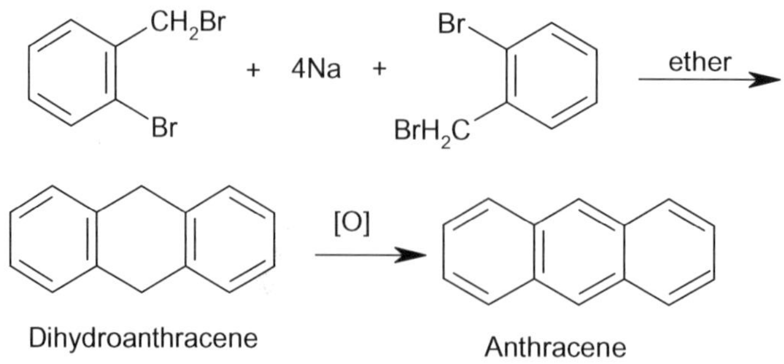

4. **Anthracene by Diels-Alder reaction:** It involves reaction of 1,4-naphthaquinone with butadiene, followed by oxidation of the product with chromium trioxide in glacial acetic acid and then distilled with zinc dust.

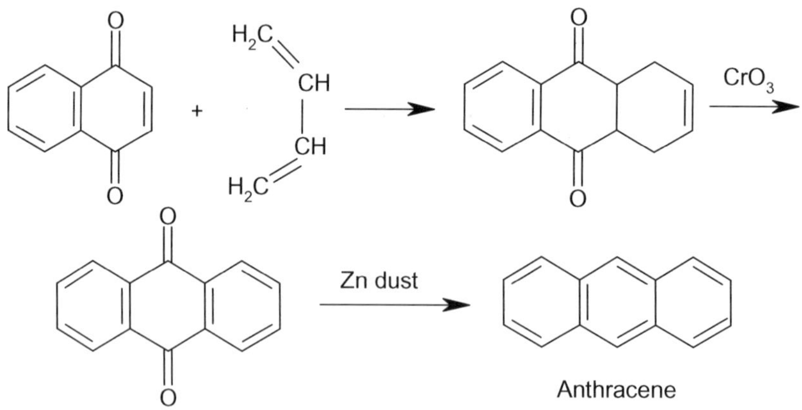

5. **Anthracene by Michael condensation**

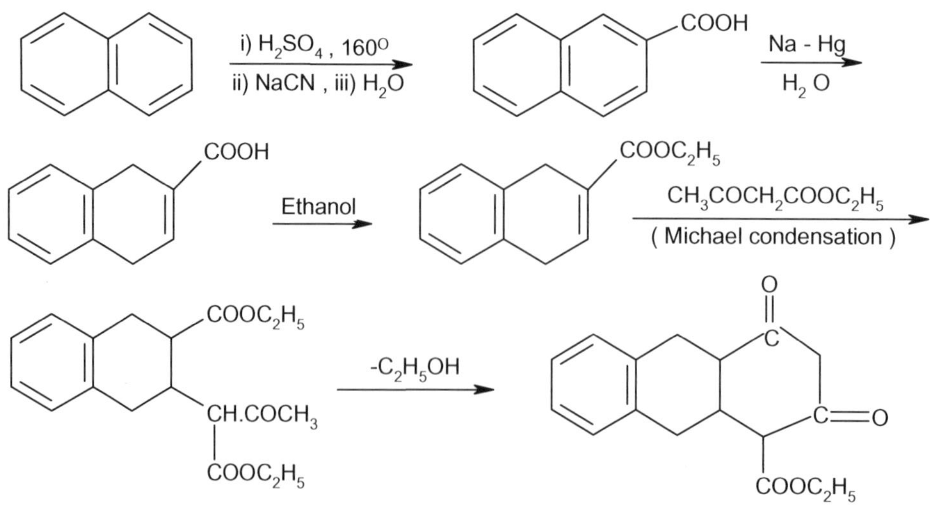

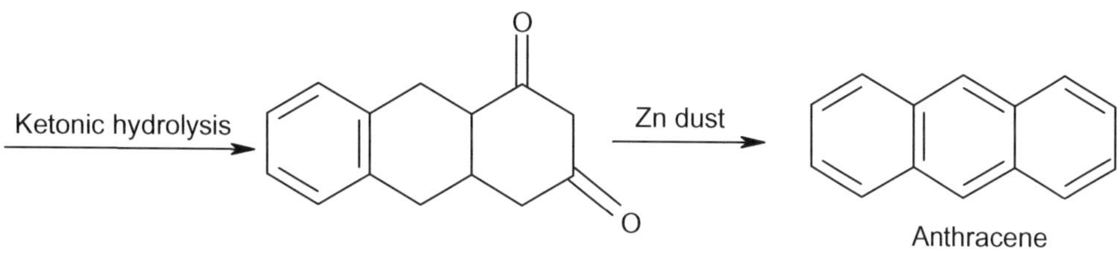

IMPORTANT REACTIONS OF ANTHRACENE

Oxidation

Oxidation of anthracene with sodium dichromate and sulphuric acid yields 9,10 anthraquinone.

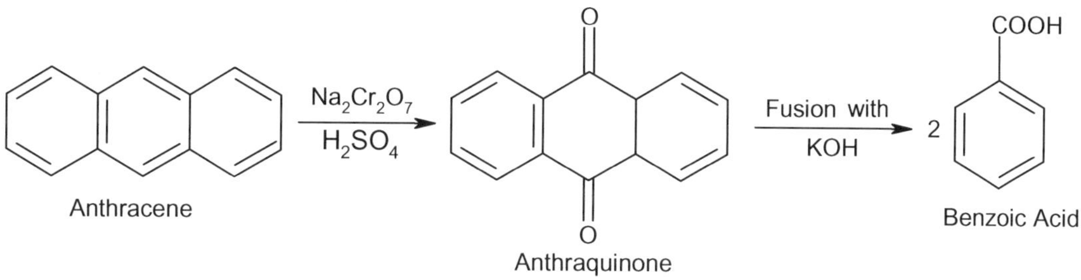

Reduction

Anthracene is reduced to 9,10-dihydroanthracene by sodium and ethanol.

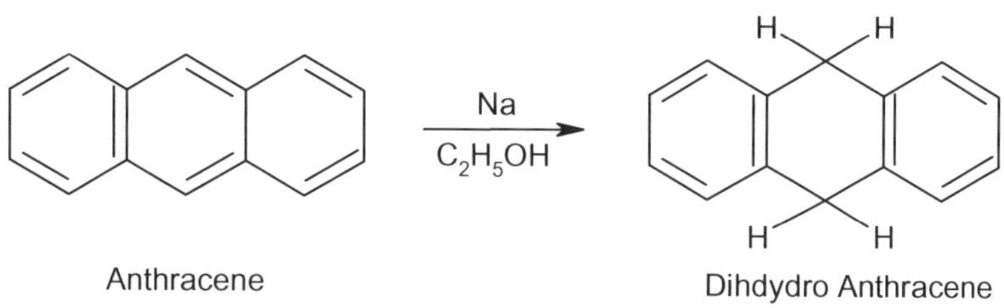

Anthracene can be completely reduced by using Nickel as a catalyst.

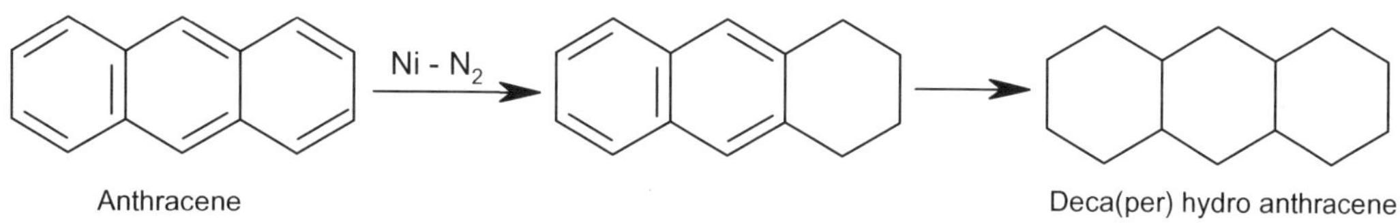

Addition of oxygen

Anthracene adds a molecule of oxygen in the presence of light to form a colourless photo-oxide in which 1,4-peroxide bridge stretches across the middle ring.

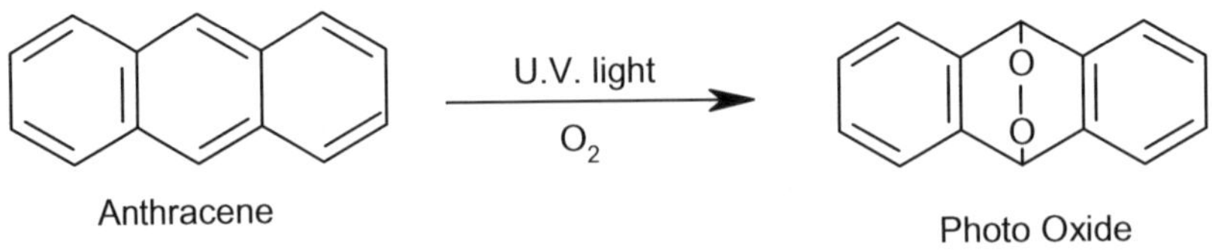

Dimerisation

Anthracene in benzene or xylene in presence of light forms dimer known as dianthracene or paranthracene.

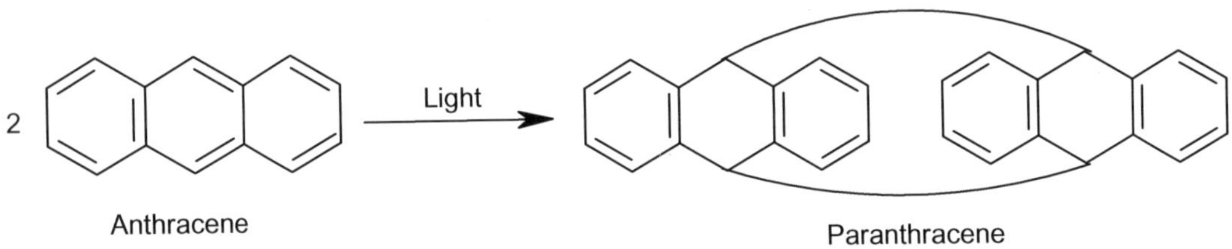

Diels-Alder reaction

Anthracene undergoes Diels-Alder reaction in the 9, 10-position to form endo anthracene maleic anhydride.

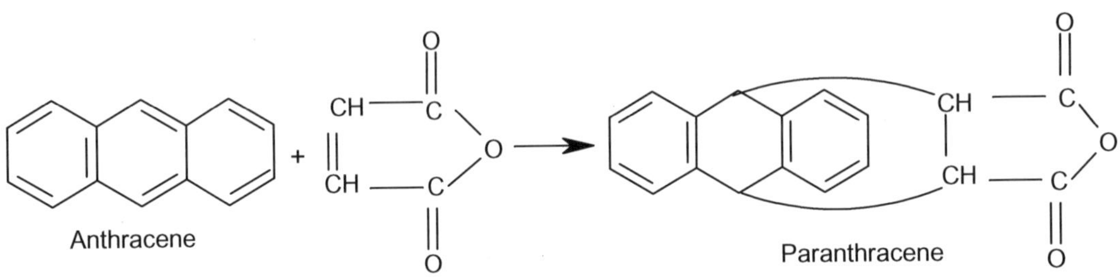

Halogenation

When chlorine is passed into a cold solution of anthracene in carbon disulphide, anthracene dichloride is formed.

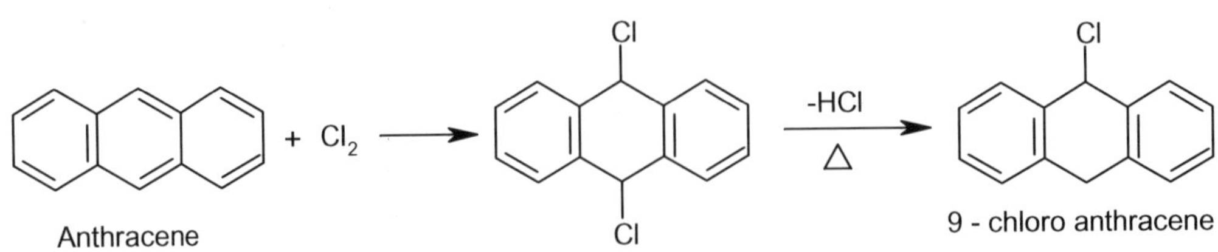

Nitration

Anthracene when treated with concentrated nitric acid in acetic an hydride, forms 9-nitroanthracene and, 10 dinitroanthracene.

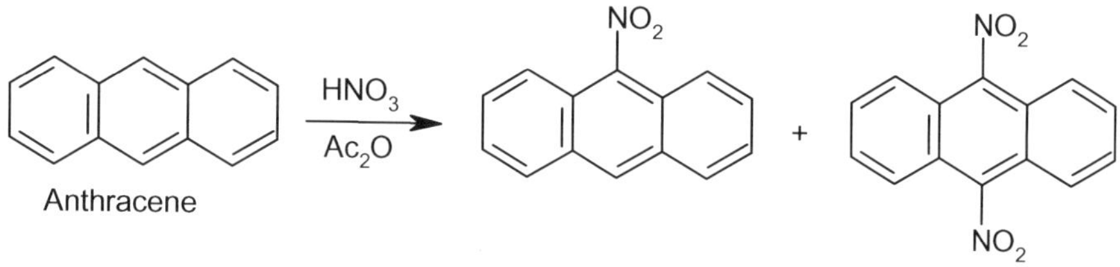

Sulphonation

Sulphonation of anthracene with conc.H_2SO_4 at low temperature gives 1-anthracene sulphonic acid and at high temperature gives 2-anthracene sulphonic acid.

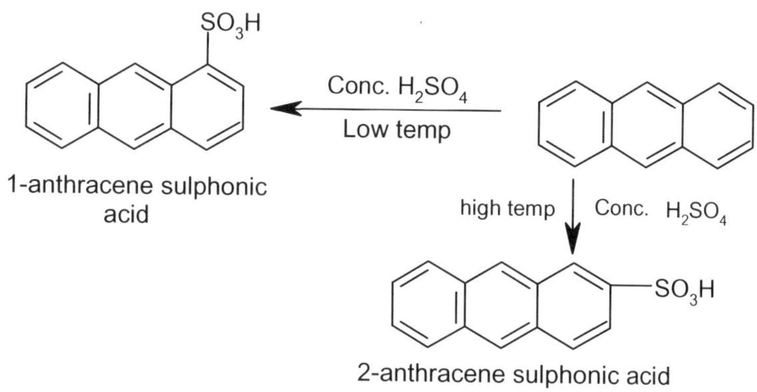

Friedel-crafts acetylation

Acetylation of anthracene by Friedel crafts reagent in different solvents give different products.

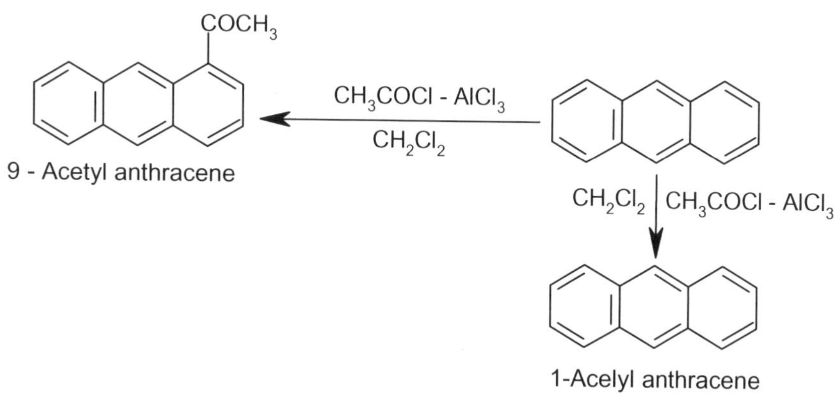

acid and copper powder Phenanthrene-9-carboxylic acid formed, on strong heating gives phenanthrene.

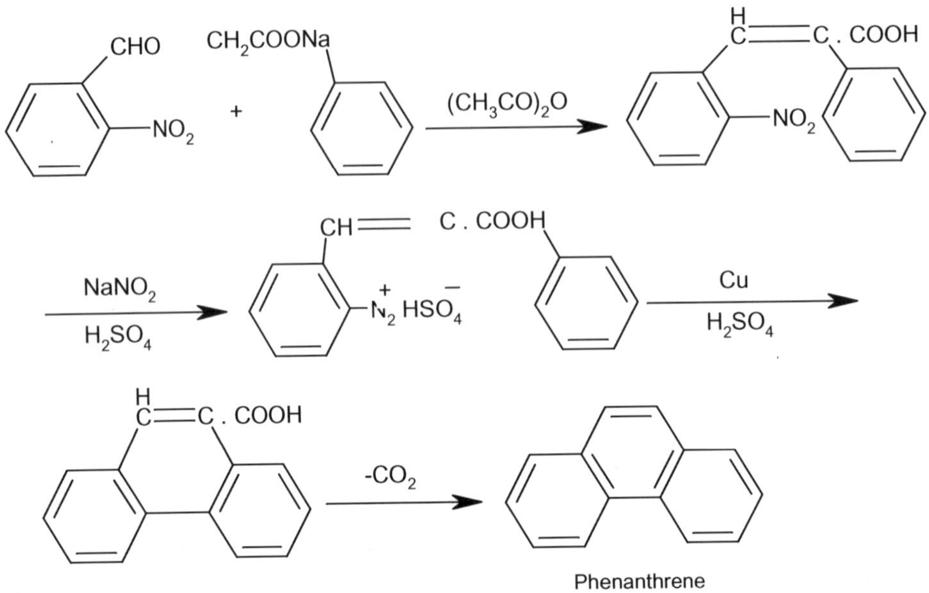

Phenanthrene by Haworth synthesis

Here naphthalene is condensed with succinic anhydride.

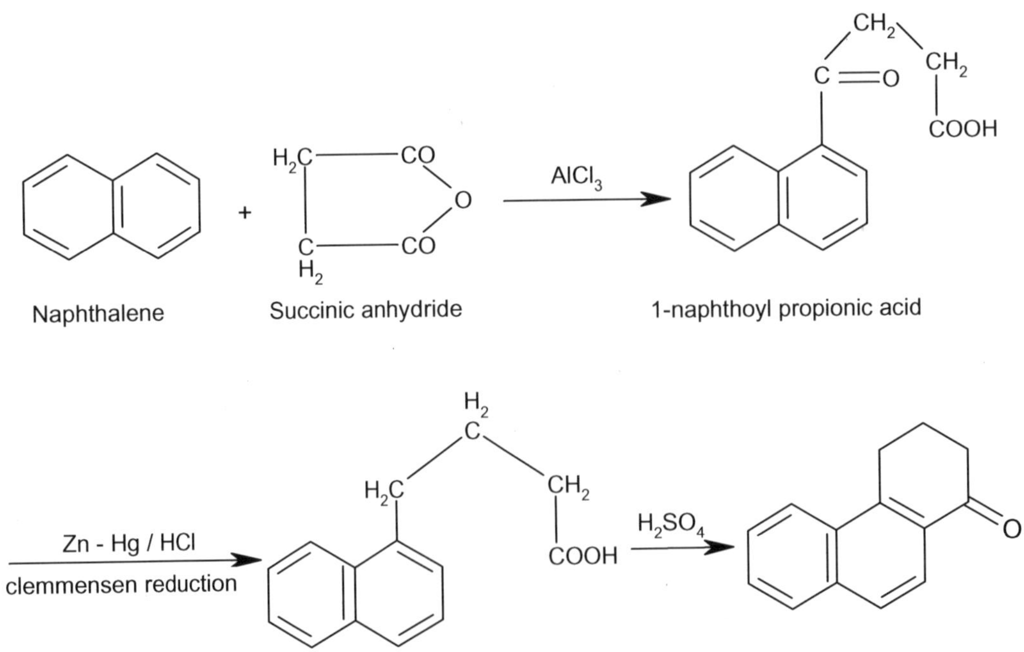

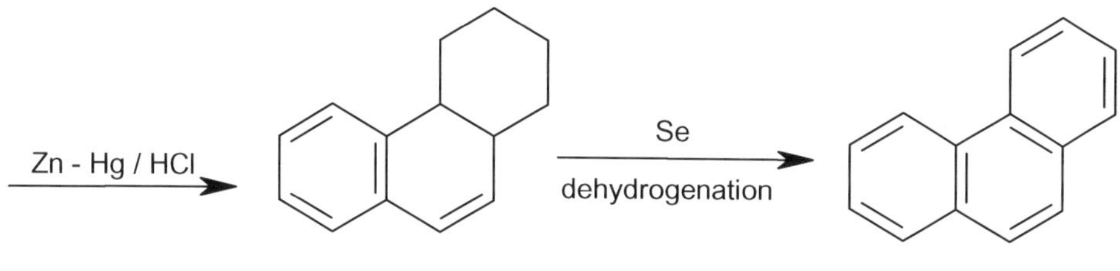

Phenanthrene

Phenanthrene Bogert-cook synthesis

In this method Phenylethylmagnesium bromide and cyclohexanone are made to react.

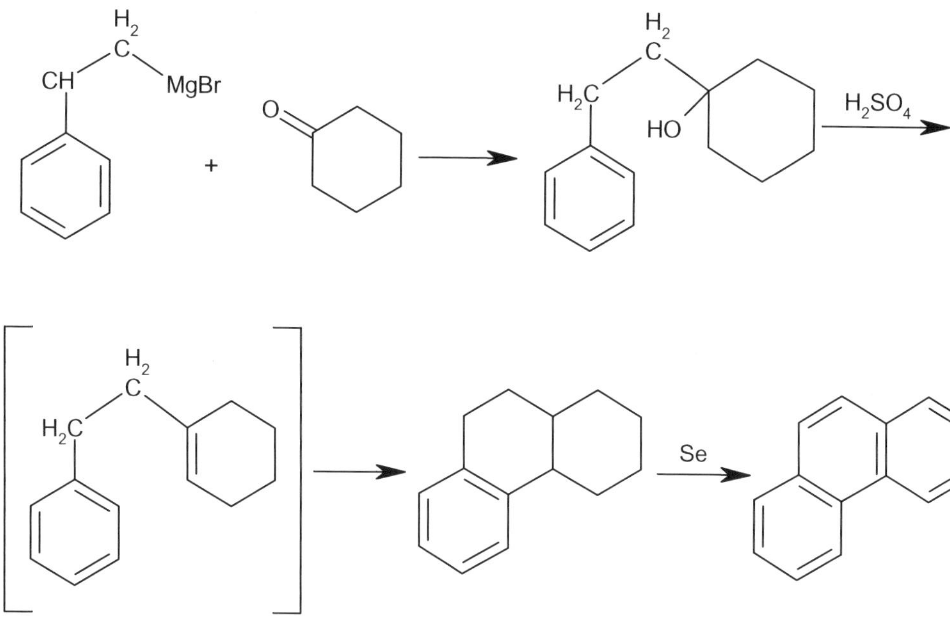

Phenanthrene from Stilbene

Both Cis and trans stilbenes can be converted to phenanthrene by irriadiation

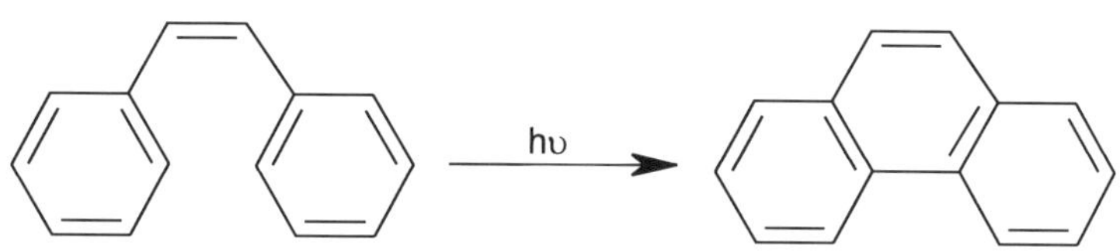

cis- stilbene　　Phenanthrene

IMPORTANT REACTIONS OF PHENANTHRENE

Ozonolysis

Phenanthrene on ozonolysis give dialdehyde which on permanganate oxidation gives Diphenic acid

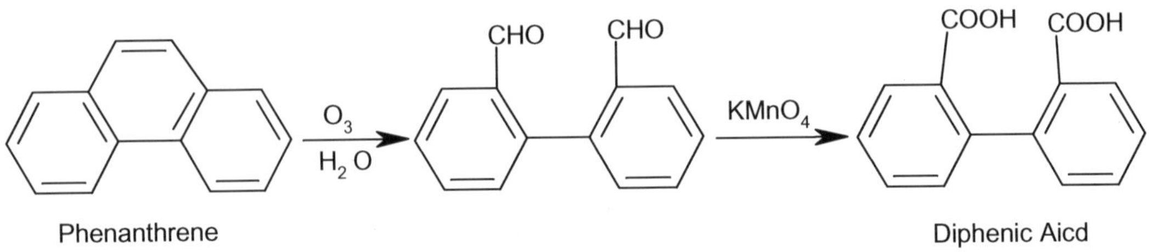

Halogenation

Phenanthrene on bromination in presence of carbontetrachloride gives 9-bromophenanthrene

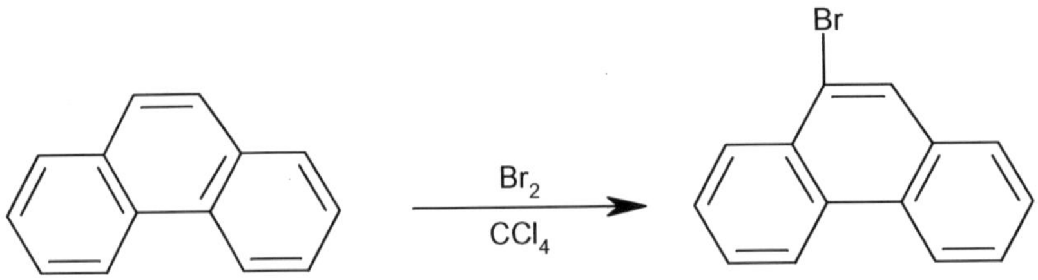

9 - bromophenanthrene

Reduction

Phenanthrene catalytically reduced to 9, 10 dihydrophenanthrene by copper-oxide-chromic oxide

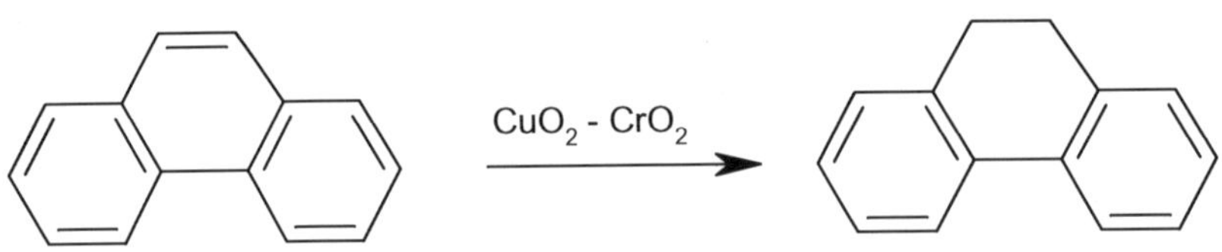

9 -10 dihydro phenanthrene

Oxidation

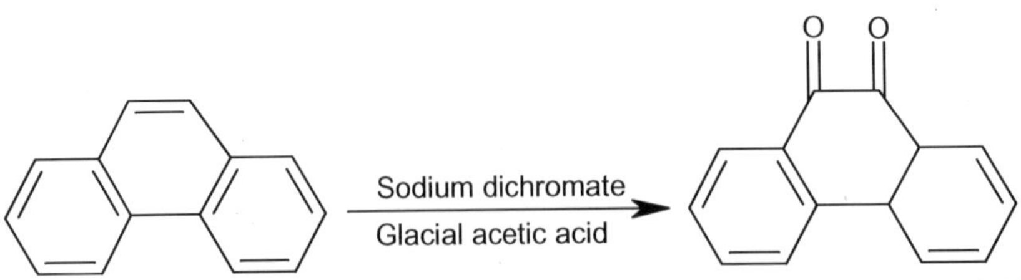

9 -10 dihydro phenanthrene - 9,10 dione

3

Drugs Containing Certain Heterocycles and Polynuclear Hydrocarbons

Some drugs containing certain heterocycles & Polynuclear hydrocarbons are given below.

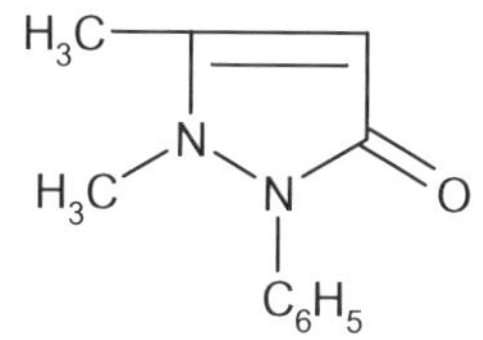

Phenazone - used as Febrifuge.

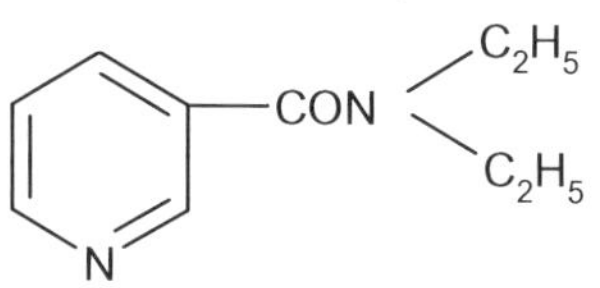

Nikethamide - used as respiratory stimulant

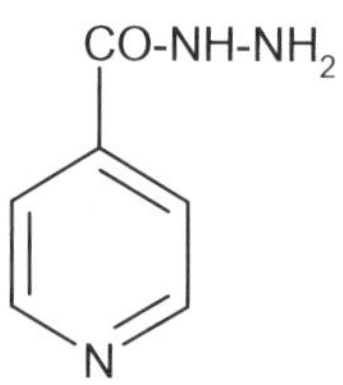

Isoniazid - used as antitubercular agent

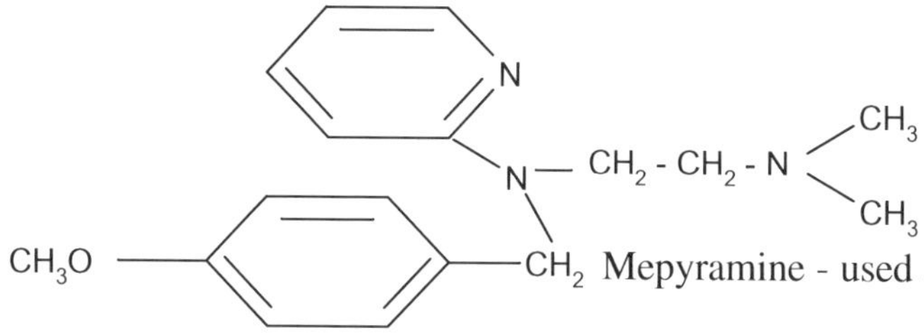

Mepyramine - used as antihistamine

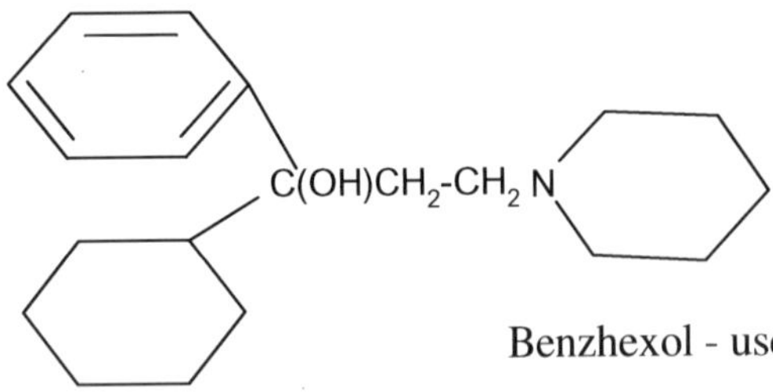

Benzhexol - used as antiparkinsonian drug

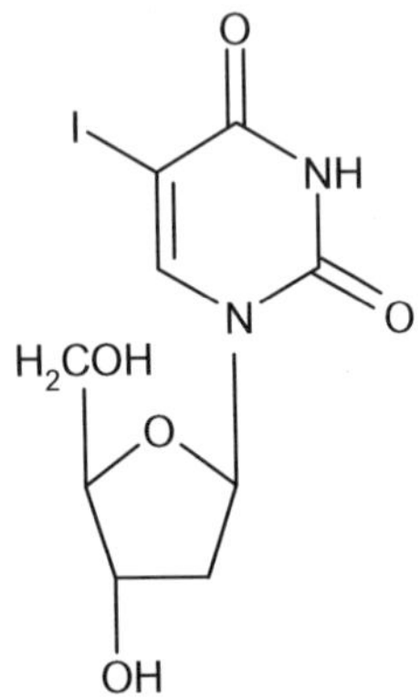

Idoxuridine - used as antiviral agent

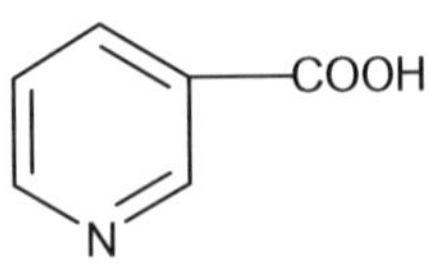

Niacin - used in treatment of pellagra

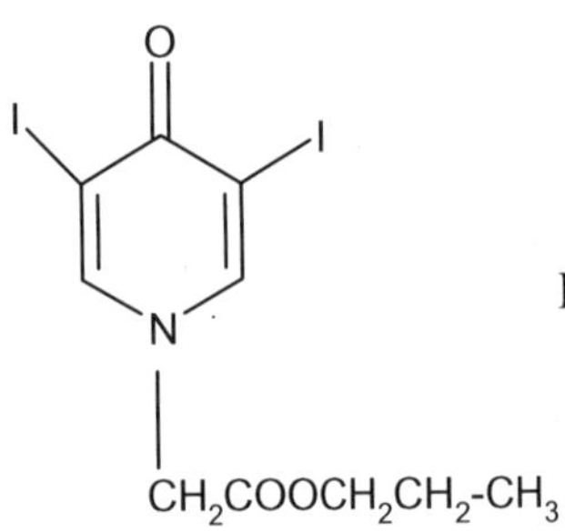

Propyl iodone - used for examining bronchial tract

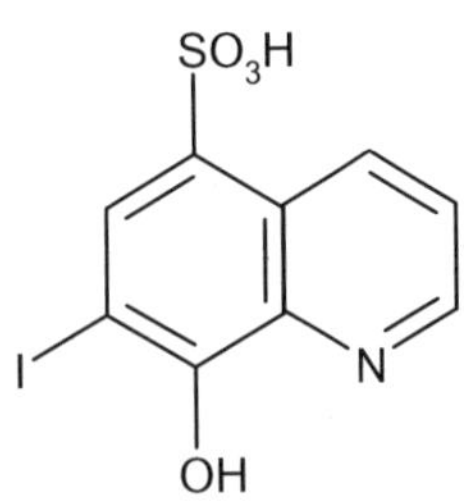

Chinofon - used as anti-bacterial drug

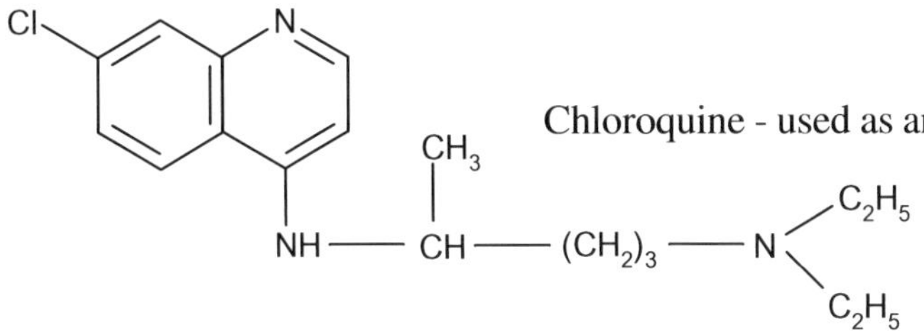

Chloroquine - used as antimalarial drug

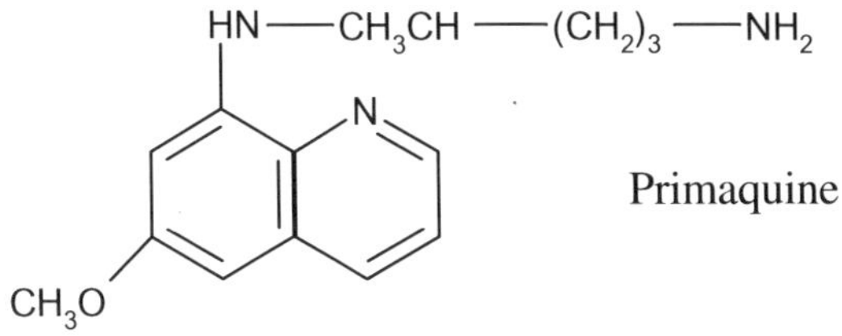

Primaquine - used as antimalarial drug

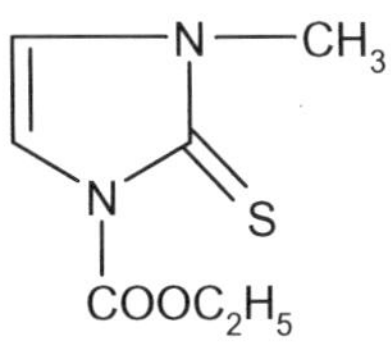

Carbimazole - used as antithyroid drug

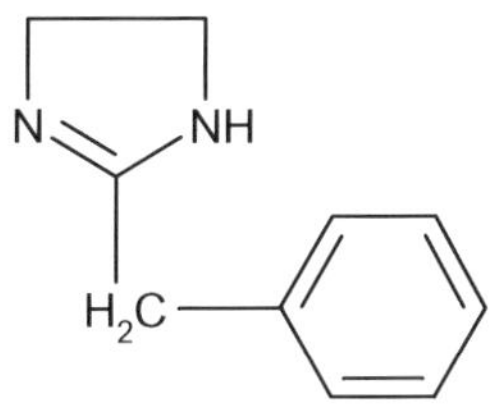

Tolazoline - used in peripheral vascular diseases

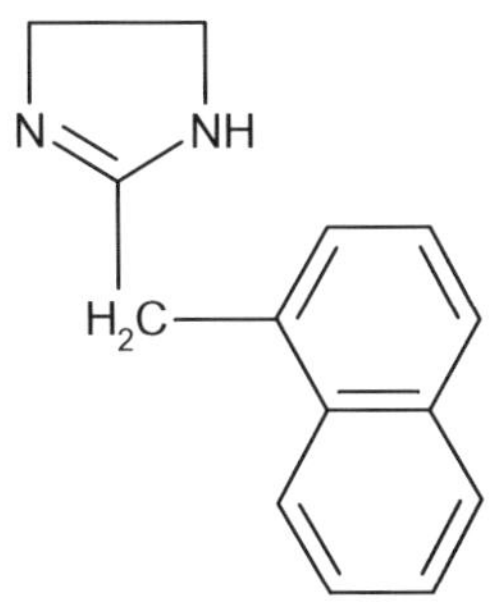

Naphazoline - used for symptomatic relief of rhinitis & sinusitis

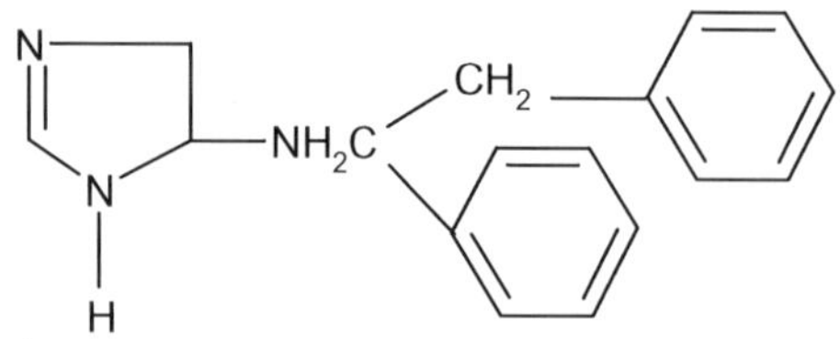

Antazoline - used as antihistamine

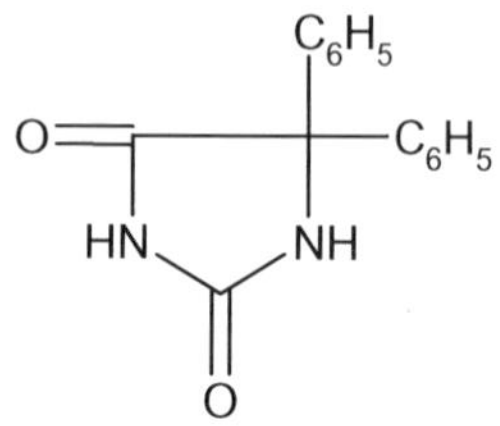

Phenytoin - used in epilepsy and cardiac arrhythmia

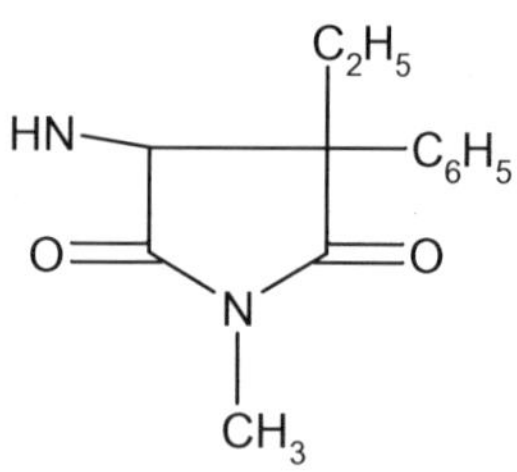

Mephenytoin - used as anticonvulsant drug

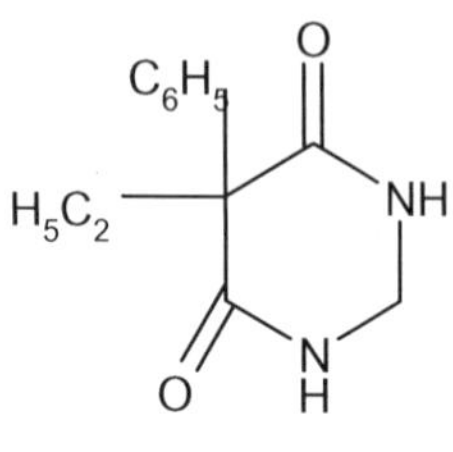

Primidone- used in epilepsy

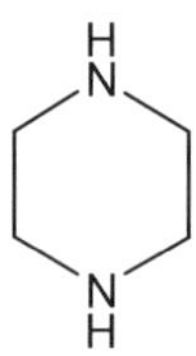

Piperazine - used as anthelmintic

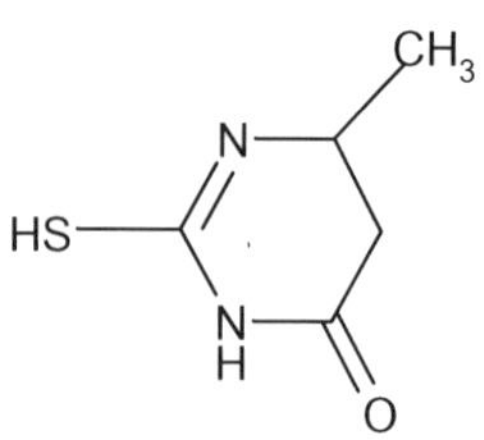

Methylthiouracil - used in thyrotoxicosis

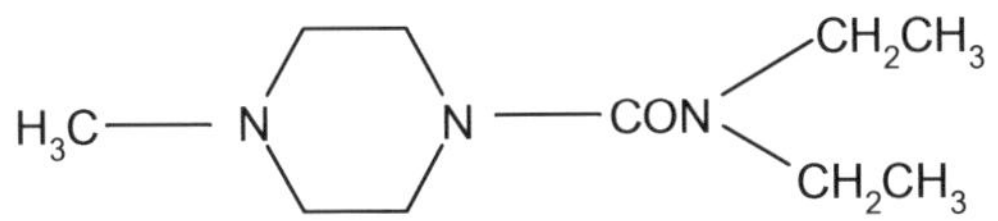

Diethyl carbamazine - used to treat Filariasis

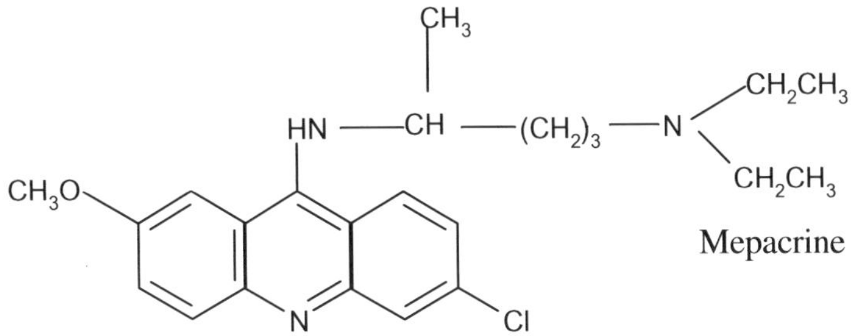

Mepacrine - used as antimalarail drug

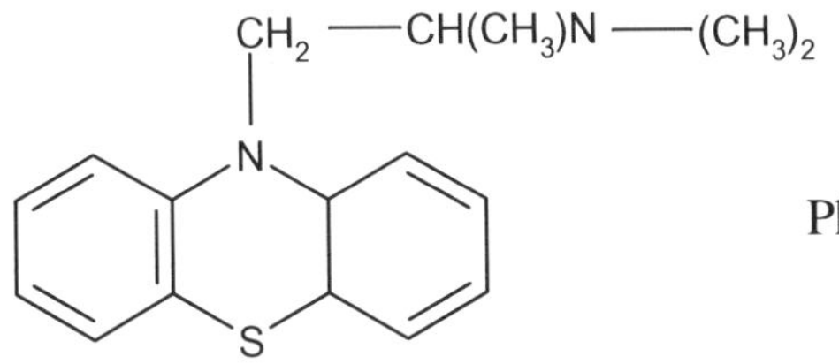

Phenergan - used as antihistaminic

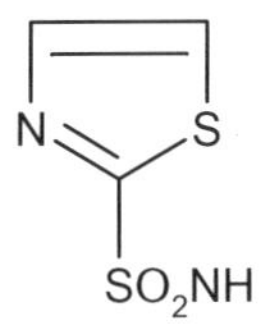

Sulphathiazole - used as antibacterial

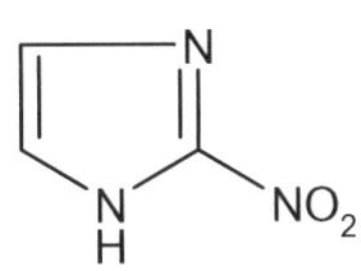

Azomycin - used as antibiotic

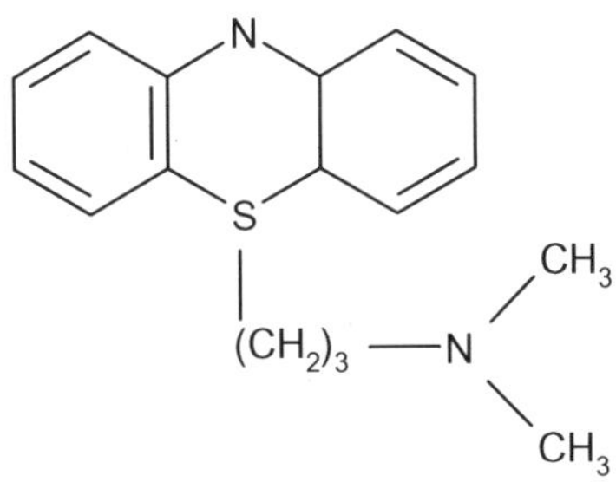

Chlorpromazine : Use as antipsychotic

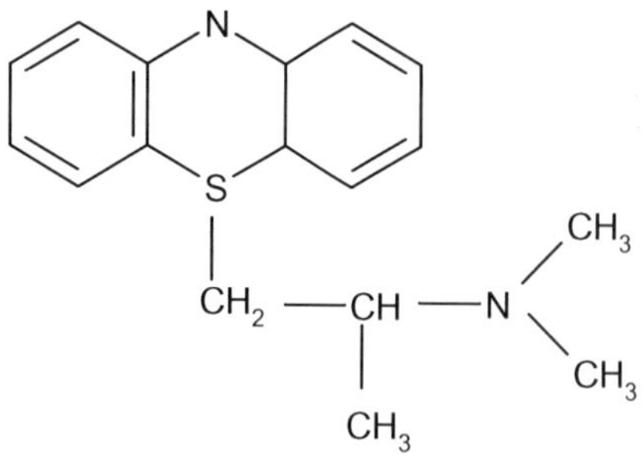

Promethazine - used as antiemetic

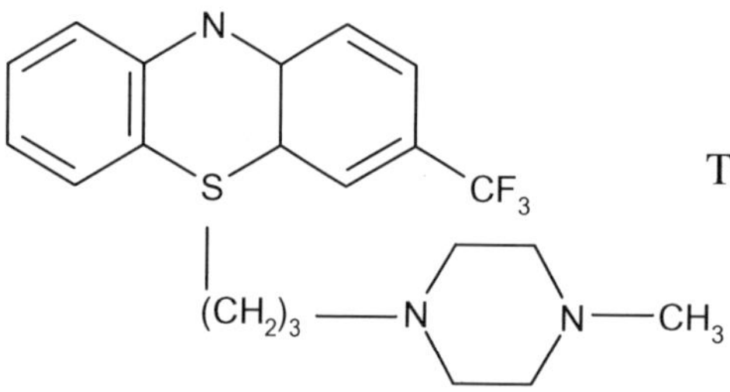

Trifluperazine - used as antipsychotic

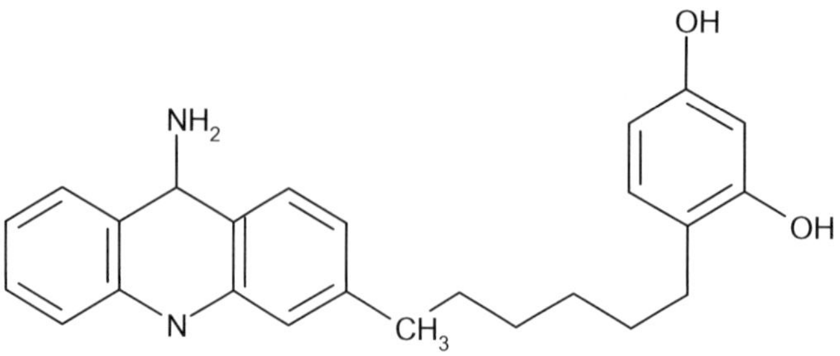

Acrisorcin - used as antimalarial

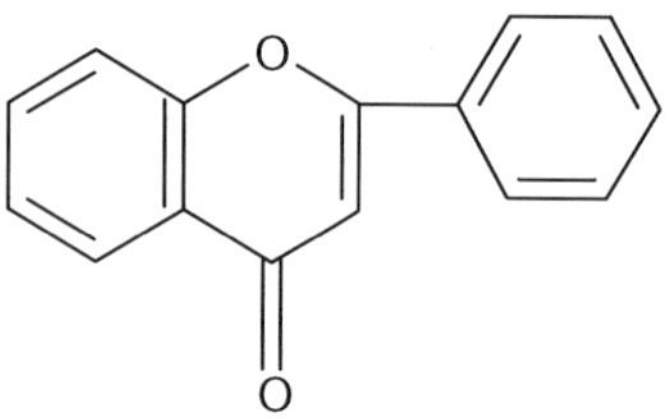

Flavone - Found to be as fungicide, Oestrogenic, antispasmodic

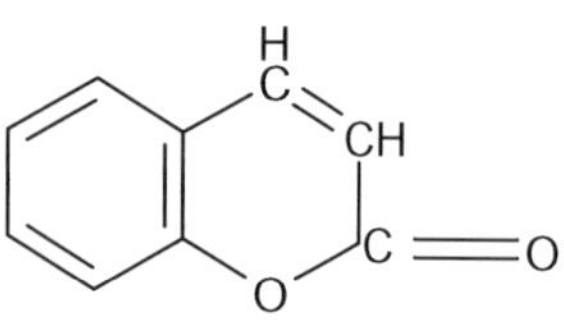

Coumarin - used as flavouring agent and fixative

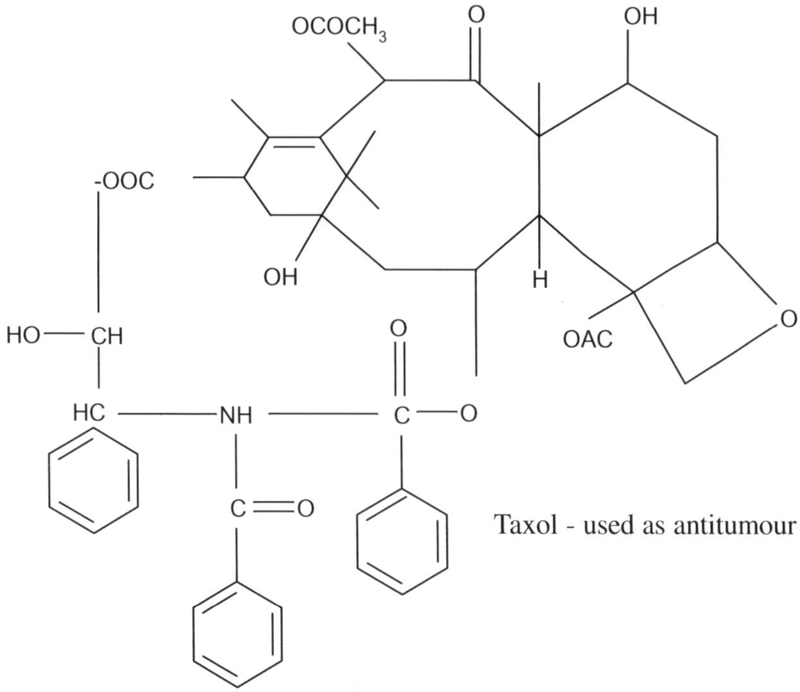

Taxol - used as antitumour agent

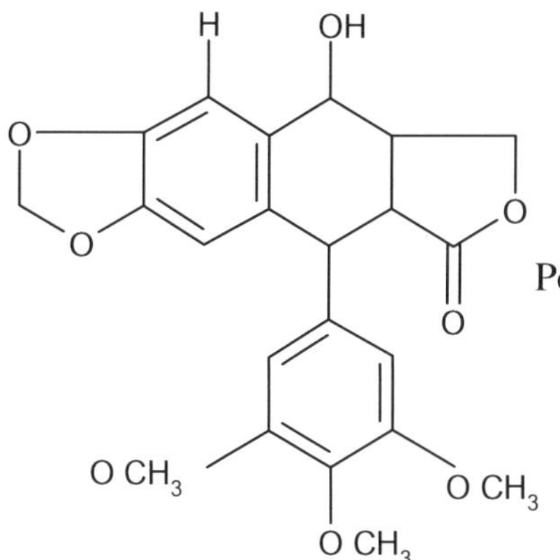

Podophyllotoxin - used as anti - cancer agent

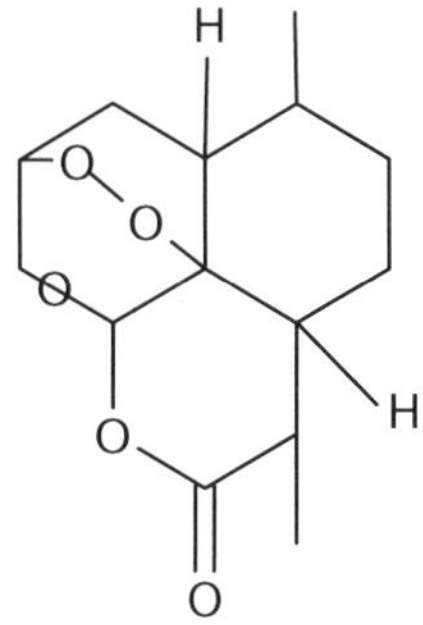

Artemisin - used as anti - malarial drug

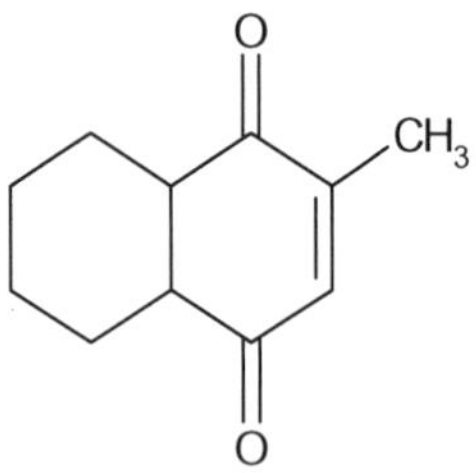

Menadione or Menaphthone - used as analogous for vitamin K

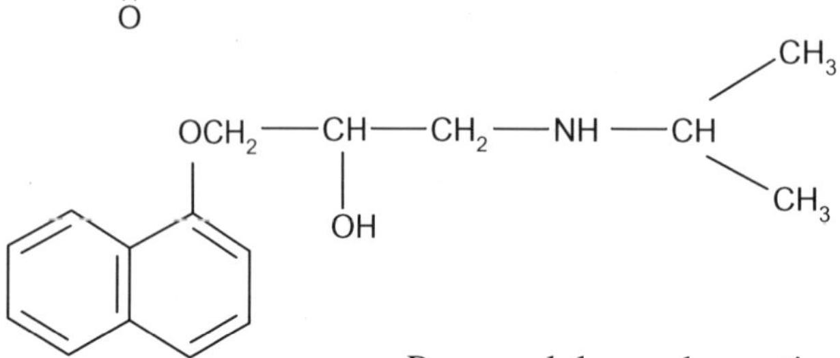

Propranolol - used as anti - arrhythmic & β-adrenergic blocker.

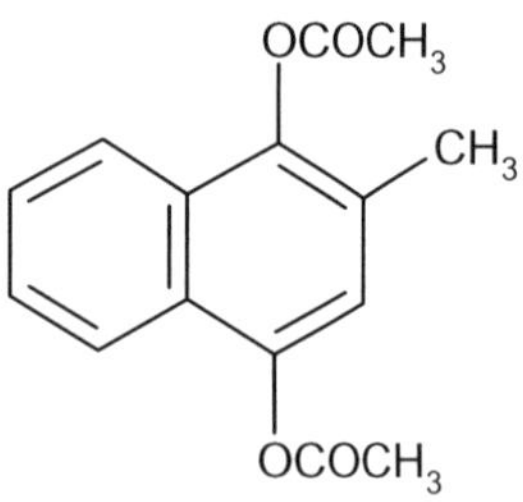

Acetomenaphthone - used as antihaemorrhagic

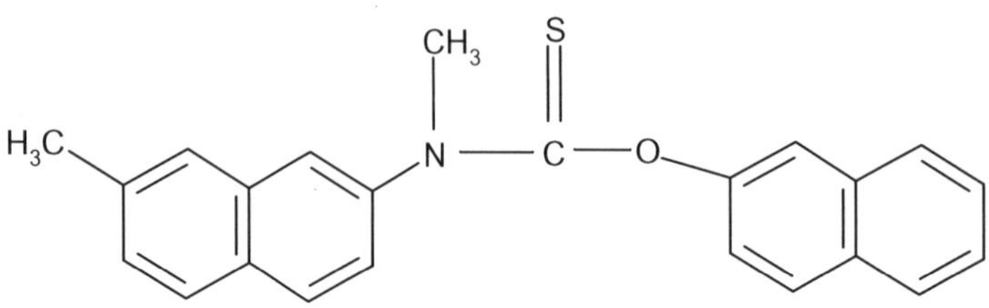

Tolnaftate - used as antifungal agent

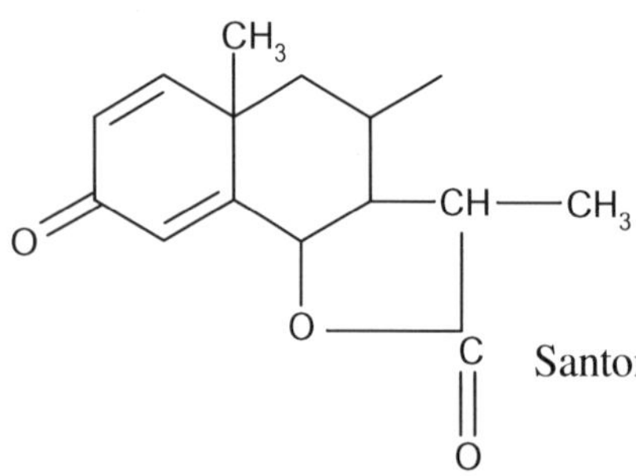

Santonin - used as anthelmintic

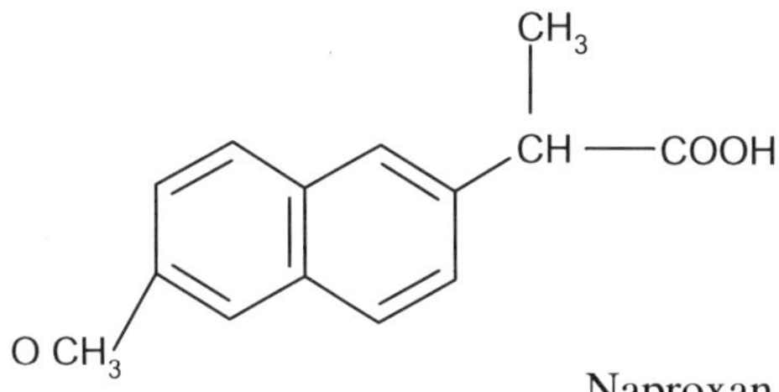

Naproxan - used for rheumatoid arthritis

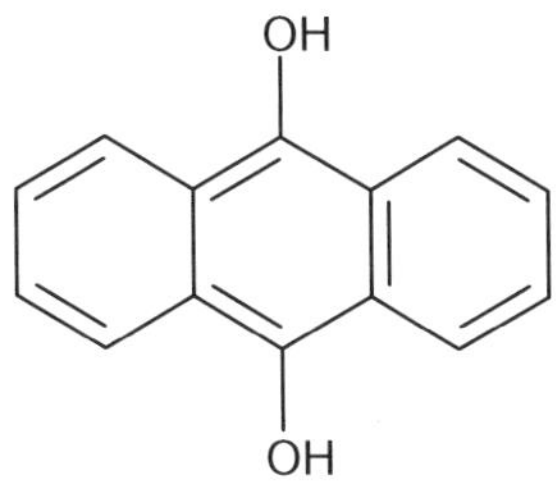

Anthraquinol - used as purgative drug

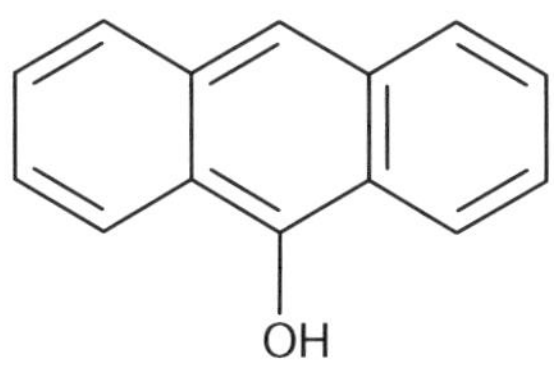

Anthrol - used as purgative

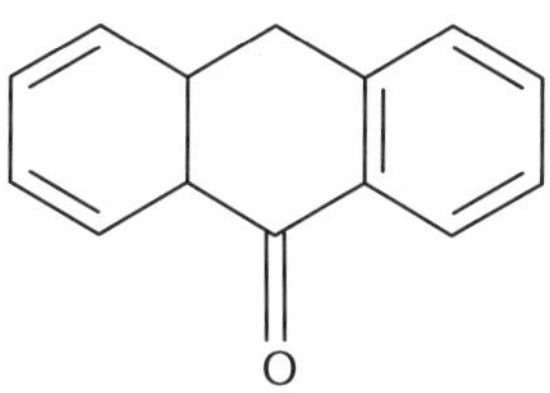

Anthrone - used as purgative

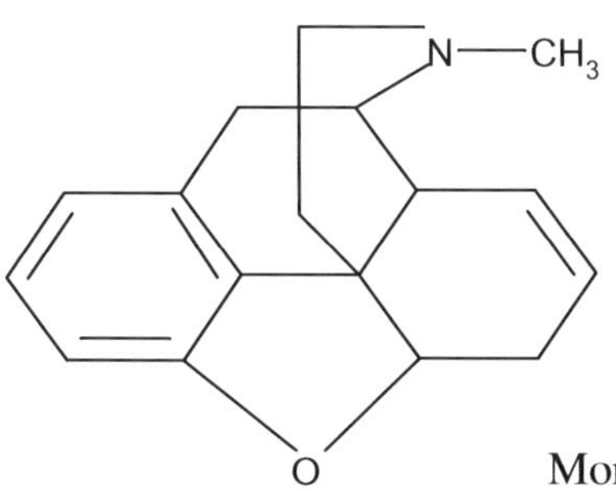

Morphine - used as analgesic and narcotic

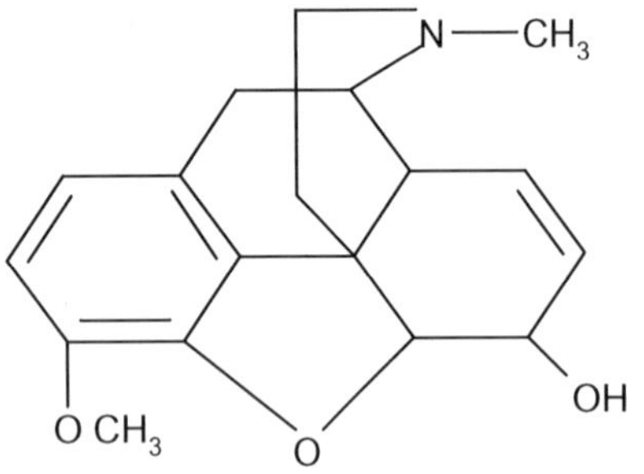

Codeine - used to suppress unproductive cough

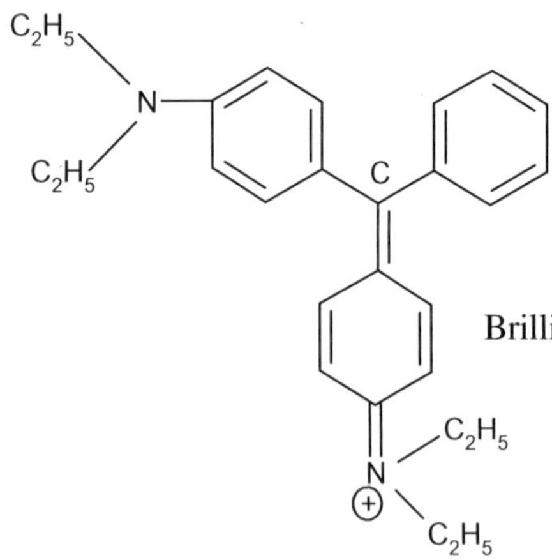

Brilliant green - used as antiseptic and Disinfectant

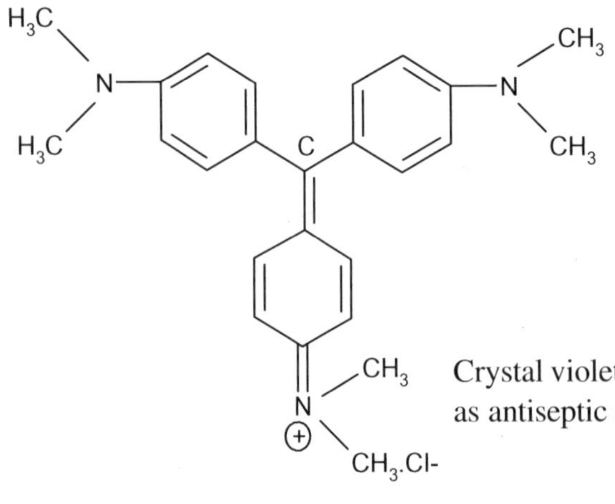

Crystal violet (Gentian violet): - used as antiseptic as well as anthelmintic

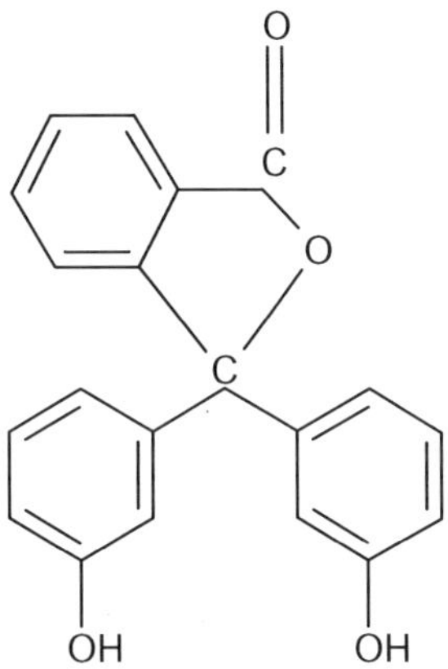

Pehenolphthalein - used as Purgative

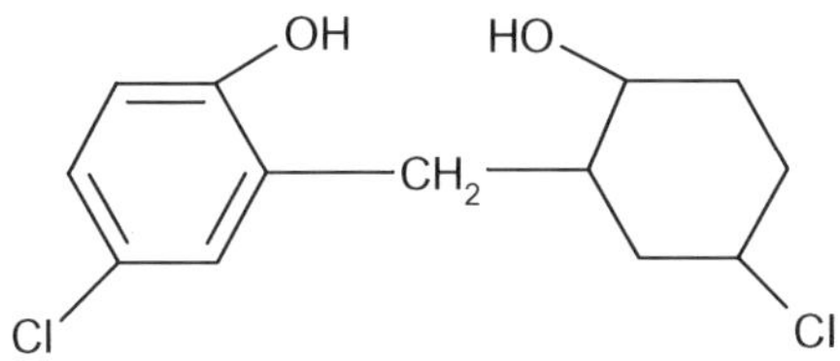

Dichlorophen - used in Tape worm infestation

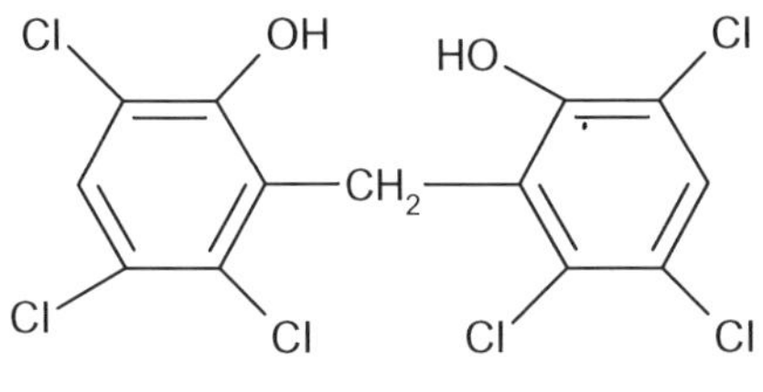

Hexachlorophen - used as antiseptic

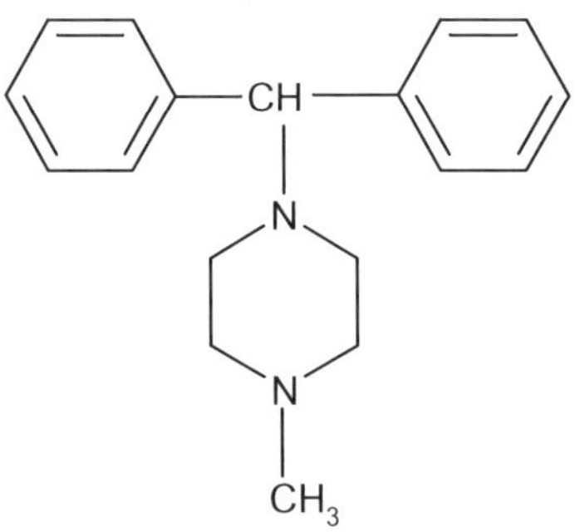

Cyclizen - used as antihistamine

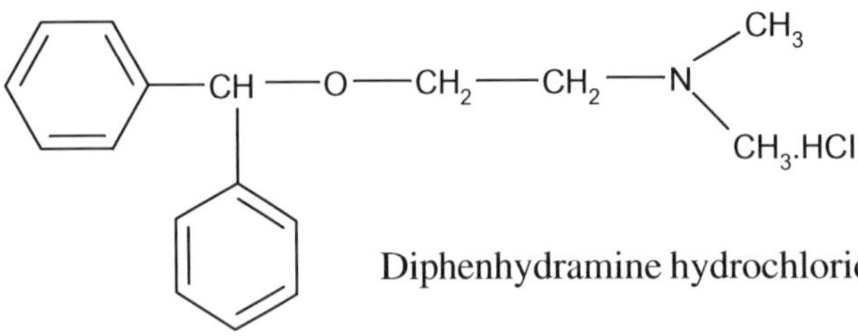

Diphenhydramine hydrochloride : Used as sedative and antihistaminic

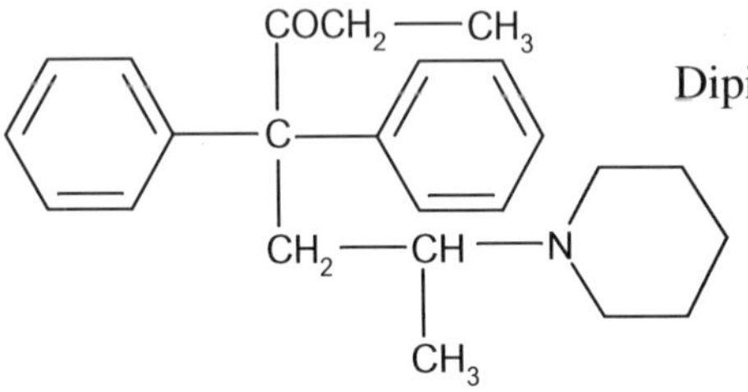

Dipipanone : Used as analgesic

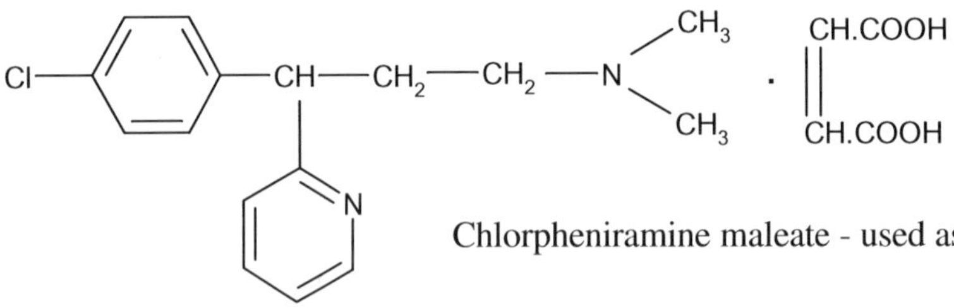

Chlorpheniramine maleate - used as antihistamine

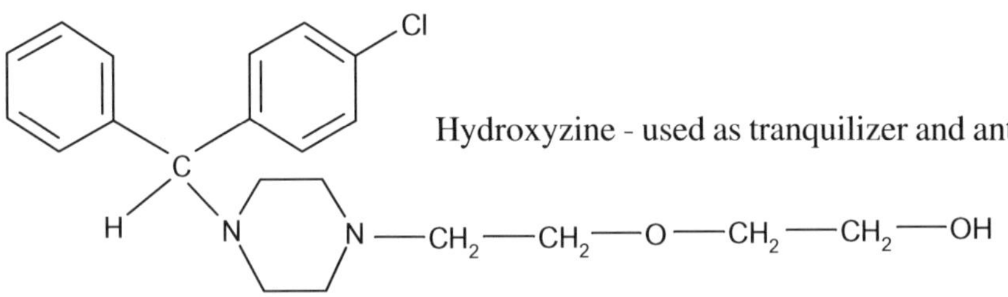

Hydroxyzine - used as tranquilizer and antihistaminic

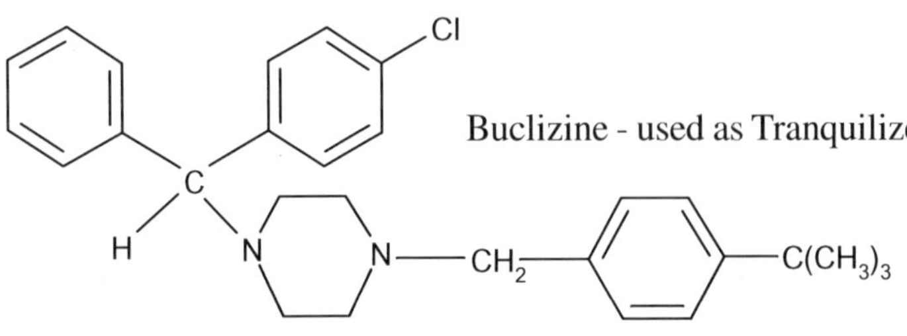

Buclizine - used as Tranquilizer

Indole Containing Drugs

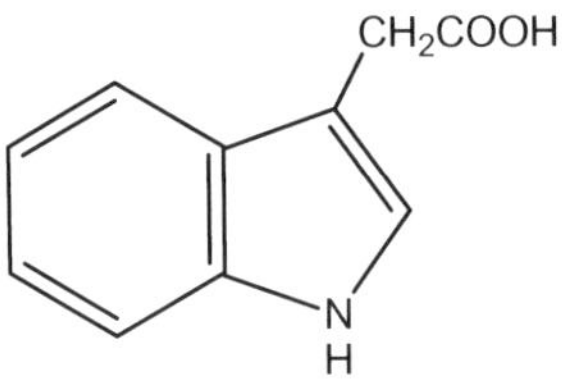

Indole 3- acetic acid - plant.growth regulating horomone

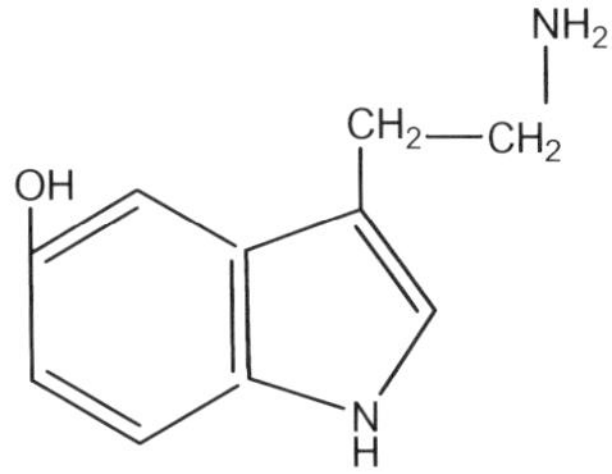

Serotonine - Vasoconstrictor

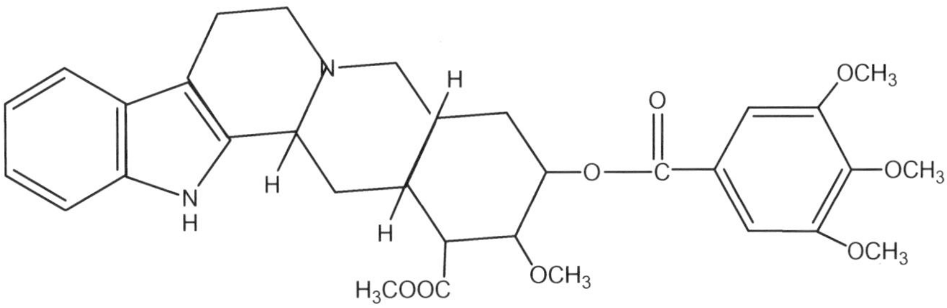

Reserpine - Tranquilizer & antihypertensive

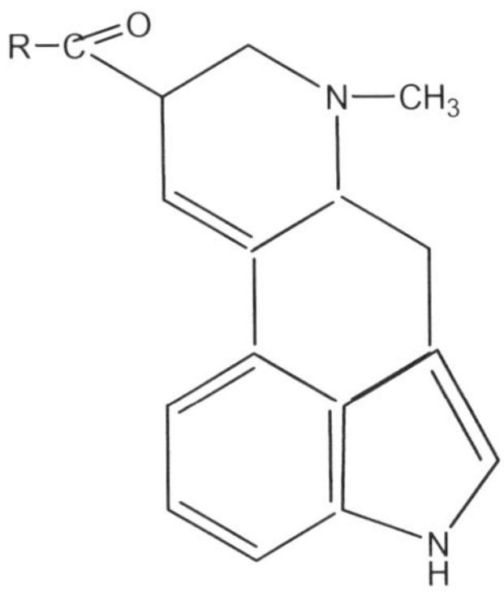

Ergotamine - Vasoconstrictor for migrain

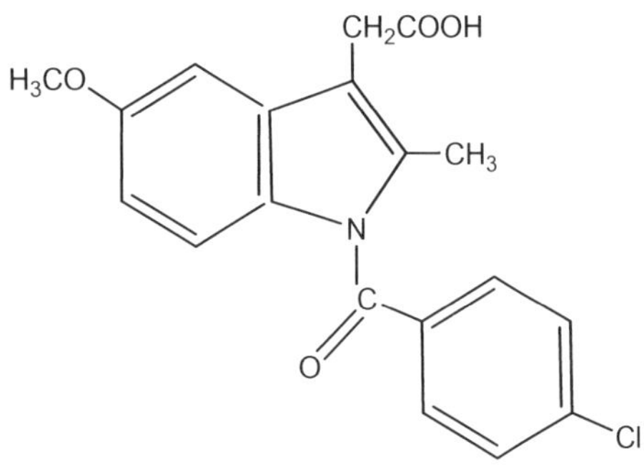

Indomethacin - anti-inflammatory agent

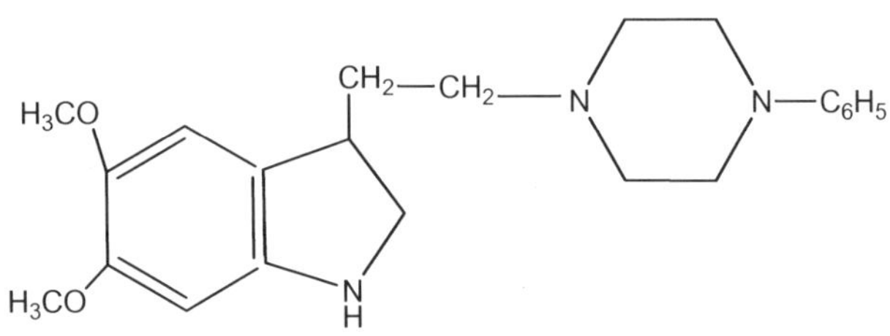

Oxypertine - tranquilizer

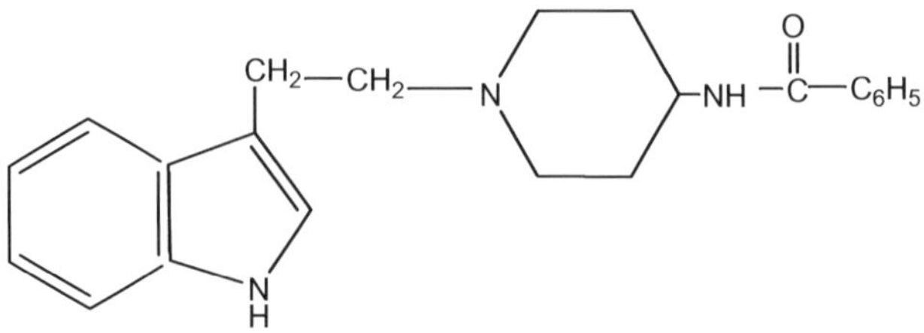

Indoramine - antihypretension

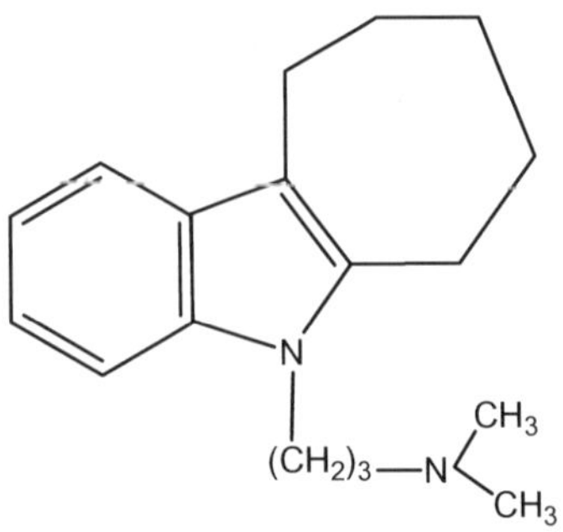

Iprindole-neurotransmitter

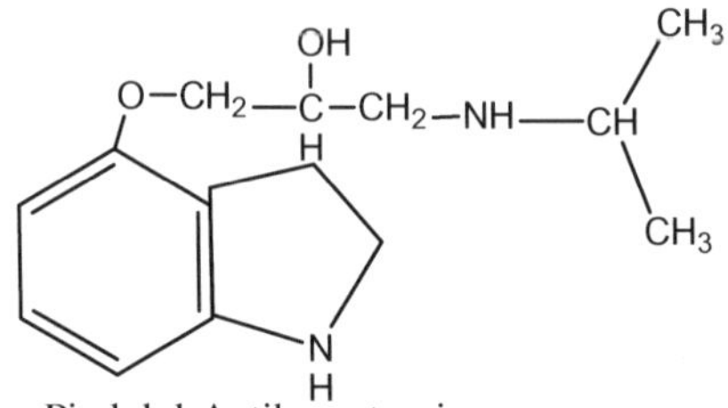

Pindolol-Antihypertensive

Imidazole Containing Drugs

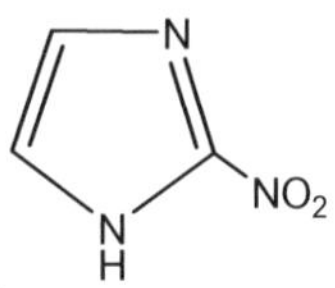

Azomycin-antibiotic

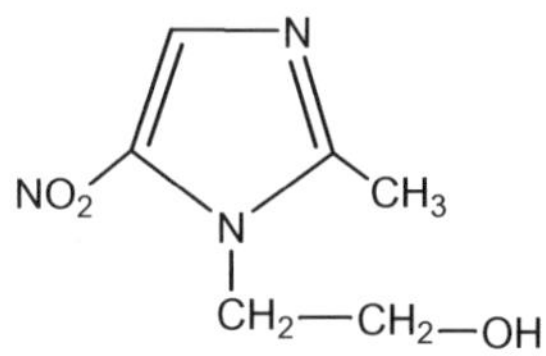

Metronidazole-Antibacterial

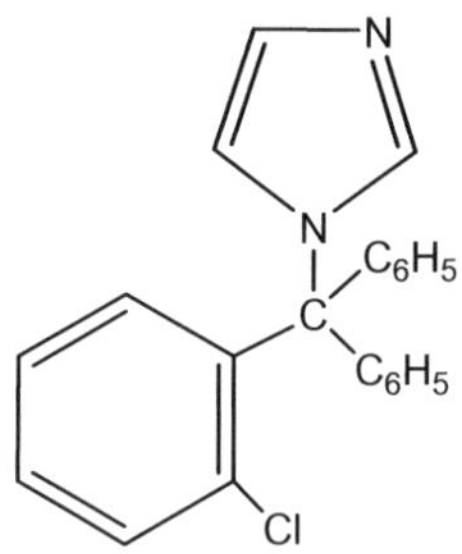

Clotrimazole-antibacterial

Thiazole

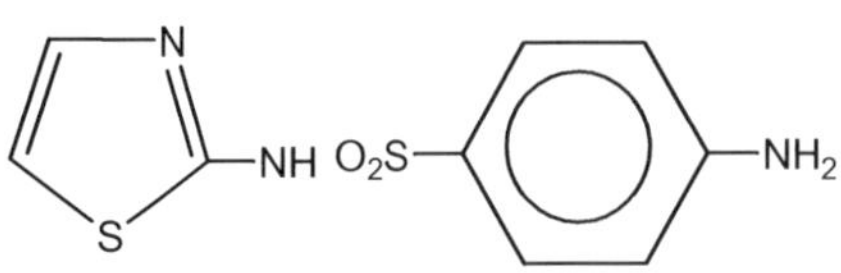

Sulfathiazole-antibiotic

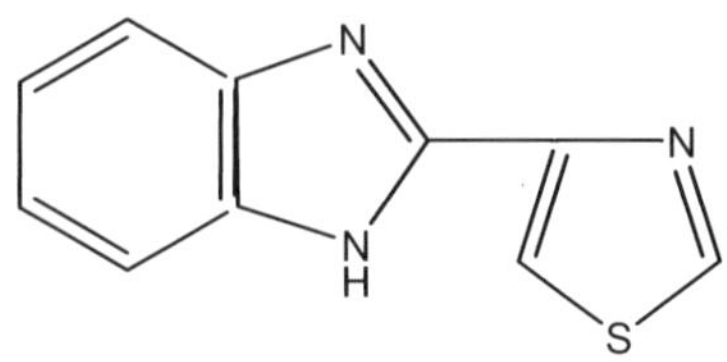

Thiabendazole-anthelmintic & fungicide

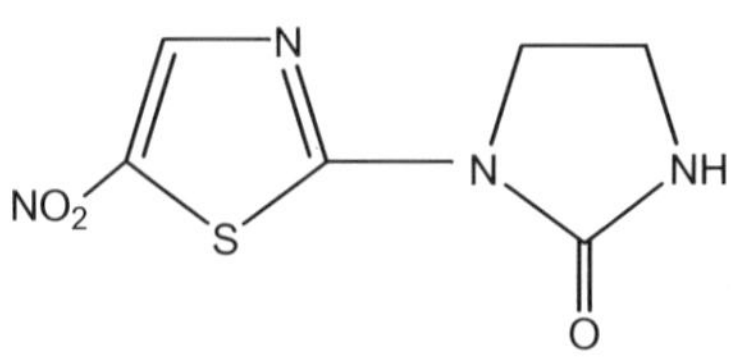

Niridazole-Schistosomicidal

4

Synthetic Tools

BECKMANN REARRANGEMENT

Beckmann rearrangement is the conversion of ketoximes to N-substituted amides by heating in the presence of acids like;

$$H_2SO_4, BF_3, P_2O_5, PCl_5, SO_3, SOCl_2, C_6H_5SO_2Cl$$

In this rearrangement shift or migration of groups is always trans (anti) to the leaving group (-OH). Trans migration can be represented as follows;

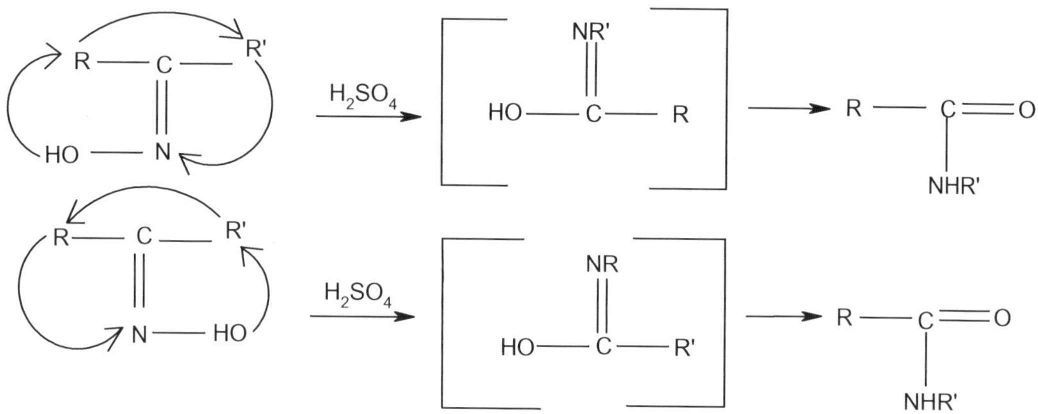

It involves migration of an alkyl or allyl group with its electron pair from C to N with the elimination of -OH. The rearrangement takes place in some intermediate, formed between the oxime and amide, and not in oxime itself. The alkyl or acyl group(R) migrates intramolecularly. The anion (-OH or -OX) migrates intermolecularly. In this reaction a carbonium ion accept hydroxyl ion or a water molecule from solvent, hence the original oxygen molecule of the oxime is completely lost during the reaction.

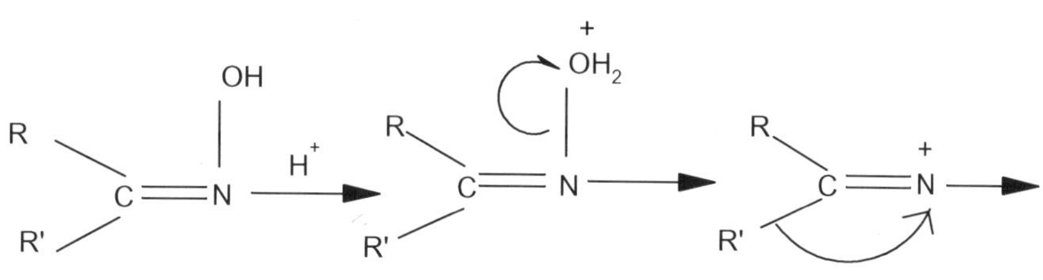

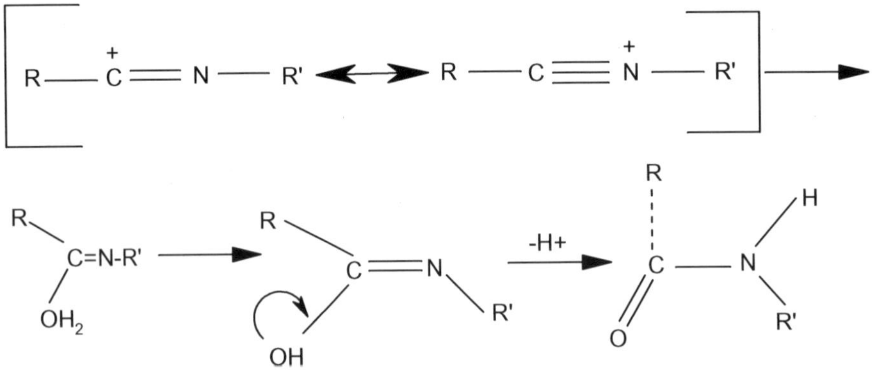

Applications of Beckmann Rearrangement

1. To determine the configuration of Ketoximes

It is based on the fact that two isomeric Ketoximes, Syn and anti give different amides by Beckmann rearrangement. The corresponding amides can be identified by their hydrolysis. For. eg:

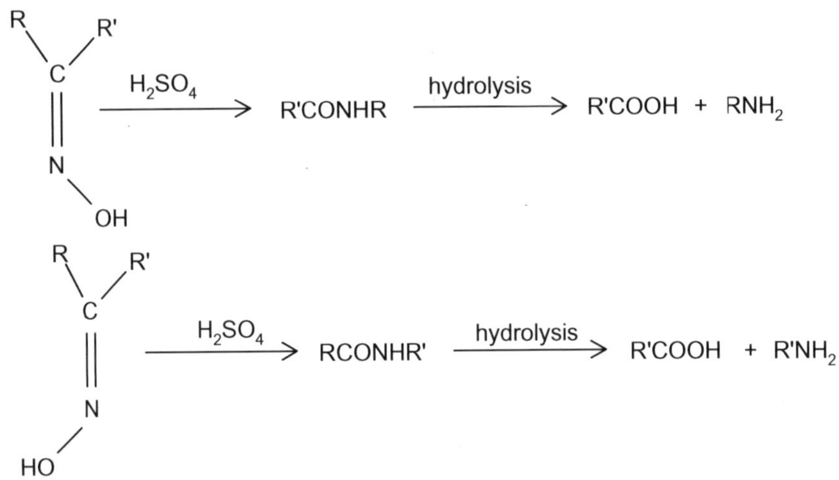

2. To synthesis isoquinoline

Cinnamaldoxime is Cyclized to isoquinoline by Beckmann rearrangement.

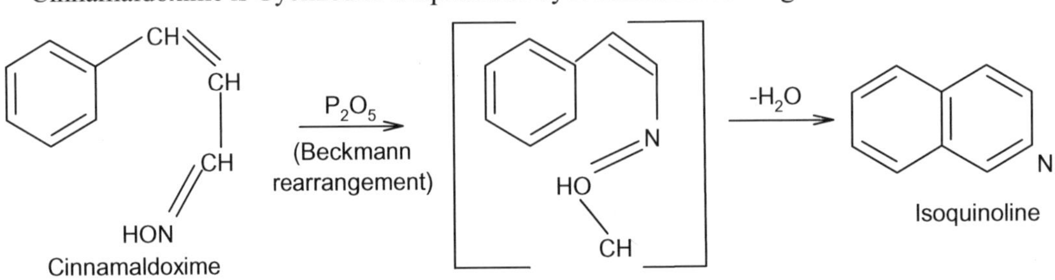

3. To synthesis-caprolactam

Caprolactam is a raw material for polymers like nylon. Cyclohexanine oxime undergo Beckmann rearrangement in the presence of Sulphuric acid to form Caprolactam.

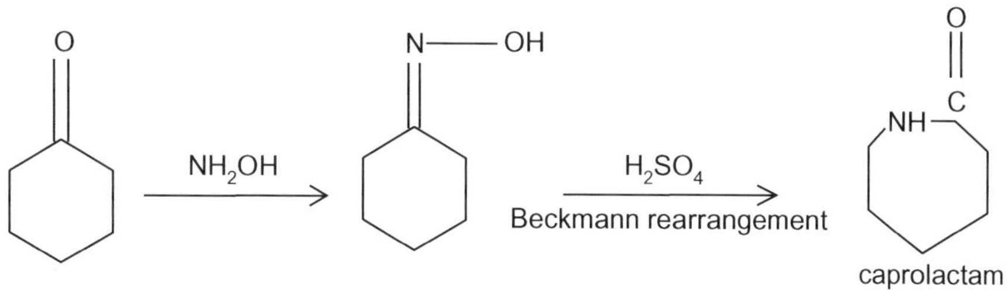

SCHMIDT REACTION

Carboxylic acids react with hydrazoic acid in the presence of concentrated Sulphuric acid give amine directly is known as Schmidt reaction.

$$RCOOH + N_3H \xrightarrow{H_2SO_4} R-NH_2 + CO_2 + N_2$$

Schmidt reaction also takesplace between aldehydes or ketones and hydrazoic acid to form a mixture of Cyanides and formyl derivatives of primary amines and amides respectively.

$$RCHO + N_3H \xrightarrow{H_2SO_4} R-CN + RNH.CHO$$

$$RCOR + N_3H \xrightarrow{H_2SO_4} RCONHR + N_2$$

Mechanism for Reaction with Acids

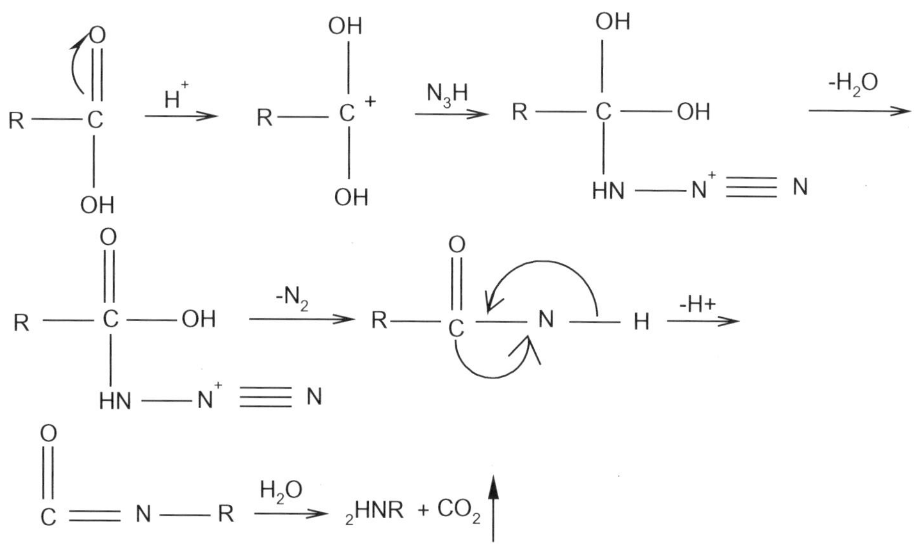

Mechanism for Reaction with Ketones

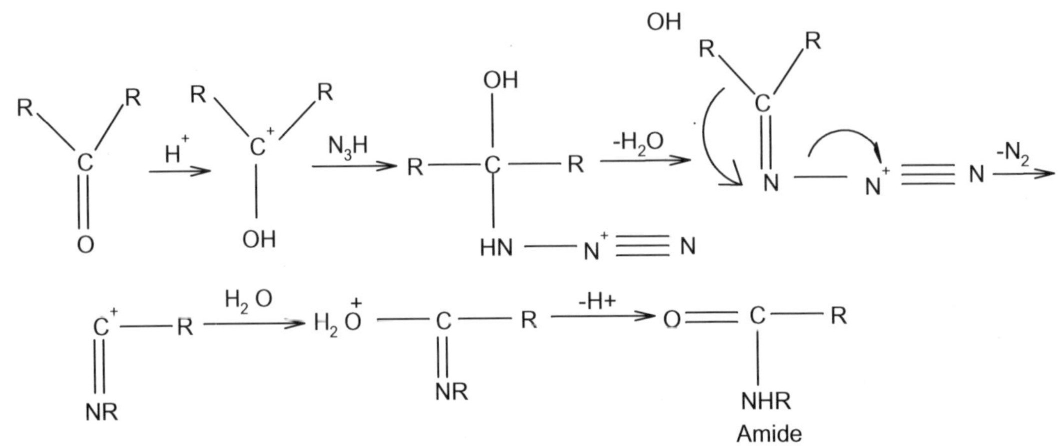

Mechanism for Reaction with Aldehydes

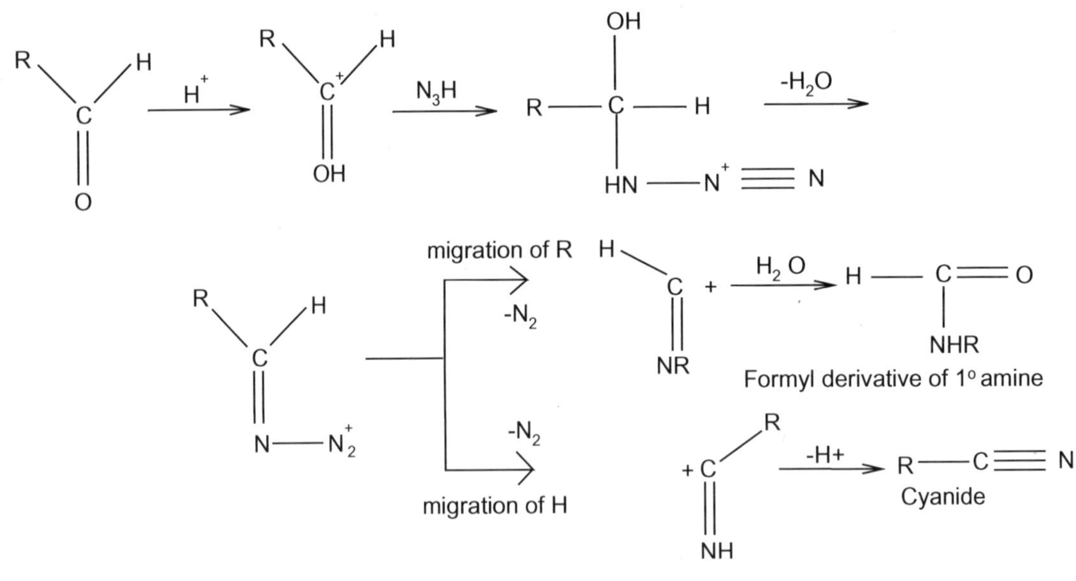

Application of Schmidt Reaction

1. Preparation of primary amines

Reaction with Hydrazoic acid is explosive and is applicable only when the Carboxylic acid used does not contain any group sensitive to concentrated Sulphuric acid.

$$C_6H_5COOH + N_3H \xrightarrow{H_2SO_4} C_6H_5-NH_2 + CO_2\uparrow + N_2\uparrow$$

2. Preparation of α amino acids

α-amino acids can be prepared from acetoacetic ester.

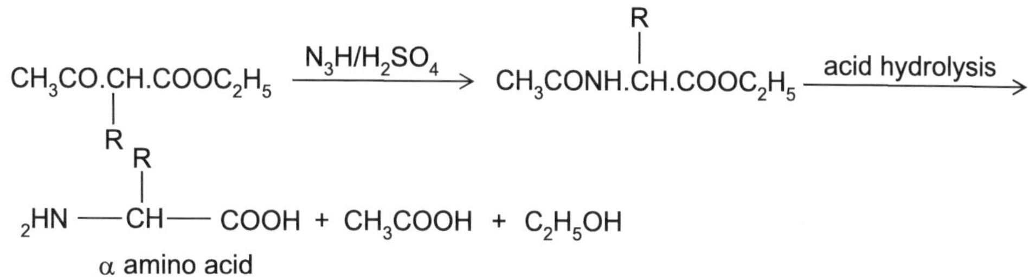

MEERWEIN-PONNDORF-VERLEY REDUCTION (MPV reduction)

Here aldehydes and ketones are reduced to respective alcohol by treatment with aluminium isopropoxide in isopropanol solution.

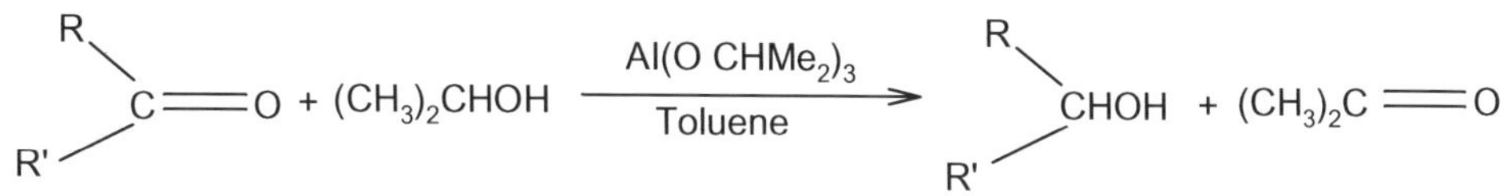

Mechanism

It involves migration of a hydride ion from the isopropoxide to Carbonyl compound.

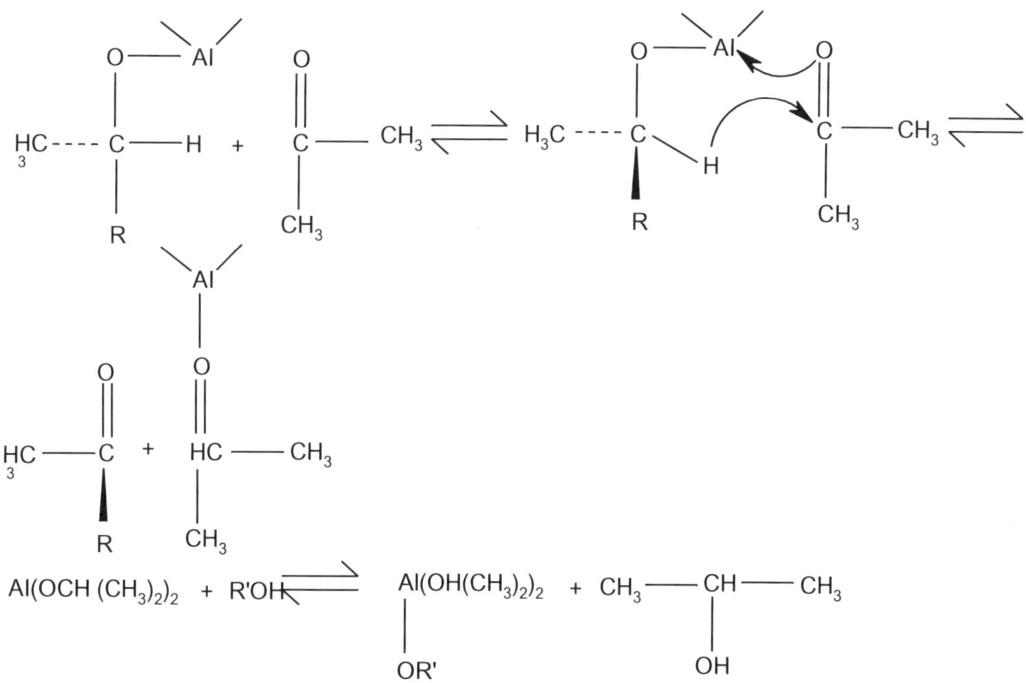

Application

1. Preparation of Chloromycetin

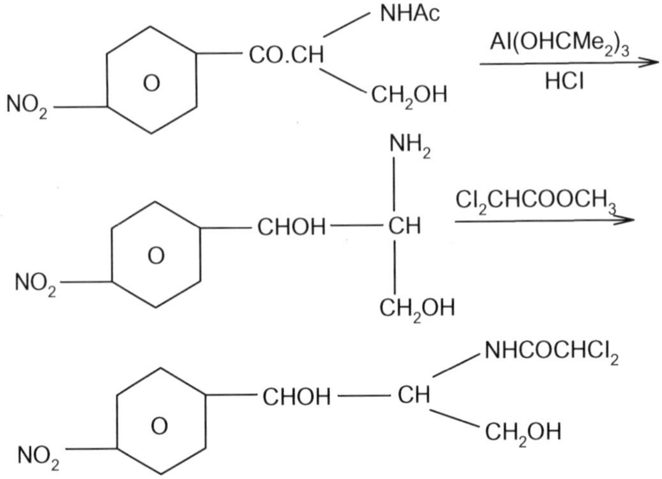

2. In the preparation of Oestradiol

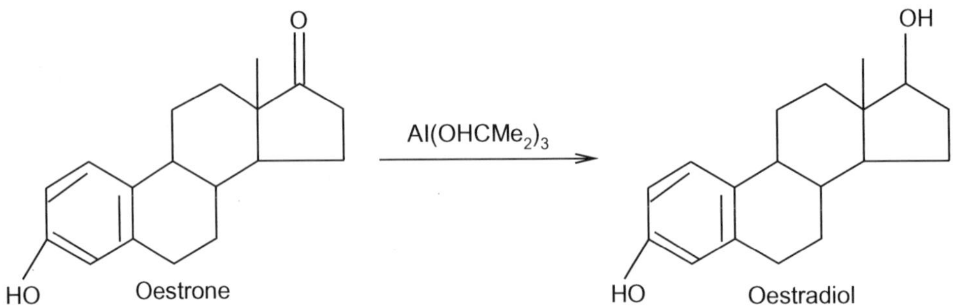

CLEMMENSEN REDUCTION

Reduction of aldehyde or ketones in the presence of zinc amalgam and hydrochloric acid is known as Clemmensen reduction. Ketones are reduced more often than aldehydes.

$$R-\underset{\underset{O}{\|}}{C}-R' \xrightarrow{ZnHg/HCl} R-CH_2-R'$$

The reaction commonly takesplace in a 3 phase mixture of toluene, aqueous hydrochloric acid and Zinc-amalgam.

Eg 1)

$$C_6H_5-CO-CH_2-CH_2-COOH \xrightarrow[\text{Tolouene}]{Zn-Hg/H_2O} C_6H_5(CH_2)_3-COOH$$

Eg 2)

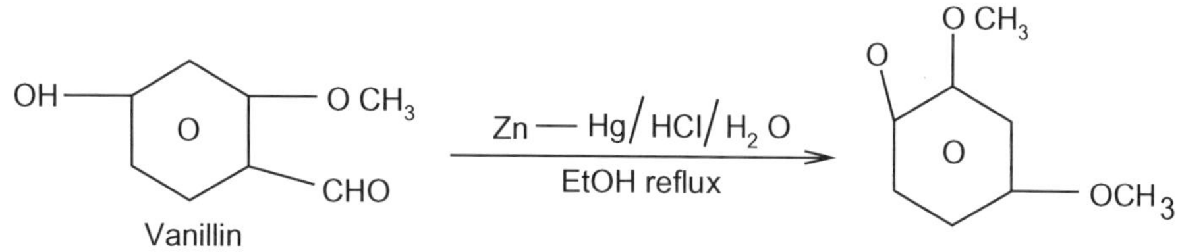

Mechanism

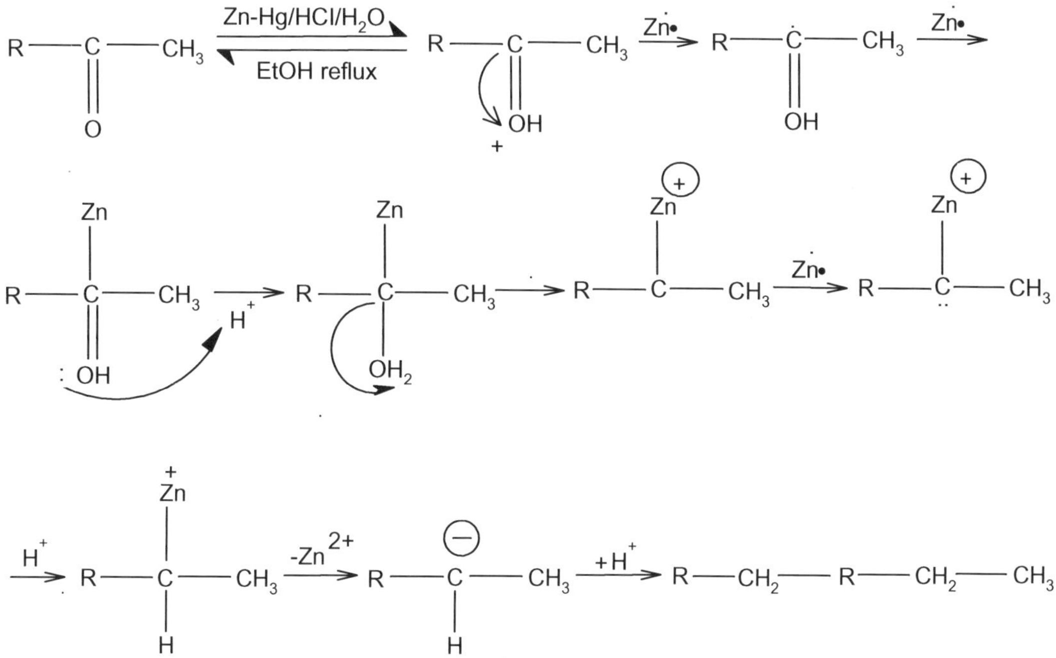

Applications

1. In the structural elucidation of Cholesterol

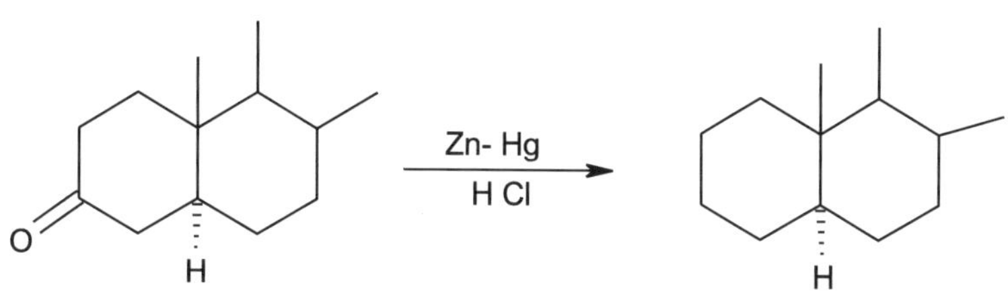

Cholestrone 5-alpha Cholestane

2. In the synthesis of phenanthrene

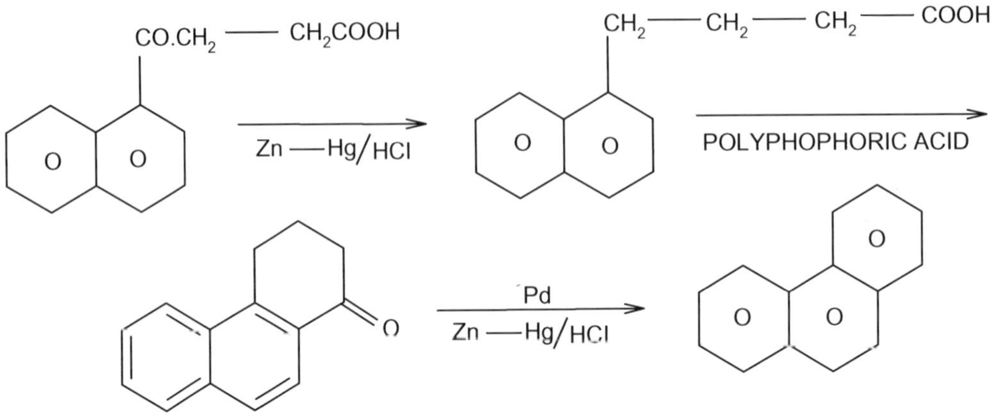

3. Reduction of cyclohexanone into cyclohexane

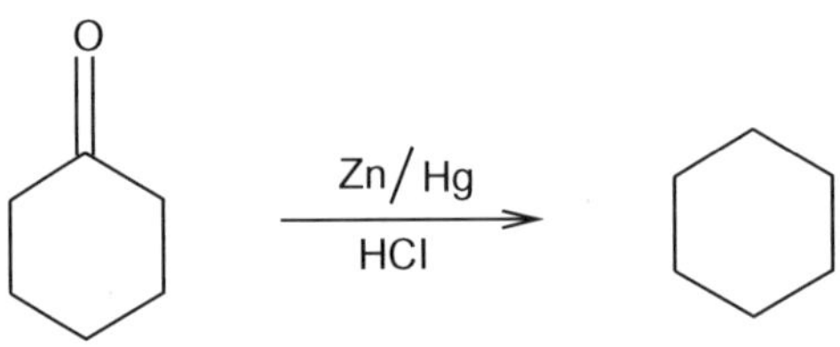

BIRCH REDUCTION

Aromatic rings are reduced by Sodium in liquid ammonia in the presence of alcohol is known as Birch reduction. Here 1, 4 addition of hydrogen takes place.

Eg : Benzene undergoes Birch reduction to form 1, 4 diene.

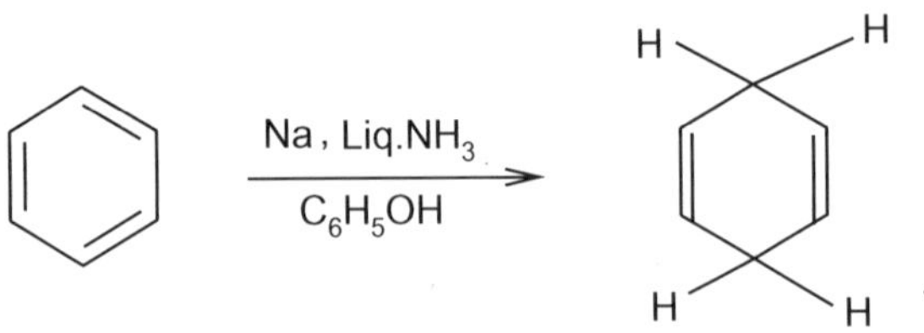

Alcohol provide the proteins and Sodium metal used to transfer electrons. Mechanism involved can be summerized as follows.

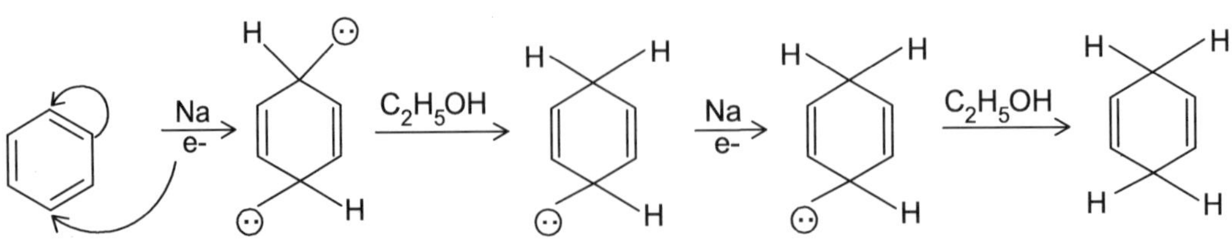

Application

1. Birch reduction can also applied to reduce terminal double bond.

$$R-CH=CH_2 \xrightarrow[C_2H_5OH]{Na,Liq.NH_3} R-CH_2-CH_3$$

2. Pyridine undergoes Birch reduction to form 1,4 dihydro pyridine.

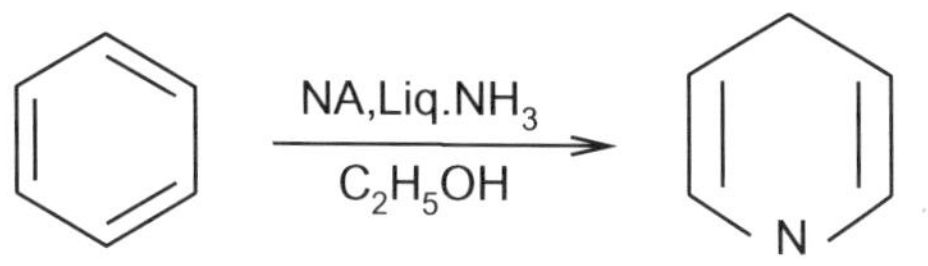

3. Mono & disubstituted alkenes are reduced more rapidly than tri or tetra substituted ones. It provides further degree of selectivity illustrated by reduction of carvone to dihydrocarvone leaving the trisubstituted double bond intact.

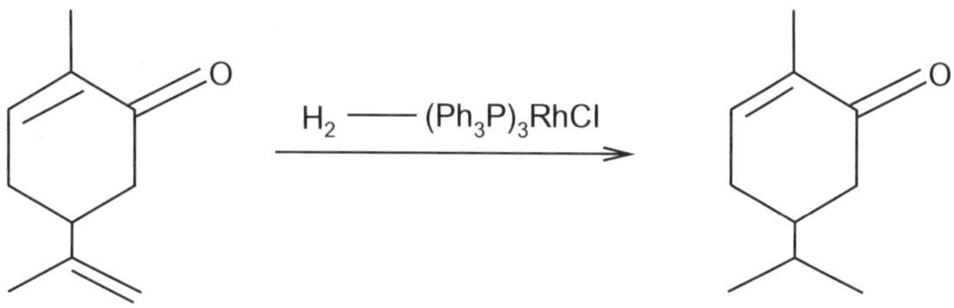

4. Hydrogenolysis does not occur. Eg: Benzyl Cinnamate gives dihydro derivative.

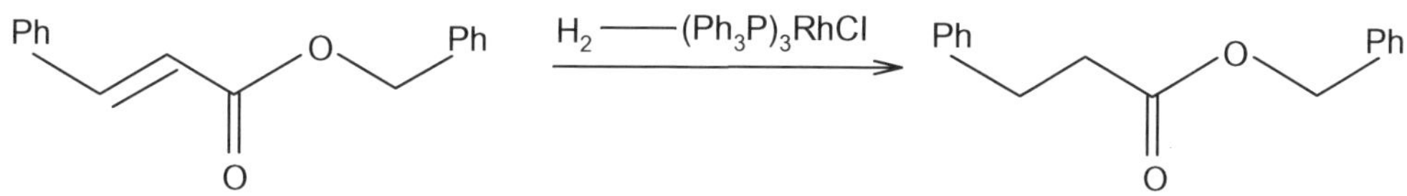

CATALYTIC HYDROGENATION

Addition of hydrogen to a compound is known as hydrogenation. Hydrogen is added to multiple bond in the presence of a catalyst. Energy liberated during the process is known as heat of hydrogenation. More substituted alkene will have more stability. The order of their stability can be written as

$$R_2C=CR_2 > {}_2RC=CHR > R_2C=CH_2RCH=CHR > {}_2HC=C\,H2$$

Mechanism involved can be represent as follows

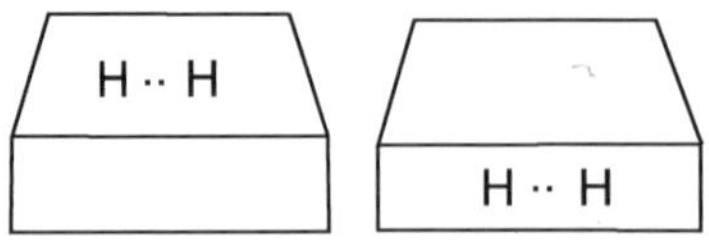

Hydrogen absorbed by catalyst

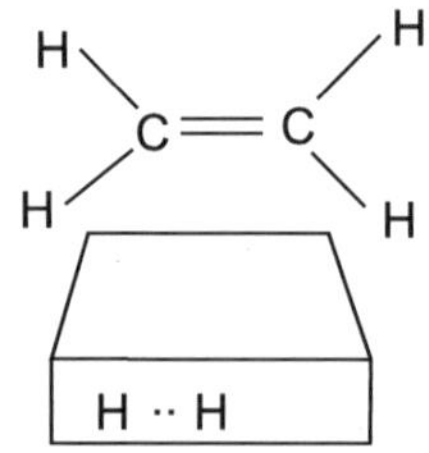

Alkane molecule approaches catalyst surface

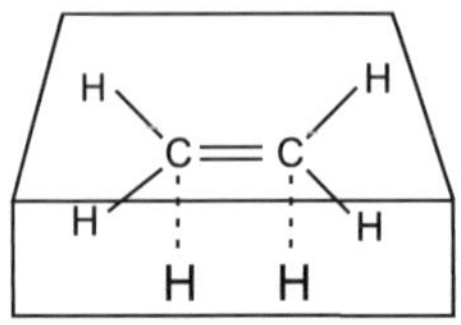

Intermediate bonding of Alkenes and cis transfer of Hydrogen

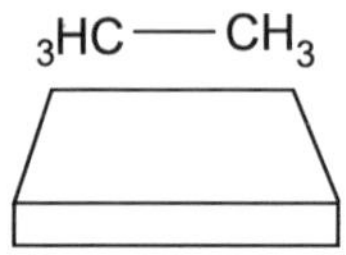

Product Leaves Surface

Catalytic hydrogenation can be used for estimating the amount of unsaturation. Catalysts used are can be divided into heterogenous catalysts and homogenous catalysts. Heterogenous catalysts are insoluble in the reaction medium. Eg: Raney nickel, Palladium, Platinum, Rhodium, Ruthenium, Zinc oxide etc. Homogenous catalysts are soluble in reaction medium.

Eg:

Wilkinson's catalyst.(Triphenyl phosphine Chlororhodium = $Rh[(C_6H_5)]_3Cl$).

Three advantages are there for using homogenous catalysts. 1) only alkane and alkynes are reduced; other common groups such as C=O,C≡N & NO_2 are unaffected. It makes possible selective reduction such as

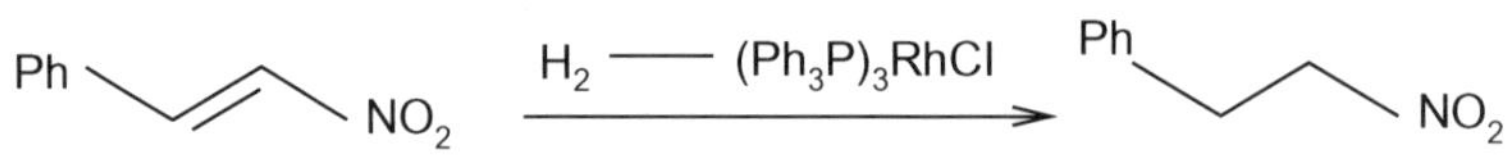

Application

1. Alkenes can be coverted to Alkanes

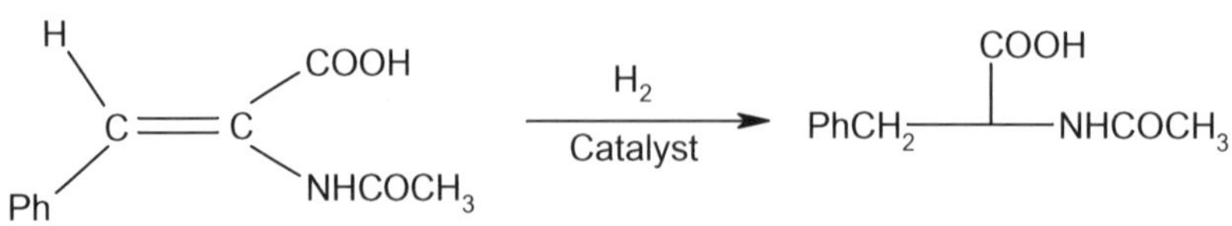

2. Aromatic compound can be converted to Aliphatic compound

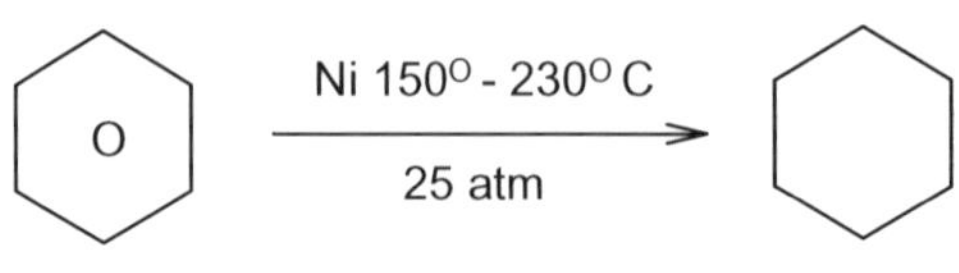

Dehydrogenation

Dehydrogenation is an elimination reaction. Elimination of hydrogen from cyclic aliphatic compounds yields aromatic compound.

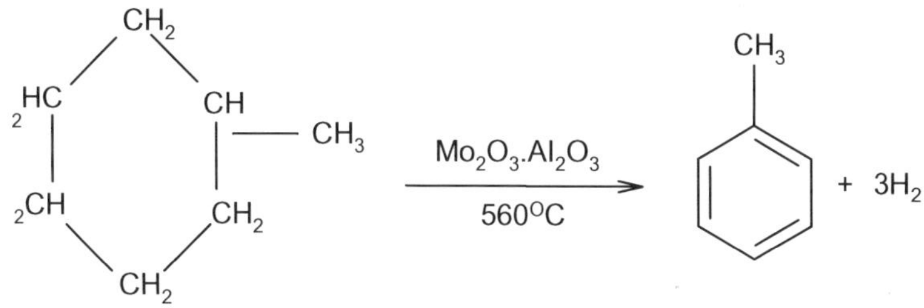

Methyl Cyclohexane Toluene

Alcohols are dehydrogenated to give aldehydes and ketones

$$R—CH_2OH \xrightarrow[\text{Chromite}]{\text{Cu}} RCHO$$

Phenols are dehydrogenated in the presence of potassium dichromate and sulphuric acid give Quinones.

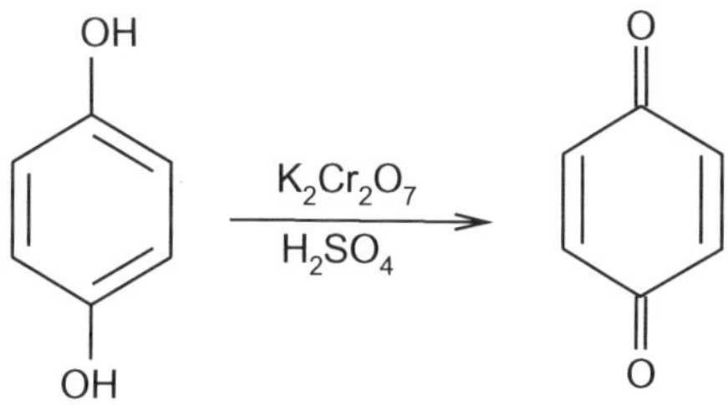

DARZEN'S REACTION

It involves the treatment of aldehyde or ketone with α-halgon ester in the presence of sodium ethoxide and sodamide gives epoxy ester also known as glycidic ester, Generally we can represent the reaction as

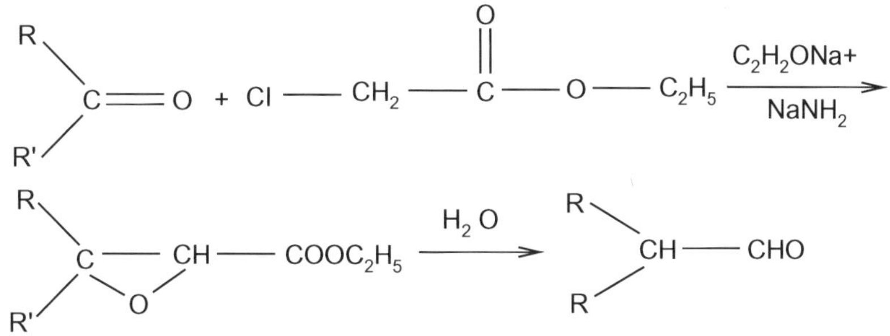

α , β epoxy ester

By Darzen condensation, higher carboxyl group can be obtained from lower carboxyl group like

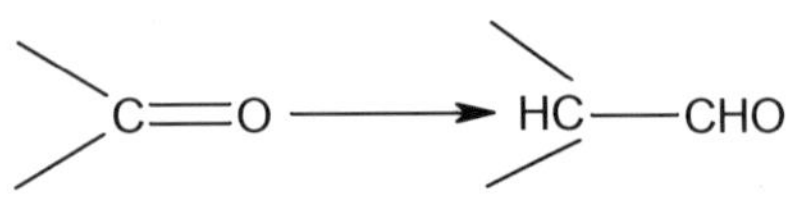

The condensation reaction follows the pattern as

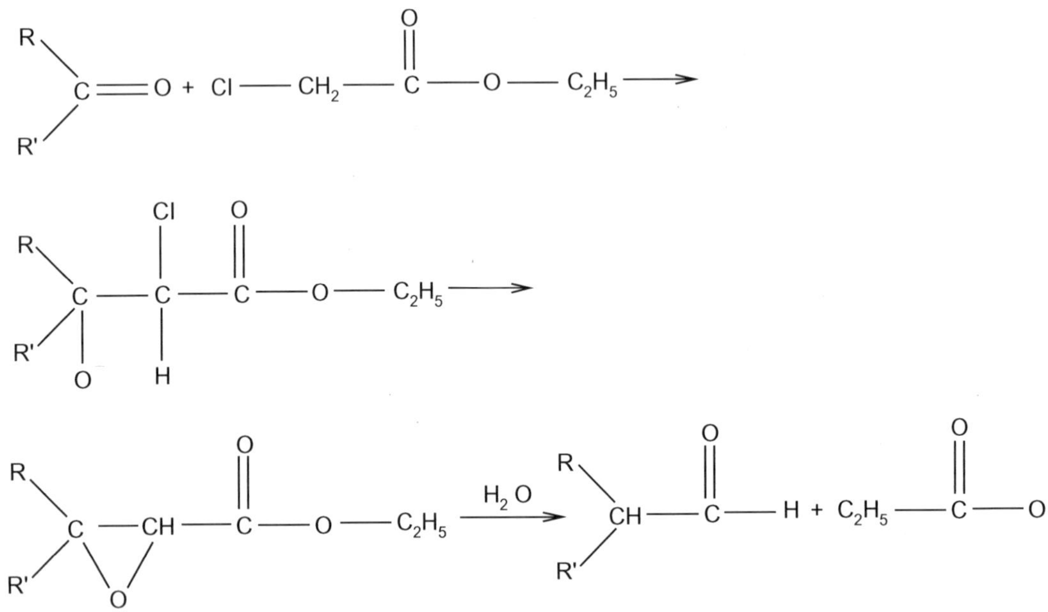

α, β epoxy ester

Applications

1. In the synthesis of Vitamin A

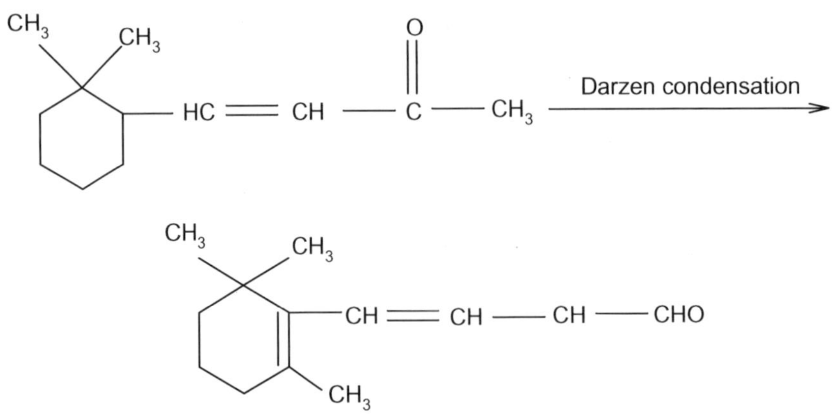

Vit.A

2. Synthesis of α-pinene also involves Darzen reaction

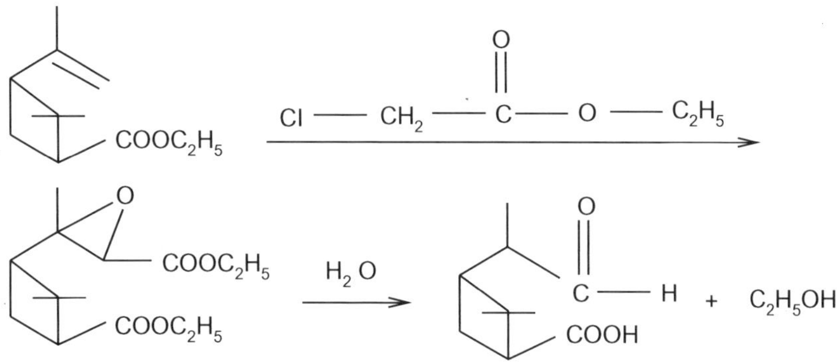

α , β epoxy ester

Some Oxidation Reactions with Important Oxidising Agents

The reaction where electrons are wholly or partially removed is known as oxidation.

REILEY REACTION (OXIDATION WITH SELENIUM OXIDE)

In 1932, Reiley used SeO_2 as an oxidising agent for oxidation of methylene Ketones (—CH_2—CO—) to diketones (—CO—CO—)

$$\text{—}CH_2\text{—}CO + SeO_2 \longrightarrow \text{—}CO\text{—}CO + H_2O + Se$$

This oxdising agent can oxidise aldehydes and ketones of various types into 1, 2-dialdehydes, aldoketones and 1, 2-diketones.

Preparation and properties

SeO_2 is prepared by heating metallic selenium in an atmosphere of oxygen. NO_2 may be used as catalyst for the reaction. It is a white crystalline solid, sublimes at 300°C and dissolves in water forming selenious acid, H_2SeO_3, which is also a powerful oxidising agent.

Applications

1. Selenium dioxide exhibits specific oxidation of methylene ketones to α-diketones.

$$\underset{\text{Acetophenone}}{C_6H_5COCH_3} \xrightarrow[\text{Dioxan}]{SeO_2} \underset{\text{Phenyl glyoxal}}{C_6H_5CO.CHO} + Se + H_2O$$

50°-55°C

2. Compounds containing active methyl or methylene group can also oxidise by SeO_2
   eg: 1)

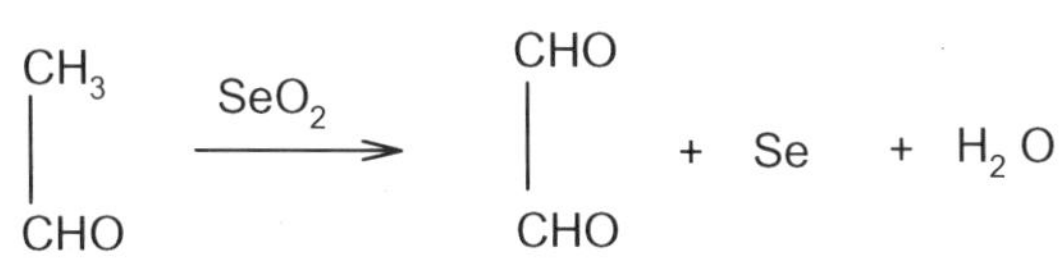

Acetaldelyde Glyoxal

eg: 2)

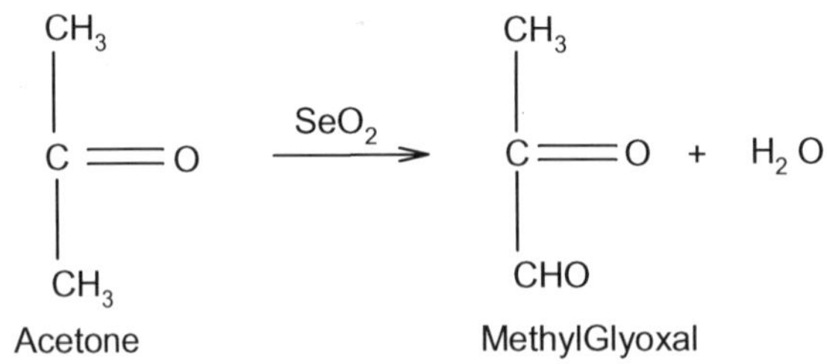

eg: 3)

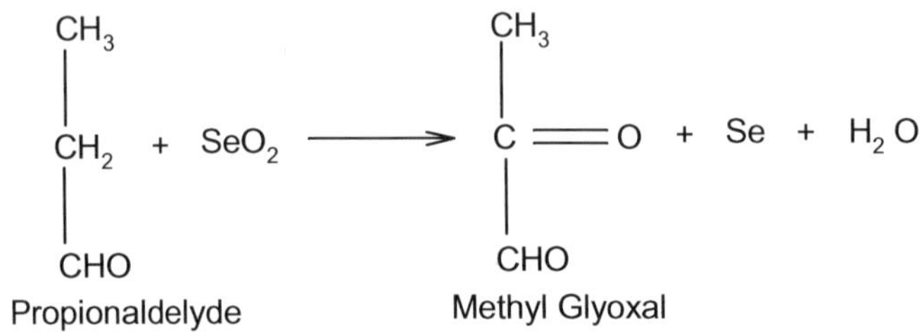

eg: 4)

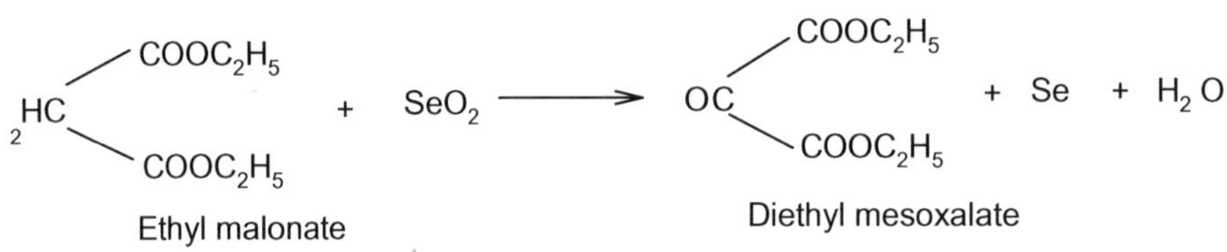

eg: 5)

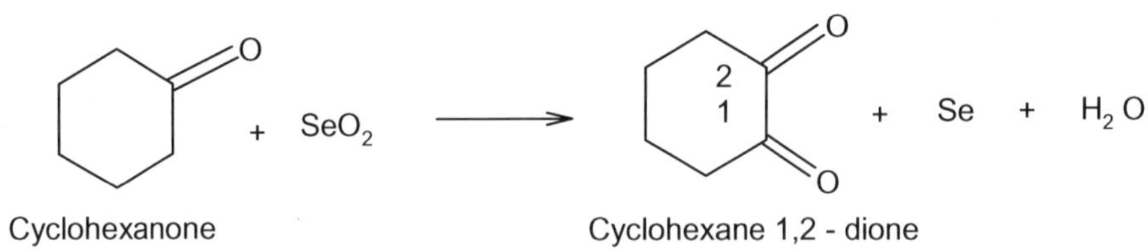

eg: 6)

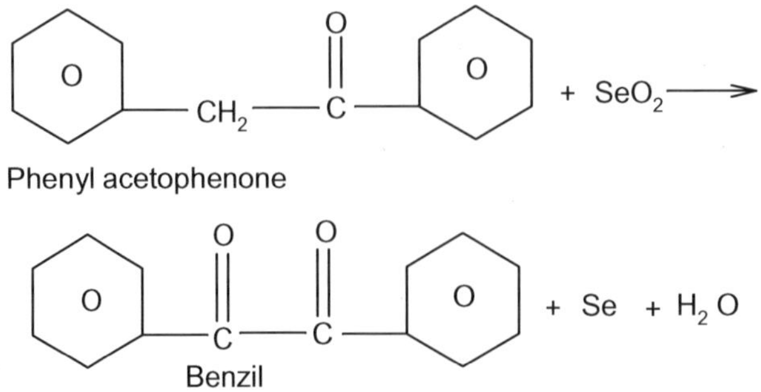

eg: 7)

$$C_6H_5CH_2COOH + SeO_2 \longrightarrow C_6H_5-\overset{O}{\overset{\|}{C}}-COOH + Se + H_2O$$

Phenyl acetic acid → Benzoyl formic acid

eg: 8)

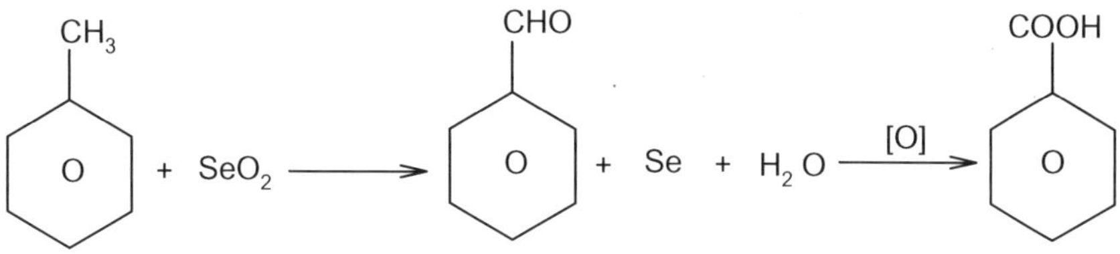

Toluene, Benzaldehyde, Benzoic acid

eg: 9)

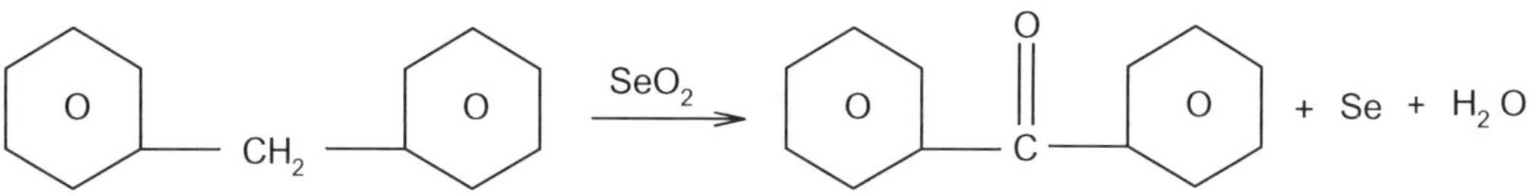

Diphenyl methane, Benzophenone

OXIDATION WITH MERCURIC ACETATE

Mechanism involved can be generally represented as

$$R_3C-CH=CH_2 + Hg(CH_3COO)_2 \xrightarrow{THF}$$

$$R_3C-\underset{\underset{COOCH_3}{|}}{CH}-CH_2-HgCOOCH_2 \xrightarrow[NaBH_4]{NaOH} R_3C-\underset{\underset{OH}{|}}{CH}-CH_2 + Hg$$

Applications

1. Mercuration reaction

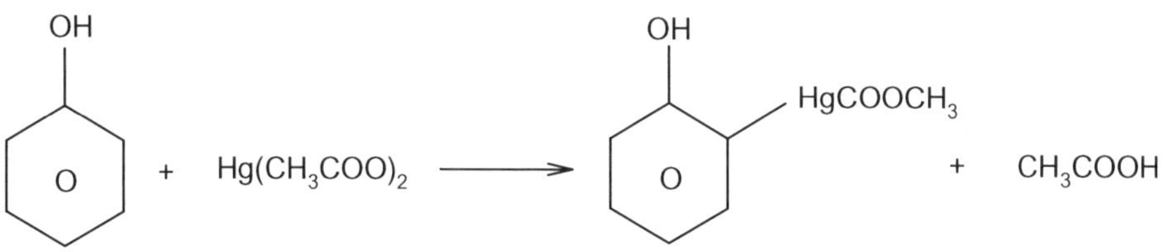

Phenol, acetoxy mercuric phenol

2. Mercuric acetate is used in vinyl ester interchange

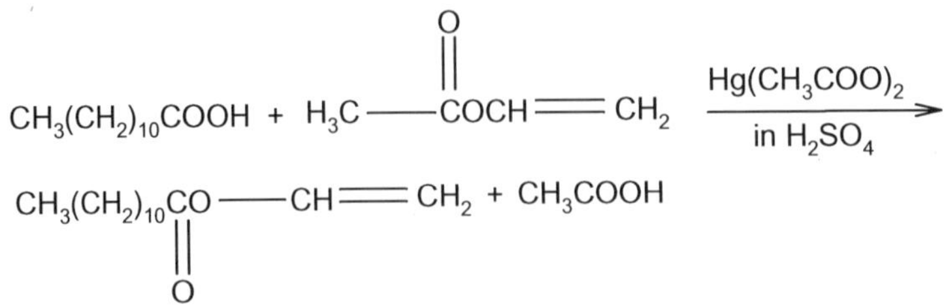

3. Mercuric acetate can be used to convert vinyl halides to ketones.

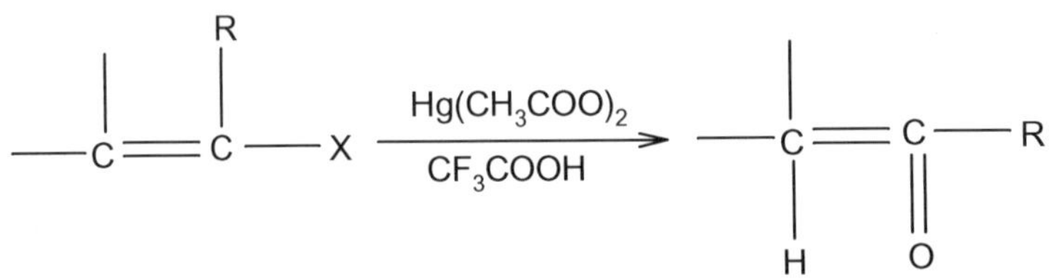

4. Dehydrogenation of aliphatic compound in presence of mercuric acetate yield carbon. carbon double bond

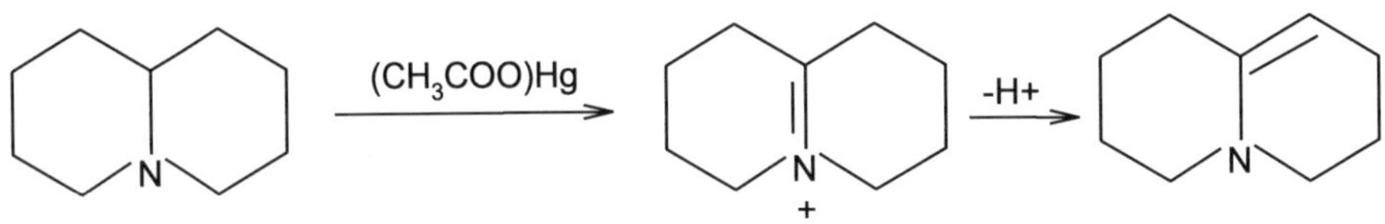

OXIDATION WITH LEAD TETRA ACETATE

Lead tetra acetate ($(CH_3COO)_4Pb$) is a powerful oxidising agent.

Preparation

Red lead oxide (Pb_2O_4) added in portions to a mixture of acetic acid and acetic anhydride with stirring. Temperature is maintained between 55°C-80°C. On cooling crystalline lead tetra-acetate separated out, which is washed and re-crystallised from acetic acid

$$8CH_3COOH + Pb_3O_4 \xrightarrow{(CH_3CO)_2O} (CH_3COO)_4Pb + 2(CH_3COO)_2Pb + 4H_2O$$

Mechanism can be generally written as

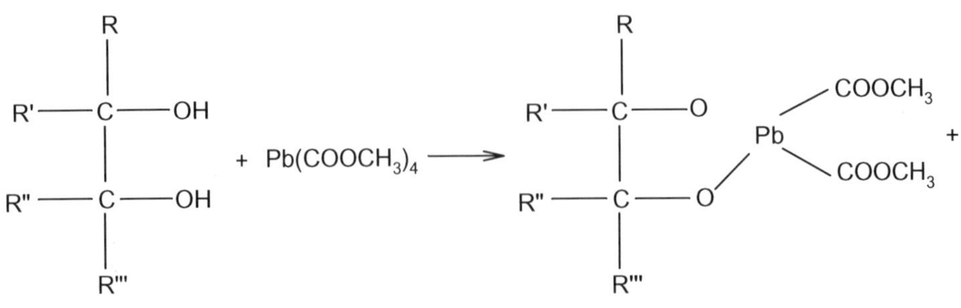

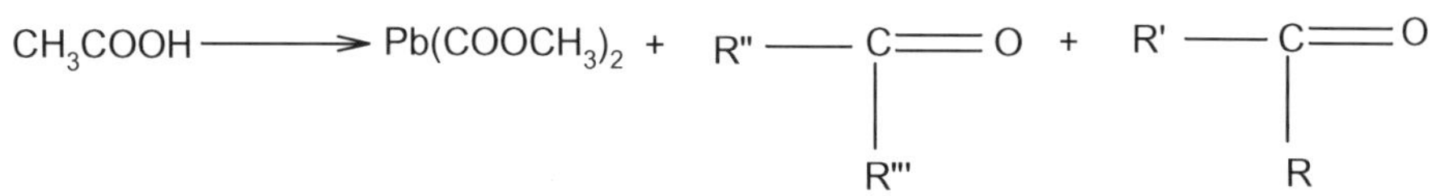

Applications

1. Dibutyl tartrate reacts with lead tetraacetate give butyl glyoxylate

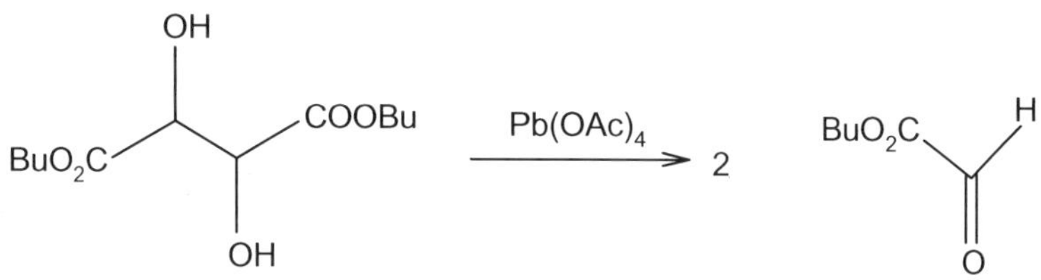

2. Lead tetraacetate effects bisdecarboxylation of succinic acids

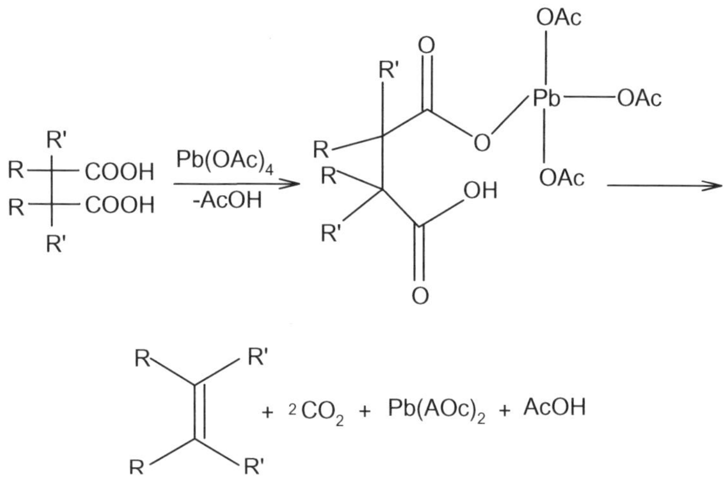

3. Hydroquinone can be oxidised to Quinone by lead tetra-acetate

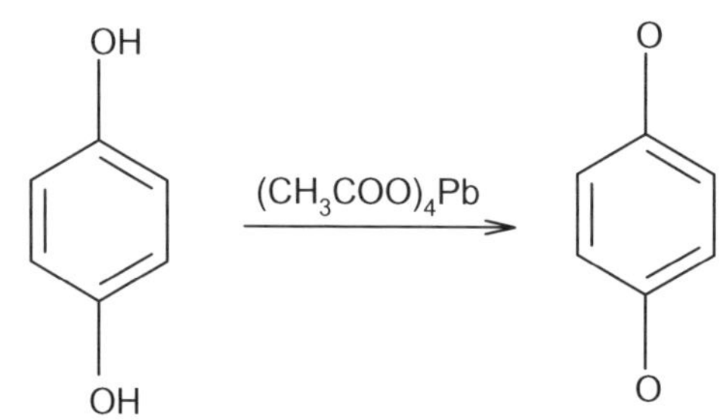

Hydroquinone Quinone

4. Lead tetra-acetate in oxidative rearrangement

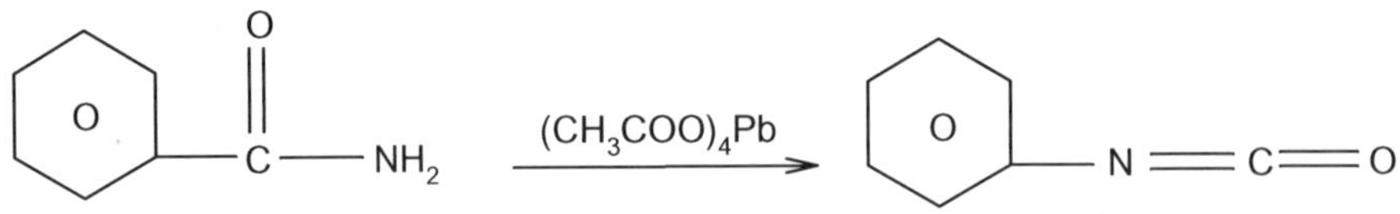

Benzoic amide   Benzoic isocyanate

5. Oxidation of Ethylene glycol by lead tetra-acetate

$$\begin{array}{c} CH_2OH \\ | \\ CH_2OH \end{array} \xrightarrow{(CH_3COO)_4Pb} HCHO + HCHO$$

6. Lead tetra-acetate oxidise 2, 6 Dihydroxy naphthalene

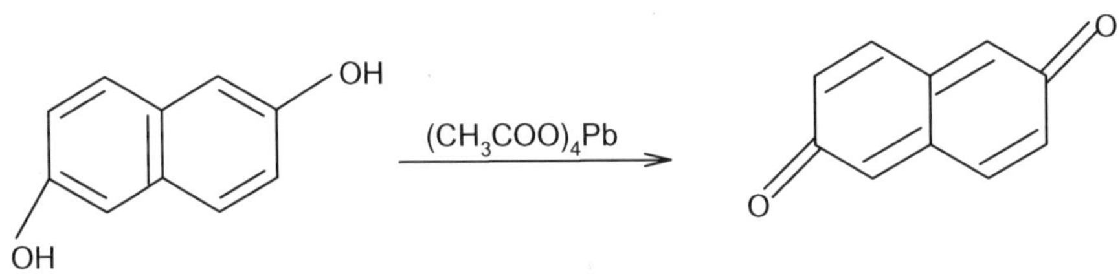

OXIDATION WITH PERCHLORIC ACID ($HClO_4$)

Perchloric acid is a strong acid which on ionisation give $H_3O^+ + ClO_4^-$. It is unstable and decomposes with explosion on heating and sometimes merely on standing for a few days even in dark. On dehydration with P_2O_5 at -10°C, it gives Cl_2O_7 which is the anhydride of $HClO_4$.

$$2HClO_4 + P_2O_5 \longrightarrow Cl_2O_7 + 2HPO_3$$

The metals like Zn , Fe dissolve in aqueous solution of the acid forms soluble percholrates

$$Zn — 2HClO_4 \longrightarrow Zn(Clo_4)_2 + H2 \downarrow$$

When a suspension of Iodine is heated with perchloric acid para-periodic acid is obtained.

$$2HClO_4 + I_2 + 4H_2O \longrightarrow 2H_5IO_6 + Cl_2$$

The aqueous solution of the perchloric acid is used for estimation of Potassium gravimetrically.

Mercuration of nitrobenzene with mercuric acetate in perchloric acid predominantly give meta product.

$$Hg(COOCH_3)_2 + HClo_4 \longrightarrow CH_3COOH + CH_3COOHg^+ \, Clo_4^-$$

Reduction with Some Important Reagents

Reduction is a process can be carried out by three ways,the removal of Oxygen, the addition of Hydrogen and the gain of electrons.

Addition of Hydrogen can be again subdivided into 'Hydrogenation' and 'Hydrogenolysis'. Hydrogenation means addition of Hydrogen to an unsaturated system.

Eg:

$$CH_2 = CH_2 + H_2 \xrightarrow{\text{Catalyst}} CH_3\text{-}CH_3$$

Hydrogenolysis means, addition of Hydrogen with concomitant bond rupture.

Eg:

$$ArCH_2\text{-}NMe_2 + H_2 \xrightarrow{\text{Catalyst}} Ar\text{-}CH_3 + HN(CH_3)_2$$

REDUCTION WITH HYDRAZINE

Hydrazine (H_2N - NH_2) is a powerful reducing agent

1. Applications

In wolf kishner reduction hydrazine is used as reducing agent. Here Aldehyde or ketone is converted to hydrazine, which is then treated with Sodium ethoxide to give hydro carbon.

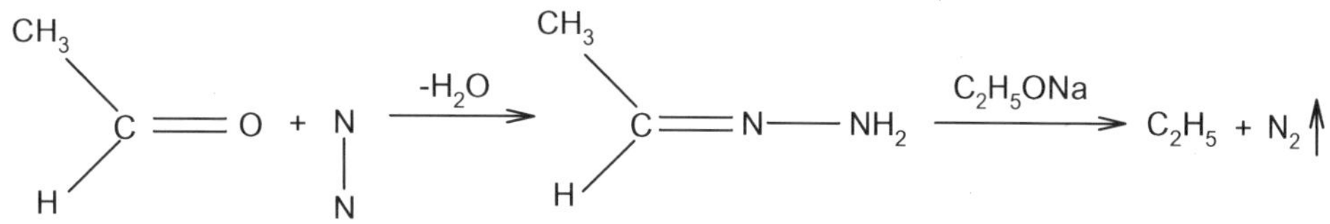

2. Ester or acyl chloride on reaction with hydrazine forms acid hydrazides.

Eg: 1. $RCOOC_2H_5 + N_2H_4 \longrightarrow RCONHNH_2 + C_2H_5OH$

2. $RCOCl + N_2H_4 \longrightarrow RCONHNH_2 + HCl$

3. In the presence of palladized charcoal , hydrazine reduces aromatic nitro compounds.

Eg: 1. 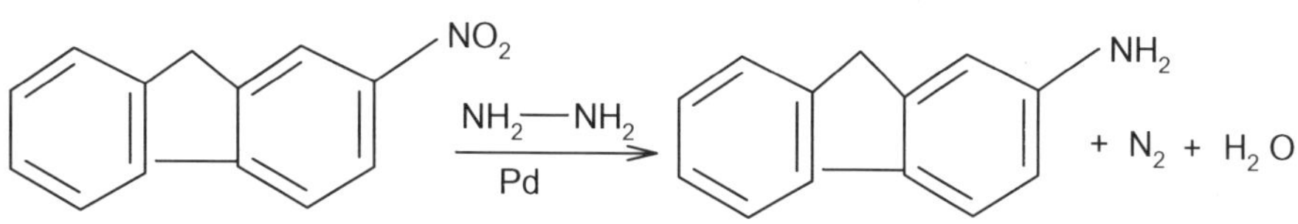

2. 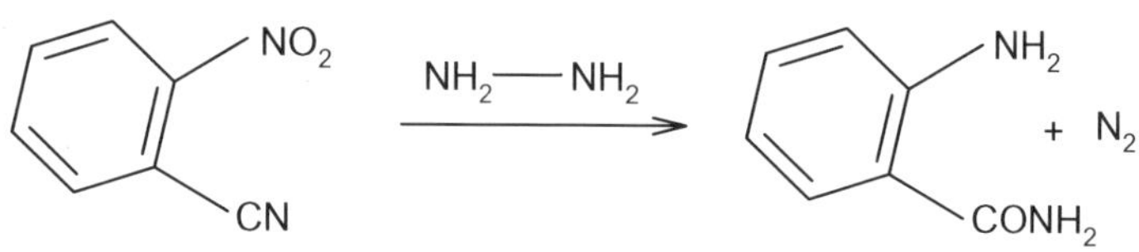

4. Epoxy ketones can be reduced to allyl alcohols.

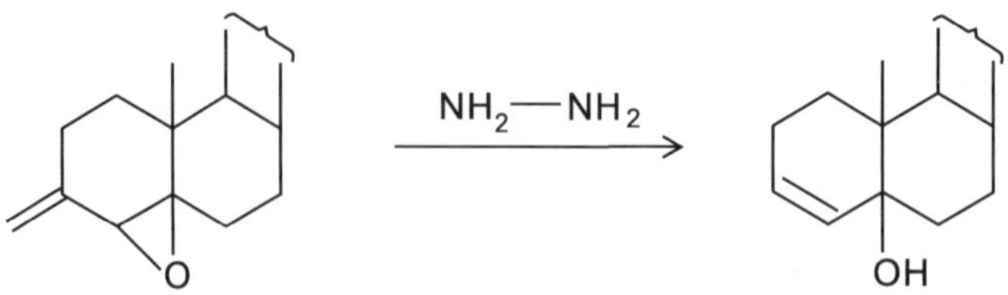

The important substituted hydrazine is phenyl hydrazine. It is prepared by reduction of benzenediazonium chloride with stannous chloride and hydrochloric acid.

$$C_6H_5\overset{+}{N_2}\overset{-}{Cl} \xrightarrow{SnCl_2/HCl} C_6H_5NHNH_2.HCl$$

The important reaction of phenyl hydrazine is with carbonyl compounds to form phenylhydrazones and with simple sugars to form osazones.

METAL HYDRIDE REDUCTION

Many complex metallic hydrides reduces various functional groups and the most versatile metal hydride is Lithium Aluminium Hydride.

Lithium Aluminium Hydride = $LiAlH_4$

Lithium Aluminium Hydride can reduce aldehydes, ketones, esters, acids, acid chlorides ...etc. to alcohols in a very good yield without affecting the ethylenic double bond. It does not affect the asymmetric centres.

Preparation

Finely devided anhydrous $AlCl_3$ is added to a slurry of Lithium hydride in dry ether. The solution is filtered to remove LiCl and excess LiH.

$$4\,LiH + AlCl_3 \longrightarrow LiAlH_4$$

Applications

1. Lithium Aluminium Hydride reduces aldehydes to primary alcohols

$$R\text{—}CHO \xrightarrow{LiAlH_4} R\bullet\ CH_2OH$$

2. Lithium Aluminium Hydride reduces ketones to secondary alcohols.

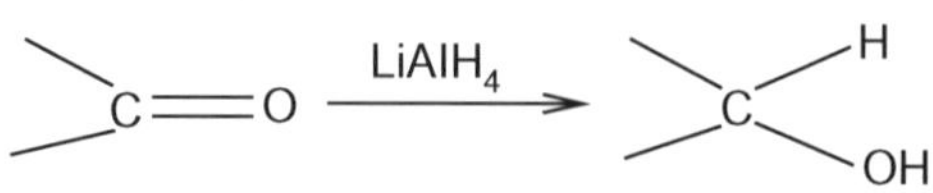

3. Lithium Aluminium Hydride reduces carboxylic acids and other esters to 1° alcohols.

$$R\text{—}COOH \xrightarrow{LAH} R\text{—}CH_2OH$$

$$R\text{—}COOR' \xrightarrow{LAH} R\bullet\ CH_2OH + R'\text{—}OH$$

Eg:

$$CH_3-CH=CH.COOH \xrightarrow{LAH} CH_3-CH=CH.CH_2OH$$

Crotonic acid → Crotyl alcohol

$$C_6H_5CH=CH-COOH \xrightarrow{LAH} C_6H_5-CH=CH-CH_2OH$$

Cinnamic acid → Cinnamyl alcohol

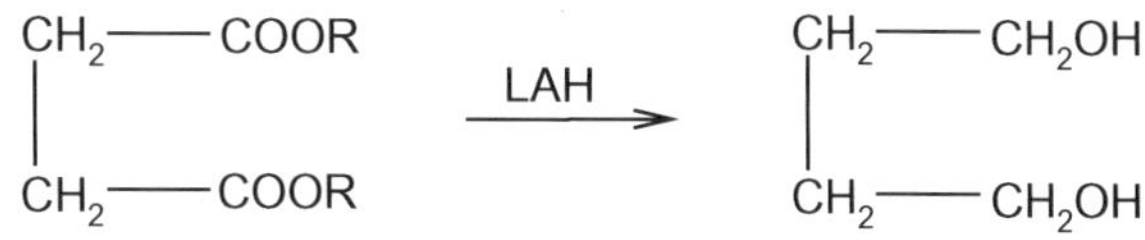

Succinic acid ester → Butane diol

In aromatic compounds, if amino group is present ortho or para to acid or ester, then -COOH & -COOR reduced to $-CH_3$ instead of $-CH_2OH$.

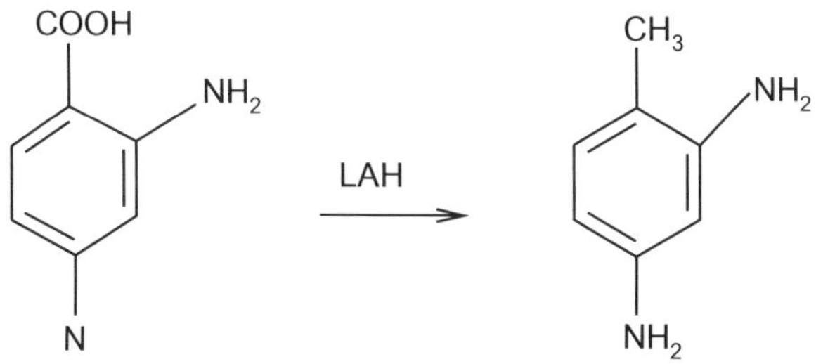

1,4 diaminobenzoic acid → 2,4 diamino toluene

4. LAH reduces amide group into amine.

$$R-CONH_2 \xrightarrow{LAH} R-CH_2-CH_2-CH_2-NH_2$$

5. LAH reduces nitrite group into amine.

$$R-C\equiv N \xrightarrow{LAH} R-CH_2NH_2$$

$$CH_3-CH_2-CH_2-CN \xrightarrow{LAH}$$

Butyronitrile

$$CH_3-CH_2-CH_2-CH_2-NH_2$$

n-Butylamine

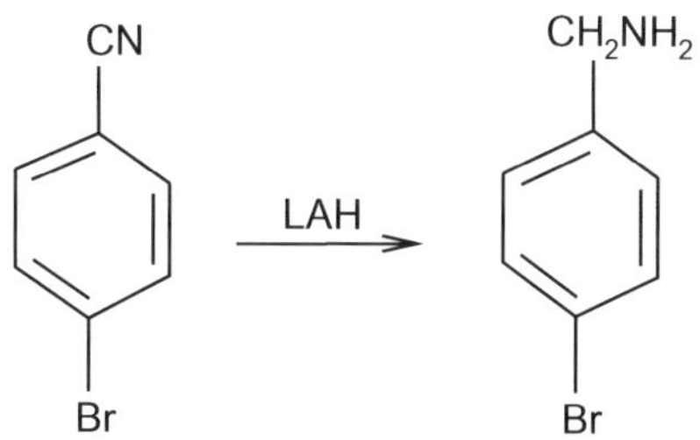

6. LAH reduces acid chlorides into alcohol.

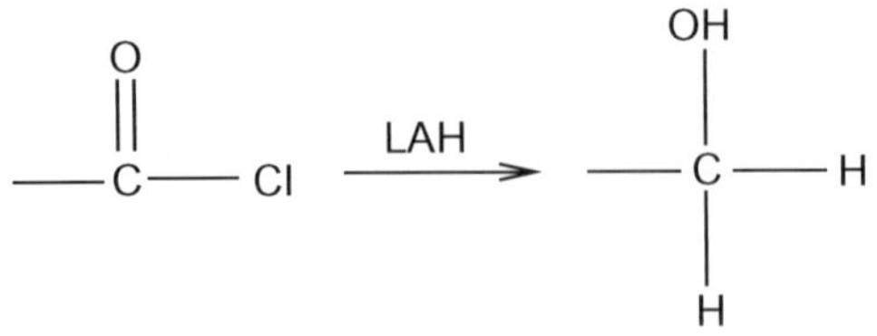

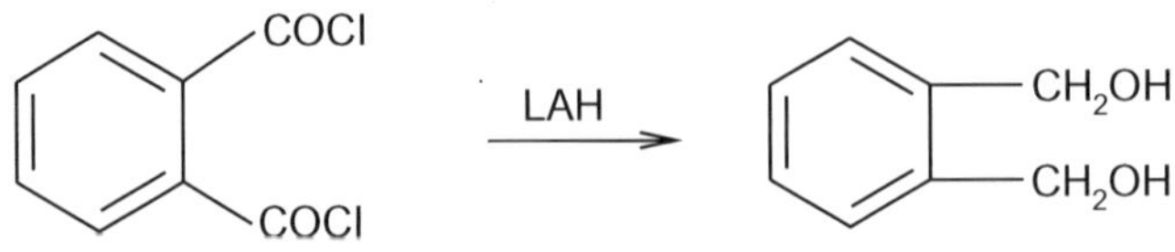

Phthaloyl chloride — Phthaloyl alcohol

7. From aliphatic primary and secondary halides, halogen can be replaced by hydrogen.

$$CH_3Cl \xrightarrow{LAH} CH_3 - H + LiCl + AlH_3$$

8. LAH reduces aliphatic nitro compounds into amines, whereas aromatic nitro compounds give azo derivatives.

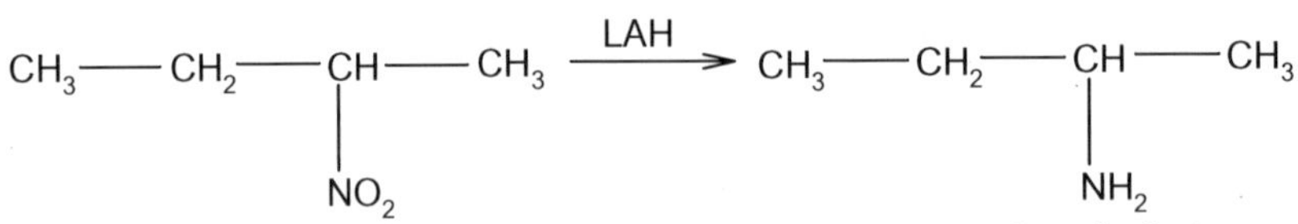

2-nitrobutane — 2-aminobutane

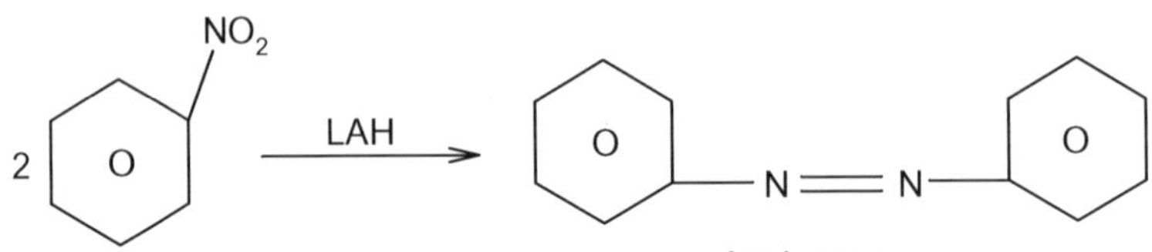

Nitrobenzene — Azobenzene

9. β-α unsaturated aliphatic aldehydes, ketones and cyclic ketones can be reduced without affecting the double bond.

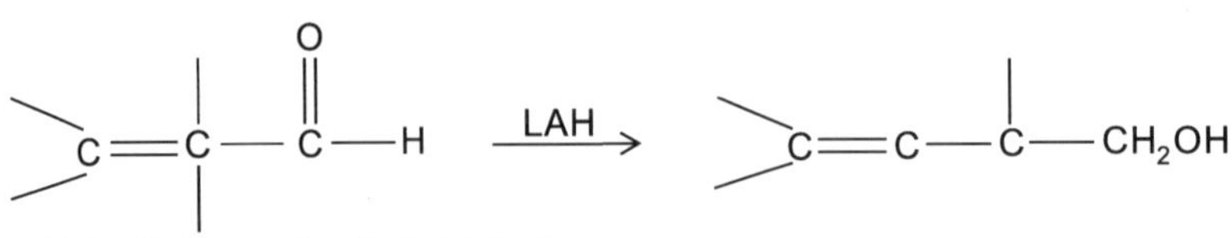

Alpha Beta unsaturated aldehyde

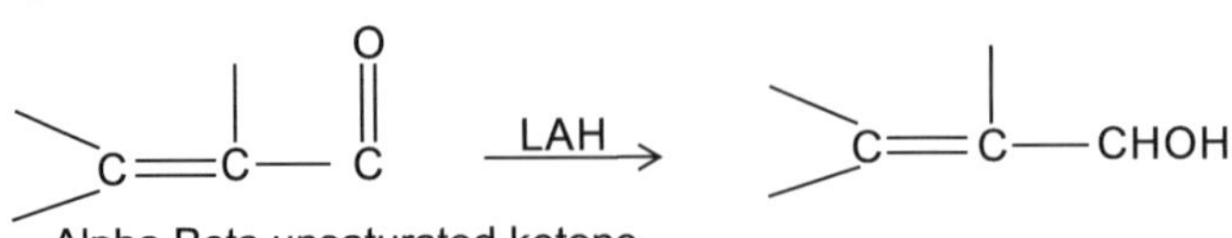

Alpha Beta unsaturated ketone

10. Carbonyl group present in compounds containing two or more double bonds in conjugation, can also be reduced without affecting the double bonds.

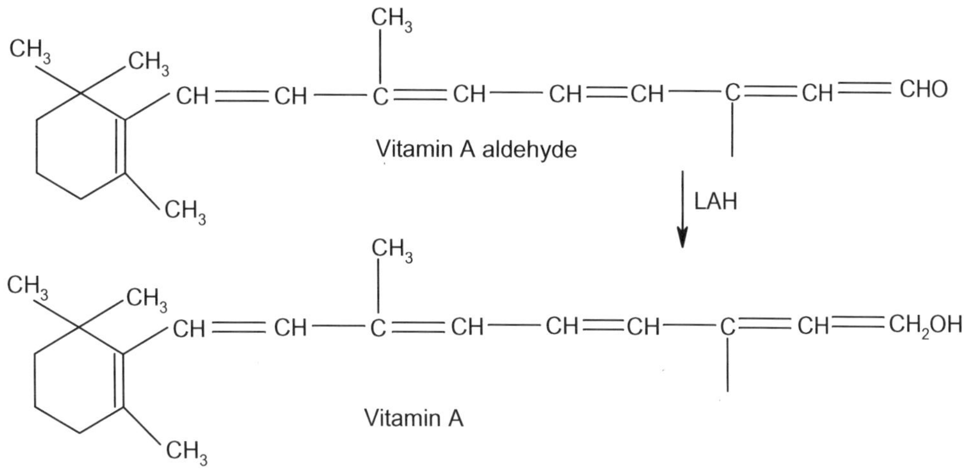

REDUCTION BY SODIUM BOROHYDRIDE ($NaBH_4$)

SBH reduces carbonyl compounds, as that of LAH, but is selective, SBH reduces only aldehydes, ketones and acid chlorides. SBH reduces unsaturated aldehydes and ketones without affecting the double bond. SBH reduction can be carried out even in water.

$$\underset{\text{Crotonaldehyde}}{CH_3-CH=CH-CHO} \xrightarrow{NaBH_4} \underset{\text{Crotyl alcohol}}{CH_3-CH=CH-CH_2OH}$$

$$\underset{\text{Ethyl aceto acetate}}{CH_3-CO-CH_2-COOC_2H_5} \xrightarrow{NaBH_4} \underset{\text{Ethyl-}\beta\text{-hydroxy butyrate}}{CH_3-\overset{\overset{\displaystyle O}{|}}{CH}-CH_2-COOC_2H_5}$$

$$\underset{\text{6-cyanohexanal}}{NC-CH_2-(CH_2)_3-CH_2CHO} \xrightarrow{NaBH_4} \underset{\text{6-cyanohexanol}}{NC-CH_2-(CH_2)_3-CH_2-CH_2OH}$$

$$\underset{\text{Benzaldehyde}}{C_6H_5CHO} \xrightarrow{NaBH_4} \underset{\text{Benzyl alcohol}}{C_6H_5-CH_2OH}$$

FRIES REARRANGEMENT

It is a mixed type of aromatic rearrangement. The reaction of aryl esters with Lewis acids to give ortho and para-hydroxy ketones is known as Fries rearreangement.

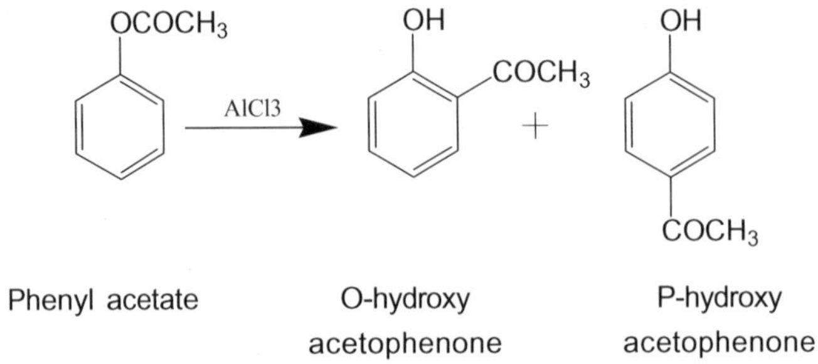

Mechanism is believed to be a combination of intermolecular and intramolecular mechanism. Intermolecular mechanism explains formation of complex between the ester and lewis acid eliminates an acylium ion which substitutes at ortho and para positions.

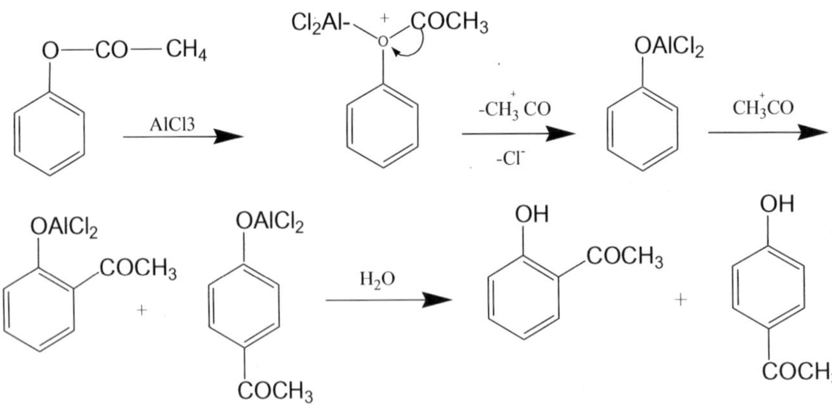

As a result of the rearangement, generally forms a mixture of P- and O- isomers. The relative amount of each isomer depends upon many factors like temperature, solvent, amount of the catalyst and structure of the ester. Low temperature favours the formation of P- isomer, while high temperature favours the formation of O- isomer.

Eg:

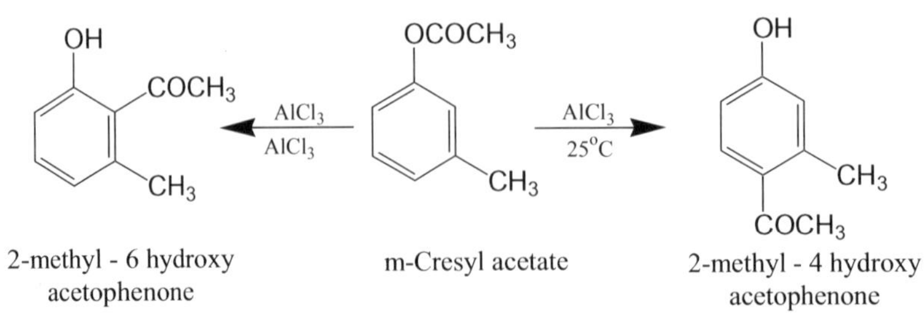

Fries rearrangement generally does not require any solvent, but sometimes use of some solvent reduces the temperature at which reaction proceeds at a useful rate. E.g.:

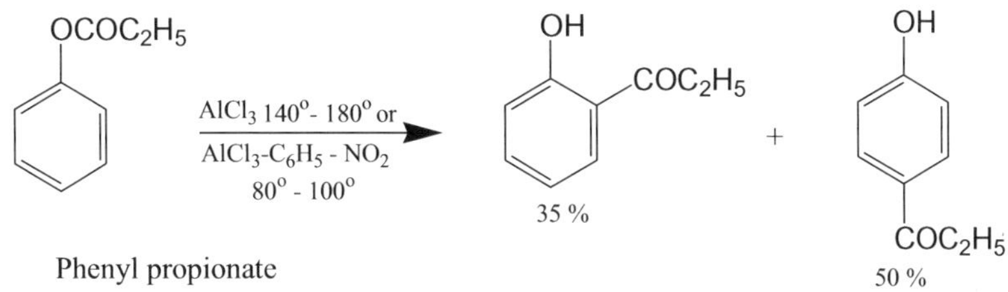

Generally the esters and Lewis acids are used in equimolar amounts. But in some cases two moles of $AlCl_3$ are used per mole of the acetate. E.g.: in the rearrangement of Guaicol acetate.

Nature and position of substituent in aromatic nucleus of ester is also a key-factor. E.g.: Presence of m-directing group generally retards the reaction.

Applications of Fries Rearrangement

Fries rearrangement provides an important route for preparation of hydroxy ketones. Amount of required isomers can be varied by making changes in reaction conditions as explained in the factors influenzing reaction.

Fries rearrangement can be applied to the esters of enols to give 1,3-diketones. E.g.: isomerization of isopropenyl acetate to acetyl acetone by heating at about 500°C.

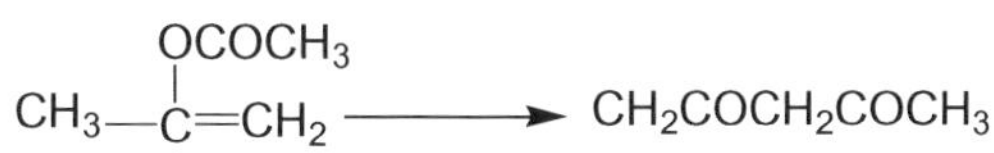

An important application in Fries arrangement is the synthesis of adrenaline.

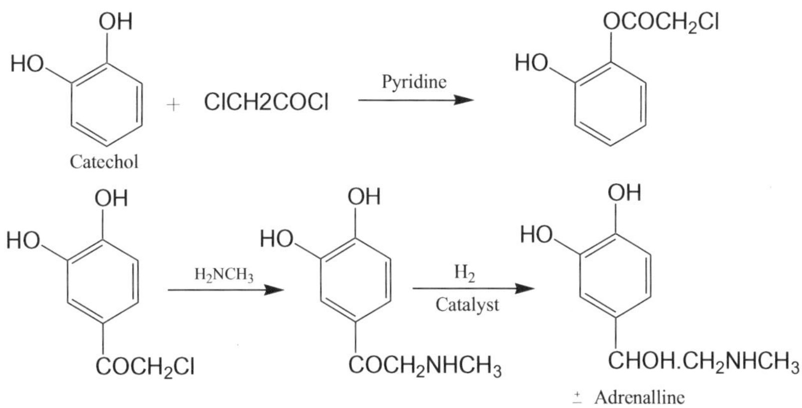

MANNICH REACTION

This is the condensation between a compound containing at least one active hydrogen atom, formaldehyde and ammonia, a primary or a secondary amine. During the reaction one active hydrogen atom is replaced by an aminomethyl group or substituted amino methyl group. So the base formed is known as Mannich base usually isolated as hydrochloride. Important reactants mainly are,

a. Compounds containing active hydrogen atom.

b. Amines

c. Aldehydes are explaining briefly.

a. Compounds containing active hydrogen atom.

(i) Ketones:

Ketones are compounds containing ‾CO. CH< group. E.g.: acetophenone, acetone...... etc. Unsymmetrical ketones predominantly at more highly substituted α position.

(ii) Acids and its esters

Specially aceto acetic, malonic, β-Cyano and β-Keto-acids with ethyl malonic acid.

$$C_2H_5.\,CH(COOH)_2 + HCHO + (CH_3)_2NH \longrightarrow C_2H_5C(COOH)_2.CH_2N(CH_3)_2$$

(iii) Phenols

In the case of Phenols , basic group enters O and /or P to the Phenolic group.

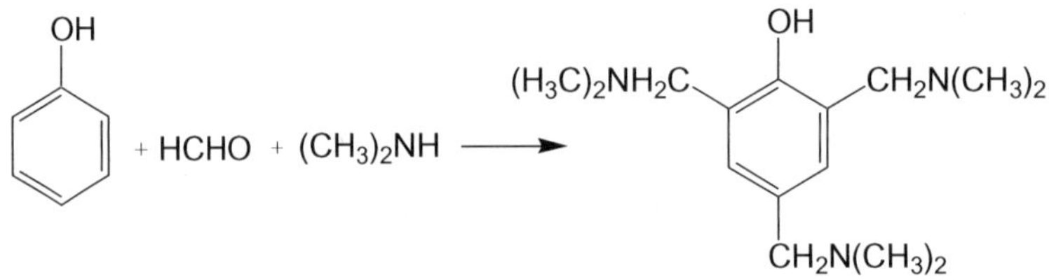

(iv) Heterocyclic compounds and their derivatives

Compounds like Pyrrole, Furan and Indole are sensitive to acids and hence the reaction must be carried out in presence of weak acids like acetic acid, Formic acid.

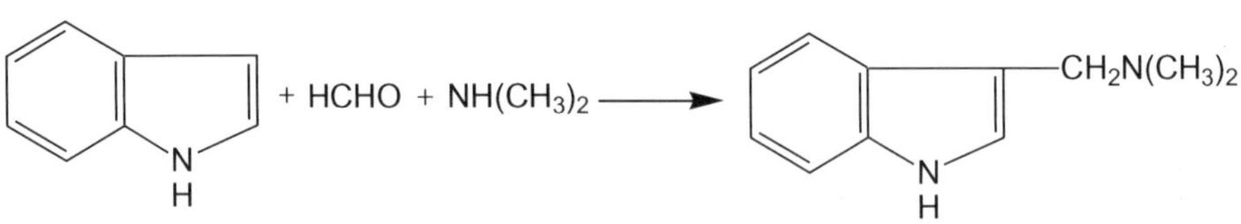

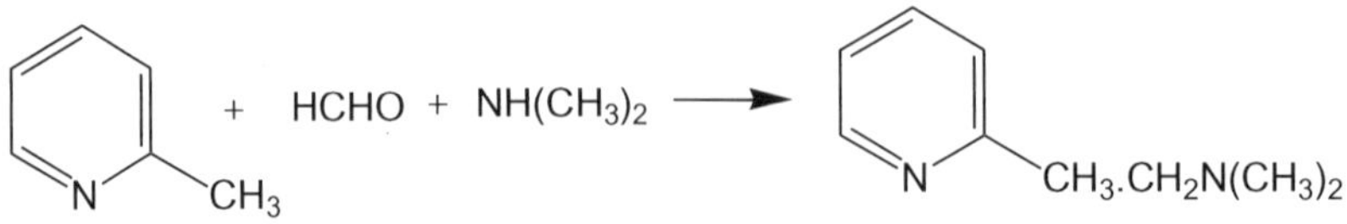

(v) Nitro compounds

Primary as well as secondary nitro compounds undergo mannich reaction.

$$R_2CH.NO_2 + HCHO + NH_4Cl \longrightarrow R_2C(NO_2)—CH_2—NH_2.HCl + H_2O$$

(vi) Acetylenes

Phenylacetylenes and some of its nuclear substituted derivatives undergo mannich reaction.

$$C_6H_5C\equiv CH + HCHO + (CH_3)_2NH \xrightarrow[-H_2O]{H^+} C_6H_5.C\equiv C.CH_2N(CH_3)_2$$

Amines

Amine can be primary or secondary. Most convenient will be secondary amines since they posses only one replacable hydrogen atom. (R_2NH)

$$CH_3.CO.CH_2CH_2NH.CH_3 + HCHO + CH_3\text{-}CO\text{-}CH_3 \longrightarrow CH_3.CO.CH_2.\underset{}{\overset{CH_4\atop |}{C}}H_2N.CH_2.CH_2.CO.CH_3$$

Aldehydes

Commonly formaldehyde is used is mannich reaction.

Mechanism of Mannich reaction

The probable mechanism can be as that the lone pair of electrons of hydrogen attacks on the carbonyl group of formaldehyde to form an ion which is protonated and finally eliminates a molecule of water to produce an ion, which is attacked by carbanion derived from ketone to yield the mannich base.

$$(C_2H_5)_2\ddot{N}H + CH_2{=}O \longrightarrow (C_2H_5)_2\overset{+}{N}H{-}CH_2\overset{-}{O} \xrightarrow{H^+}$$

$$(C_2H_5)_2\overset{+}{N}H{-}CH_3OH \xrightarrow{-H_2O} \left[(C_2H_5)_2\overset{+}{N}{=}CH_2 \rightleftharpoons (C_2H_5)_2N{-}\overset{+}{C}H_3\right]$$

First ion

Formation of second carbon ion

$$C_6H_5{-}CO{-}CH_3 \xrightarrow{H^+} C_6H_5{-}CO{-}\overset{-}{C}H_2$$

Formation of first carbon ion

$$(C_2H_5)_2N{=}CH_2 + C_6H_5{-}CO{-}\overset{-}{C}H_2 \longrightarrow$$

$$C_6H_5{-}CO{-}\overset{-}{C}H_2{-}CH_2{-}N(C_2H_5)_2 \longrightarrow$$

Mannich base

Applications of Mannich reaction

1. Synthesis of alkaloids

   Eg: Tropinone (For synthesis atropine), Cocaine, Pseudopelletierine.

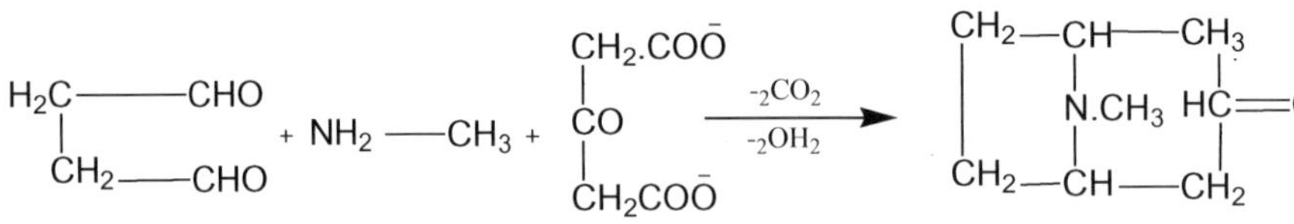

Succinaldehyde Acetone dicarboxylate Tropinone

Synthesis of Pseudopelletierine

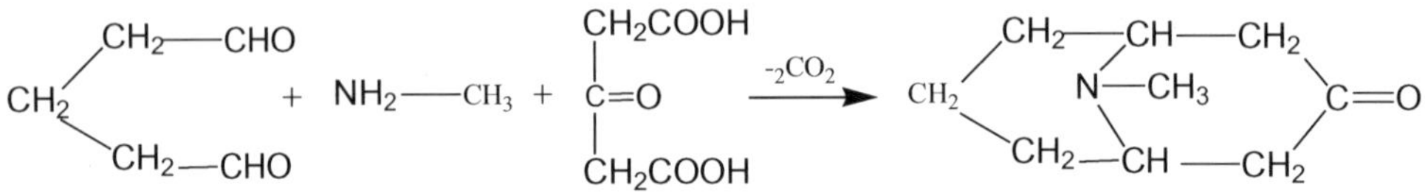

Pseudopelletierine

2. Synthesis of Local anaesthetics

   Mannich reaction can be applied to synthesise certain local anaesthetics. Eg: Tutocaine.

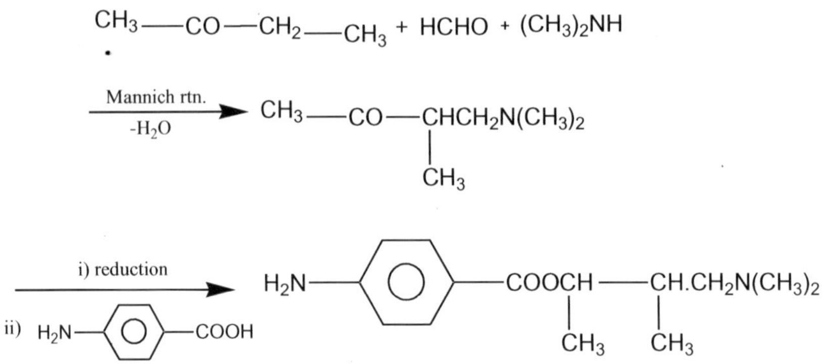

Tutocaine

3. Woodward's Synthesis of Cholesterol utilized mannich reaction.
4. Mannich reaction also involved in synthesis of epiandrosterone.
5. α, β-unsaturated compound can be prepared by mannich reaction.

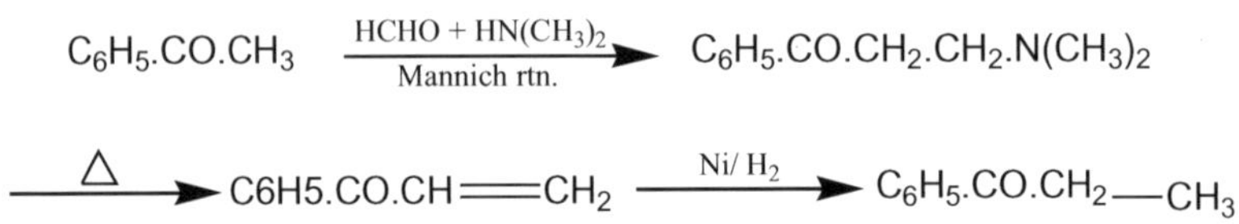

By this catalytic reduction of unsaturated produt gives the next higher homologue of the ketone from which mannich base was derived.

6. Mannich reaction used in synthesis of indole-β-acetic acid.

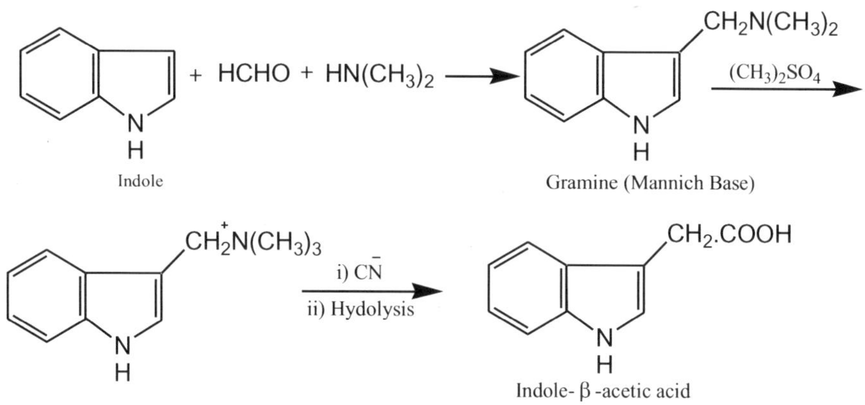

7. Mannich reaction in synthesis of Quinine

Mannich base is prepared from 7-hydroxy isoquinoline formaldehyde and piperidine.

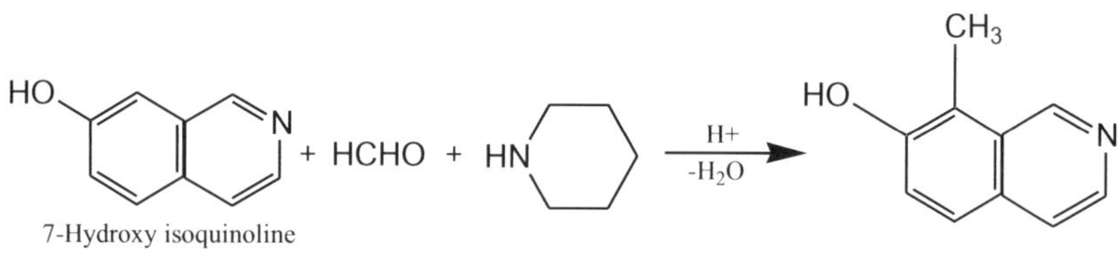

MICHAEL REACTION

It is an addition reaction between an α, β-unsaturated compound (acts as acceptor) and a compound with an active methylene group (acts as addendum) in the presence of a base.

$$C_6H_5.CH{=}CH.COOC_2H_5 + \underset{\text{Addendum}}{CH_2(COOC_2H_5)_2} \xrightarrow{C_2H_5ONa} C_6H_5\underset{\displaystyle CH(COOC_2H_5)_2}{\underset{|}{CH}}{-}CH_2.COOC_2H_5$$

Acceptors in Michael addition

All α, β-unsaturated compounds having a carbonyl or nitrile group in conjugation with double bond constitute acceptors.

a) Ketones

$C_2H_5CH{=}CH.COOC_2H_5$	Ethyl Cinnamate
$C_2H_5CH{=}CH.CO.CH_3$	Benzylidene acetine
$(CH_3)C{=}CH.CO.CH_3$	Mesityl oxide

Addendum in Michael addition

All compounds containing an active methylene group ie. which can ionise to a proton and a carbon ion.

Eg: Malonic ester, acetoacetic ester, Cyanoacetic esters, Phenyl acetic esters, aliphatic nitro compounds, Benzyl cyanide, cyanacetanide, Cyclopentadine, indene, Fluorene, sulphones.

Catalysts used in Michael addition

Basic catalysts are mainly used.
Eg: Sodium ethoxide, Potassium tertiary-butoxide.

Mechanism of Michael addition

The basic catalyst facilitates anion formation of addendum. Then carbon ion adds on β-carbon atom of acceptor. The product formed thus takes up a portion from alcohol present to give enol compound which finally tautomerises to keto form.

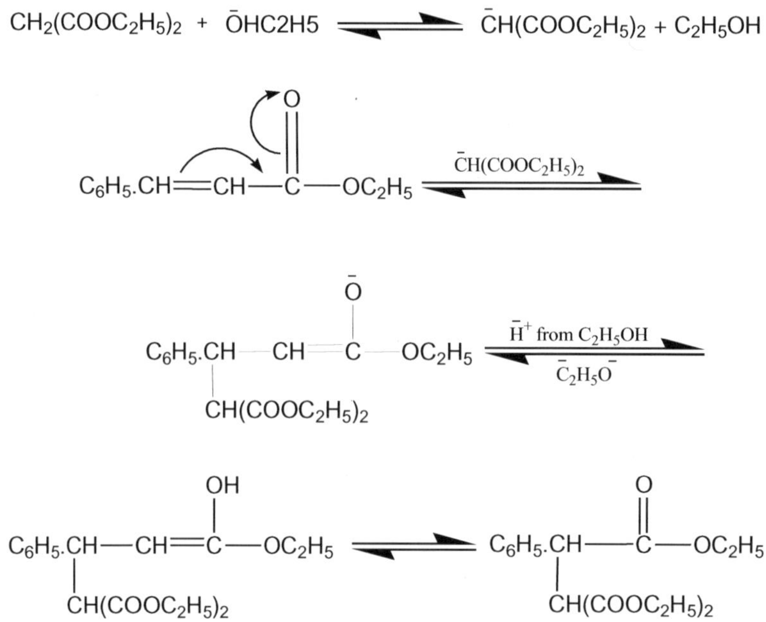

Applications of Michael addition

1. Synthesis of dicarboxylic acids

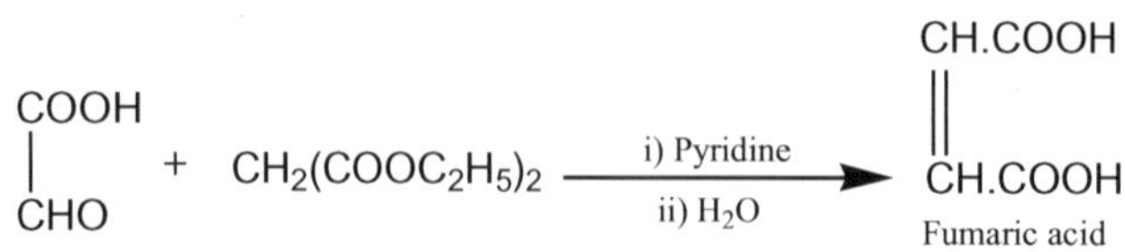

2. Synthesis of tricarboxylic acids
   Eg: Propane-1,2,3-tricarboxylic acid (Tricarballylic acid). Its esters are used as plasticizers.

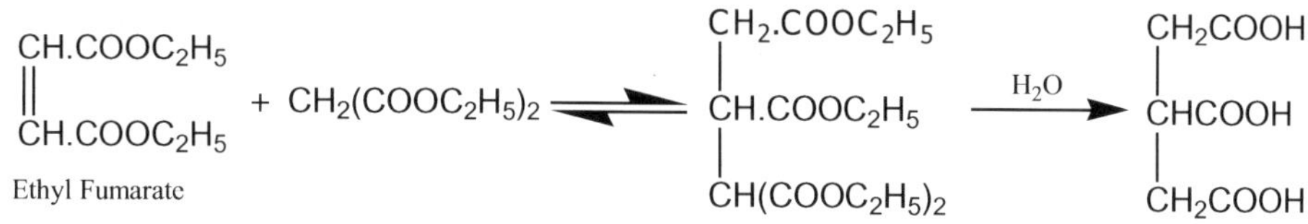

Eg: 2 synthesis of propene-1,2,3-tricarboxylic acid. (aconitic acid). Its derivatives are medicinally used as febrifuge. It's esters are used as plasticizers and in the manufature of wetting agents.

3. Synthesis of Dimedone

Dimedone can be synthesized from mesityl oxide and malonic ester in the presence of C_2H_2ONa. Dimedone is an important reagent for characterizing aldehydes.

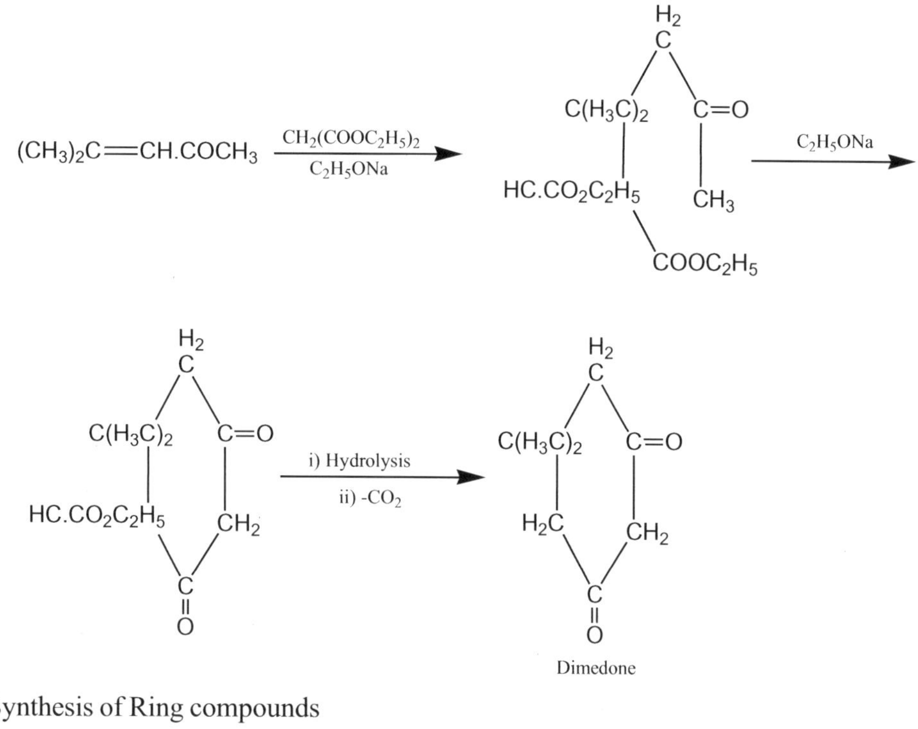

Dimedone

4. Synthesis of Ring compounds

Double Michael additions are employed for synthesising ring compounds.

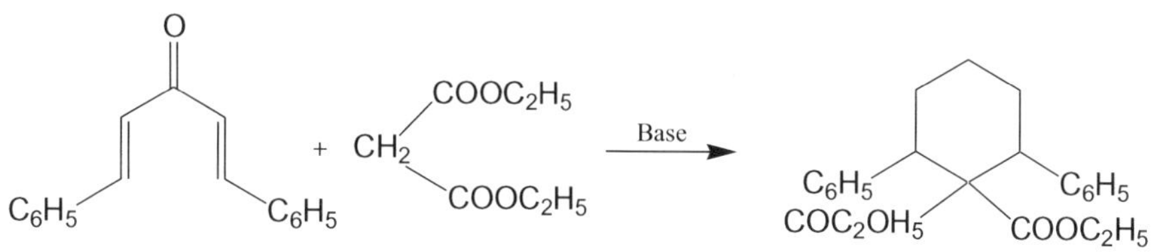

5. Michael addition frequently employed to prepare alicyclic system of steroids. Eg: In the synthesis of Cholesterol.
6. Michael addition is also applied in the synthesis of Morphine.
7. Synthesis of Cincholoiponic acid.

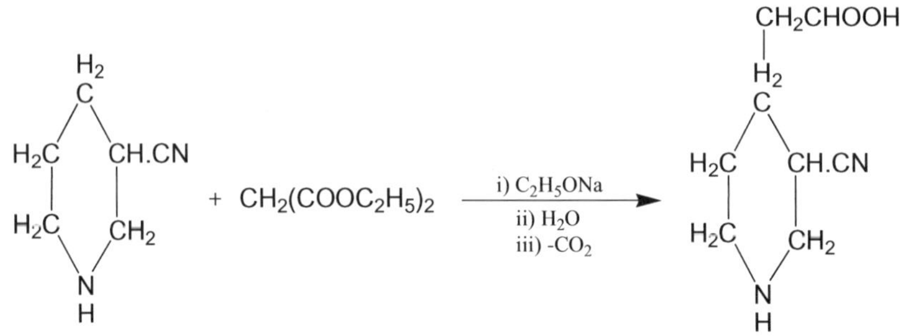

5

Stereo Chemistry

INTRODUCTION

Stereo Chemistry is a branch of chemistry, which deals with three dimensional structure of molecule. Isomers are compounds having different structures but same molecular formula. Isomers having identical structures, but different spatial arrangement of atoms or groups of atoms within the molecule are termed as stereo-isomers and this phenomenon is termed as stereo isomerism. Stereoisomerism is further classified into optical isomerism and Geometrical isomerism.

TETRAHEDRAL CARBON ATOM

In the tetrahedral arrangement of carbon atoms, the carbon is situated at the centre of tetrahedron and four valencies of carbon atom are directed towards the four apex. When four groups are identical, the bond angle becomes 109°-28". The tetrahedral arrangement for a molecule like Cabde is shown below;

Four valencies of carbon are distributed in three dimensions and if we join the ends of these four valencies by straight lines, we get what we call as regular tetrahedron. Tetrahedral nature of the carbon is evidenced by theoretical considerations and various physical measurements such has bond length, bond angles, dipole moments, X-ray, spectroscopy, electron diffraction ....etc. Tetrahedral nature of carbon, can be strongly support by the reduction of dextro & laevo rotatory lactic acid to optically inactive propionic acid, which is possible only with tetrahedral arrangement.

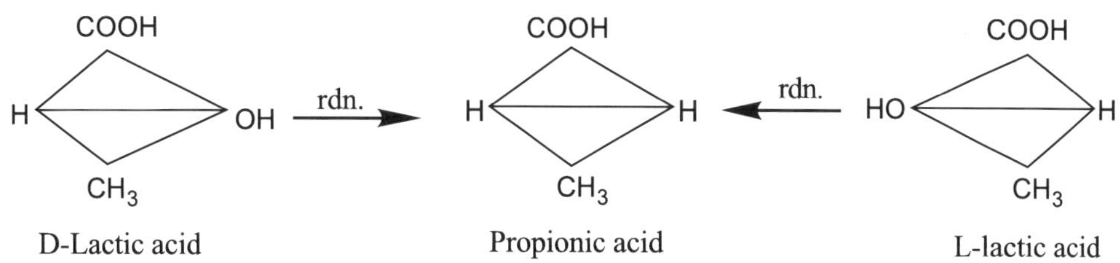

The validity of the tetrahedral carbon atom is shown as the compound like Cabde can exists in two possible forms which are related to each other as an object and its mirror image, a situation where in they are not superimposable. Such a Carbon atom to which four different groups are attached becomes a chiral centre and carbon, a chiral carbon.

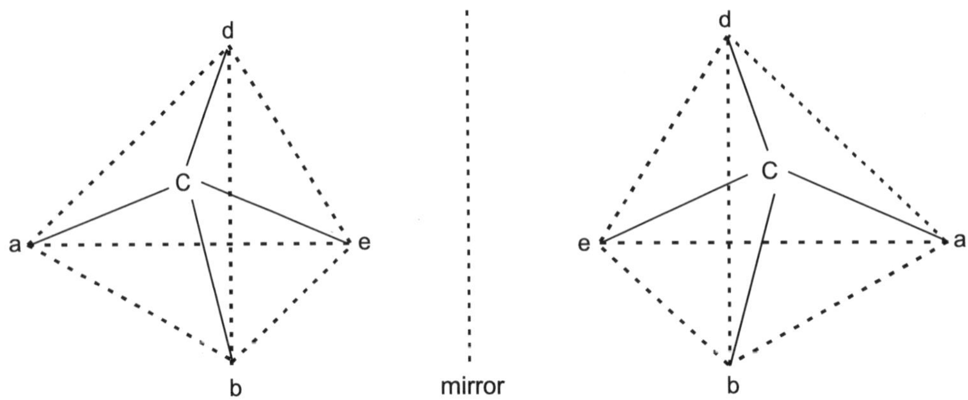

Practically it is found to be true as they have different configurations. Theory also predicts that two isomers of the compound cabde can be converted to one and the same compou nd Ca_2bd with the loss of optical activity, as we have seen in the reduction of lactic acid.

ELEMENTS OF SYMMETRY (CONDITIONS OF MOLECULAR ASYMMETRY)

When a molecule and its mirror image become super-imposable, they will have elements of symmetry, such as;

1,a plane of symmetry
2,a centre of symmetry
3,an alternating axis of symmetry

Plane of Symmetry

A molecule is said to have a plane of symmetry if it divides the molecule in such a way that atoms or groups on one side of the plane become mirror images of those on the otherside. eg: Meso tartaric acid. CH(OH)COOH. CH (OH) COOH.

Centre (Point) of Symmetry

A centre of symmetry is an imaginary point in the centre of a molecule from which if lines are drawn to any group, on both sides to an equal distance, it divides the molecule into two equal halves which are the mirror images of each other. Centre of symmetry is possibly present in even-membered ring systems eg; (1,) trans form of dimethyl ketopiperzine eg; (2,) 2,4, dimethyl cyclobutane-1, (3)-dicarbboxylic acid.

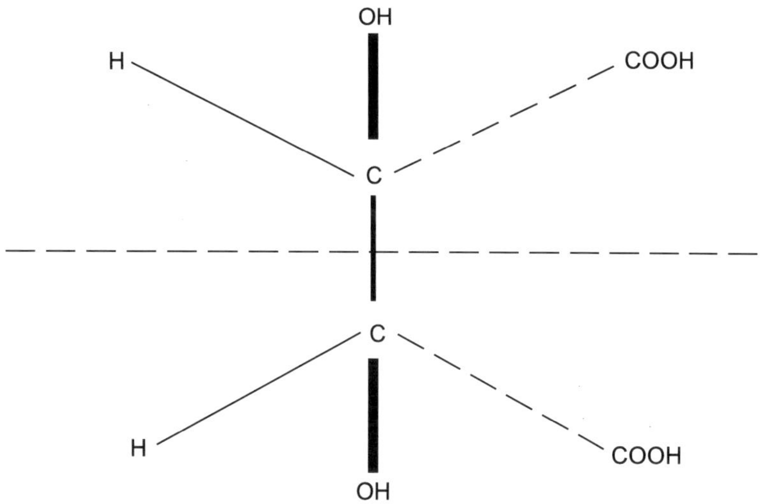

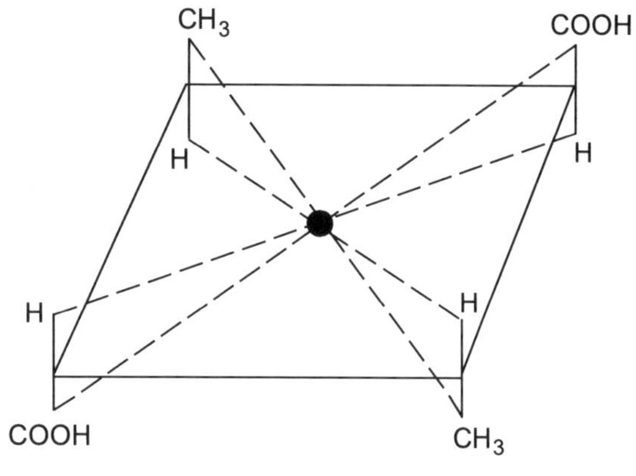

An alternating axis of Symmetry

A molecule said to posses n fold alternating axis of symmetry, if when rotated through an angle of 360°/n about the axis and then reflected in a plane perpendicular to the axis, gives back the original molecule. eg: an imaginary molecule 1,2,3,4 tetramethyl cyclobutane. It shows a fourfold alternating axis of symmetry. On rotating this molecule (a) through 360°/4 about the axis AB (passing through the centre of the ring perpendicular to its plane, gives (b) and reflection of (b) in a plane perpendicular to the axis gives back (a).

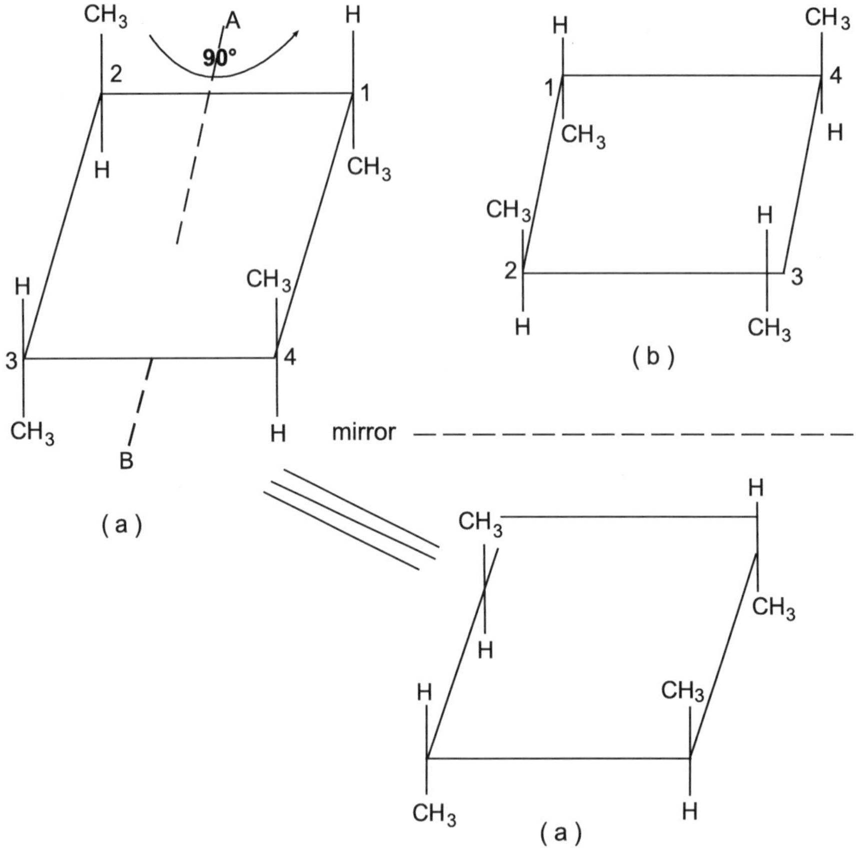

OPTICAL ACTIVITY

A beam of ordinary light may be regarded as a bundle of electromagnetic waves vibrating in all directions perpendicular to the axis of beam. When such beam is passed through a specially cut crystal of minerals or a sheet of special plastic known as polaroid, all vibrations except those in one plane are eliminated. This is known as plane polarized light. When such a beam of plane polarized light is paased through a solution of an optical isomer, if the plane polarized found to rotate to the left, is described as levorotation; if it is to the right is known as dextro-rotation.

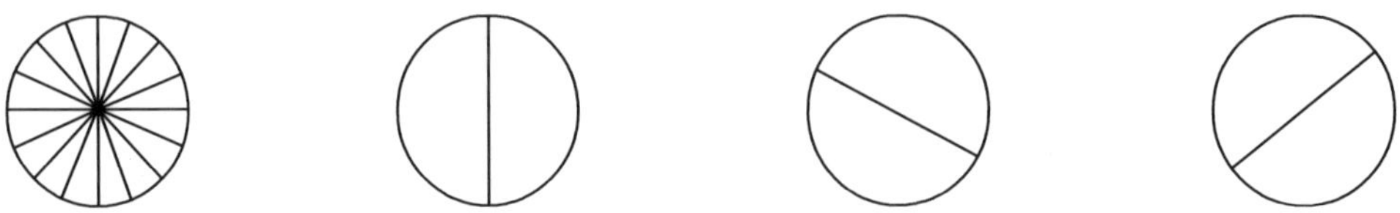

Ordinary light Oscillations in all - planes of beam.	Plane polarized light Oscillations in one - plane of beam.	Plane polarized light rotated anticlockwise - or levo.	Plane polarized light rotated clockwise - or dextro.

The phenomenon of rotating the plane polarized light towards left or right is known as optical activity and the compounds exhibiting this property are known as optically active compounds. Cause of optical activity is chirality in the molecule. A carbon atom having four different monovalent atoms or groups is known as chiral carbon or a chiral centre or assymmetric.

Optical Isomerism in Lactic Acid

A molecule which has anyone of the symmetry is superimposable with its mirror image and hence becomes optically inactive. In contrast, if a molecule has no elements of symmetry is not superimpossable with its mirror image and hence becomes optically active. eg: optical isomers of lactic acid.

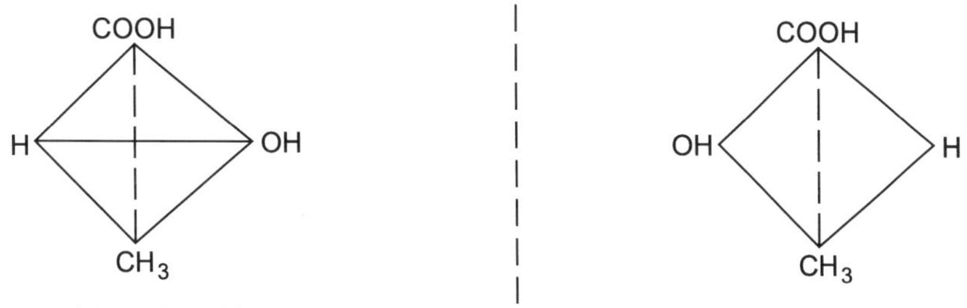

D(+)Lactic acid   Mirror   L(–)Lactic acid.

Lactic acid formed in the muscle is dextro-rotatory. Lactic acid formed by fermentation, of lactose, is a mixture containing equal amounts of dextro and laevo lactic acid. By inoculating suitable micro-organism +or-lactic acid can be isolated. The two isomers of lactic acid ie. object and its mirror image are called enantiomers or optical antipodes or antimers. They have the same chemical structure but different configurations. They have the same physical and chemical properties except in their sign of optical rotation. Both rotates plane of polarised light to same extent but in opposite directions.

Optical Isomerism of Tartaric Acid

Tartaric acid contains two chiral centres and hence it is expected to have $2^2 = 4$ - tartaric acid exists in four different forms like

1 (+) tartaric acid,
2 (–) tartaric acid,
3 Racemic tartaric acid.
4 Meso tartaric acid.

(+) and (–) are optically active whereas racemic and meso are optically inactive.

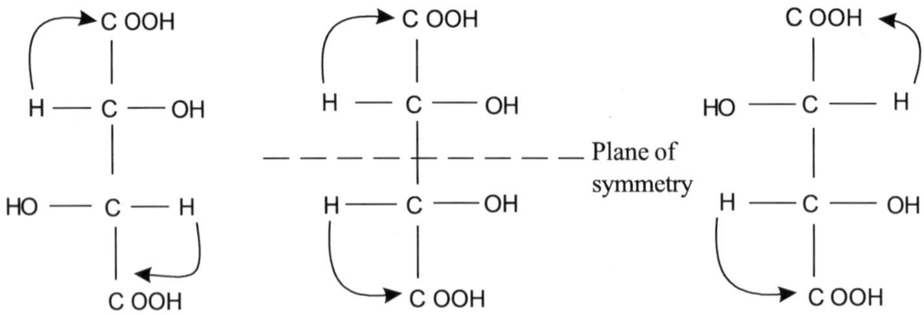

(+) Mesotartaric acid (–)

A(+) tartaric acid naturally occur in grape juice. Racemate of tartaric acid is optically inactive due to external copensation while meso form have a plane of symmetry which makes the molecule inactive. In meso form both upper and lower asymmetric carbon atoms have same value of rotation but opposite signs & this is why total rotation becomes zero. Meso tartaric acid is a diastereoisomer of enantiomers and shows difference in physical properties such as melting point, density, water solubility & dipole moment. The melting point of enantiomer of tartaric acid is 170°C, of racemate is 206°C and that of meso is 140°C.

Racemic Modification

Racemic modification is and equimolecular mixture of a pair of enantiomers and is optically inactive due to external compensation. Such a mixture is generally denoted by (+/–) or dl

Preparation of Racemic Modification

I. By mixing of enantiomers

This is done by intimate mixing of exactly equal amounts of two enantiomers.

II. By Synthesis

The synthesis of assymmetric compounds from symmetric compounds in the absence of optically active agents or circularly polarised light always produce a racemic modification.

Eg. Formation of lactonitrile from acetaldehyde.

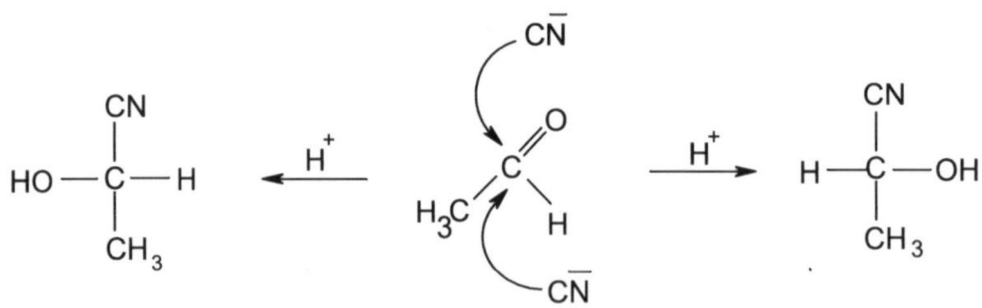

L-Lactonitrile Acetaldehyde D-Lactonitrile

III. By racemisation

Racemisation is the process of converting an optically active (d/l) compound into the racemic modification.

Important mechanisms for racemisation are (a) Thermal racemisation (b) By anion formation (c) By cation formation (d) By reversible formation of stable inactive intermediates, (e) By walden inversion (f) By chemical transformation.

(a) Thermal racemisation

Heating at a higher temperature make homolytic splitting of one of the four bonds attached to the asymmetric carbon atom Eg: on heating 6-6 difluorodiphenic acid easily racemises.

(b) By anion formation

Since the carbanions are generally planar, they are optically inactive. The formation of carbanion intermediate is the common practice of racemisation. The ease of racemisation depends upon the acidity of hydrogen atom: the more labile and acidic the hydrogen atom, then greater will be the case of racemisation.

(c) By cation formation

Cation formation also results in racemisation. In such cases,the group X (which is usually a halogen) is reversibly removed with its bonding pair of electron with the help of Lewis acid like $AlCl_3$,

$SbCl_5$..........etc.

Eg:(+)α-Cholroethylbenzene racemises on treatment with antimony pentasulphide.

(d) By reversible formation of stable inactive intermediates

Mechanism is same as that of anion and cation formation,but here symmetrical,non-ionic stable intermediate is formed

Eg: Optically active α-chloroethyl benzene racemises easily in liquid SO_2 by a dehydrohalogenation-hydrohalogenation process.

(e) By walden inversion

Certain SN^2 reactions involving symmetric centres proceed with inversion of configuration (walden inversion) and thus may cause racemisation of the original optically active compound

Eg:Treatment of optically active iodides in presence of iodide ion yields racemic modification.

(f) By chemical transformation

In this method, an enantiomer is converted into racemic modification without breaking any of the bond.

Eg: 5-methyl-2-cyclohexenyl acid phthalate has been racemised in aqueous acetone at 100°C.

PROPERTIES OF RACEMIC MODIFICATION

A racemic modification generally has the same boiling Point, density and refractive index as that of pure enantiomers. But in solid state racemic modification have some properties different from that of pure enantiomers. Thus three solid states possible for racemic modification are as follows:

(i) Racemic mixture (Conglomerate)

It is a mechanical mixture of the crystals of two enantiomers (+) and (–). These are formed when enantiomers have greater affinity for the molecules of its own type than that for opposite enantiomer. Its melting point will be lower than that of pure components and solubility will be higher than that of pure component. Eg: Sodium ammonium (+/–) tartarate crystallised from water below 27°C.

(ii) Racemic compounds (Racemates)

When each enantiomer has greater affinity for molecules of the other enantiomer than for its own kind, such type molecular compound formed is known as racemic compound. Most of the physical properties of racemate are different from that of pure enantiomers. A racemic mixture is converted to racemic compound at a particular temperature which is known as transition temperature.

(iii) Racemic solid solution (pseudo racemic compound)

When a pair of isomorphous enantiomers crystallises together, the product formed is known as racemic solid solution.

RESOLUTION OR SEPARATION OF RACEMIC MODIFICATION

The process of separation of racemic modification into its pure enantiomers is known as resolution. Following are the different methods of resolution.

1. Mechanical Separation or spontaneous resolution

Sodium ammonium tartarate crystallises out in the form of racemic mixture below 27°C. Here the crystals of two forms have different shapes, can be seperated using magnifying lens and a small forceps

2. Preferential crystallisation by inoculation

This method involves seeding of a saturated solution of racemic mixture with a pure crystal of one of the two enantiomers. The solution now becomes supersaturated with respect to the added enantiomer. After cooling for sometime, it begins to crystallises out.

Eg: Resolution of free α-amino acid with the aid of l or d isomers of the corresponding amino acid.

3. Bio chemical separation

In this method, certain micro-organisms such as bacteria,yeast,mould and fungi are allowed to grow in dilute solution of racemic modification. They assimilate one enantiomer rapidly than the other.

Eg: The mould penicillium glauccum perferentially destroys + isomer of racemic ammonium tartarate and thus leaves – ammonium tartarate in solution.

4. By Diastereoisomers(chemical method)

This is the best method for resolution of racemic modification. Principle involved in this is the formation of salts. It is easy to convert enantiomer of racemic modification to diastereoisomers with the aid of a pure enantiomer of another compound. Since diastereoisomers (optical isomers, which doesn't have mirror images and the configuration of upper asymmetric part is different, but lower symmetrical part has identical configuration) are non-identical, they have different physical properties and can be separated easily by fractional crystallisation. Each diastereoisomers can be converted back to its original parent component by appropriate reacion. Success of this method can be pointed out as

1. Diastereoisomers easily formed in crystals.
2. By Suitable reactions, they can be easily converted back to parent components.
3. The resolving agent either be cheaper, readily prepared or even quantitatively recoverable after resolution.

Acids

Resolution of racemic modification of acid is carried out with the aid of optically active bases. Various naturally occuring optically active alkaloids are used for the resolution of racemic acids; some of them are brucine, strychnine, Quinine, Morphine

Alcohols

Racemic alcohols are separated as their acid phthalate or as succinate ester,formed by treating the alcohol with phthalic or succinic anhydride in presence of pyridine. The acid esters are then resolved in normal manner with an optically pure base to two enantio meric acid esters. Now the resolved acid ester are converted into their respective alcoholos and acid either by hydrolysis or by reduction with Lithium Aluminium Hydride

Aldehydes and Ketones

Carbonyl compounds can be resolved by means of optically active carbonyl reagents such as menthyl hydrazine, menthyl semicarbazide and tartramide acid hydrazide.

Another method involves conversion of carbonyl compounds into their 4-carboxy phenyl semicarbazone by means of 4-carboxyphenyl semicarbazide. The semicarbazones are acidic in nature and hence can be resolved with optically active base (brucine) and then hydrolysed to give back optically active carbonyl compounds.

5. By complex formation

Sometimes a racemic modification forms crystalline diastereomeric complexes with a disymmetric reagent. If the two diastereomeric complexes posses different solubilities, one will precipitate out in preference to the other. After this the two original enantiomers can be obtained from the two complexes by decomposition with heat, dissolution,chromato graphic or chemical treatment.

6. By chromotogrophy

This process involves addition of a solution of the racemic modification over an optically active adsorbent and collecting the two enantiomers from the adsorbates. Since the adsorbates formed by the combination of enantiomers and adsorbents are diastereoisomers, they are not equally stable and hence one of them will pass through the column faster than the other. The two enantiomers are then obtained from the two diastereoisomers by means of careful elution.

7. By kinetic method

This method based on the fact that one of the enantiomer of racemic modification reacts faster than the other with an optically active compound.

8. By asymmetric transformation

The phenomenon of asymmetric transformation is exhibited by optically unstable compound ie. when the enantiomers are readily interconvertable.

If an equimolecular amount of an optically stable (+) and an optically unstable (+/–) acids are dissolved in a solvent, the solution will have equal amounts of two possible disastereoisomers. But since the acid is optically unstable at the time of equilibrium, the two diastereoisomers will be present in unequal amounts. This establishment of equilibrium in solution between the two diastereoisomers having a real existence is known as first order asymmetric transformation.On the other-hand whenever either of the diastereoisomers crystallises out from solution ie. they need not have a real existence in solution, the phenomenon is termed as 2nd order asymmetric transformation.

Conformational Analysis

Conformation may be defined as the term used to denote any one of the infinite number of spatial arrangements of the atoms of a molecule that can arise from rotation about a single bond. So conformation is the interconversion by rotation of one part of the molecule with respect to the rest of the molecule about a single bond joining these two parts.

Eg. 1) Conformation of Ethane.

If one of the methyl group is allowed to rotate along the c-c axis keeping the rest of molecule undisturbed, an infinite number of possible arrangements of the related methyl group with respect to the undisturbed methyl group is generated. Each of these possible arrangement represents a conformation. So six possible conformations are obtained. Out of which three of them are staggered form in which two hydrogen atoms on the different carbon atoms are arranged as far apart as possible (1, 3 & 5). The other three are eclipsed in which the two hydrogen atoms on the different carbon atoms are very close as much as possible. (2, 4 & 6).

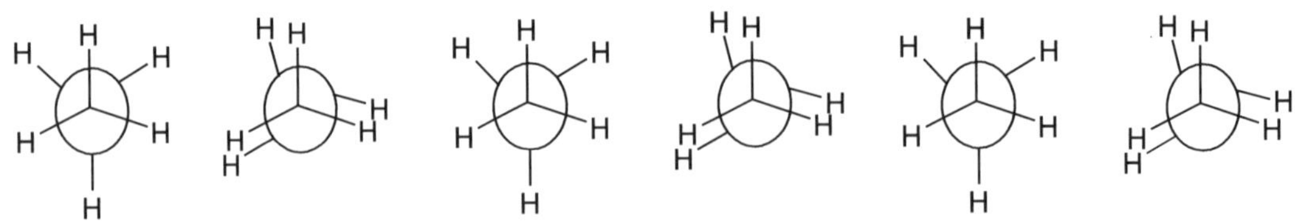

(1) (2) (3) (4) (5) (6)

Eg:2) Conformation of cyclohexane.

In cyclohexane, there are two strainless or puckered conformations in which all the angles are tetrahedral. These are chair or Z form and boat/flexible/form. Comparatively chair form is more stable than boat form.

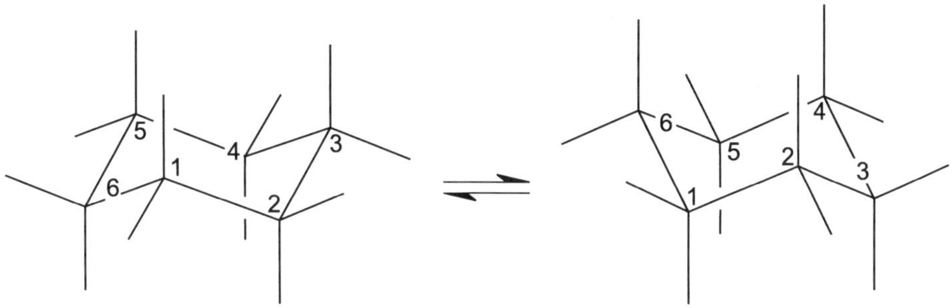

Chair form/Z form

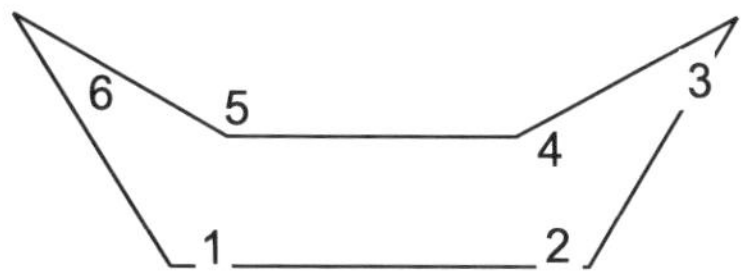

Boat form

Eg. 2) Conformation of fused ring compounds

Fused ring compounds are those in which the adjacent rings have two atoms in common. They may be either bicyclic or polycyclic.

Bicyclic system- eg: Decalin

In decalin two cyclohexane rings fused in two manners either cis or trans.So there are cis-decalin and trans-decalin.In both decalins cyclohexane rings are joined together in chair conformations.

Polycyclic system-eg: perhydrophenanthrene

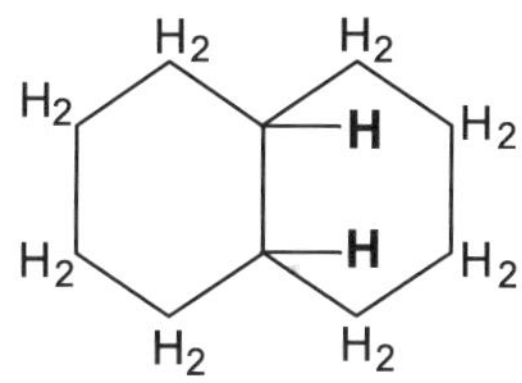

Cis decalin

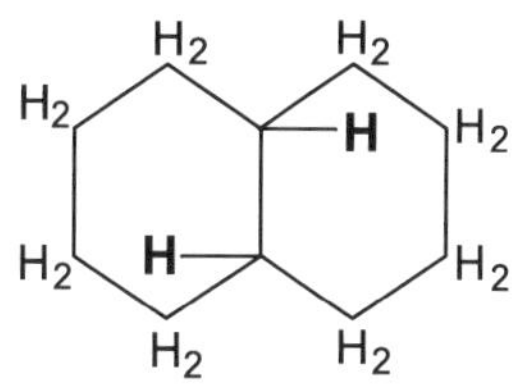

Trans decalin

Polycyclic system-eg: perhydrophenanthrene

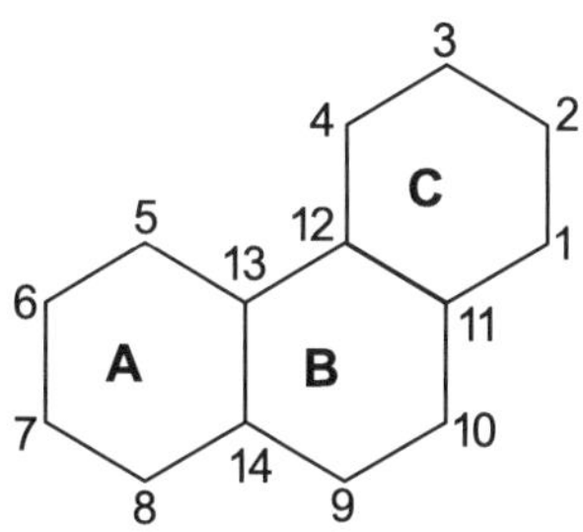

In perhydro phenanthrene, the two rings A&B are linked at 13th and 14th positions. Similarly B&C are at 11th and 12th positions. If the hydrogens at these junctions C_{13}& C_{14} or C_{11}& C_{12} are present on the same side of the ring a cis configuration is obtained.If hydrogens at C_{13}& C_{14} or C_{11} & C_{12} are present on opposite sides, then trans configuration is obtained.

CONFIGURATION

Configuration means the arrangement of atoms or groups around the asymmetric centre. Two system have been developed.

(i) Relative configuration (D-, L-, nomenclature)

(ii) Absolute configuration (R & S system)

Relative configuration: by Rosanoff

The configuration of a compound with - reference to arbitarily assigned configuration of a reference substance is known as its relative configuration.

The enantiomer having hydroxyl group in the right, when the aldehyde group placed at the top is called 'D' configuration. If the hydroxyl group is at the left called 'L' configuration.

Any compound that can be prepared from, or converted to D (+) glyceraldehyde will belongs to D-series & similarly any compound that can be prepared from or converted to L(–) glyceraldehyde will belongs to L-series.

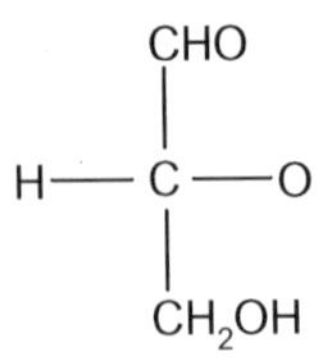

D (+) -glyceraldehyde
(having- OH group at right)

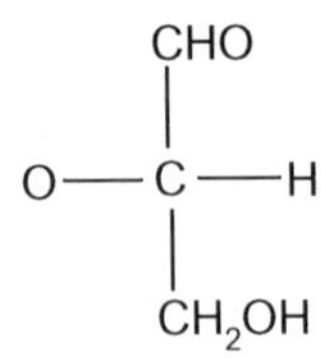

L (-) - glyceraldehyde
(having- OH to the left)

Other compounds are assigned 'D' or 'L' configuration as follows

(i) compounds similar in structure to glyceraldehyde

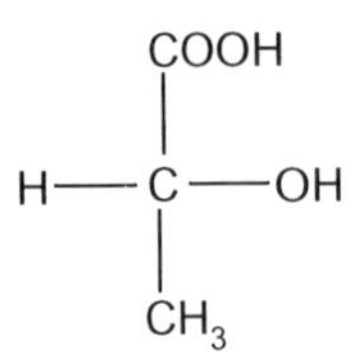

D (-) -Lactic acid

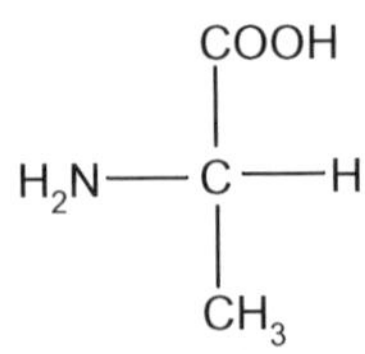

L (+) -Alanine

(ii) When representing , relative configurational relationship of molecules containing more thane one asymmetric Carbon atom, the asymmetric Carbon atom of glyceraldehyde is always drawn at the bottom & rest of the molecule is then built up.

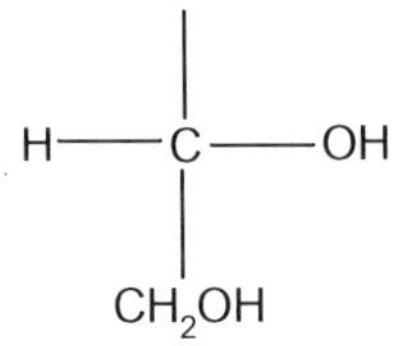

D series

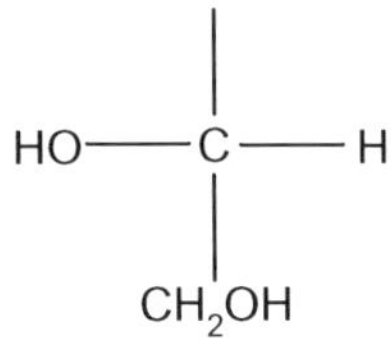

L series

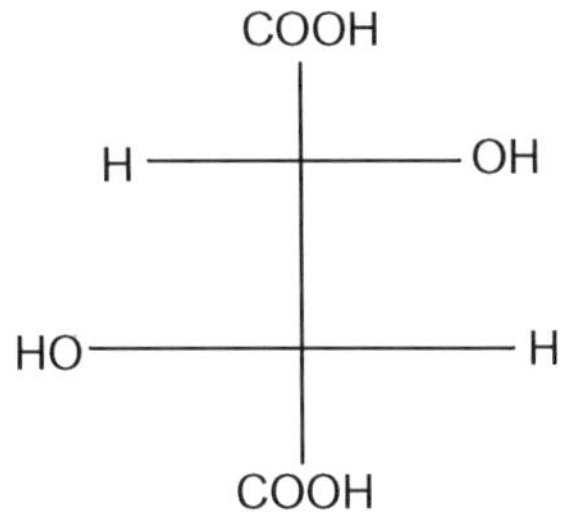

L (+)tartaric acid

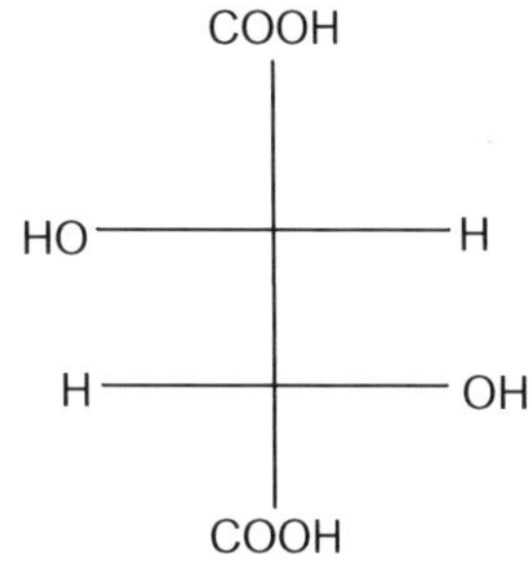

D(–) tartaric acid

It should be noted that 'D' & 'L' are configurational symbols & there can be D(+) & D(–) Compounds, similarly L(+) & L(–) Compounds.

In the sugar series, the configuration is assigned with respect to the highest asymmetric Carbon atom (next to the primary alcoholic group; the glyceraldehyde Carbon atom)

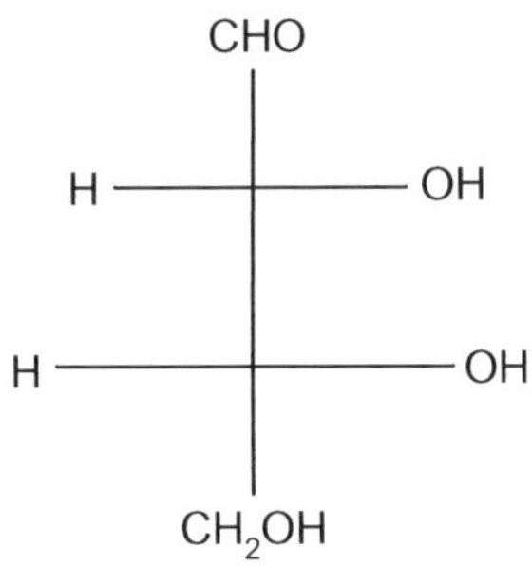

D(-) Erythrose

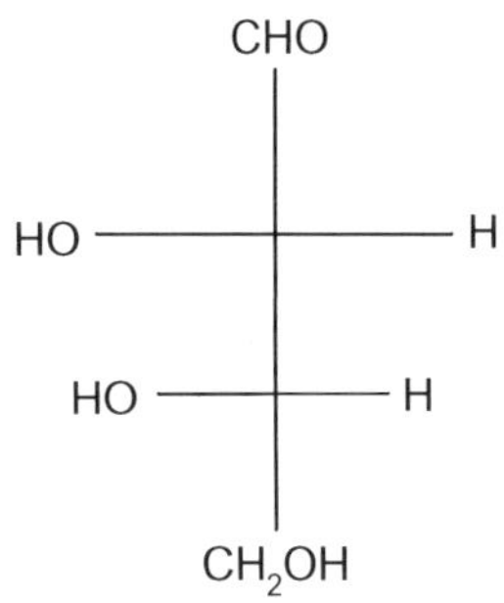

L(+) Erythrose

Absolute Configuration

Absolute configuration is also known as R& S system of nomenclature; Abolute configuration can be determined by X-ray technique or electron diffraction.

The important features of R & S system of nomenclature are as follows;

(i) The four different groups attached to the asymmetric carbon atom are arranged in priority sequence. To indicate the structure about an asymmetric carbon atom x,in xabced,the groups a, b, c, & d are arranged in priority sequence based on the sequence rules given below.

(ii) If the priority is established as a > b > c > d. 'a' has the highest priority & 'd' the lowest.

(iii) The molecule is then represented by projection formula in such a manner that the lowest priority groups is at the bottom. If the sequence a → b → c is in clockwise direction, it is designated as S.

(iv) When there are more than one asymmetric centres the above procedure is applied to each asymmetric atom.

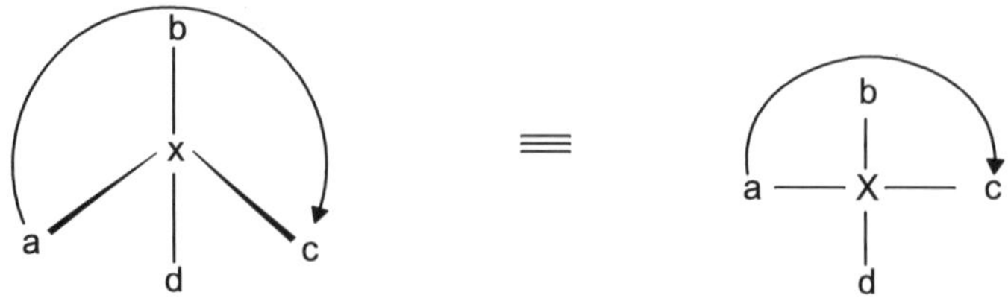

Three Dimensional formula   fischer projection formula

R - Configuration

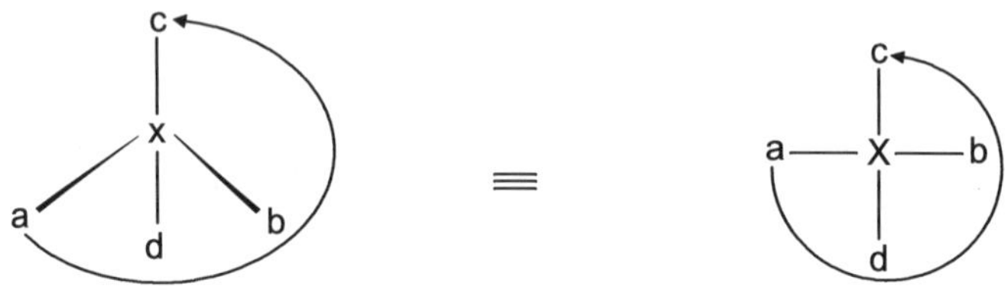

3 Dimensional formula   fischer projection formula

S - Configuration

Sequence rule (Rules to decide priorities)

(i) The substituent atom having highest atomic number given priority. On this basis, the order of priority for halogens decreases in the order I, Br, Cl, F.

(ii) For substituent group of atom, same rule is applicable. The group in which the first atom has the highest atomic number gives I[st] priority. In this case the sequence is I, Br.Cl, SO_3H, F, OH, NH_2-------- etc.

(iii) Isotopic atoms of higher mass number proceed that of lower mass number.

(iv) The Cis group takes precedence over 'trans' groups

Eg: 1) Bromo chloro acetic acid

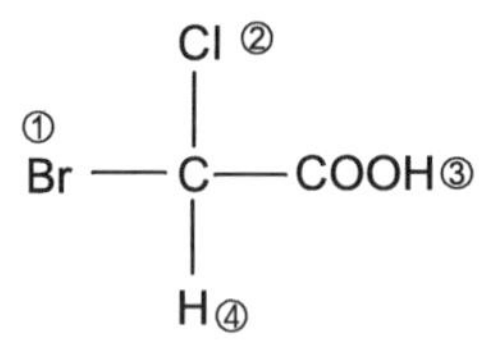

The movement is clockwise from Br ⟶ Cl ⟶ C. Hence is assigned as R-Configuration with dextro rotation.

Eg: 2)

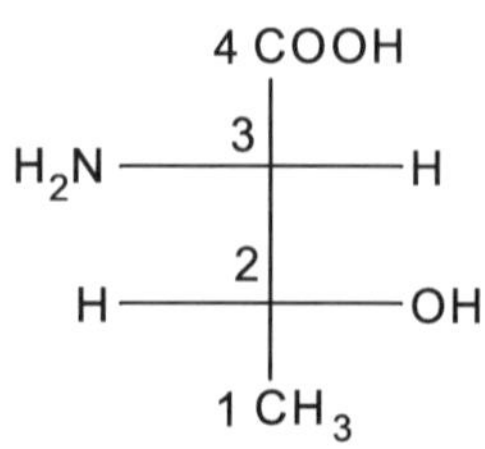

(2S, 3R), Threonine

Methods of Determining Configuration

In order to determine configuration of unknown we have to relate that compound with a compound. having known configuration.

1. Conversion of the unknown to, or formation of the unknown from, a compound of known configuration without disturbing the chiral center since the chiral center was not disturbed, the unknown obviously have the same configuration of known.

Glyceraldehyde ⟶ Glyceric Acid.

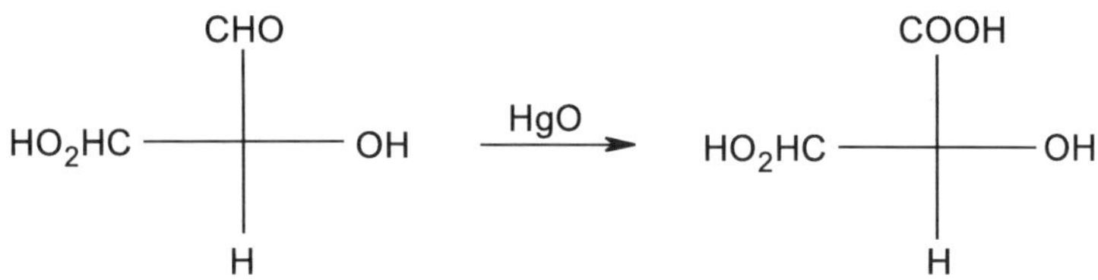

(S) (S)

2. Bio chemical methods

In a series of similar compounds such as amino acid or certain types of steroids,a given enzyme will usually attack only molecules with one kind of configuration. If the enzyme attacks only the L form of eight amino acid, say then attack on unknown 9th assume will be a L form.

3. Optical comparison

In a homologous series, the rotation usually changes gradually & in one direction. If the configurations of enough members of the series are known, the configurations of the missing ones can be determined by extrapolation.

4. X-ray methods, optical rotatory dispersion, circular dichroism, N.M.R & asymmetric synthesis can also used to determine absolute configuration.

(S) - 2 - Iodo butane (R) - Iodo butane

By the application of all rules priority sequence for common substituents are as follows; I → Br, Cl, SO_3 H, SH, F, COR, OR, OH, NO_2, NHCOR, NHR, NH_2, CCl_3, COCl, CO_2 R, COOH, $CONH_2$, COR, CHO, CH_2OH, CN, (R_3) C_6H_5, CHR_2, CH_2R, CH_3, D, H

CONFIGURATION OF THE BIPHENYL MOLECULE

Configuration is the term means the arrangement of atoms or groups around the asymmetric centre, which is most commonly a carbon or nitrogen atom. 6, 6-dinitrodiphenic acid can be synthesised by means of ullmam reaction ethyl ester of 2-chloro-3-nitro benzoic acid and hydrolysing the product.

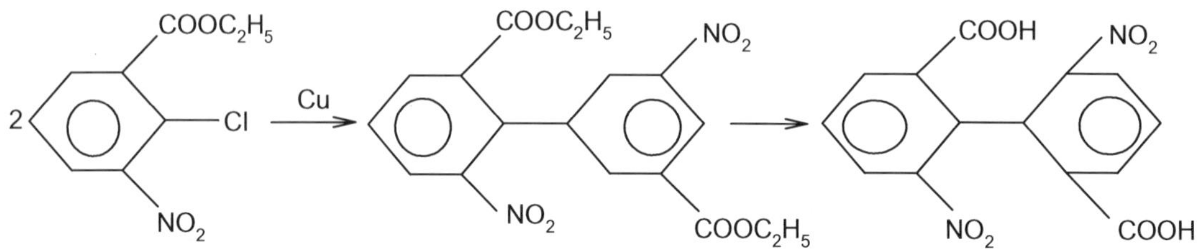

The product is found to be optically active & opticat activity can be accounted due to co-axial structure, more than that the two benzene rings do not lie in one plane.

Physico-chemical methods also used to determine the configuration of biphenyl Eg: The crystal structure 4,4'-biphenyl derivatives shows a centre of symmetry. This is possible only for co-axial formula. Dipole moment also confirm this configuration. eg. the dipole moment of 4,4'-dichlorobiphenyl is zero this again is only possible if the two benzene rings are co-axial.

Optical activity of biphenyl compounds

Two conditions were necessary for biphenyl compounds to exhibit optical activity.

(i) Neither ring must have a vertical plane of symmetry so among the following compounds. I is not resolvable & II is resolvable.

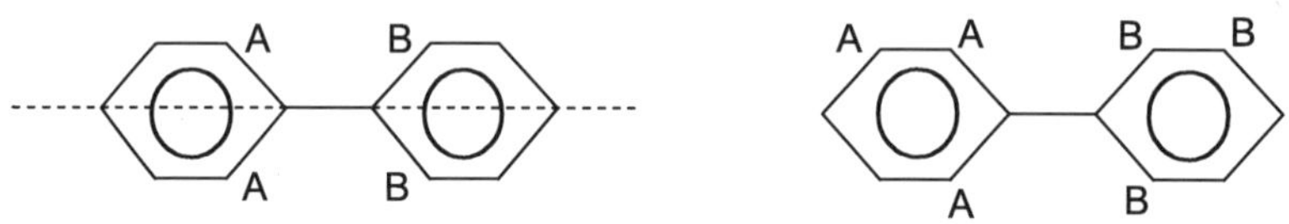

I II

(ii) The substituents in ortho-position must have a large size.

In biphenyl the two benzene rings are Co-axial, & in optically active biphenyl derivatives, the rings are inclined to each other due to steric & repulsive effects of groups. In ortho-positions. The actual angle of inclination of the two rings depends on the nature of the substituent groups,but it appears to be usually in the vicinity of 90°.ie. the rings tend to be approximately perpendicular to each other. Thus in order to exhibit optical activity, the substituent groups in the ortho-positions must be large enough to prevent the two rings from becoming co-planar, in which case the molecule would posses a plane or a centre of symmetry. eg: Diphenic acid is not optically active.

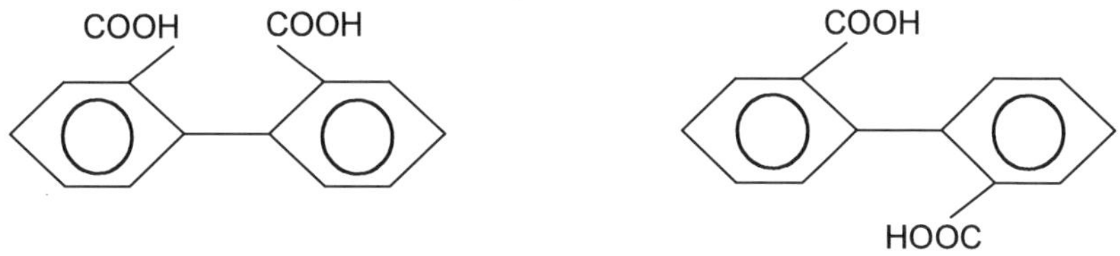

(a) (b)

The molecule represented in 'a' have a plane of symmetry, & in the case of (b) centre of symmetry present. So the configuration of Diphenic acid, can be most probably (b) because of the repulsion between the two carboxyl groups.

ATROPISOMERISM (OPTICAL ISOMERISM IN BIPHENYLS)

In the crystal, both benzene rings of biphenyl lie in the same plane. However in solution & vapour phase the two rings are twisted with respect to each other by an angle of 45°due to steric interactions between 2, 2' & 6, 6' pairs of hydrogens. These interaction effects are further enchanced by orthosubstituents larger than hydrogen.

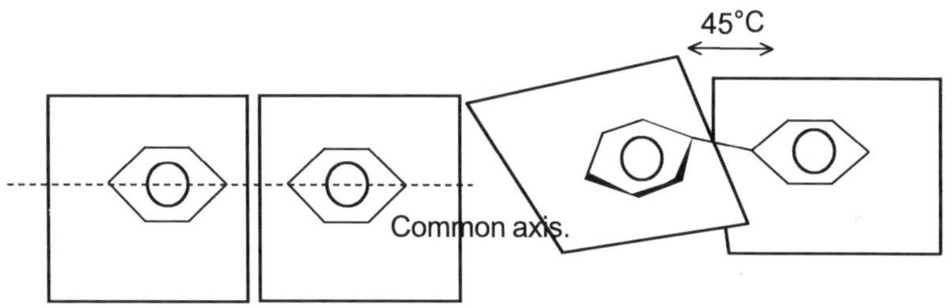

The rotation about the bond linking the two phenyl rings does not occur due to steric hindrance between the bulky ortho substituents.

Isolable sterioisomers resulting from restricted rotation about single bonds are called atropisomers, while rotamers are sterioisomers obtained by rotation about a single bond.

Asymmetric Synthesis (Asymmetric Induction)

The direct (with out resolution) synthesis of an optically active compound from a symmetric compound (Optically inactive) with or without the use of optically active reagent is known as asymmetric synthesis. These are of two types-partial asymmetric synthesis & absolute asymmetric synthesis.

Partial asymmetric synthesis

An optically active compound synthesised directly (without resolution) from a symmetrical compound by the intermediate use of semi optically active compound is known as partial asymmetric synthesis. Eg. preparation of -valeric acid from methyl ethyl molonic acid with the aid of brucine.

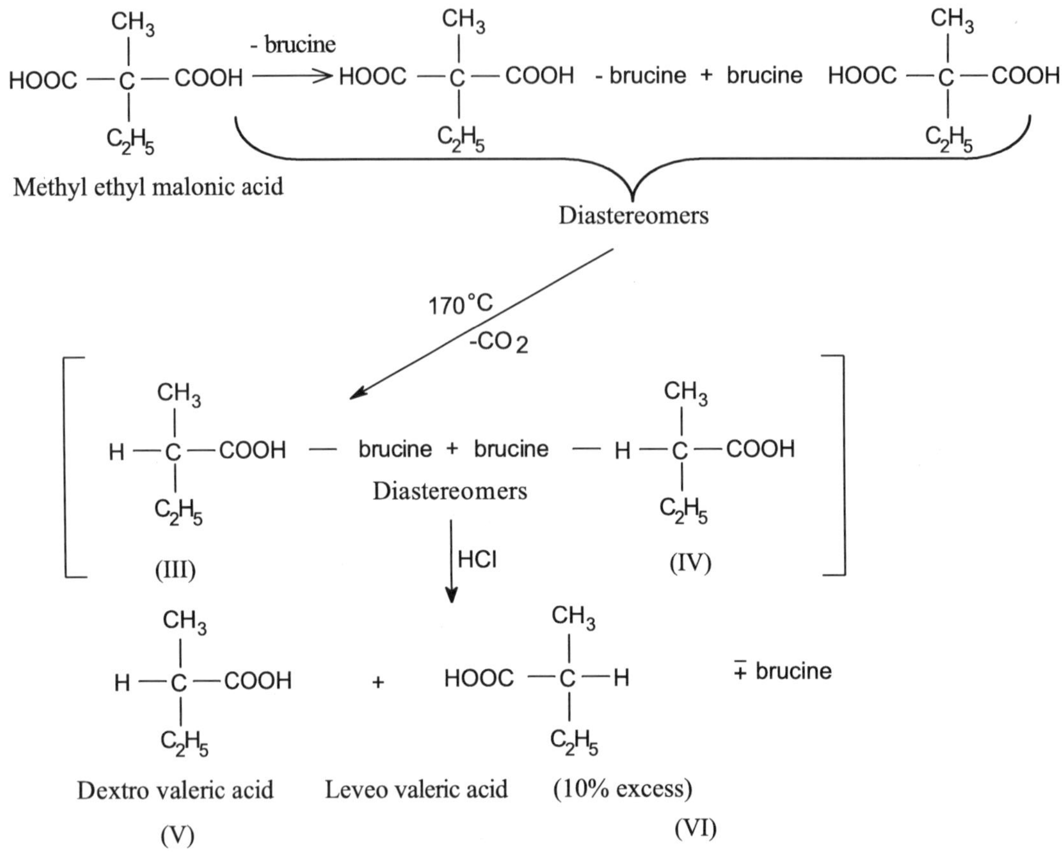

Here Levorotatory product forms more, so, the two enantiomers must be present in unequal amounts.

The difference in quantity of Leavo & dextro forms can be attributed by various points as follows;

(a) The unequal amounts was due to the different rate of decomposition of diasteromers I & II to give III & IV and hence V & VI are in unequal amounts.

(b) Another point is some of the less soluble diastereomer crystallises out during evaporation, which results the conversion of some of the more soluble diastereomer into the less soluble diastereomer and hence the product after the evaporation will contain unequal amounts of two forms.

A typical example of asymmetric synthesis is the reduction of benzoyl formic acid to mandelic acid in the presence of - menthol.

$$C_6H_5CH.COOH + - C_{10}H_{19}OH \longrightarrow C_6H_5CO.COOC_{10}H_{19} \xrightarrow{Al/Hg}$$

Benzoyl formic a   menthol

$$C_6H_5CH(OH).COOC_{10}H_{19} \longrightarrow C_6H_5CH(OH).COOH + C_{10}H_{19}OH$$

- mandelic a

Other examples of partial asymmetric sysnthesis are

Reduction of 3, 3 - dimethylbutan -2-one into + 3, 3 dimethyl butan -2-ol in presence of + -2 - methyl butyl magnesium chloride

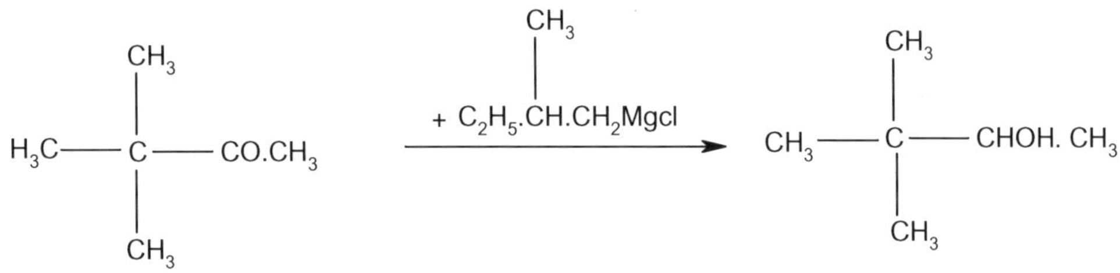

Reduction of butan -2-one with $LiAlH_4$ in presence of (+) camphor to (+) isoborneol & (+) butan -2-0l

$$CH_3\text{-}CO.\,C_2H_5 \xrightarrow[\text{(+) Camphor}]{\text{LAH}} CH_3CH(OH).\,C_2H_5 + \text{(+) Isoborneol.} + \text{butan-}_2\text{-ol}$$

Reformatsky reaction between acetophenone, (–) menthyl bromoacetate and Zinc to form (+) β-hydroxy β-phenyl butyric acid

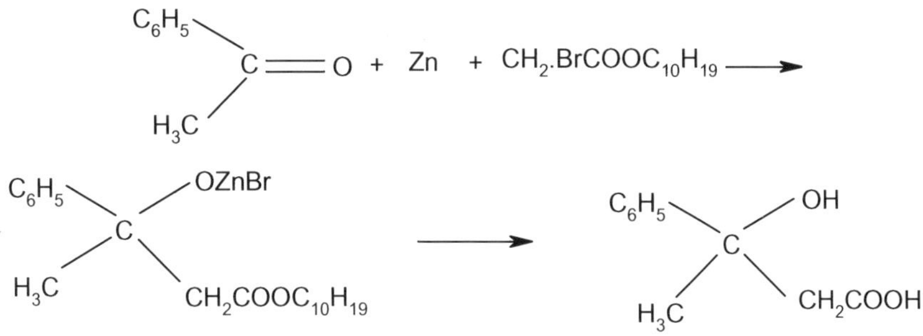

(+) β -hydroxy β phenyl butyric acid

Asymmetric synthesis can also affected by means of enzymes. Product will be almost optically pure unlike chemical partial asymmetric synthesis.

eg.

1. $C_6H_5CHO + HCN \xrightarrow{\text{emulsin (enzyme)}} C_6H_5CH(OH).CN$
   Benzaldehyde → + mandelonitrite

2. $C_6H_5COCH_3 \xrightarrow{\text{reductas}} C_6H_5\,.CHO$
   acetophenene → α-phenyl ethanol

3. 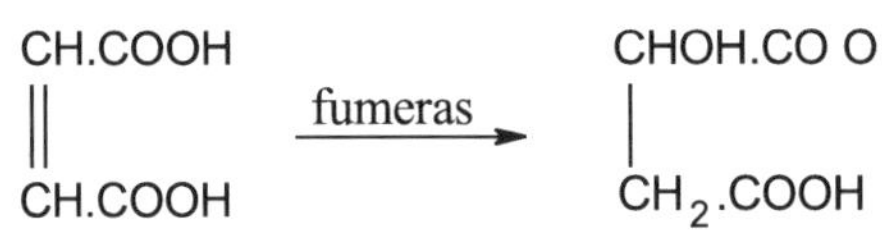
   Fumaric acid → malic acid

Absolute asymmetric synthesis

The formation of an optivally active compound from inactive one, without the intermediate use of optically active reagent is known as absolute asymmetric synthesis. In these case some sort of physically dissymmetric influence is necessary such as circularly polarised light.

Eg. Addition of bromine to 2, 4, 6-trinitro stilbene in a beam of circularly polarised light gave a feebly dextro-rotatory product.

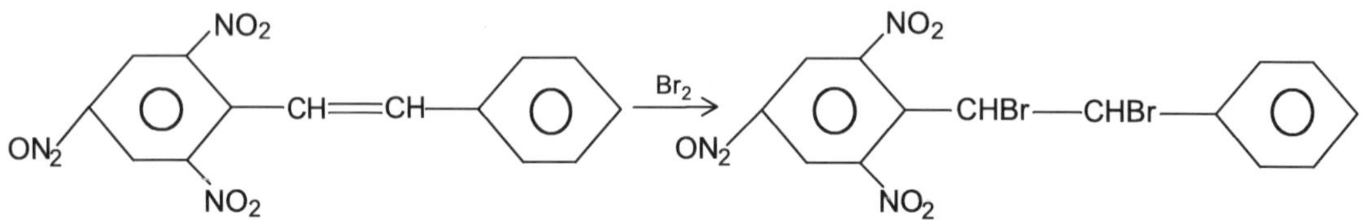

Eg. 2) Substituted tartaric acid having very small +ve rotation can be synthesised from ethyl fumarate and H_2O_2 under the influence of dextro-circularly polarised light

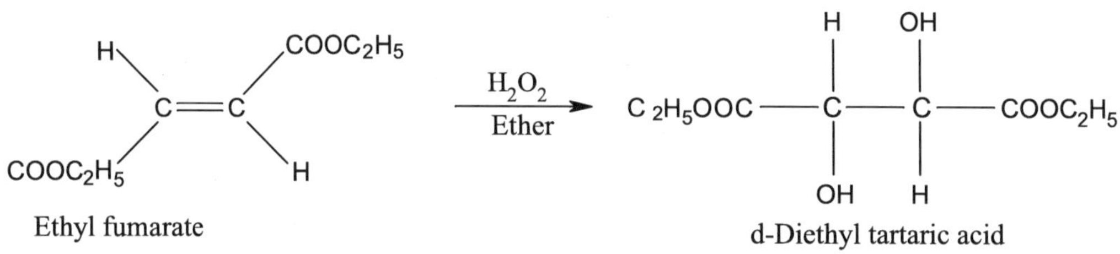

OPTICAL ISOMERISM IN NITROGEN CONTAINING COMPOUND AMINES

Teritary amine molecule (Nabc) is planar and is superimpossible on its mirror image and therefore cannot be optically active. But physico chemical method like dipole moment ,measurements and I.R spectral studies shown conclusively that, configuration of ammonia and tertiary amine is tetrahedral. Ammonia shown to have dipole moment of 1.5D. If the molecule was planar, then dipole mement would have been zero. The nitrogen valency angle eg. in triethyl amine have been found to be 108°, thus again showing that amine molecule is not planar. Still tertiary amines cannot resolve, because in the teriary amine molecule the nitrogen atom oscillates rapidly at right angles above and below the plane containing the groups a, b & c.

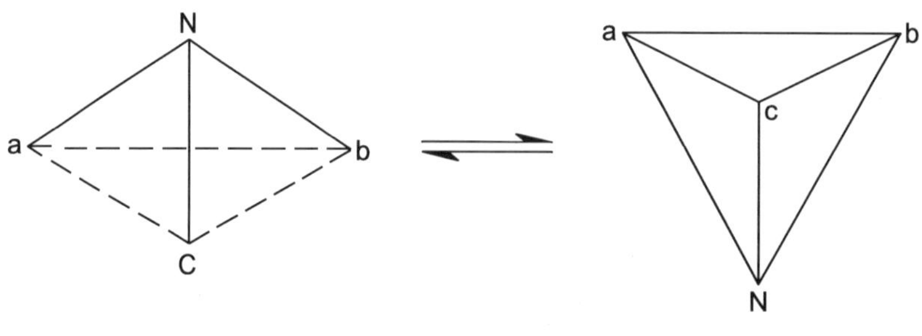

These are mirror images of each other and are not superimpossible. Thus this oscillation bring about very rapid optical inversion. This oscillation theory supported by evidence obtained from absorption spectrum of ammonia and frequency of oscillation (therefore the inversion) has been calculated to be 2.3×10^{10}/second. So the bond lengths remain unaltered and only the Nitrogen valency angles changes. From this it is clear that, if the groups a, b and c increase in weight,the frequency of the inversion of molecule decreases. So the tertiary amines are incapable of resolution because of the ease of racemisation, but if the Nitrogen atom form a part of the ring system, then the compuond would be sufficiently optically stable to be isolated.

Eg: Troger's base which is obtain from p-toludine and formaldehyde can be resolved by chromatographic adsorption on (+) lactose.

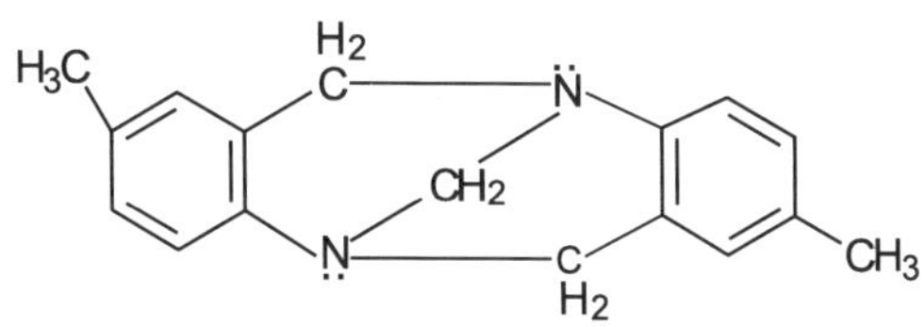

In Troger's base, since all the three valencies of Nitrogen atom forms part of the rings, the frequency of oscillation (hence optical conversion) becomes zero and therefore the compound can exist in optically active forms

Walden Inversion

Walden inversion is a molecular equivalent of an umbrella turning inside out in a high wind. The term inversion refers to the local symmetry of the abcC fragment & does not imply change of configuration from R → S or S → R between the substrate & product. Inversion of configuration takes place usually in SN[2] reaction.

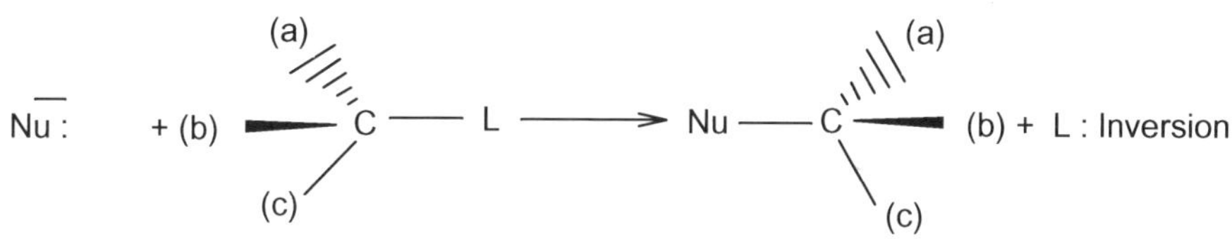

Inversion of configuration occurs when SN[2] reaction takes place with a chiral substrate. Eg: R (–)-2-Bromo-octane reacts with NaOH to yield S-(+)-2-Octanol. It is a second order reaction & occurs with complete inversion of configuration.

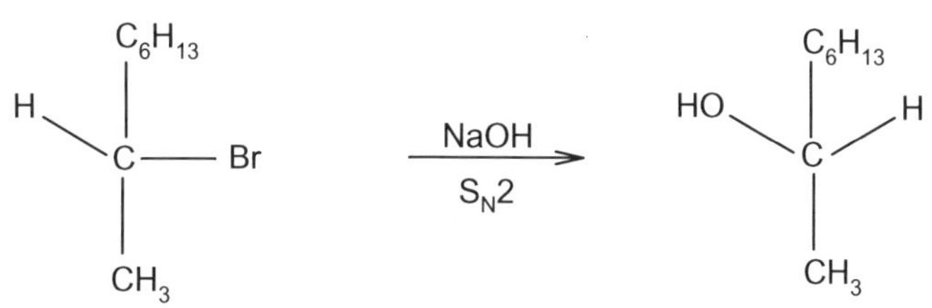

R-(-) 2 bromooctane.

S (+) 2 Octanol.

Mechanism

In the Walden inversion nucleophile attacks the Carbon atom bearing the leaving group from the opposite side. The bond making & bond breaking are simultaneous processes & in the transition state the Carbon appears to be pentavalent.

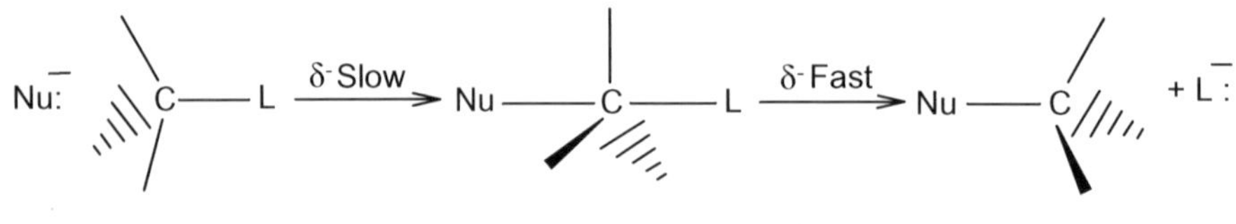

Rate determining step. Transition state.

Evidence for inversion of configuration during SN^2 reaction

Eg: No:1) Reaction between optically active 2-iodo-octane & radio active iodide ions. It is a bimolecular substitution reaction & involves replacement of iodide ions by radioactive iodide ions.

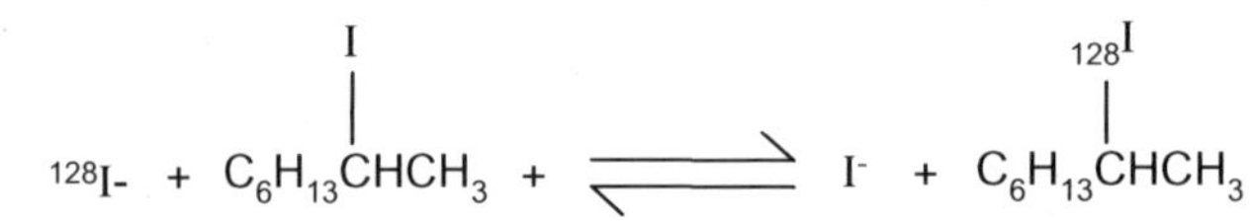

Optically active 2-iodo Octane.

Eg: No: 2) Conversion of phenyl-2-propanol, an optically active alcohol to its enantiomers, through 3 steps.

1st step

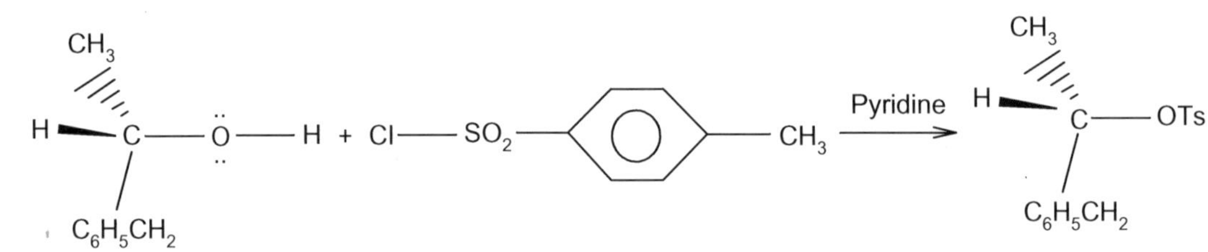

1-phenyl-2-propomol

$OTs = -OSO_2C_6H_4CH_3$-

tosylate

2nd step

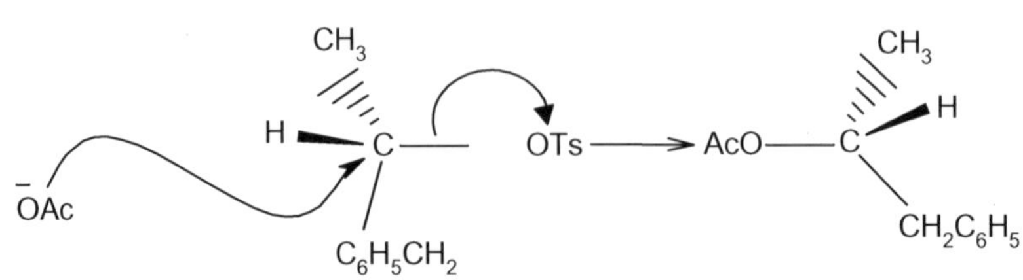

3rd step

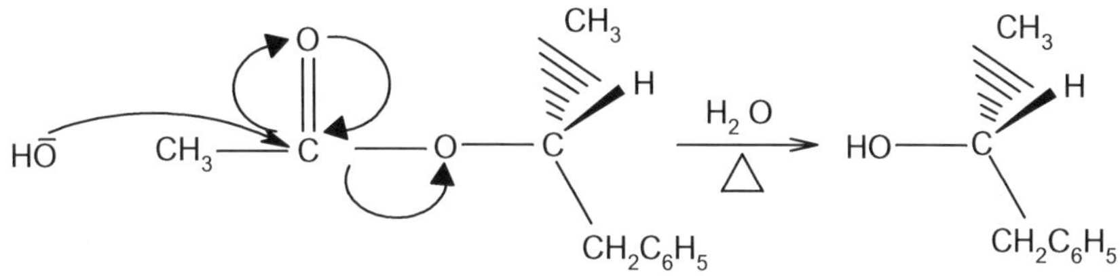

Formation of tosylate (1st step) & hydrolysis of ester (3rd step) do not involve reactions at chiral centre.In the second step substitution of acetate for tosylate occurs at chiral Carbon. Their inversion takes place.

Eg : No: 3) Reaction of 2-bromo propanoic acid with concentrated solution of a strong nucleophile like hydroxide ion. The anion of this acid reacts by normal SN^2 process with inversion of configuration.

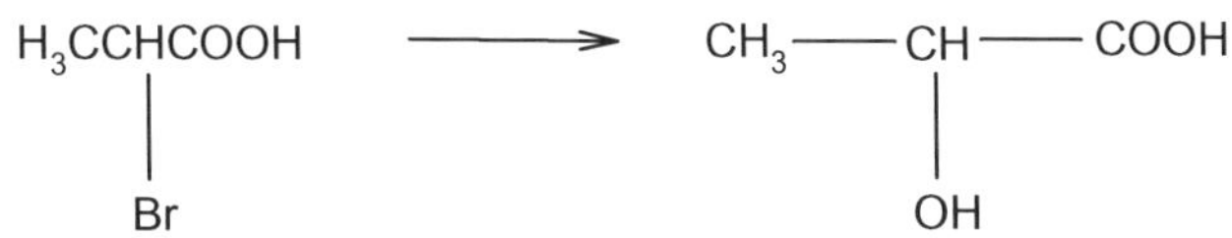

2-Bromopropanoic acid

Lactic acid.

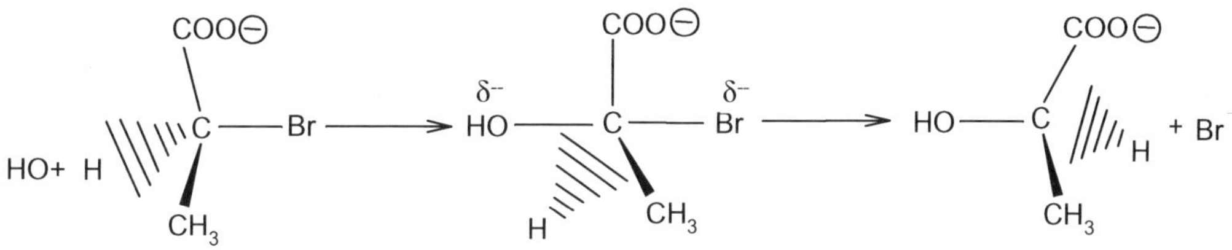

(S)-2 Bromopropanoate ion.

(R)-Lactate ion.
Inversion of configuration.

If the attack of nucleophile is initialised from the side opposite to the departing group (Chlorine) the reaction always leads to an inversion of configuration. Walden inversion is symbolized by a loop in the arrow $\underset{\text{O}}{\longrightarrow}$

GEOMETRICAL ISOMERISM

An isomer having similar groups on the same side called Cis and having similar groups on opposite side called Trans isomer and the phenomenon on the whole was known as Cis-trans isomerism. Isomerism in which failure of rotation about a double bond makes the molecule a rigid one and fixes the position of various groups is known as geometrical isomerism.

Eg :1) Maleic acid and Fumaric acid

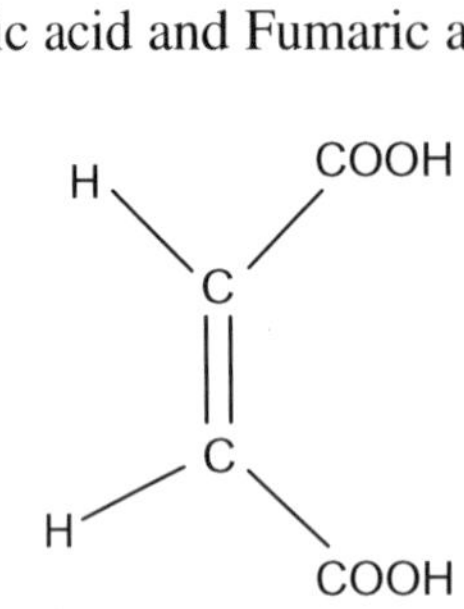

Maleic acid

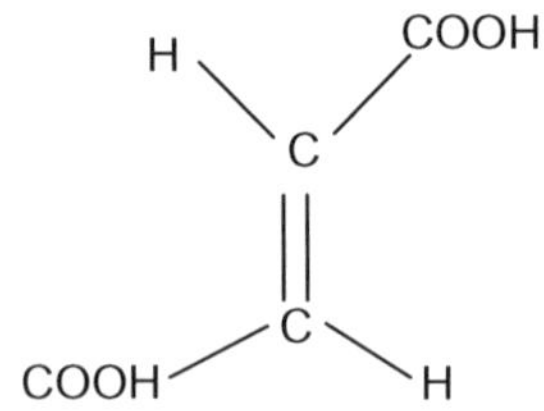

Fumaric Acid

Eg : 2) Cis-dimethyl ethylene and Trans-dimethyl ethylene

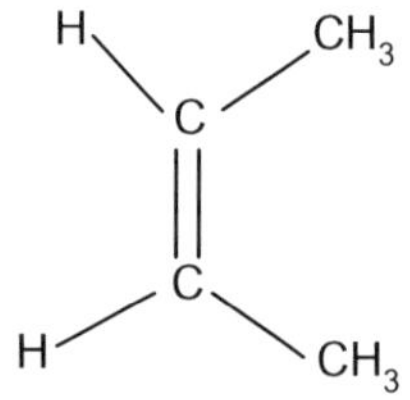

Cis-dimethyl ethylene

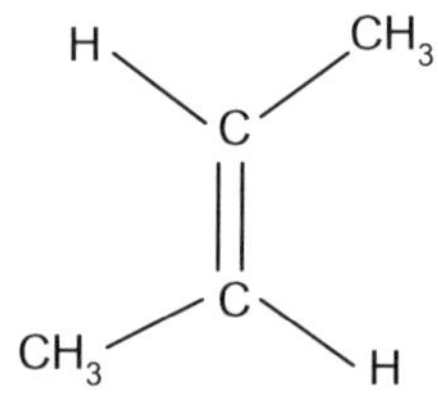

Trans-dimethyl ethylene

Common properties to both Fumaric & Maleic acid.

1. Both acids have same molecular formula- $C_4H_4O_4$.
2. On reduction both give succinic acid.
3. Oxidation by alkaline $KMnO_4$ both give tartaric acid.
4. Both of them add one molecule of HBr to form Bromo succinic acid.

Both of them differ in their density, solubility and action of heat.

Presence of a double bond or a ring restricts the rotation and also a change from one form to another.

Modern theories of double bond

One modern theory suggests, four valency bonds of a Carbon atom are distributed tetrahedrally only in saturated compounds. In such compounds the Carbon atom is in tetrahedral hybridisation and all four SP^3 bonds are sigma bonds.

In Olefenic compounds, the two Carbon atoms exhibit trigonal hybridisation. In this there are three coplanar valencies (3 sigma bonds from SP^2 hybridisation) and fourth bond (pi bond) right angles to trigonal hybrids. Pi bonds which are weaker than sigma bonds, tends to overlap as much as possible in order to make the bond as strong as possible. It is therefore this tendency to produce maximum overlap of pi electron in the pi bond give rise to resistance of rotation about a double bond.

High reactivity of unsaturated compound is based on electromeric and resonance effects. In ethylene $_2HC{=}CH_2$ one of the bond is sigma bond and other is pi bond which is perpendicular to sigma bond. Pi electron (mobile electron) undergo electromeric and resonance influence. They are held less firmly than sigma electrons and are more exposed to external influences. High reactivity of unsaturated compound is due to this.

SP^3 hybridisation describe Carbon-Carbon multiple bond; this treatment give rise to banana shaped orbitals that is bend bonds. So this method points out into rigidity of the molecule and there is no free rotation about the double bond.

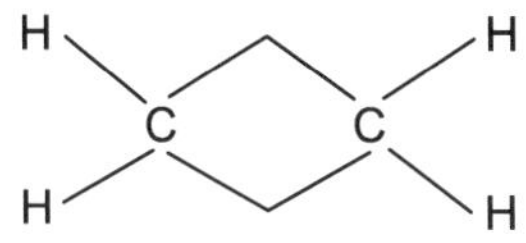

Bend Bonds

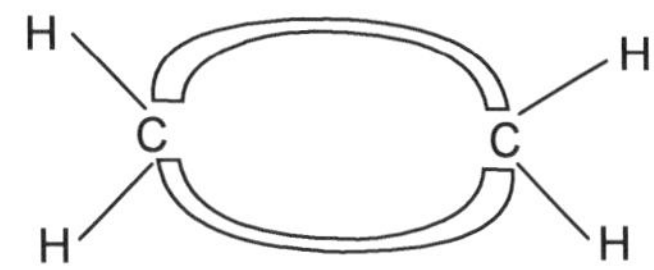

Banana Shaped Orbitals

Nomenclature of Geometrical Isomers

If a compound contains ‘n’ dissimilarly substituted double bonds, the number of geometrical isomers is 2^n. However, if some double bonds are identical, it will decrease the number of isomers. Such isomers are named on the basis of longest Carbon chain rule. The terms Cis and trans are placed before the numbers indicating the position of double bond

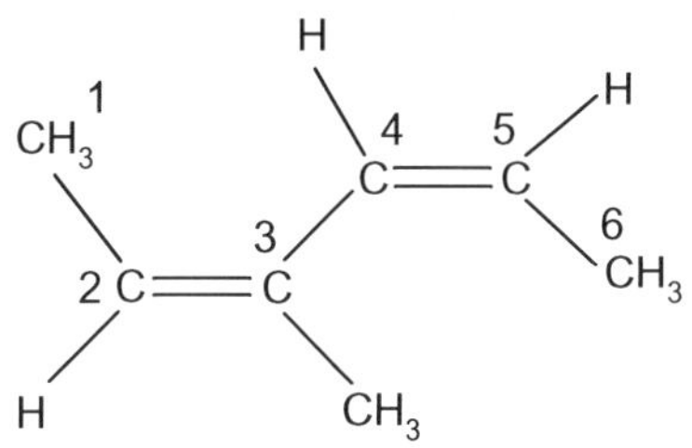

3-methyl hexa - Cis-2-cis-4-diene

E & Z nomenclature

Geometrical isomers can be of following three types.

Type: 1

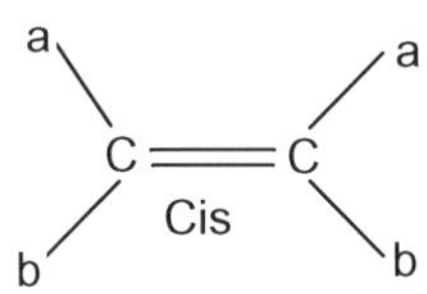

&

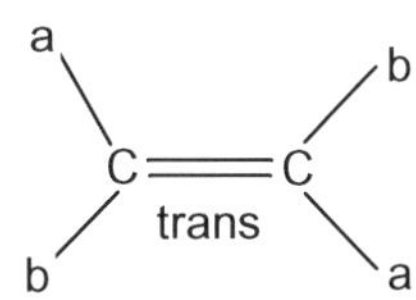

Type: 2

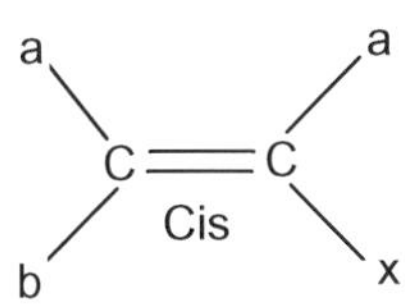

&

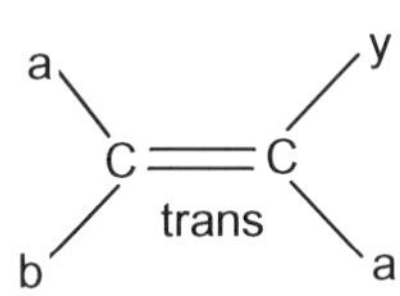

Type: 3

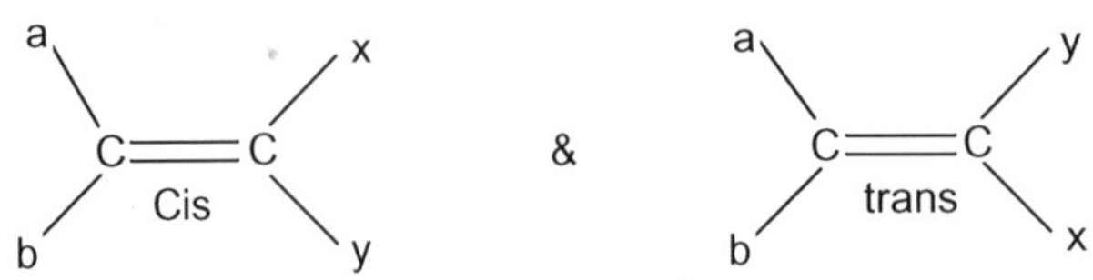

The compound is named as per following rules.

(i) The four groups attached to the double bond are assigned priority in accordance with the sequence rule.

(ii) If the higher priority atom or group on each Carbon atom is on the same side of double bond its configuration is 'Z'. If these atoms or groups of higher priority on two Carbon atoms are on opposite side of double bond, the isomer is E.

Eg:

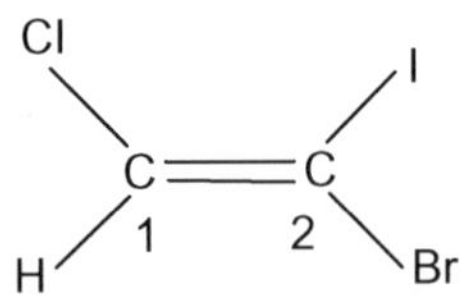

The C_1 is having Cl and hydrogen,so the priority of Cl is higher. Similarly on C_2 the priority of I is higher. Now since Cl and I atoms of higher priority are on the same side of double bond, so this compound is assigned the configuration 'Z'.

Determination of Configuration of Geometrical Isomers

1. Method of cyclisation

This method is based on the fact that, intramolecular reactions are more likely to takeplace if the reacting groups are closer. Eg: In case of maleic acid, anhydride is formed under mild conditions because the two -COOH groups are closer (Cis) but fumaric acid does not give an anhydride under ordinary conditions. Under vigorous conditions it forms maleic anhydride, so in this case the two -COOH groups are in opposite direction (trans).

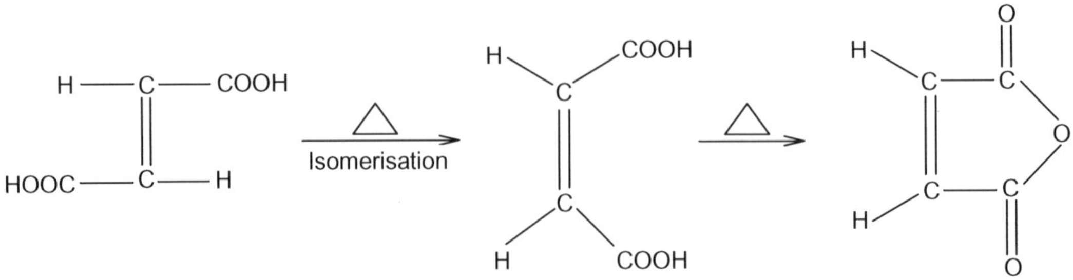

Fumaric acid　　Maleic acid　　Maleic anhydride.

Other example for determination of configuration of geometrical isomer is hexahydroterphthalic acid.

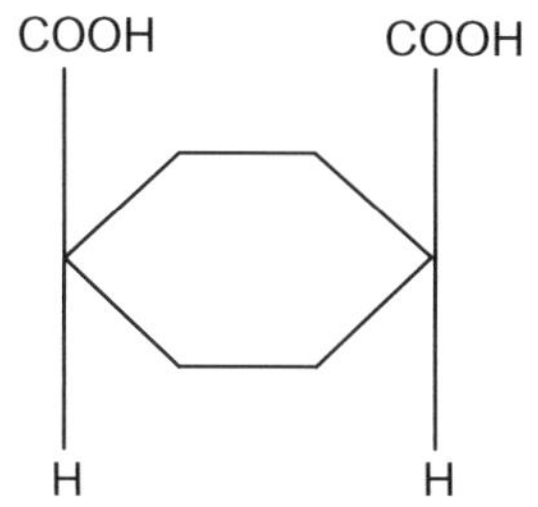

Cis - acid

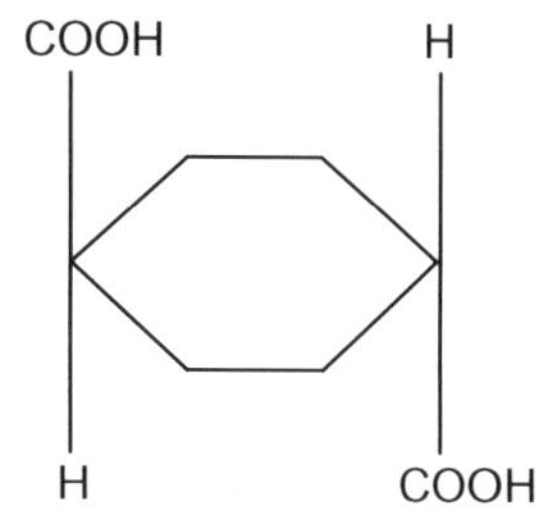

trans-acid

2. By converting into compounds of known configuration

This method is applicable in those cases in which one of the two isomers can be converted into a compound of known configuration. Assuming that there is no isomerisation during the process of conversion, then the configuration of product and that of starting material will be same.

Eg: One form of trichlorocrotonic acid can be hydrolysed to give fumaric acid, so this form of trichlorocrotonic acid must be the trans-isomer. The other form of acid does not give fumaric acid on hydrolysis and forms isocrotonic acid on reduction. Hence this form of trichlorocrotonic acid and isocrotonic acid are cis-isomers.

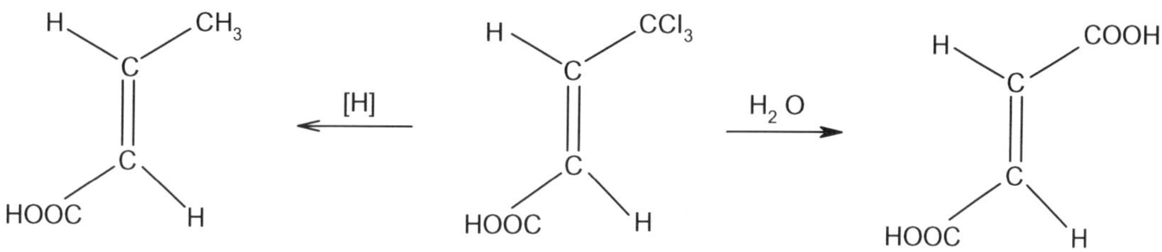

Crotonic acid (trans) Trichloro crotonic acid (trans) Fumaric acid (trans)

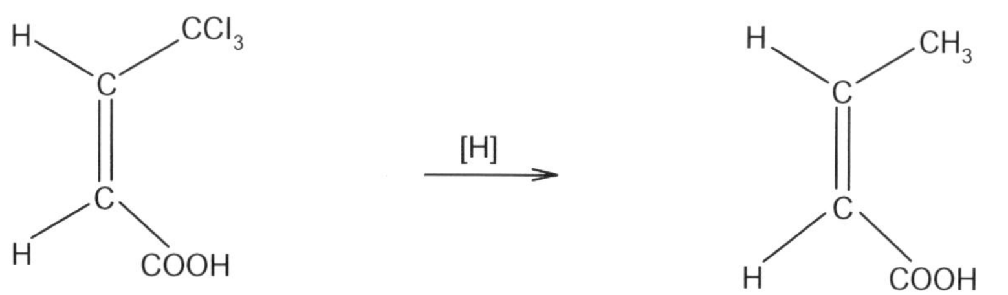

Trichloro crotonic acid Isocrotonic acid (Cis)

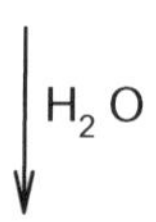

No Fumaric acid (trans)

3. Method of Optical activity

In geometrical isomers if one is optically active and other is optically inactive, then optically active compound can easily resolved.

Eg: Trans form of hexahydrophthalic acid can be resolved.

4. Methods based on Physical properties

(a) Dipole moment

The dipole moment of cis form is generally higher than that of trans form. Eg: In the case of 1,2 dichloroethylene cis isomer have 1.80 D and trans isomer have zero dipolemoment.

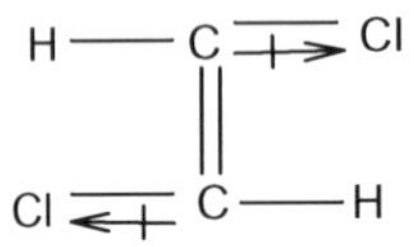

Trans1,2-Dichloro ethylene

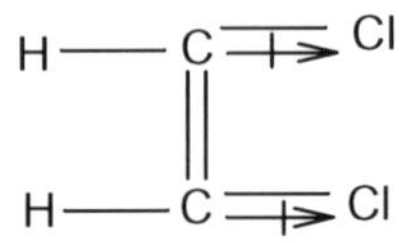

Cis 1,2-Dichloro ethylene

When a group on one Carbon atom is electron withdrawing and group on the other is electron attracting, the trans isomer has the higher dipole moment than cis form eg: 1-Chloropropene.

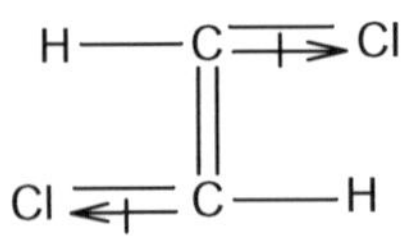

Trans form ($\mu = 1.97$ D)

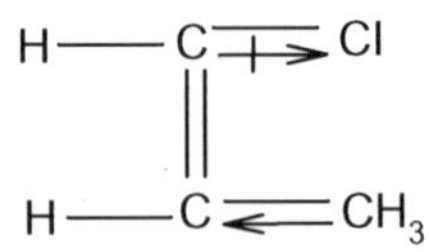

Cis form ($\mu = 1.71$ D)

(b) Melting point, Boiling point, Solubility, Density & Refractive index

How the physical constants are varying in cis and trans isomer is shown in the following table.

Physical constants	*Cis - isomer*	*Trans - isomer*
Melting point	Lower	Higher
Boiling point	Higher	Lower
Solubility	Higher	Lower
Density	Higher	Lower
Dipole moment	Higher	Lower
Refractive index	Higher	Lower
Heat of combustion	Higher	Lower
Thermal stability	Lower	Higher

(c) Acid strength

Among monobasic ethylenic acids, the cis isomer is usually more stronger than corresponding trans.The acid strength of dibasic acid strongly dependent on configuration. There is a large difference in thre ratio of 1st to 2nd dissociation constants.

eg: Maleic acid k_1/k_2=40,000 & Fumaric acid k_1/k_2=32. k_1=1st dissociation constant and k_2=2nd dissociation constants.

(d) X-ray and electron diffraction

Configuration can be determined using X-ray crystallography. X-ray crystallographic analysis of sorbic acid gave its trans configuration.

(e) Spectroscopic method

Spectroscopic method based upon trans isomer will have higher λ-max than corresponding cis isomer.

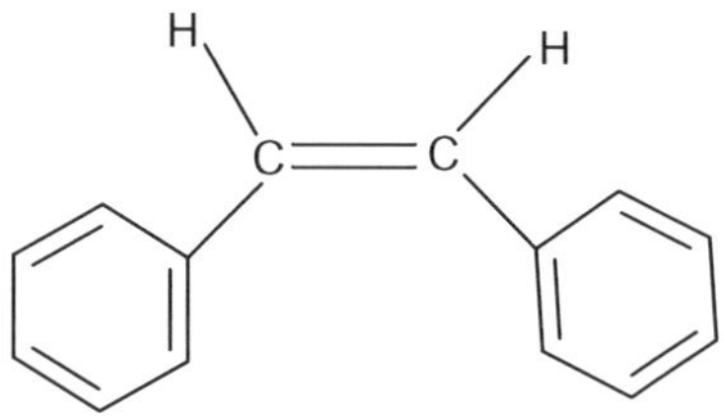

Cis - stilbene λ-max=278 n.m

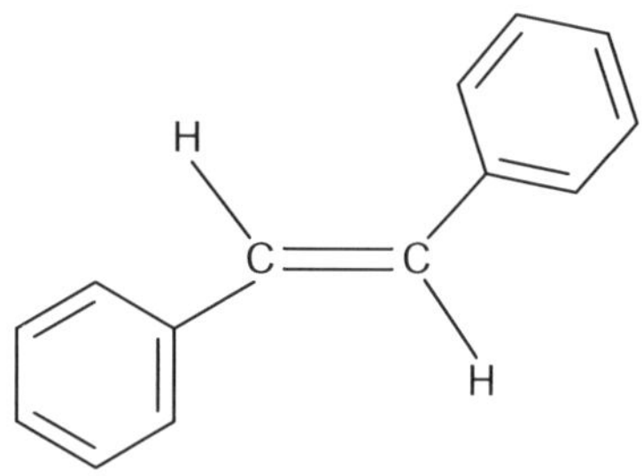

trans stilbene λ-max = 294 n.m

NMR spectroscopy also used to distinguish geometrical isomers, because trans vinyl protons are more strongly coupled to each other than cis vinyl protons.

Eg: Stibenes

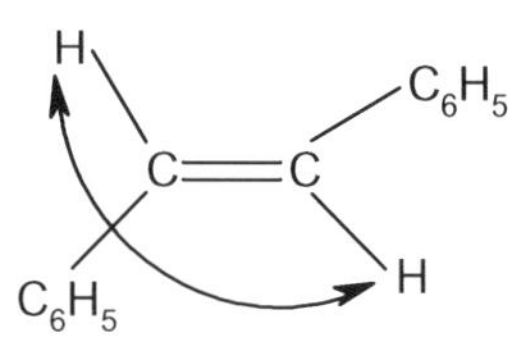

trans - stilbene
coupling constant 15.8

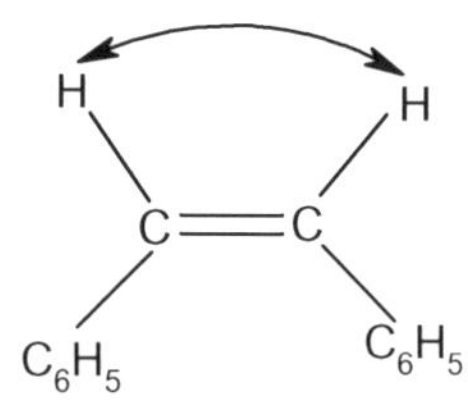

Cis - stilbene
coupling constant 12.3

5. By stereoselective reaction

In these reactions one stereoisomer is formed in more amount than the other. Hydrogenation of alkyne with sodium or Lithium in liquid ammonia gives a mixture of trans and cis alkenes in which trans isomer predominates. On the otherhand hydrogenation of alkyne using palladised charcoal gives cis alkene with a small amount of trans alkene.

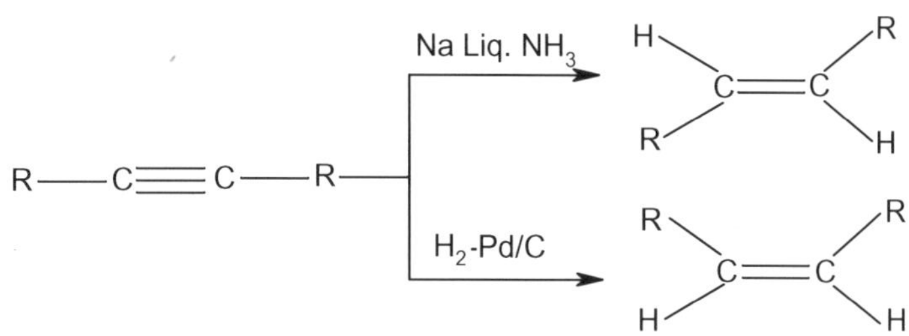

Reactions which yield predominantly one stereoisomer of several possible stereoisomers are called stereo selective reactions.

6. Stereospecific reactions

In these reactions, the formation of product is specific with respect to the stereoisomer. That is different stereoisomeric starting materials give rise to different stereoisomeric products.

Eg: In Reduction

The catalytic hydrogenation of olefins or acetylenes give rise to cis addition and a meso product is obtained if starting material is cis-isomer. A(±) product is obtained if starting material is trans isomer.

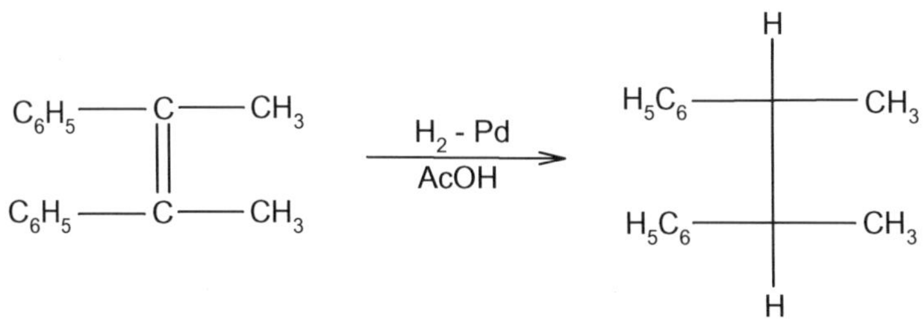

Cis-2, 3 Diphenyl butene — meso-2, 3 Diphenyl butane

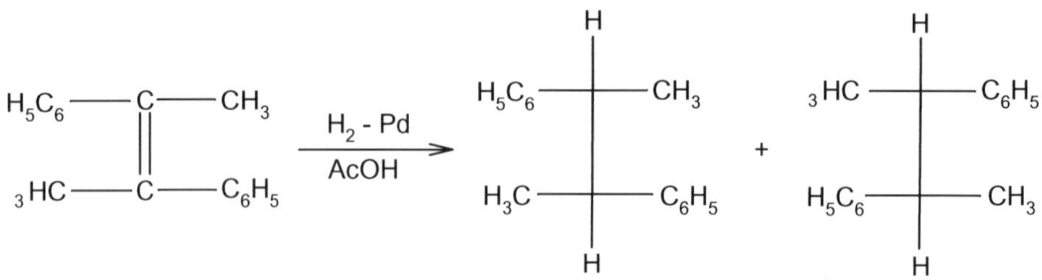

trans-2, 3 Diphenyl butene — (±) 2, 3 Diphenyl butane.

In Hydroxylation

The hydroxylation of alkenes if carried out by means of OsO_4, $KMnO_4$, H_2O_2 proceeds in cis fashion. Eg: Maleic acid (cis) and Fumaric acid (trans) give meso and (±) tartaric acid respectively.

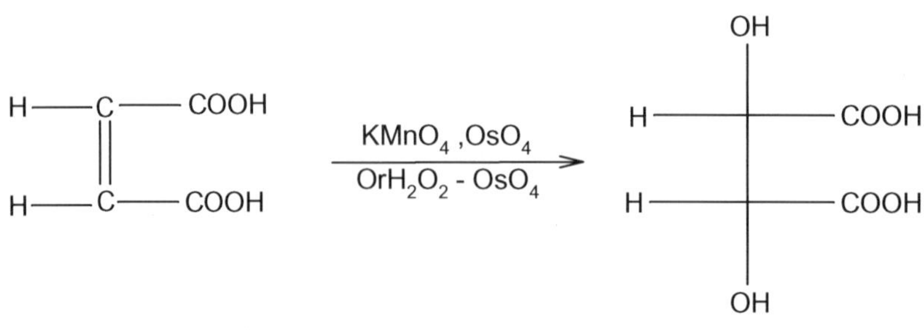

Maleic acid — Meso tartaric acid.

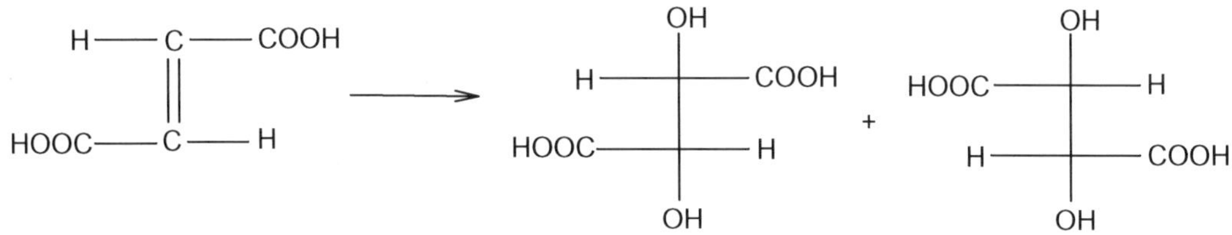

Fumaric acid (±) tartaric acid

However if hydroxylation is carried out with per acids or H_2O_2 in presence of SeO_2 a trans addition takesplace. Thus maleic acid and fumaric acid produce (±) and meso tartaric acid respectively.

Free radical addition

These additions on multiple linkage proceed in trans fashion.This type of addition is shown by addition of HBr to 1-methyl cyclohexene systems.

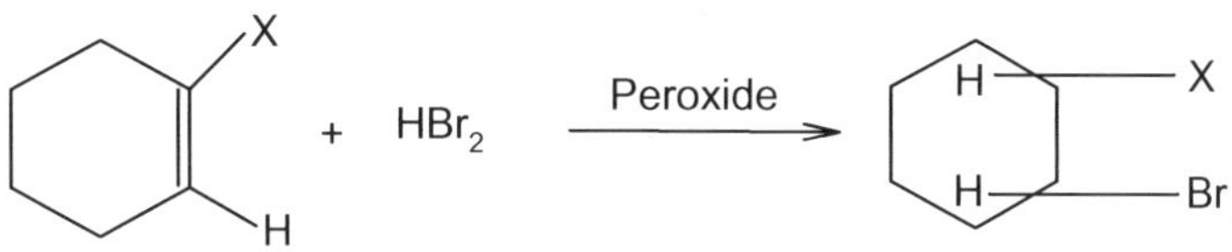

X $\equiv$ CH_3 / Br / Cl Trans - addition.

Diel's Alder reaction

Reaction of addition of a dienophile to a diene to form a cis-cyclic adduct is known as Diel's Alder reaction. The configuration of the adduct formed can be easily determined. So this reaction is used to determine the configuration of dienophile. Eg: The cis & trans Cinnamic acid with butadiene gives different adducts. So adducts are used to establish configuration of two Cinnamic acid.

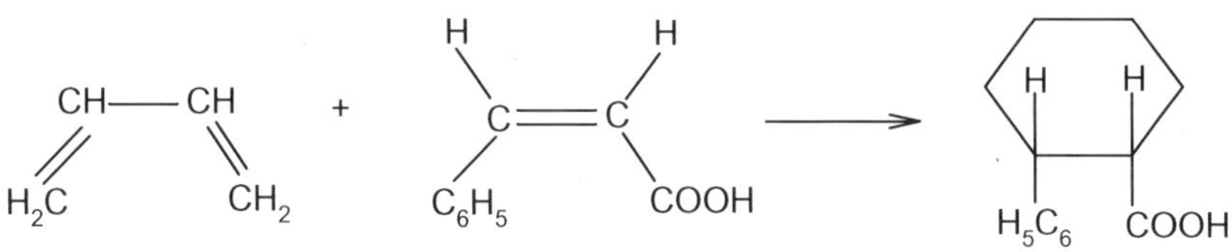

Butadiene Cis - Cinnamic acid Cis

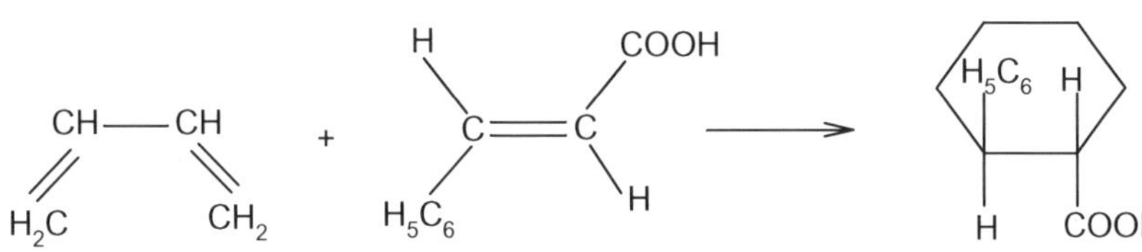

Butadiene trans - Cinnamic acid trans

Addition of Carbenes and Methylenes

Carbenes add on the double bond of alkenes in cis fashion. The two non-bonded electrons in: CR_2 may have paired or unpaired spin.If the spin is paired, the compound is in singlet state and known as 'Carbene'. If the spin is unpaired, the compound is in triplet state and called methylene. The addition of Carbene is stereospecific and a trans olefin will produce trans 1,2 disubstituted Cyclopropane.

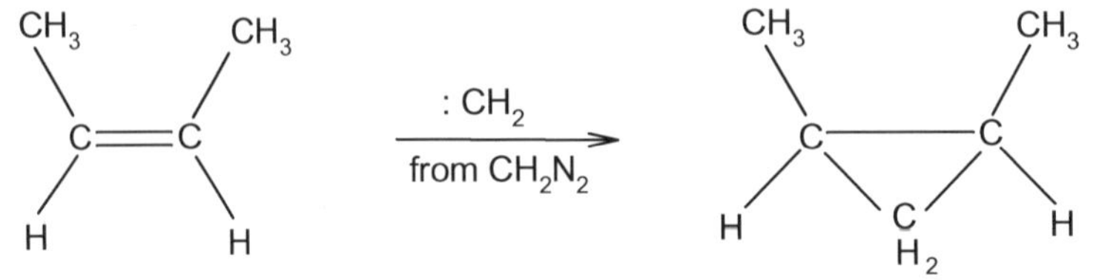

Cis Cis

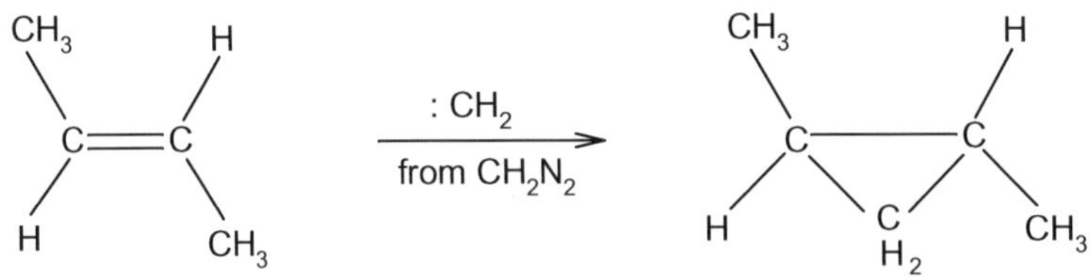

trans trans

Elimination reaction

The important stereospecific elimination reactions are the formation of acetylenes or olefines. When the atoms or groups to be eliminated are in trans position with respect to each other the reaction proceeds rapidly as compared to that when two groups are cis to each other.

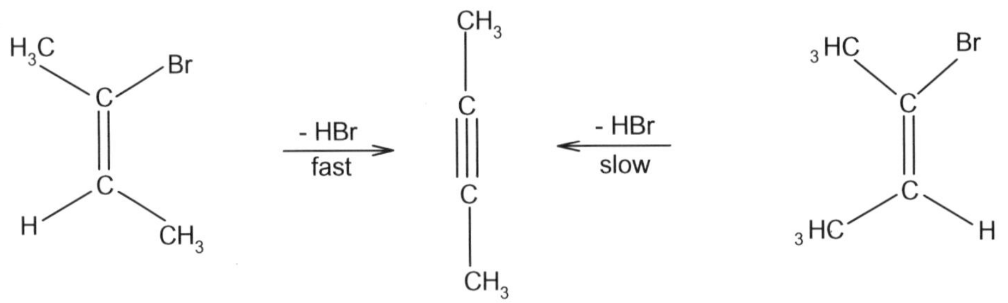

trans - 2 bromo - but -2ene bute-2-yne Cis-2-bromo-but-2ene

GEOMETRICAL ISOMERISM OF NITROGEN CONTAINING COMPOUND OXIMES

In Oximes geometrical isomerism is due to C=N bond.Free rotation in Oximes is restricted due to the presence of C=N bond (analogous to C=C bond in ethylenic compound) the Oximes may exist in two forms, quite analogous to cis and trans forms of ethylene compounds.

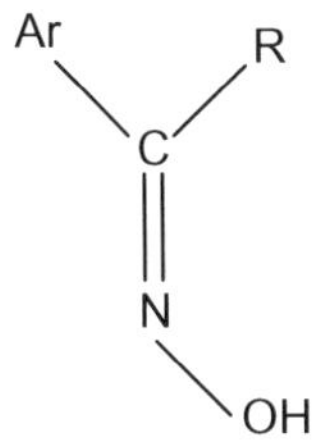

analogous to cis

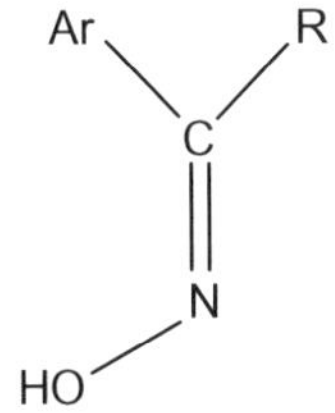

analogous to trans

Geometrical isomerism in Oximes, will disappear as soon as the two alkyl groups become similar, that is when Ar=R. In aldoximes when hydrogen and hydroxyl groups are on same side, the isomer is syn (analogous to cis) and when these groups are on opposite sides, the isomer is anti (analogous to trans)

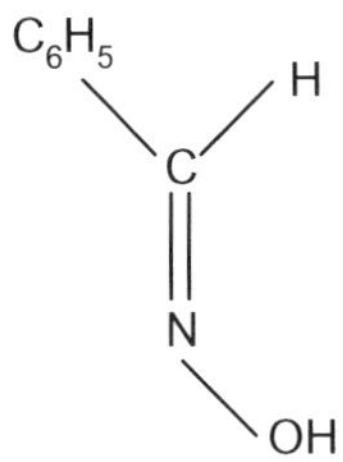

Syn-benzaldoxime

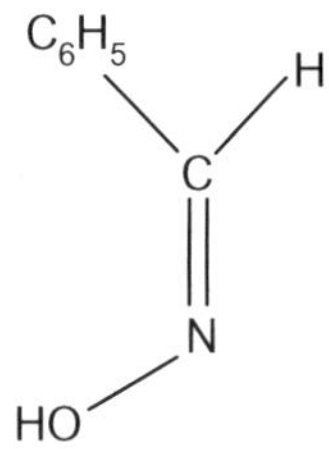

anti-benzaldoxime

In ketoximes the prefixes syn and anti indicate which group of ketoximes is syn (on the same side) or anti (on the opposite side) to hydroxyl group.

Oximes undergo rearrangement under acidic conditions to yield substituted amides.

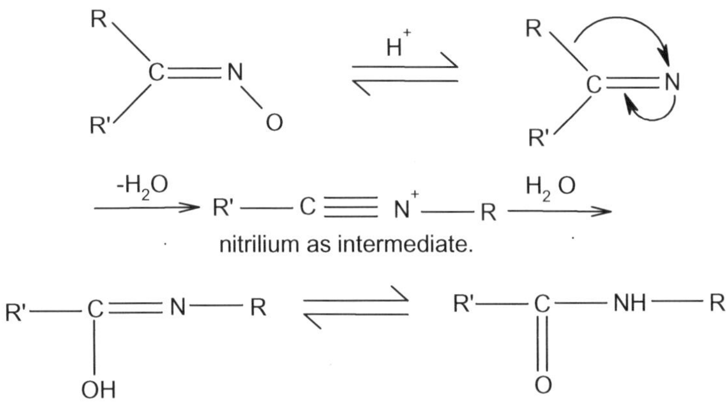

Beckmann rearrangement of oximes of 1-acetyl-2-hydroxy naphthalene-3-Carboxylic acid is antifashion. The anti-methyl oximes is resolvable as the hydroxyl group of the oxime interferes with that of the ring hydroxyl group and produces restricted rotation. The syn methyl oxime is not resolvable since rotation about the bond attached to C_1 atom of the ring is not sufficiently restricted.

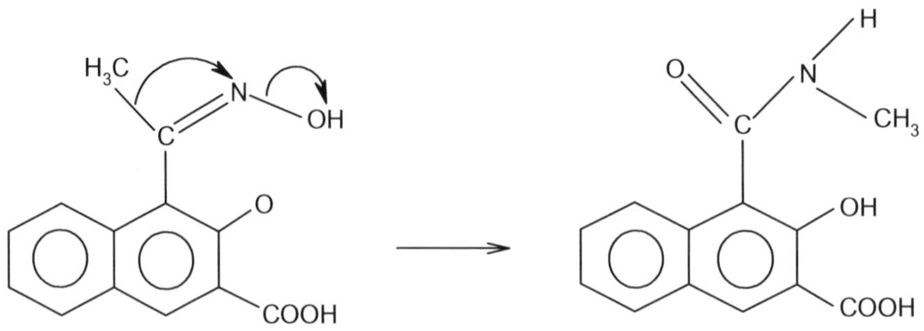

resolvable

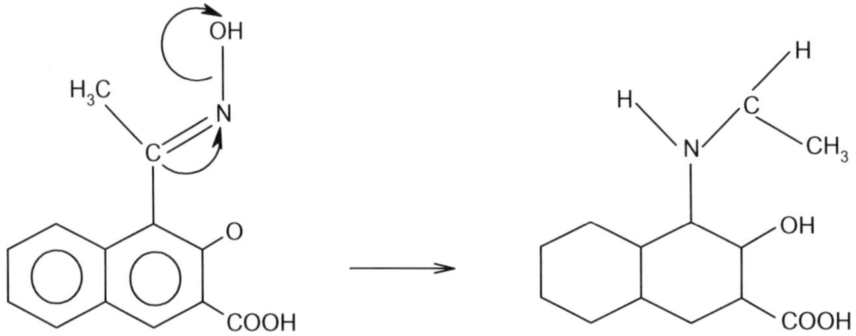

not resolvable

Stereo Chemistry of Cyclic Compounds

Consider 1-2 dimethylcyclopentane, it has two stereocentres & can exist in four stereoisomeric forms. However, it has only 3 stereoisomeric forms, the trans compound exist as a pair of enantiomers while cis-1,2 dimethyl cyclopentane is a meso compuond. It has a plane of symmetry that is perpendicular to the plane of ring.

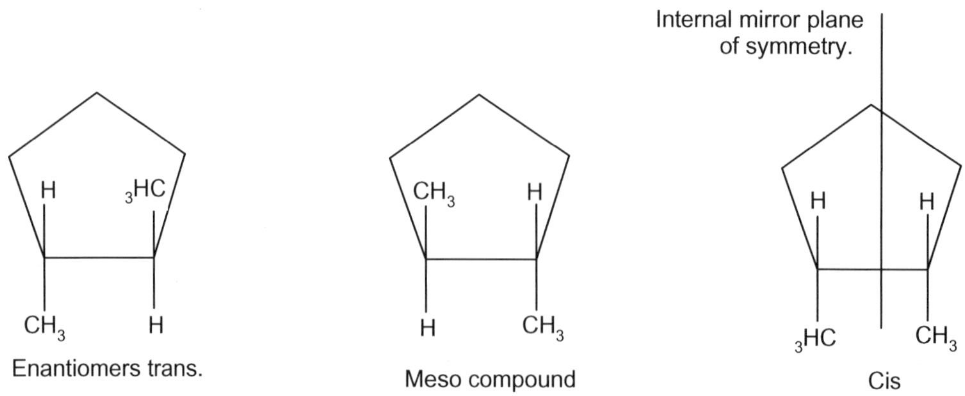

1,2 dimethyl cyclopentane have two stereocentres

In the case of 1,4 Dimethylcyclo hexane there is no tetrahedral atoms with four different groups 1,4 Dimethylcyclohexane exist as cis-trans isomers. The cis & trans forms are diastereomers. Neither compound is chiral & both forms have a plane of symmetry.

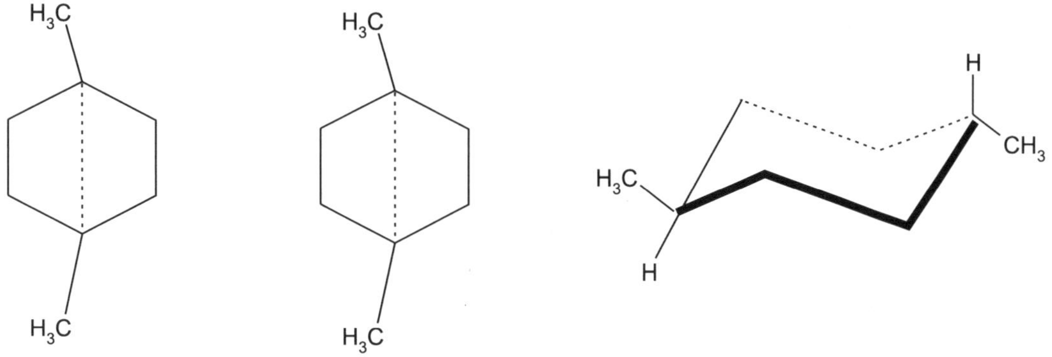

Cis 1,4 Dimethylcyclohexane   trans 1,4 - Dimethylcyclohexane

In Carbohydrate chemistry,pyranose sugars substituted with an electron withdrawing group such as halogen or alkoxy at C-1 are often more stable when the substituent occupies an axial orientation, rather than an equitorial one. The phenomenone is known as anomeric effect, since it involves substitutent at the anomeric position in Carbohydrate pyranose rings.

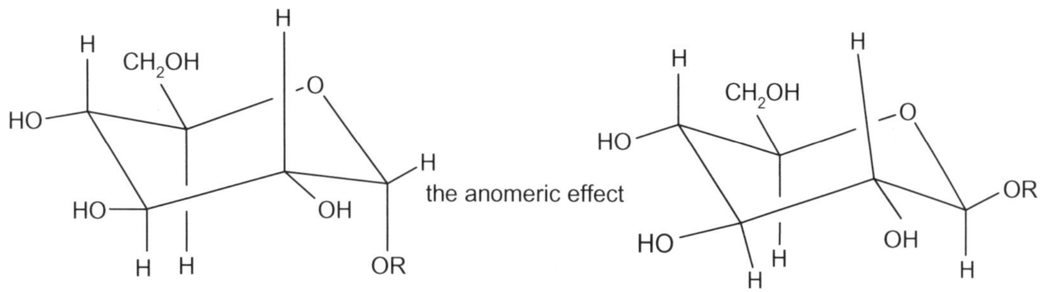

α-D glucoside   β-D glucoside

A polar group located on a Carbon alpha to a hetero atom prefers the axial position. An example of this phenomenon, known as the anomeric effect is the greater stability of alpha-glucosides over beta glucosides.

α-D glucose & β-D glucose are interconverted fairly rapidly in solution through the open chain tautomer, the beta-form predominates, as all the substituents are in equatorial positions. When crystalline α-D glucose is dissolved in H_2O, the initial specific rotation of the solution (111°) falls gradually to an equilibrium value of 52°30; the β-form has specific rotation 19°. The phenomenon is known as mutarotation.

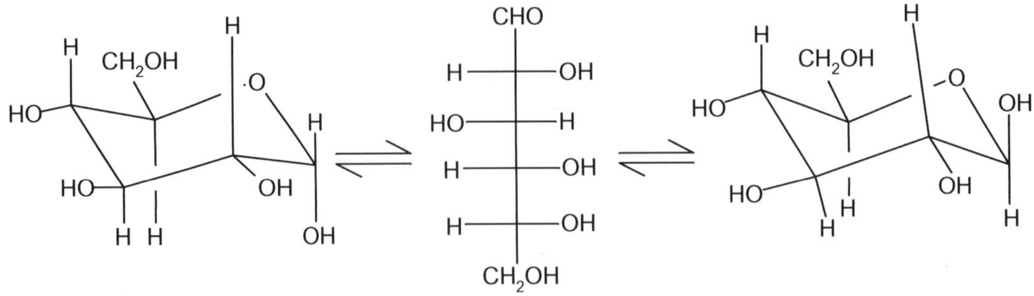

α-D glucose β-D glucose

Stereochemistry of Fused Rings – THE DECALINS

Decalin exists in two diastereoisomeric forms depending on the way in which the two cyclohexane rings are fused together. These diastereoisomers cannot be interconverted by bond rotations. Decalin can be considered as a fusion of four Carbon chain, that is CH_2-CH_2-CH_2-CH_2-to the chairs form of cyclohexane. Trans decalin is fused with this four Carbon chain in equatorial positions while in cis-decalin this fusion involves equatorial-axial positions. As a result in cis-decalin the two hydrogen atoms attached at the point of fusion between two rings lie in the same side of the ring while in trans-decalin, they are on opposite sides.

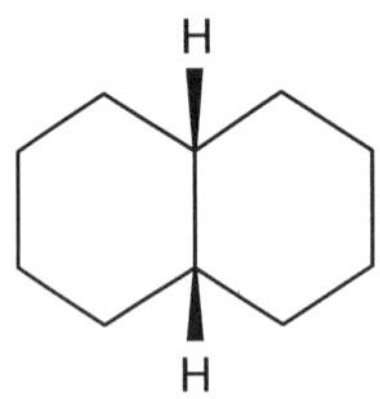

Cis -decalin

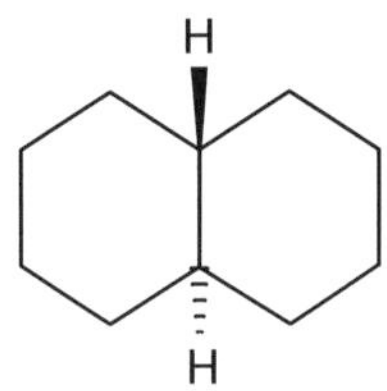

trans - decalin

Cis-decalin exists as an equilibrium between two enantiomeric all chair conformations which are interconvertable as a result of conformational flipping. As a result, any substituent attached to cis-decalin system is more or less free to adopt the equatorial orientation. Cis-decalin is disymmetric in both conformations which are non-superimpossible mirror images of each other. Because of rapid ring flipping between these forms, the compound is a non-resolvable dl-pairs.

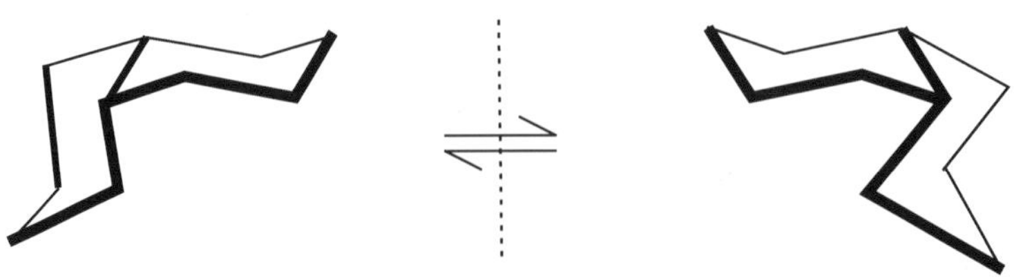

Cis Decalin
Two enantiomeric conformations

Trans-decalin has a unique & rigid conformation,interconversion of which is not possible, as it would otherwise afford a highly strained system with one ring attached to the other by two axial bonds. Trans-decalin has a centre of symmetry & is therefore optically inactive.

Simple rotation of group about Carbon-Carbon bonds cannot bring about inter-conversion of cis & trans decalins. Therefore in this respect,in decalins, the 1-2-substituents are the two ends of four Carbon chain. Trans-decalin as a result is stable by about 2.7 Kcal/mole compound to cis form.

HYBRIDISATION

Hybridisation is defined as the concept of mixing or merging of orbitals of an atom having nearly equal energy, to produce entirely new orbitals which have same energy content and identical shapes.

Atomic orbitals of an atom undergo hybridisation should satisfy following conditions,

(i) Only the orbitals of an isolated single atom can undergo hybridisation.

(ii) The hybridising orbitals must differ only slightly in their energy content.

The 3 types of hybridisation encountered in organic chemistry are SP^3, SP^2 & SP hybridisation.

Tetrahedral or SP^3 hybridisation

This type of hybridisation involves mixing of one S & three 2P pure orbitals of excited Carbon atom.The bond angle is 109° 28'.

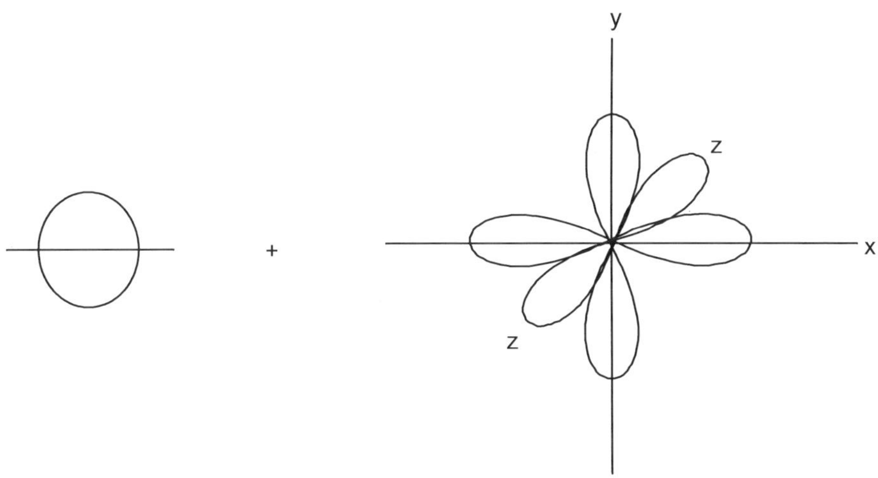

An individual SP^3 hybrid orbital has following shape.

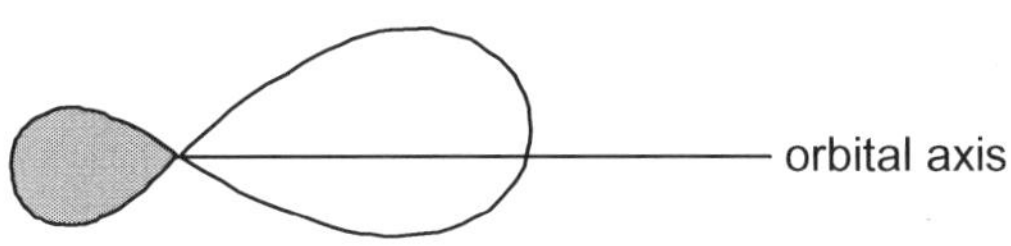

Here whole of the hybrid orbitals is concentrated on one side of the nucleus with a small tail extending in the opposite direction.This distribution of the orbital allows it to overlap more efficiently than an individually S or P orbital an orbital of another atom placed on the orbital axis on the heavy side (called head) to form a strong covalent bond.

Eg: Methane

In methane 4 hybridised orbitals of Carbon overlaps with 1S orbital of hydrogen atom to form four sigma bonds between Carbon and hydrogen by the overlapping of orbitals along the internuclear axis (head to head overlapping sigma bond)

Thus methane molecule can be represented as

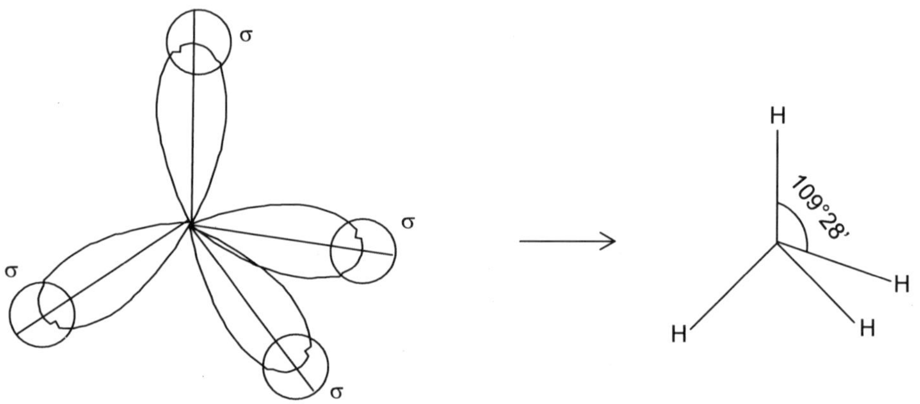

So SP^3 hybridisation takesplace in the formation of alkanes.

Trigonal or SP^2 hybridisation

This type of hybridisation involves mixing of one S orbital and two P orbitals (2Px & 2Py) to give three equivalent orbitals known as SP^2 hybrid orbitals. It's bond angle is 120°.

Here one Porbital is not involved in hybridisation & pure 'P' orbital directed at right angles to the plane of SP^2 orbitals.

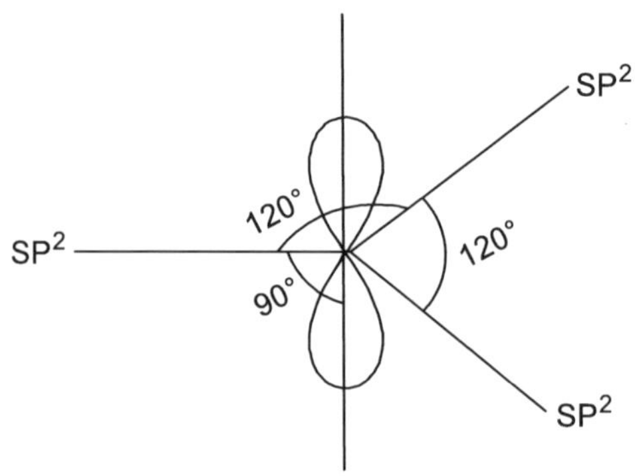

This type of SP^2 hybridisation takes place to form C=C & C=O bonds.

Eg: ethylene.

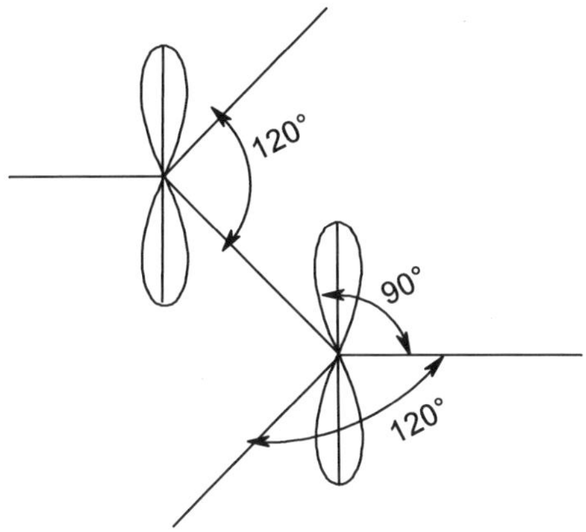

The two unhybridized (pure) P orbitals are in the same plane with each other.

Diagonal or SP hybridisation

This type of hybridisation involves, mixing of one S and one P orbitals to form two equivalent collinear orbitals which are directed in a straight line with an angle of 180° & the unhybridised two P orbitals remains pure.

This type of hybridisation takes place in the formation of Carbon-Carbon triple bond. Eg: acetylenes.

6

Chemistry of Biomolecules

CARBOHYDRATES

INTRODUCTION

Carbohydrates are polyhydric alcohols having potentially active aldehyde and ketone groups.

Carbohydrates are widely distributed in plants and animals having vital roles in day to day life. Some of them serving as source of energy while some are storage of energy. Some fruit sugars yield alcohol on fermentation. Many of their products, and derived products are valuable like cotton, linen, jute, straw, grass, paper, Iaquer, paints and explosives. Ribose of RNA and deoxyribose of DNA are carbohydrates.

NOMENCLATURE

The suffix- 'ose' is employed for naming sugars.

According to the type of carbonyl groups that is Aldoses for aldehyde and ketoses for ketone groups have been assigned. Some individual names reflects origin and history of them eg: Milk sugar namely lactose is derived from latin word lactis means milk.

CLASSIFICATION

Carbohydrates are broadly classified into sugars and non-sugars (polysaccharides). Sugars are again classsified into monosaccharides, Disaccharides & oligosaccharides.

Monosaccharides

Monosaccharides contain only one molecule of sugar and they cannot be broken into simpler substances by hydrolysis. Monosaccharides are again classified according to the number of carbon atoms present is as follows:

Diose: having two carbon atoms, Eg: Glycolaldehyde
Triose: having three carbon atoms, Eg: Glyceraldehyde

Tetrose: having four carbon atoms, Eg: Erythrose

Pentose: having five carbon atoms, Eg: Ribose

Hexose: having six carbon atoms, Eg: Glucose

Heptose: having seven carbon atoms, Eg: Glucoheptose.

Disaccharides

Disaccharides are sugars which on hydrolysis give two moles of same or different monosaccharides.

Eg: 1) $\underset{\text{Maltose}}{C_{12}H_{22}O_{11}} + H_2O \longrightarrow \underset{\text{Glucose}}{C_6H_{12}O_6} + \underset{\text{Glucose}}{C_6H_{12}O_6}$

2) $\underset{\text{Sucrose}}{C_{12}H_{22}O_{11}} + H_2O \longrightarrow \underset{\text{Glucose}}{C_6H_{12}O_6} + \underset{\text{Fructose}}{C_6H_{12}O_6}$

Oligosaccharides

Oligosaccharides are sugars which on hydrolysis give three to 10 moles of same or different monosaccharides.

Eg: For Trisaccharide: Raffinose $C_{18}H_{32}O_{16}$

For Tetrasaccharide: Stachyose $C_{24}H_{42}O_{21}$

For pentas accharide: Verbascose $C_{30}H_{52}O_{26}$

Non Sugars or polysaccharides

Polysacchaccharides are long chains or polymers of monosaccharides. These are usually tasteles amorphous solids and either insoluble in water or form colloidal suspension. On hydrolysis by dilute acids, polysaccharides yield sweet monosaccharides.If they proudce same types of monosaccharides, then known as homopolysaccharides. If they produce different types of monosaccharides then known as heteropolysaccharides.

Eg: Starch, Glycogen, Cellulose, Inulin etc.

CHEMICAL PROPERTIES OF MONOSACCHARIDES

Glucose and fructose are taking as model.

1. Oxidation

With different oxidising agents, monosaccharides give different products.

With Bromine Water

Bromine water oxidise aldose to corresponding aldonic acid, which on evaporation gives stable γ-lactone. This lactone can be reduced back into parent compound by birch reduction.

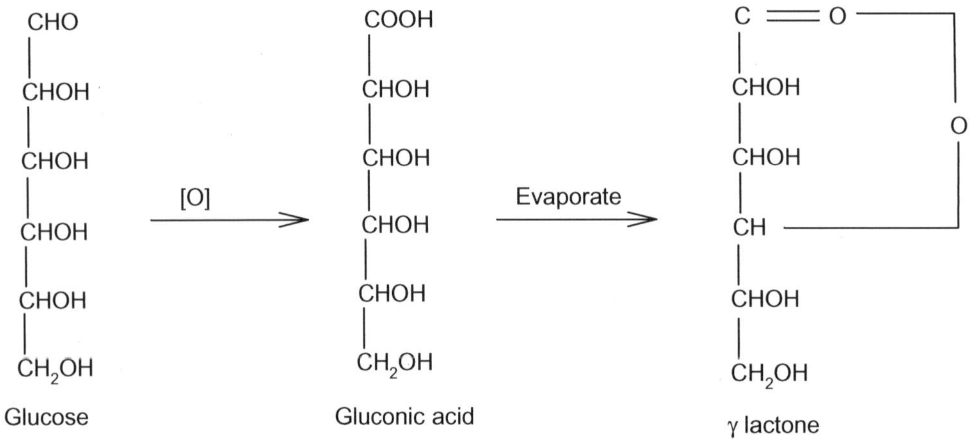

Bromine water do not oxidise ketoses.

With Nitric acid

Nitric acid oxidise aldose to dicarboxylic acid.

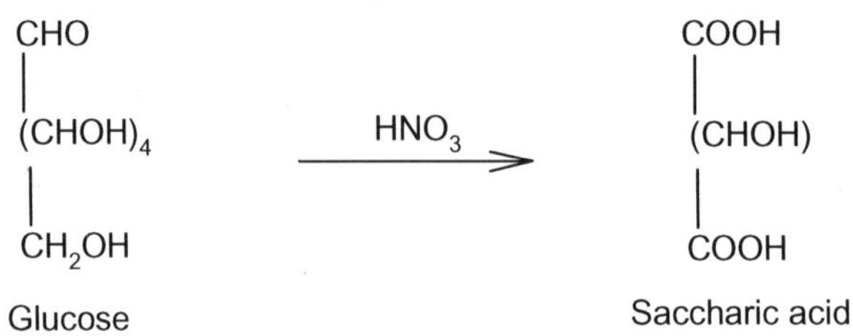

Nitric acid oxidise ketoses to a mixture of acids having fewer carbon atoms.

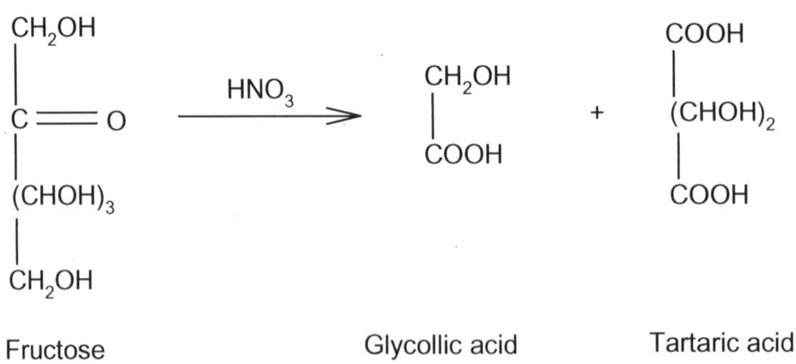

With lead tetra-acetate and periodic acids

These reagents oxidize 1,2-glycolic portions of monosaccharide molecules (except compounds devoid of two hydroxyl groups on two adjacent carbon atoms) rapture C-C bond to give dialdehydes.

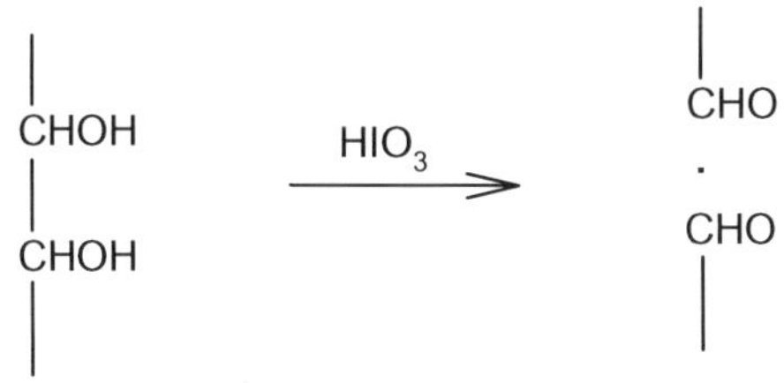

With Benedict's or Tollen's reagent

Benedicts reagent (an alkaline solution of copper sulphate complexed with citrate ion) and Tollen's reagent (alkaline silver nitrate solution) are mild oxidising agents. Both reagents (active species are $Cu(OH)_2$ & Ag_2O respectively) Oxidise aldoses to respected aldonic acid and themselves get reduced. So the sugars undergo oxidation by these reagents are known as reducing sugars.

$$R.CHO + Cu(OH)_2 \longrightarrow R.COOH + Cu_2O\downarrow$$

$$R.CHO + Ag_2O \longrightarrow R.COOH + 2Ag\downarrow$$

Both reagents oxidise ketoses having α-hydroxy ketonic group. Eg: fructose.

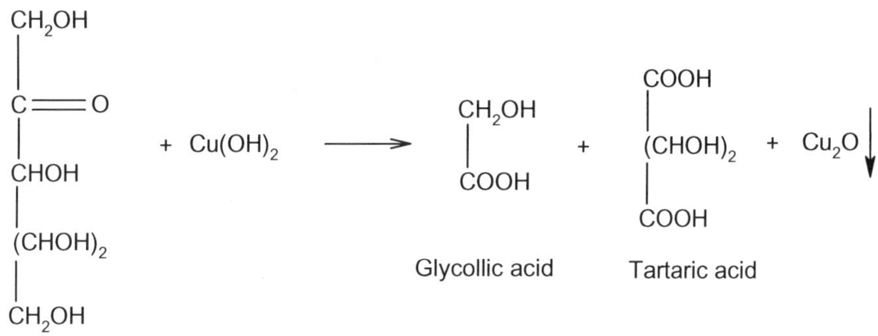

Glycollic acid Tartaric acid

Fructose

2. Reduction

Hydriodic acid and phosphorus reduces hydroxyl groups to methylene groups. Sugars undergo reduction at a high pressure inthe presence of catalysts like nickel, copper or sodium borohydride give alcohols. Aldoses give one alcohol while ketoses give a mixture of two alcohols

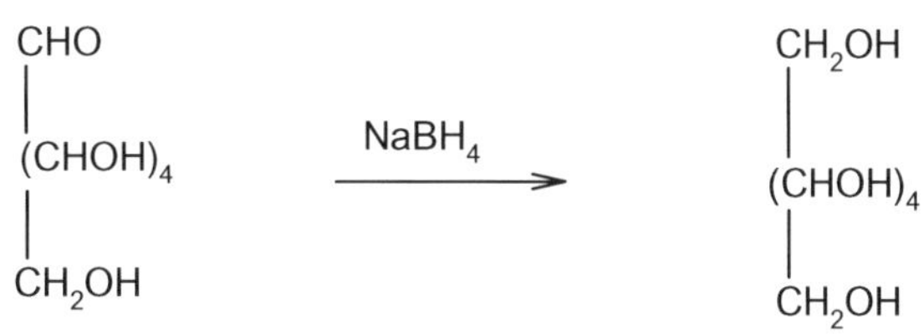

Glucose (Aldose) Sorbitol

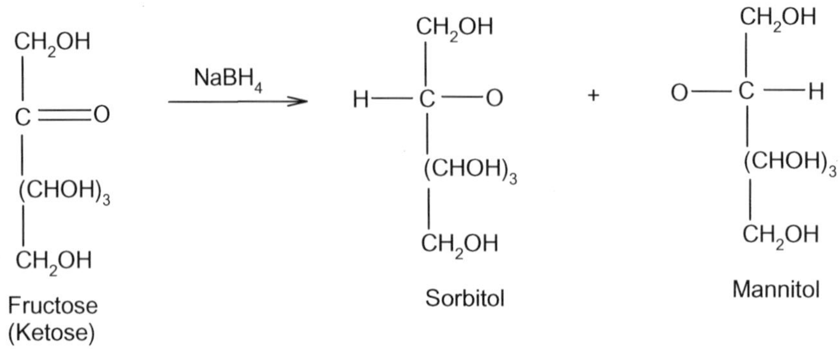

3. Acetylation

Monosaccharides on reaction with acetic anhydride, the hydroxyl groups are converted to esters; So by this reaction number of hydroxyl group present in sugar can be determined.

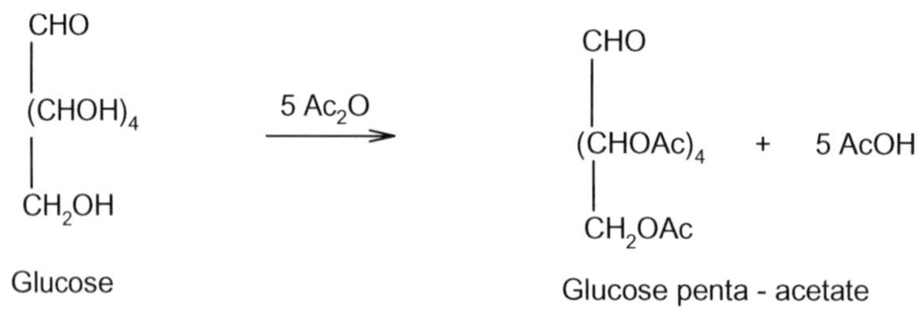

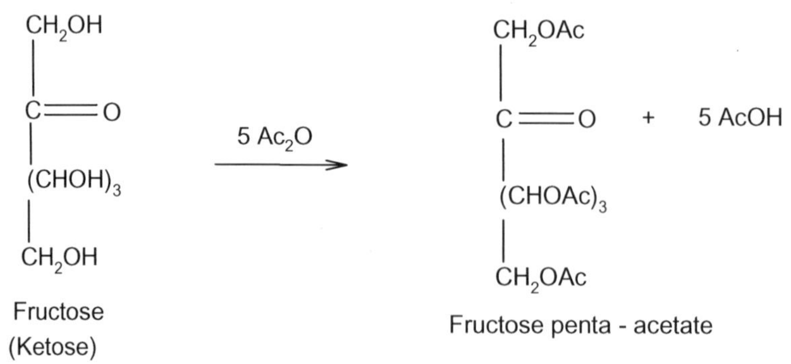

4. Glycoside Formation

Monosaccharides on treating with methanolic hydrogenchloride forms two isomeric compounds known as methyl glycosides. During the reaction aldehyde group is converted to acetal group which is stable in alkaline medium and labile in acidic medium.

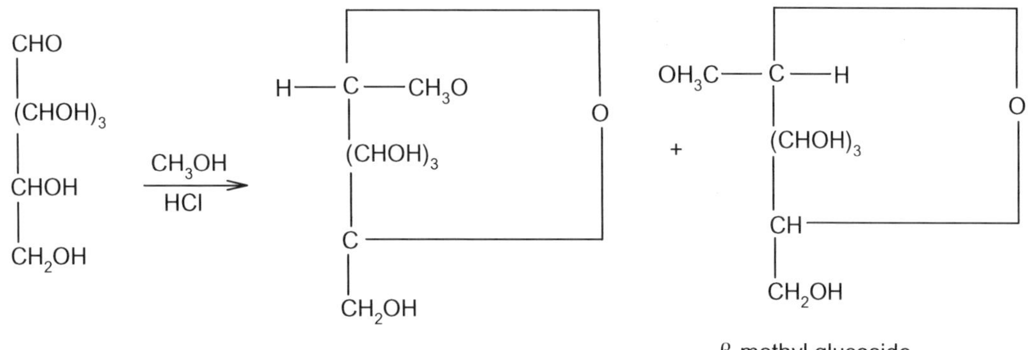

Glucose α-methyl glucoside β-methyl glucoside

5. Reacton with phenylhydrazine

Sugars react with one mole of phenyl hydrazine forms phenyl hydrazones while with excess phenyl hydrazine forms osazones. Two types of mechanisms namely Fischer's mechanism as well as weygand's mechamism are involved in the formation of Osazones.

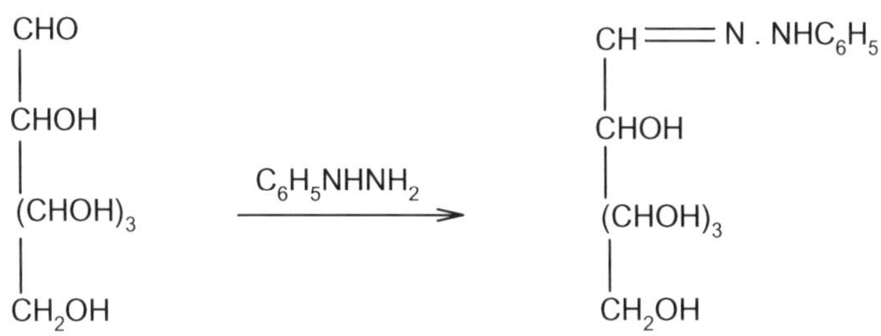

Glucose Glucose Phenyl hydrazone

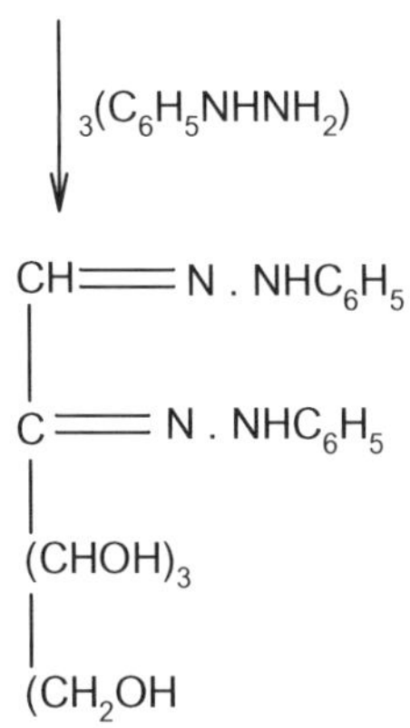

Glucosazone

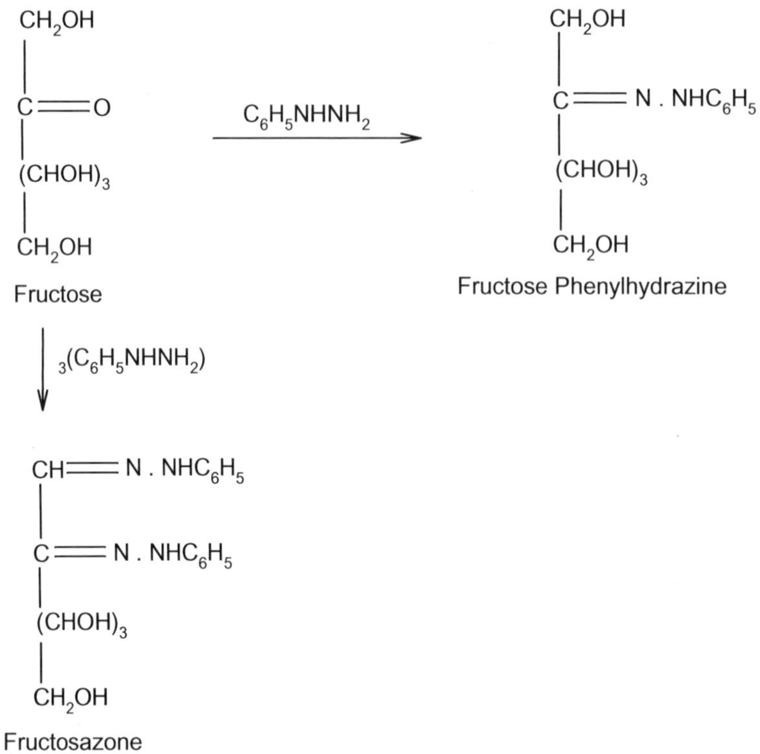

6. Epimerisation

Epimers are optical isomers which differ in the configuration at only one asymmetric carbon atom (C_2). The process of converting one epimer to other ie ...inversion of configuration at one assymmetric centre, without affecting other asymmetric centres is known as epimerisation.

To make epimer, aldonic acid is heated to 150°C in aqueous pyridine or quinoline. So that acid and epimer forms in equal amounts, which are separated.

Eg: Epimerisation of glucose to mannose.

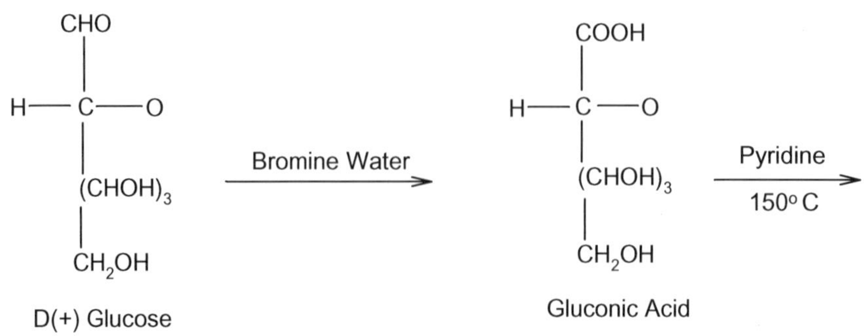

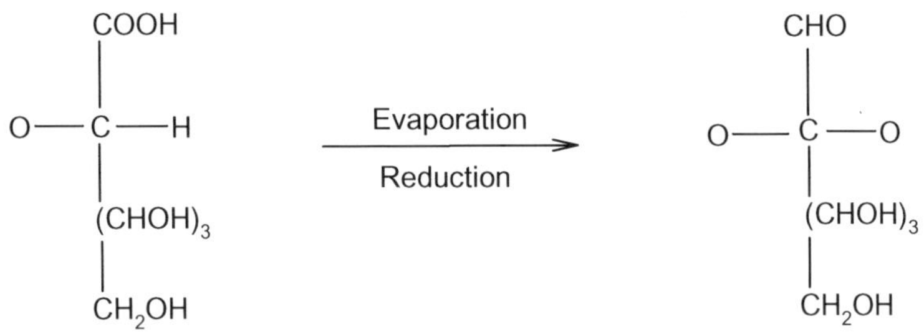

Mannonic acid D(+) Mannose

7. Action of alkali

On reaction with alkali sugars undergo rearrangement, forms mixture of sugars. This is also known as Lobry de Broyn-Van Ekenstein Reaction.

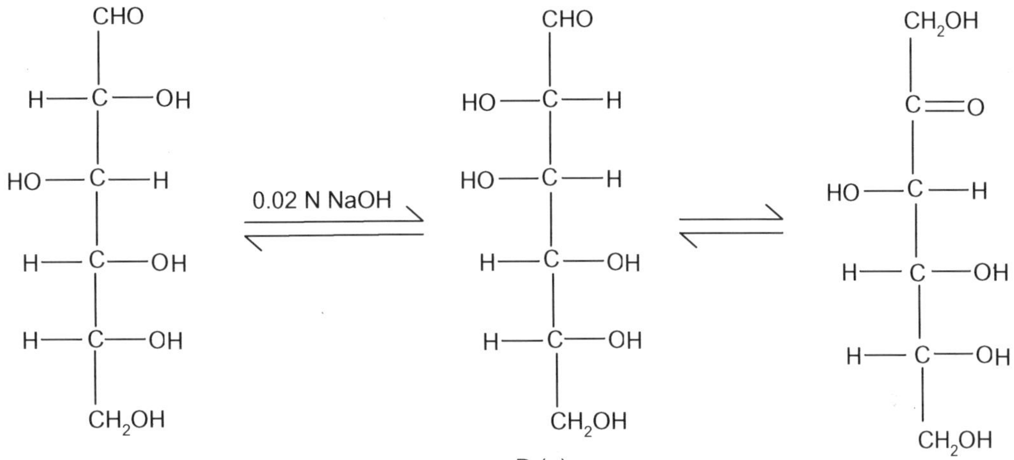

D (+) glucose D (+) mannose

INTERCONVERSIONS OCCURING IN MONOSACCHARIDES

Conversion of an aldose into respective ketose

Aldose is converted to osazone, which is treated with concentrated acid or benzaldehyde to give ozone, thus remove phenyl hydrazine residue. The ozone is reduced with zinc and acetic acid to produce ketose.

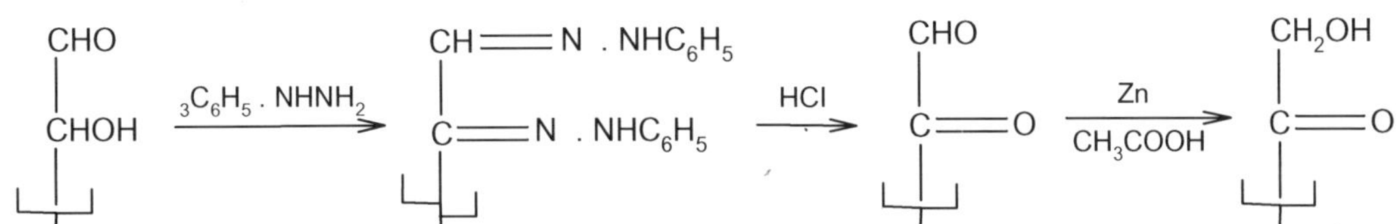

Aldose Osazine Ozone Fructose

Conversion of an aldose into the next higher ketose

This is achieved through Arndt-Eistert reaction. Eg: Arabinose → Fructose. Here arabinose is an aldopentose which is oxidised and then acetylated. Acetylated product is, Chlorinated to produce acid chloride, which undergo Arndt-Eistert synthesis to produce higher alcohol which is treated with alkali to produce fructose.

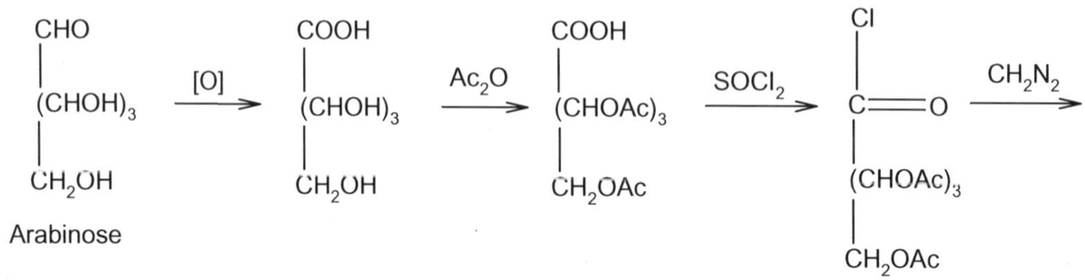

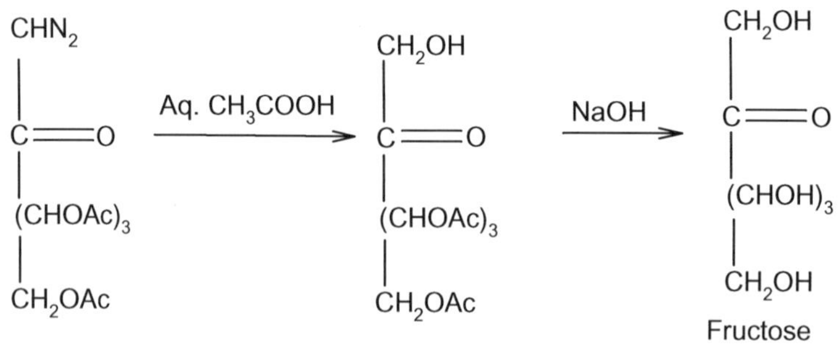

Conversion of ketose into corresponding aldose

Ketose is catalytically reduced into corresponding alcohol, which is carefully oxidised to a monocarboxylic acid, which undergo lactonization, then reduction to produce aldose.

Eg: Fructose ⟶ Glucose

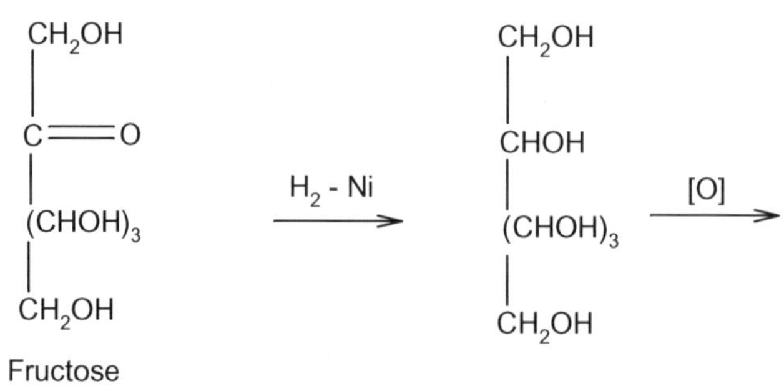

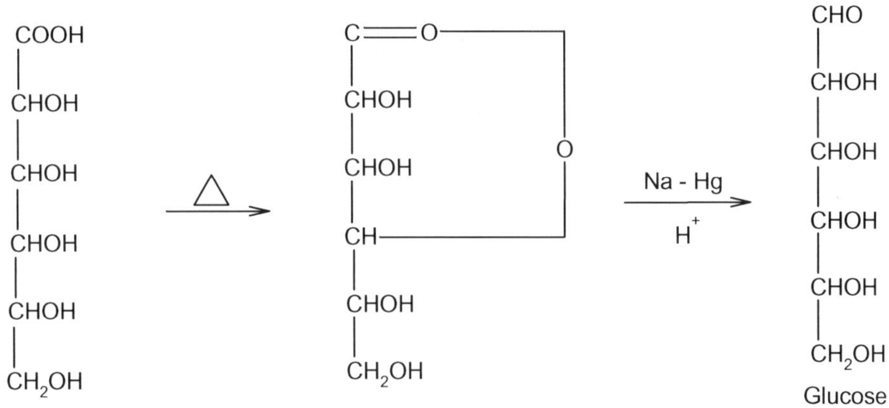

Apart from these interconversions, specified synthetic methods are there to produce same higher series compounds like Kiliani synthesis, sowden synthesis.

Kiliani Synthesis

In this lower aldose is treated with hydrogen cyanide, the cyanohydrin formed is hydrolysed to higher aldonic acid, which is lactonised and reduced to produces higher series aldose.

Eg: Arabinose ⟶ Glucose

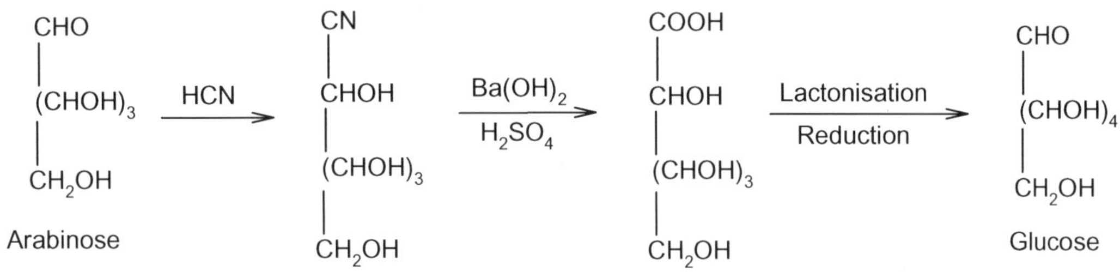

Kiliani's method can be utilized to produce having upto ten carbon atoms.

Swoden Synthesis

Nitromethane is used as an important reactant here therefore, this method is also known as Nitromethane synthesis. Here lower series aldose is condensed with nitromethane in the presence of methanolic sodium methoxide to form 1-nitro-1-deoxy compound which is converted to its sodium salt. Hydrolysis of sodium salt with cold diute sulphuric acid gives higher series aldose.

Eg: Arabinose ⟶ Glucose

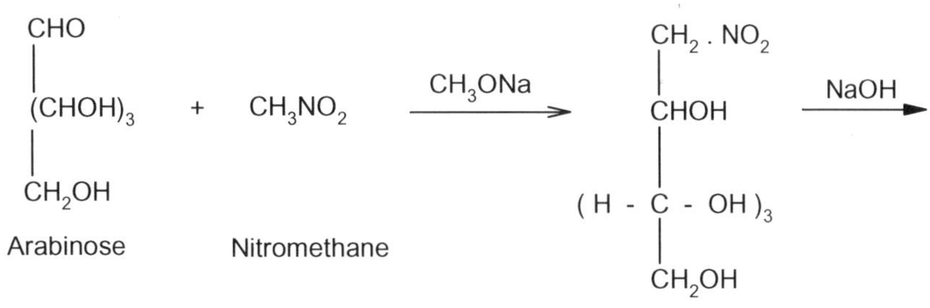

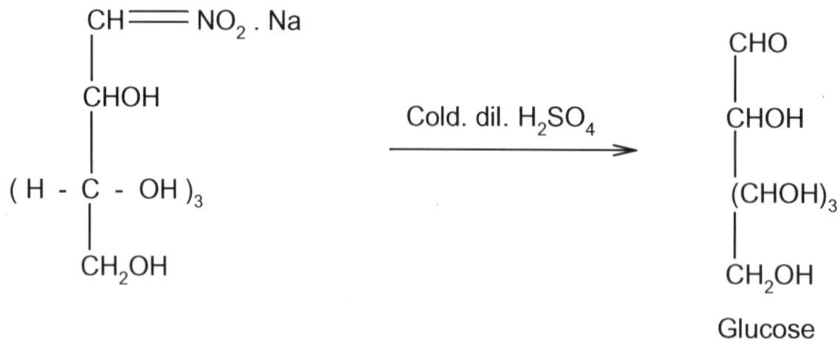

As we have seen above, higher series compound can be converted to lower series compound, by various methods like wohl's method, weygand's method, Ruff's method, weerman's, method, Macdonald method etc.

Wohl's Method

In this method higher series aldose converted to oxime, which is heated with acetic anhydride in the presence of zinc chloride or sodium acetate, so that oxime will dehydrate to nitrile group and hydroxyl groups get acetylated. This on treatment with ammoniacal silver nitrate produce lower series aldose.

Eg: Hexose ⟶ Pentose

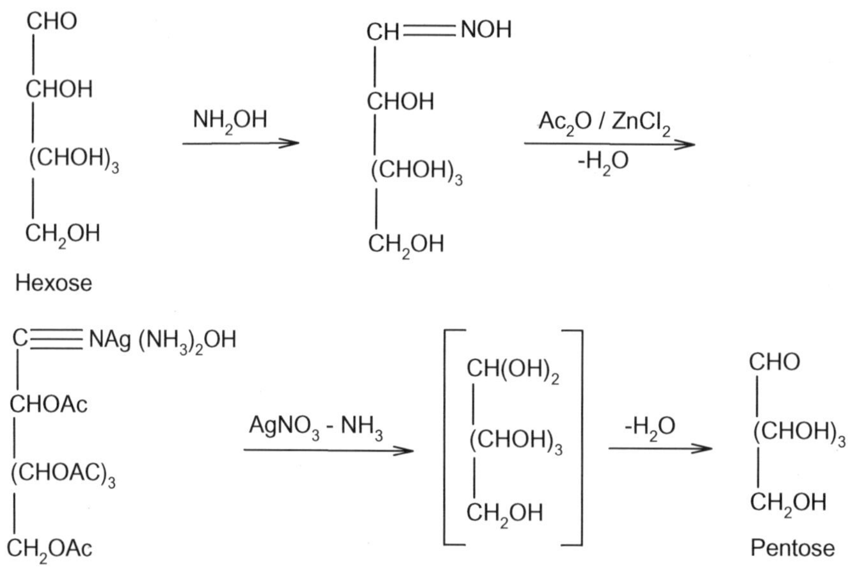

Weygand's Method

In this method oxime of the aldose is treated with 1-fluoro-2,4-dinitrobenzene and the product is again treated with warm sodium bicarbonate.

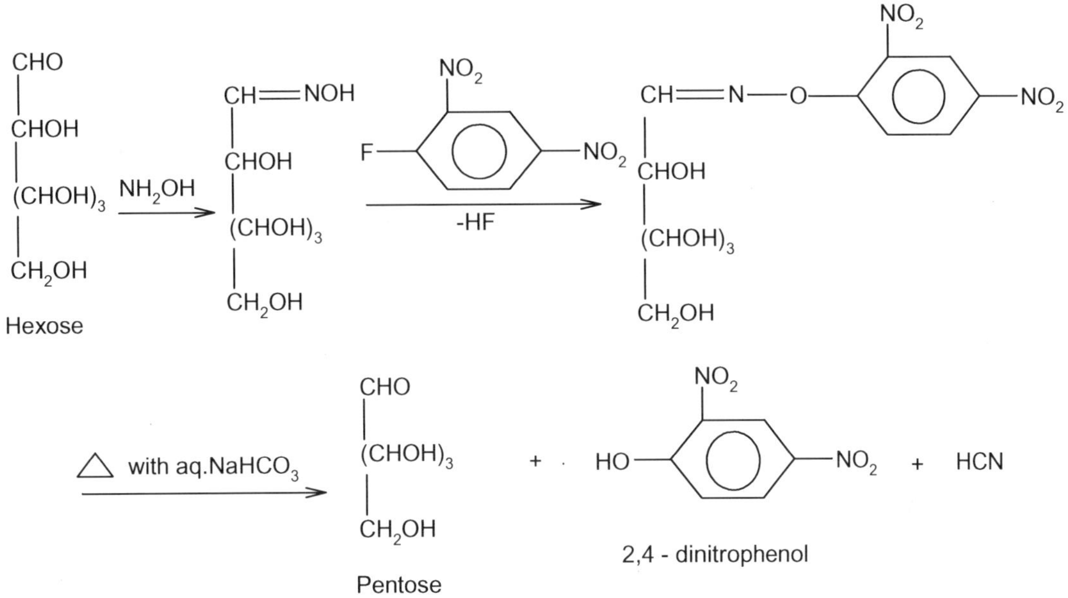

Ruff's Method

Here aldose oxidised to aldonic acid, which is conversted to its calcium salt, by lime water; then calcium salt again oxidised by H_2O_2 in the presence of $FeSO_4$ to a α-keto acid which is decarboxylated to give lower series Aldose.

Eg: Hexose ⟶ Pentose

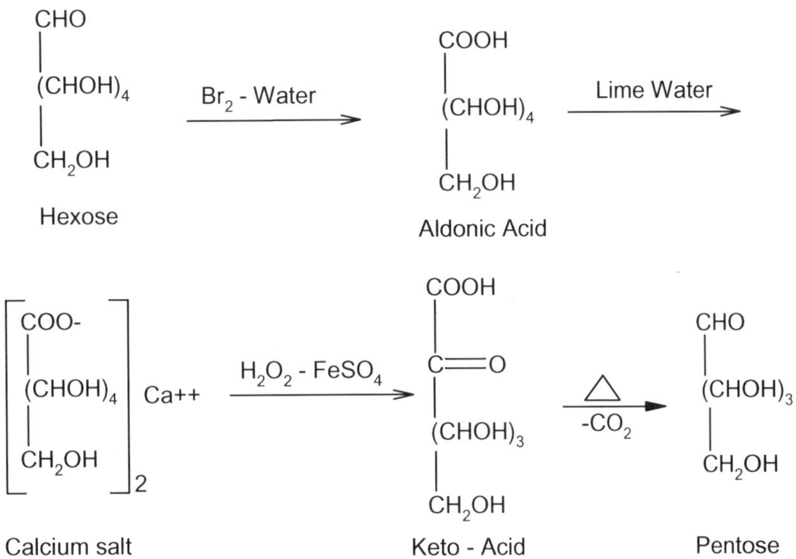

Combinaton of oxidising agent H_2O_2 in presence of $FeSO_4$ is also known as fenton's reagent.

Weerman's Method

Hof mann degradation is applied in the sugars series

Eg: Pentose ⟶ Tetrose

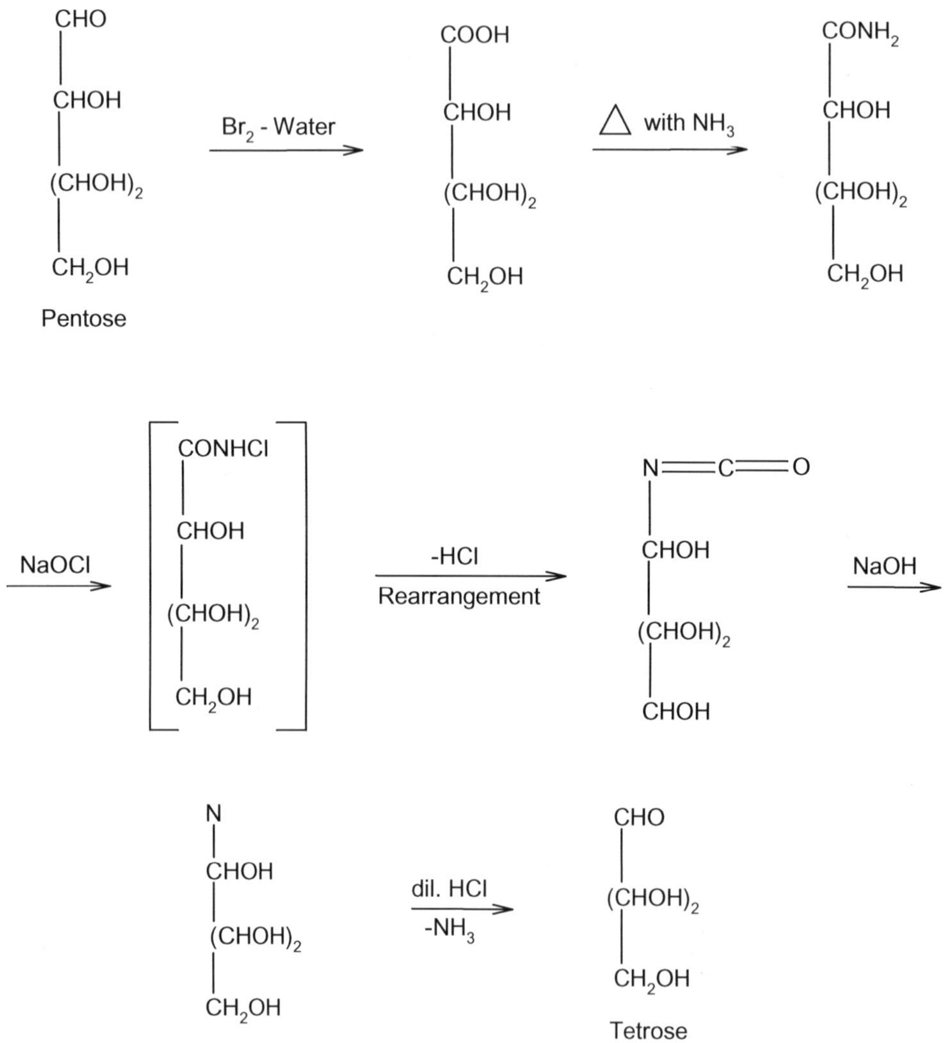

Mac Donald Method

Here aldose is treated with thiol derivative in presence of conc. HCl to give thioacetal, which is oxidised with peracid to form bis alkyl Sulphonyl derivative which on treatment with aqueous ammonia gives lower series aldose.

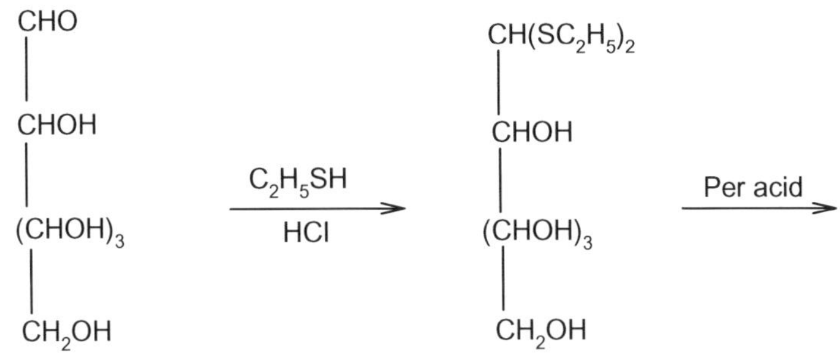

Hexose　　Mercaptal

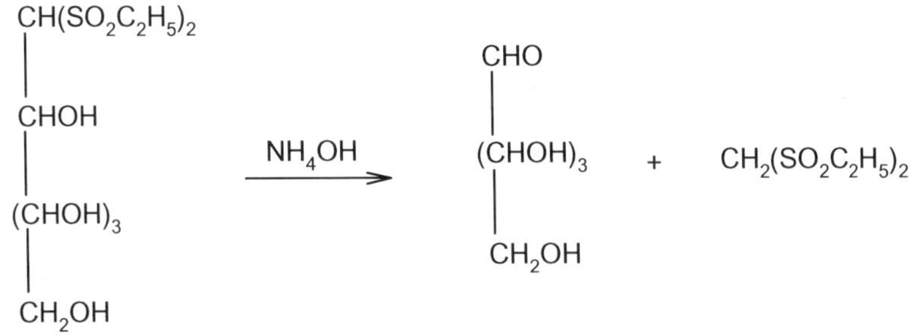

bis (ethyl Sulphonyl) derivative　　bis (ethyl Sulphonyl methane)

Configuration of Monosaccharides

Configuration means arrangement of atoms or groups at asymmetric carbon atom. For example $C_6H_{12}O_6$ is the molecular formula for hexoses. But there are sixteen different hexoses possesing similar structure as that of glucose like.

OHC—CHOH—CHOH—CHOH—CHOH—CH_2OH: Such sugars are called stereo isomers. Examples for stereoisomers are given here.

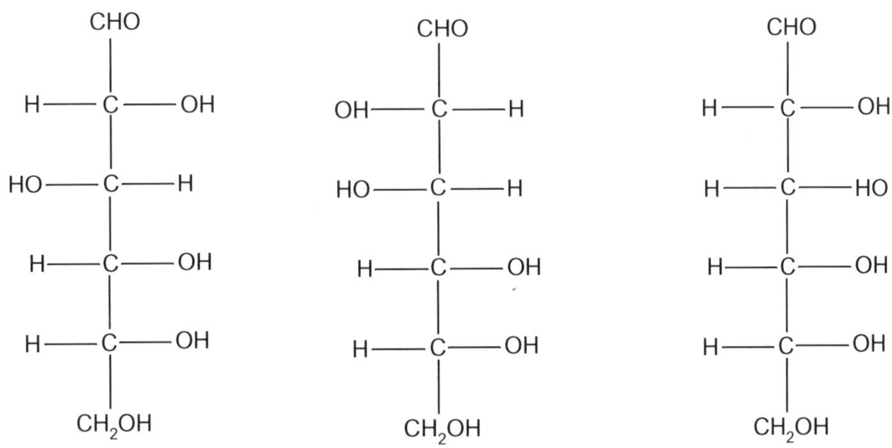

D - Glucose　　D - Mannose　　D - Allose

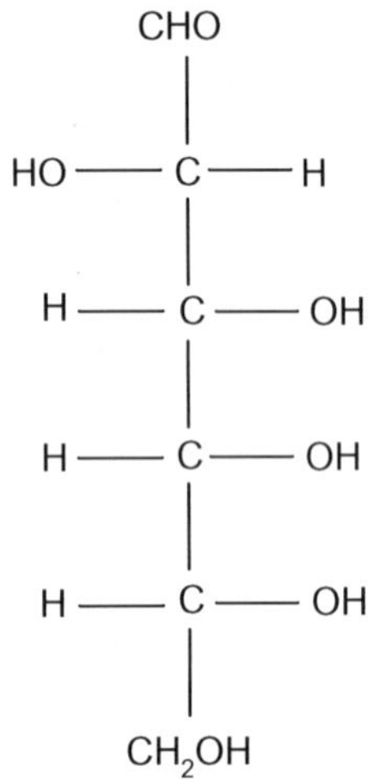

D - Attrose

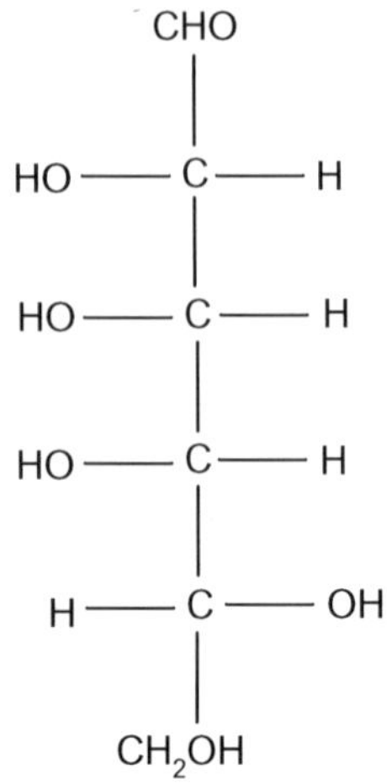

D - Talose

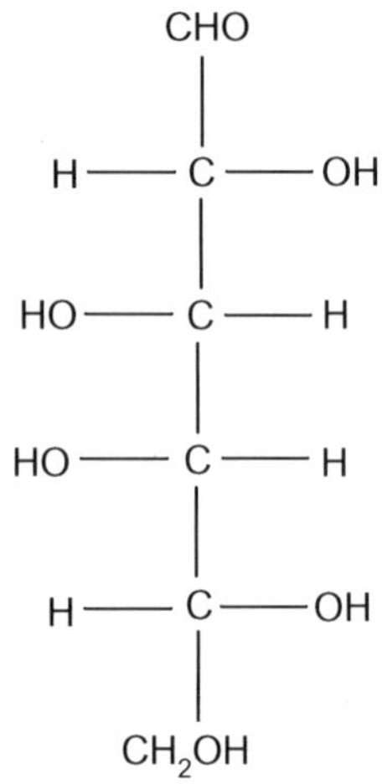

D - Galactose

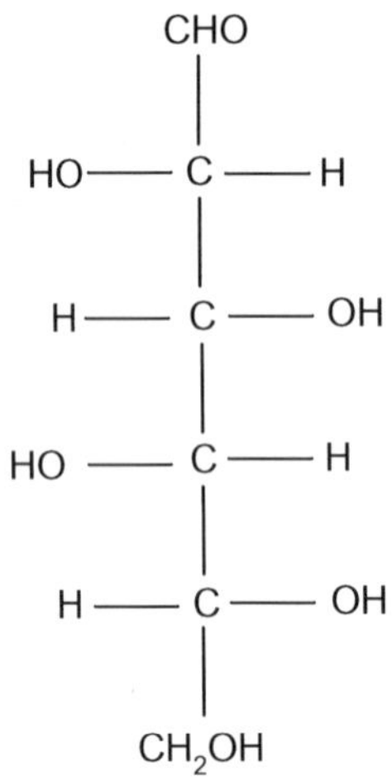

D - Idtose

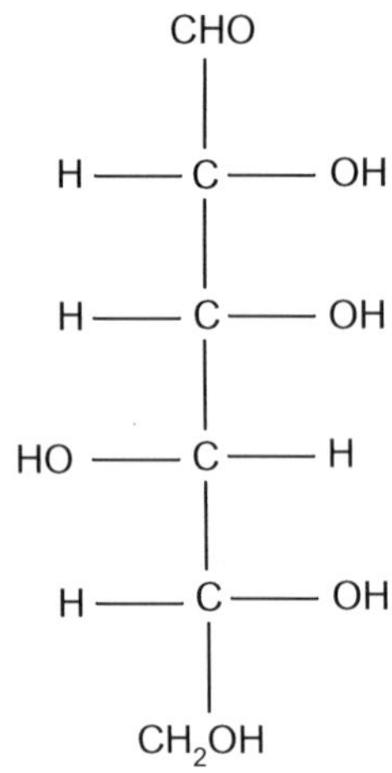

D - Glucose

Glyceraldehyde, the simplest sugar, arbitrary taken here as the standard for studying configuration of carbohydrates. If OH group of Glyceraldehyde is on right, known as D-Glyceraldehyde, while on left side is called L-Glyceraldehyde.

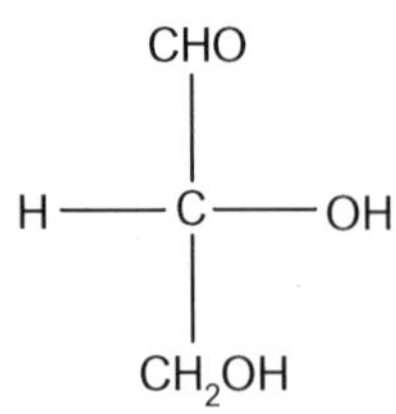

D - Glyceraldehyde

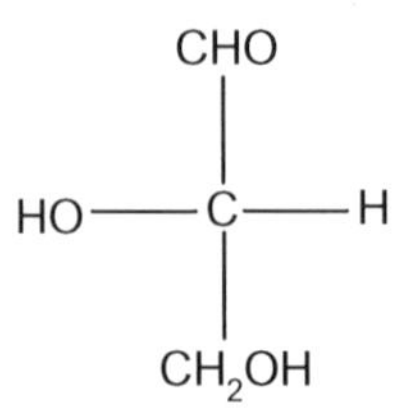

L - Glyceraldehyde

Sugars having configuration similar to that of D or L-glyceraldehyde are said to belong to D or L series respectively.

General method for determinig the configuration of a monosaccharide consisting upgrading the lower homologue of known configuration by one higher isomeric monosaccharides, the nature of which is determined by their oxidation to acids.

Cyclic Structure of Glucose

The open chain formula for glucose as polyhydroxy aldehyde fail to explain certain properties like; Glucose do not restore schiff's reagent colour. Glucose do not form a bisulphite compound. Glucose forms two isomeric penta-acetates, but neither of which react with corbonyl reagents. When Glucose is dissolved in water, its specific rotation gradually changes until it reaches a constant value. This change in specific rotation is known as mutarotation. Mutarotation and existence of Glucose in two isomeric forms cannot be explained by open chain formula. Since Glucose is not responding to weak corbonyl reagents like schiff's reagent or bisulphite, but strong carbonyl reagents like HCN, NH_2OH, $C_6H_5NHNH_2$....etc. are able to open the ring and make aldehyde group as reactive, to form products.

By various physical and chemical methods, in the α-form of D series, the hydroxyl group or substituted hydroxyl group is attached to right, while in α-form of L-series, the hydroxyl group is attached to left. The two isomers differing only in configuration of C_1 in aldoses or C_2 in ketoses are known as anomers, while such carbon atom is known as anomeric carbon atom.

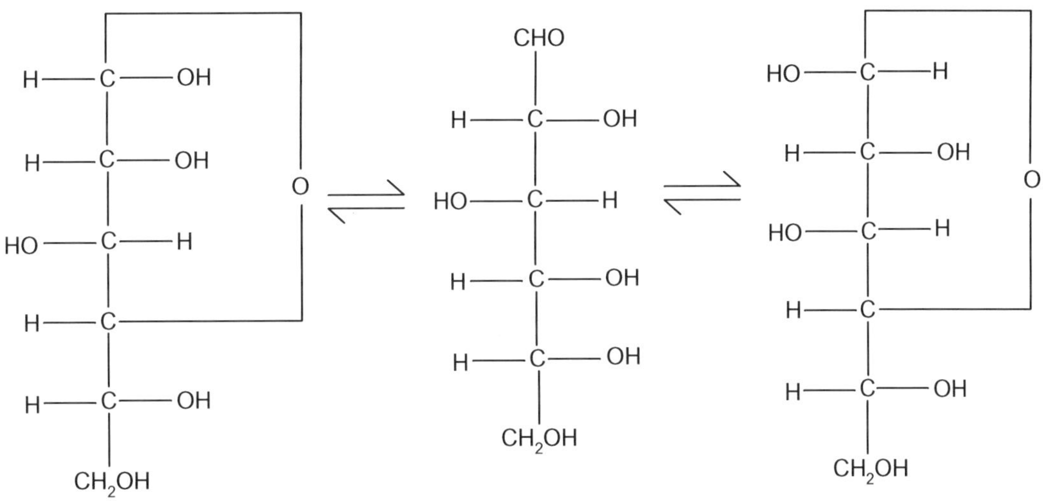

α - D - Glucose　　Aldehydic form　　β - D - Glucose

Mutarotation can be explained on the fact that interconversion of α-form (+113°) to β-form (+19.0°) and vice-versa through aldehydic structure till an equilibrium (+52.5°) mixture of both forms formed. Formation of cyclic intermediate during muta-rotation confirmed by isotopic studies, UV spectrum and polarographic studies.

Two types of ring structures are possible in sugars. γ Oxide or 5-membered ring structure and δ-oxide or 6-membered ring structure, which are shown below.

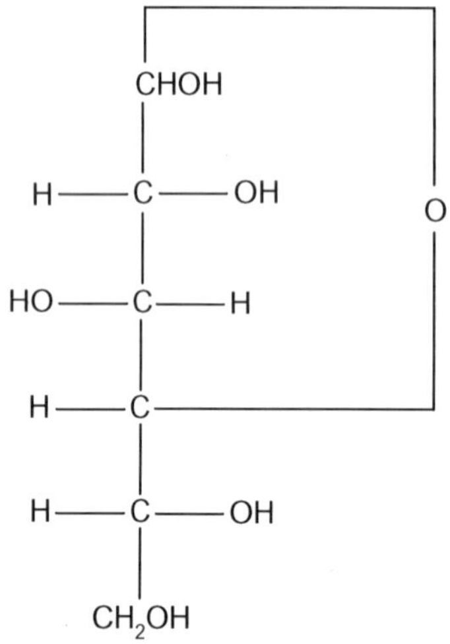

γ - Oxide or 5 membered ring structure.

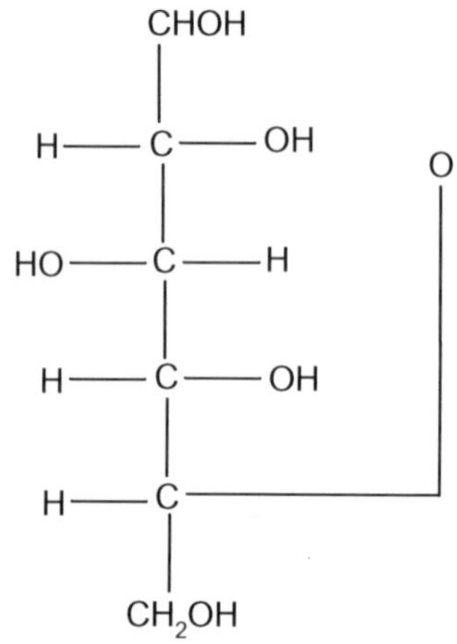

δ - Oxide or 6 membered ring structure.

Five and six-membered oxide rings of monosaccharides bear a normal relation ship to the heterocyclic compounds furan and pyran respectively. So the rings are denoted by the terms furanose and pyranose. Eg: α-D Glucopyranose & -D-L Glucofuranose.

Determination of the Size of Ring

The size of ring can be determined by methylation method and periodic acid oxidation method.

Methylation method

The sugar is com pletely methylated, then hydrolysed with dilute hydrochloric acid, so only glycosidic. Methyl group get hydrolysed and finally product is oxidised. Identification of oxidation product leads to the ring size of sugar.

Eg: Glucose.

D -Glucose is refluxed with methanolic hydro-chloric acid to get methyl glucoside which is treated with methyl sulphate in the presence of alkali to get methyl tetra-methyl -D-Glucoside -which on hydrolysis gives a tetramethyl -D-glucose which is oxidised by bromine water gives a lactone which is further oxidised by nitric acid gives a dicarboxylic acid identified as xylotrimethoxy glutaric acid, which is also obtained by oxidation of methylated xylose. All reactions can be summerized as follows;

$$\text{D - Glucose} \xrightarrow[\text{HCl}]{CH_3OH} \text{Methyl Glucoside} \xrightarrow[\text{NaOH}]{Me_2SO_4}$$

$$\text{Methyl tetra - methyl D - Glucoside} \xrightarrow{\text{HCl}} \text{D - tetra methyl glucose}$$

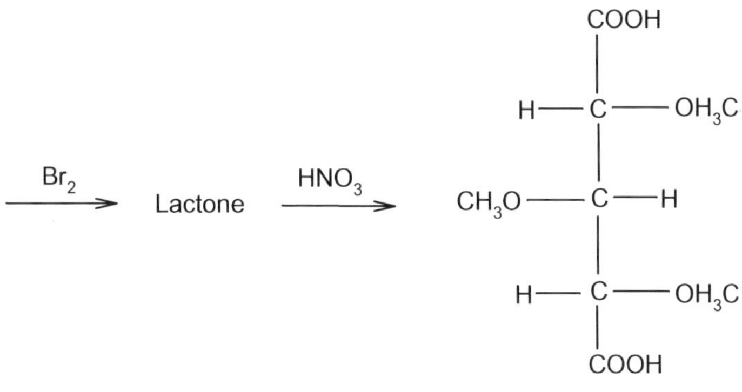

Xylotrimethoxy glutaric acid.

The above reactions indicate one of the -COOH group in acid must be derived from first carbon atom of the lactone & other from the carbon atom which is involved in ring formation in the sugar. Therefore only three hydroxyl groups are present inside the ring of glucose and the ring must be pyranose. Presence of three methoxy group in dicarboxylic indicate, three hydroxyl groups are inside the ring of glucose, & the lactone formed in between C_1 & C_5. Structurally the reactions can be drawn as;

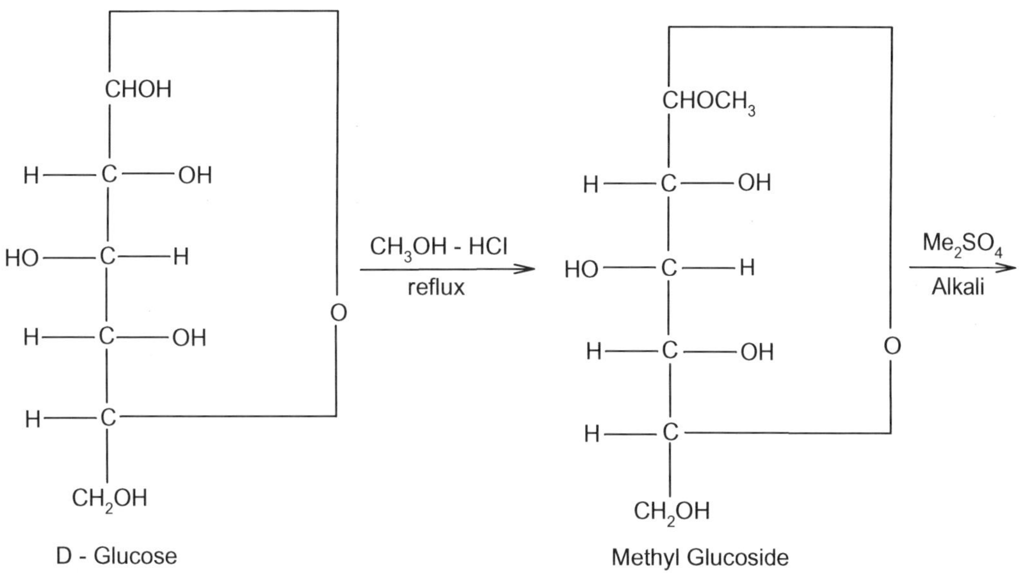

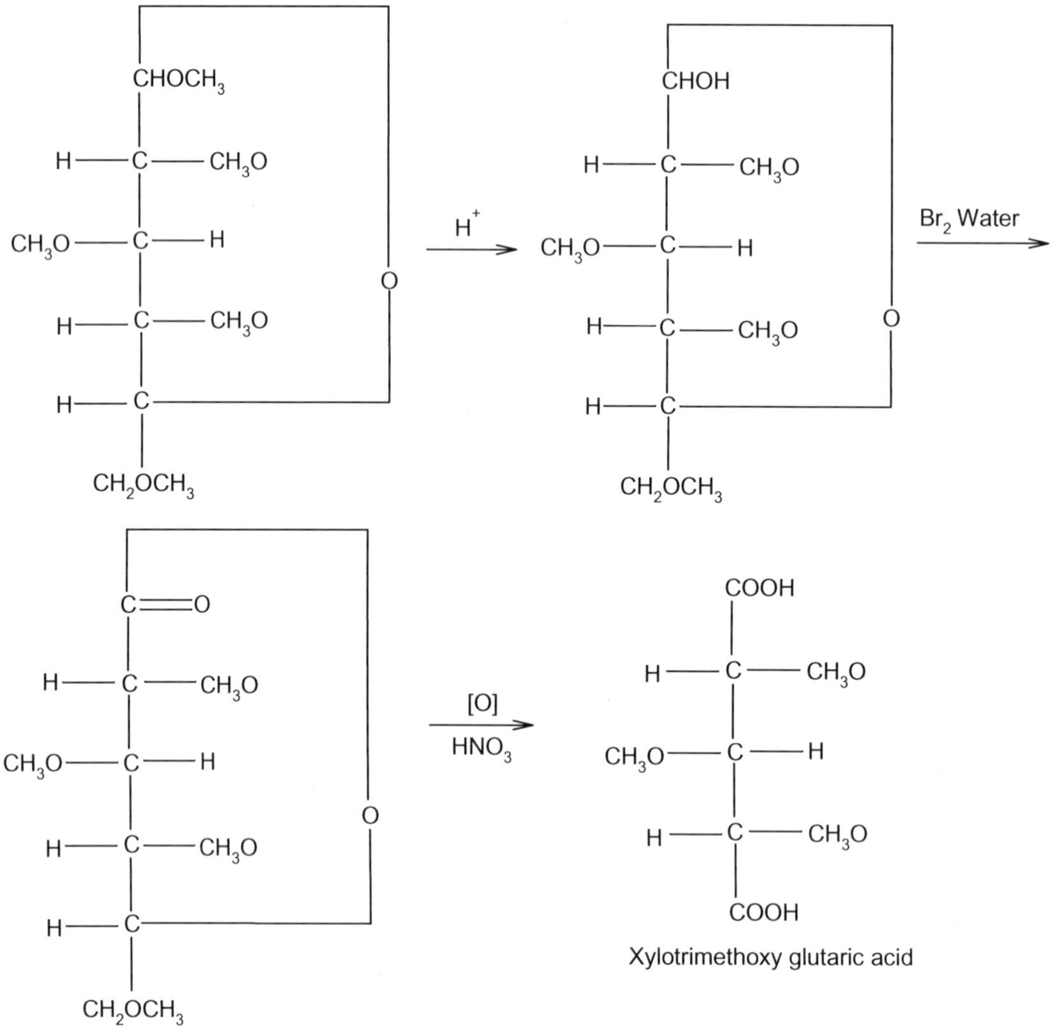

Xylotrimethoxy glutaric acid

The pyranose structure further can be confirmed by periodic acid oxidation. This method involves use of periodic acid for solutions pH <4, sodium meta periodate for solutions. pH 4-7 or potassium metaperiodate for alkaline solutions. One molecule of periodic acid is consumed between every two adjacent hydroxyl groups. When CHOH group on one sided only attacked, that is only mole of reagent utilised for forming CHO group. If one CHOH group attacked by two moles of reagent, then HCOOH will be formed. Thus by estimating the number of moles of periodic acid consumed and number of moles of HCHO & HCOOH produced the size of the ring can be determined.

Eg: Oxidation of methyl -α -D-glucopyranoside.

Methyl -α -D-glucopyranoside on oxidation, two moles of periodic acid is consumed and one mole of formic acid and a dialdehyde is formed, indicate that starting compound have three adjacent hydroxyl groups, which is possible with pyranose structure.

Fischer's projection formula

Fischer who worked out the structural configuration of the monosaccharides, formulated dextrorotatory glucose and levorotatory glucose as shown here.

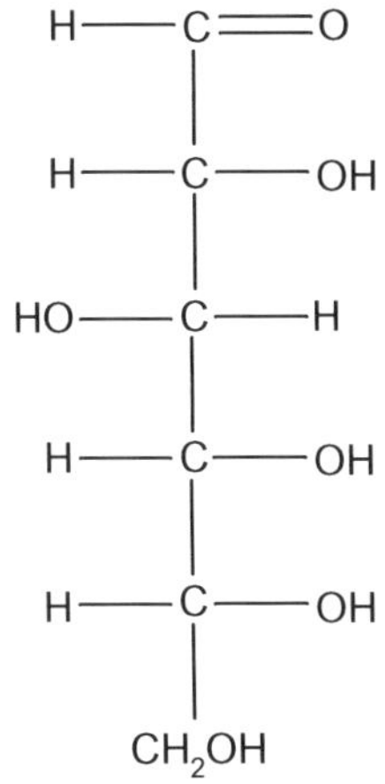

D - Glucose

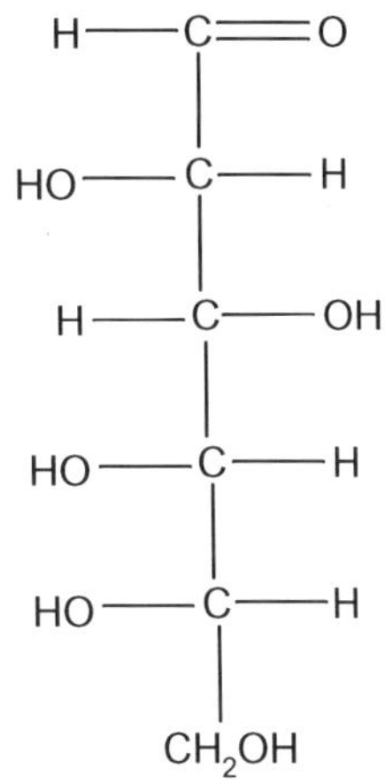

L - Glucose

In the dextrarotatory glucose the secondary alcoholic group at fifth carbon atom is on the right, where as, in the levorotatory glucose, the secondary alcoholic gorup at fifth carbon atom is on the left.

Conformation of Monosaccharides

Conformation means arrangement of atoms in space of a single chemical structure. Pyranose sugars and their derivatives assume a chair conformation in preference to boat form. Chair form is more stable because of the mininum hydrogen interactions than in boat form. Chair conformation of α-D glucose and β-D glucose is as follows;

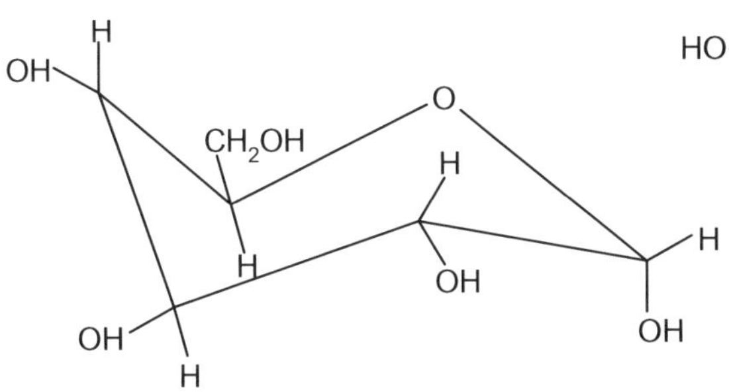

α D - Glucose

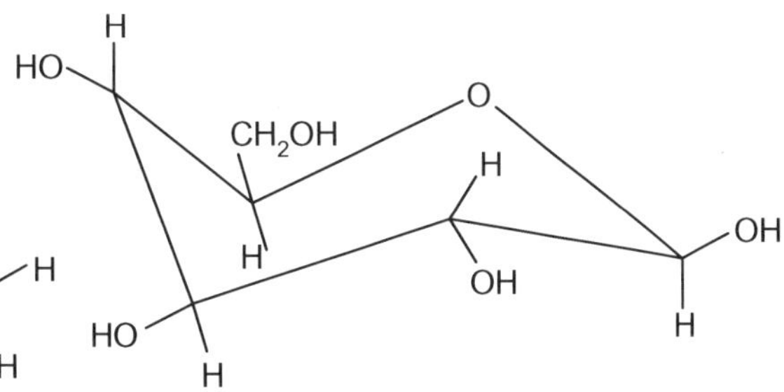

β D - Glucose

β-form is predominat over α form & β form is more stable as most of the OH groups are in equitorial position while in α-for OH at c_1 is axially oriented.

Conformations of α-L-glucose and β-L-glucose are as follows;

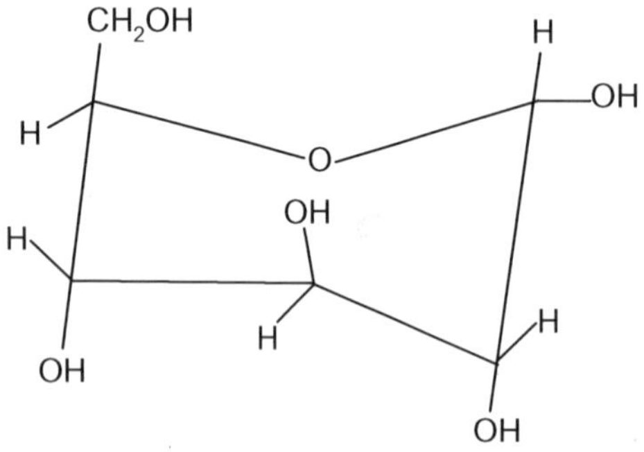

α L - Glucose

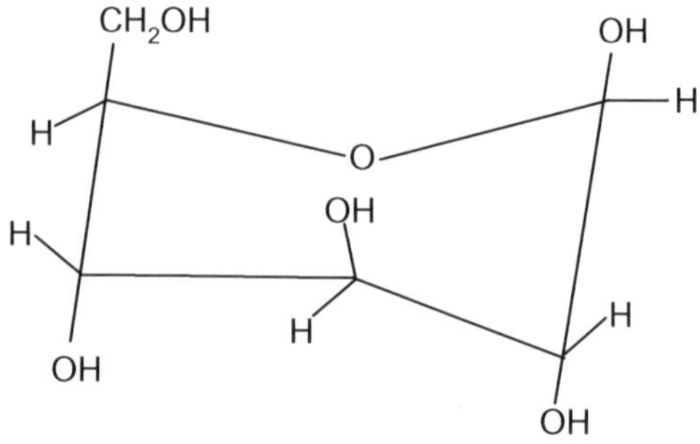

β L - Glucose

Structure of Glucose

1. Molecular formula of Glucose is $C_6H_{12}O_6$.
2. Presence and position of five hydroxyl groups.

Glucose on acetylation with acetic anhydride and sodium acetate gives penta-acetate indicate the presence of five hydroxyl groups. Glucose being a stable compound, all hydroxyl groups must be on different carbon atoms.

3. Presence of carbonyl group.

Glucose + hydrogen cyanide ⟶ Cyanohydrin

Glucose + Hydroxylamine ⟶ Mono-oxime

Formation of cyanohydrin and mono-oxime indicating the presence of a carbonyl group.

4. Nature of carbonyl group.

Glucose on oxidation gives gluconic acid having the same number of carbon atoms confirms the presence of aldehyde. It is supported by the fact that glucose reduces Fehling as well as Tollen's reagent

5. Nature of carbon skeleton.

Cyanohydrin obtaining from glucose by reacting with HCN undergo hydrolysis followed by reduction with hydriodic acid and red phosphorous gave n-heptanoic acid, indicate that glucose has a straight chain of six carbon atoms.

$$C_5H_{11}O_5 . CHO \xrightarrow{HCN} C_5H_{11}O_5 . CH(OH)CN \xrightarrow{H_2O}$$

$$C_5H_{11}OH . CH(OH) .COOH \xrightarrow{HI - P} C_6H_{13} . COOH$$

n - Heptanoic acid

So the structure of glucose can be written as a straight-chain penta hydroxy aldehyde.

$$CHO—CHOH—CHOH—CHOH—CHOH—CH_2OH$$

Structure of Fructose

1. Molecular formula of fructose is found to be $C_6H_{12}O_6$
2. Presence and position of five hydroxyl groups.

On acetylation as did in glucose, fructose also gives penta acetate indicate the presence of five hydroxyl groups on different carbon atoms.

3 Presence of carbonyl group

Formation of cyanohydrin with hydrogen cyanide and oxime with hydroxylamine indicating the presence of carbonyl group.

4. Nature of carbonyl group

$$\text{Fructose} \xrightarrow[\text{HNO}_3]{[\text{O}]} \text{Tartaric acid} + \text{Glycolic acid}$$

Both products have lesser number of carbon atoms than fructose indicate carbonyl group is ketone and present at second position.

5. Nature of Carbon Skeleton.

Fructose on reduction by sodium-amalgam and water gives sorbitol and mannitol, which on further reduction with hydriodic acid and red phosphorous gives 2-iodo-hexane and n-hexane suggests, fructose is strain chain with six carbon atoms.

6. Structure of fructose

$$\text{Fructose} \xrightarrow{\text{HCN}} \text{cyaholydrin} \xrightarrow[\text{HI-P}]{\text{H}_2\text{O}} \text{n-butyl methyl}$$

acetic acid indicate ketonic group is present at position 2. Overall reaction can be written as follows;

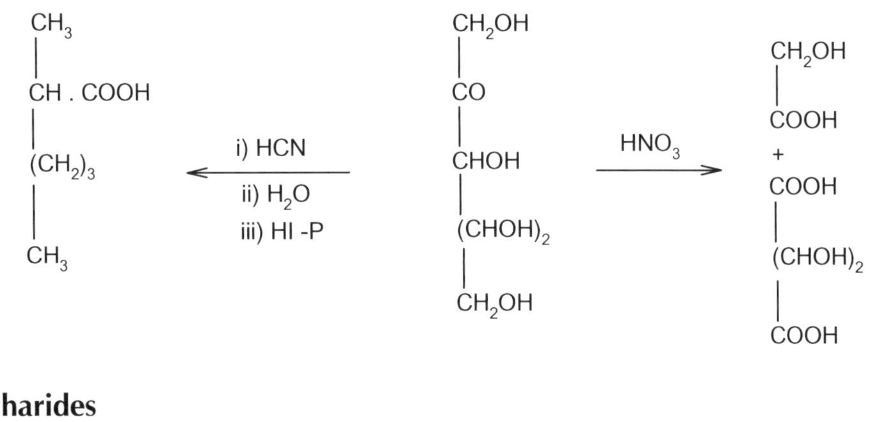

Disaccharides

Disaccharides are formed by intermolecular dehydration between two monosccharide molecules. Thus Disaccharide on hydrolysis gives two monosaccharides. Monosaccharide units can be linked by C_1,C_4 or C_6. On this basis Disaccharides can be divide in to three groups.

$C_1 \longrightarrow C_1$, $C_1 \longrightarrow C_4$, $C_1 \longrightarrow C_6$

$C_1 \longrightarrow C_1$

In this category reducing carbon of each monosaccharide is involved in linkage, the disaccharide have no latent carbonyl group and are called non reducing disaccharides. So these are unable to react with carbonyl reagents like phenyl hydrazine, Tollen's reagent, Fehling's solution. These are stable in alkaline and neutral conditions, so do not mutarotate in alkaline or neutral medium.

$C_1 \longrightarrow C_4$

In this category C_1 of the first is linked to $C_4$of the second monosaccharide. Since C_1 of the second monosaccharide is free, these type of disaccharides are able to react with carbonyl reagents and also undergo mutarotation in solution. These are also known as reducing disaccharides.

$C_1 \longrightarrow C_6$

Here C_1 of the first monosaccharide is linked to C_6 of the second monosaccharide. Therefore reducing carbon ie. C_1 of second monosacchrides available for reaction with carbonyl reagents.

Examples for important disaccharides are maltose, Lactose and Sucrose.

Maltose

It is also known as malt sugar and is obtained by the action of diastase enzyme upon starch. It's molecular formula is $C_{12}H_{22}O_{11}$. Monosaccharide units present is only D-glucose. Maltose can be hydrolysed by different enzymes like maltase and emulsin. Maltose is oxidised by bromine water to maltodic acid. Maltose reduces Fehling's Benedict's and Tollen's reagents. Maltose exhibits mutarotation.

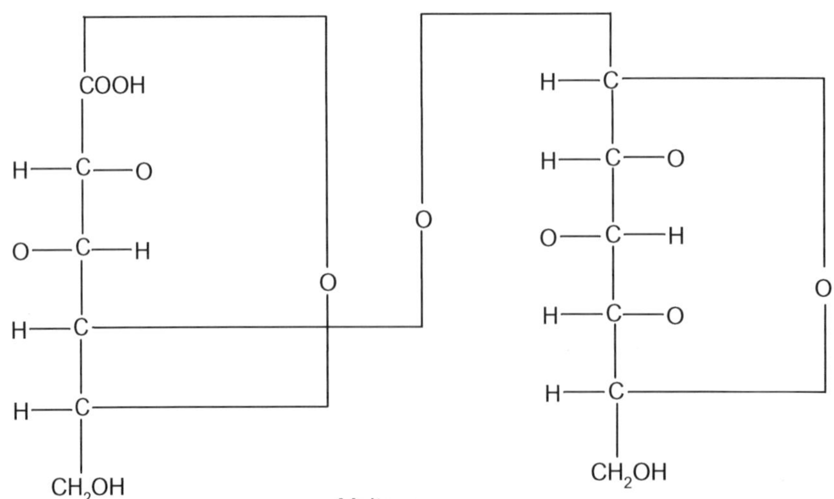

Maltose

Lactose

Lactose is milk sugar and its molecular formula is $C_{12}H_{22}O_{11}$. Lactose hydrolysed by the enzyme Lactase Hydrolysis of Lactose by acid or enzyme gives two types of monosasccharides namely glucose and galactose Bromine water oxidise Lactose to Lactobionic acid.

Lactose exhibits mutarotation also.

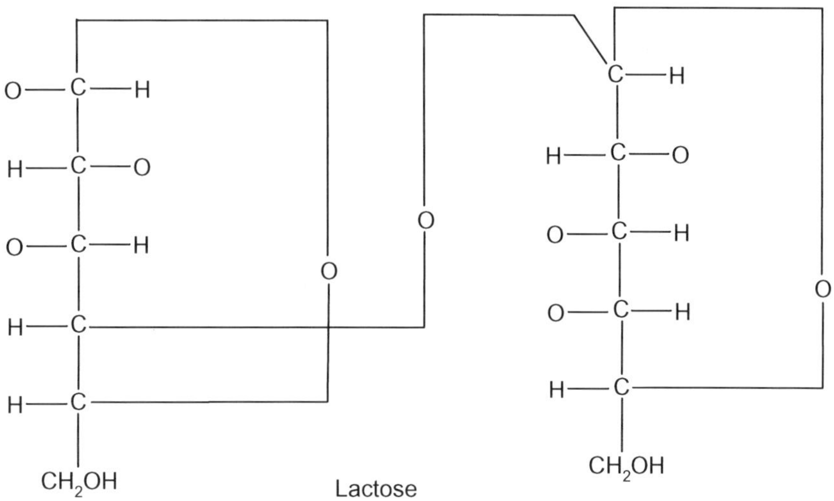

Lactose

Sucrose

Sucrose is the commonest sugar, mainly found in sugar cane, sugar beets, saps, honey and fruit Juices. It's molecular formula is C_{12} H_{22} O_{11}. Sucrose can be hydrolysed by two enzymes maltase and takaimertase. Sucrose on hydrolysis by enzymes or acids give D-glucose and D-fructose.

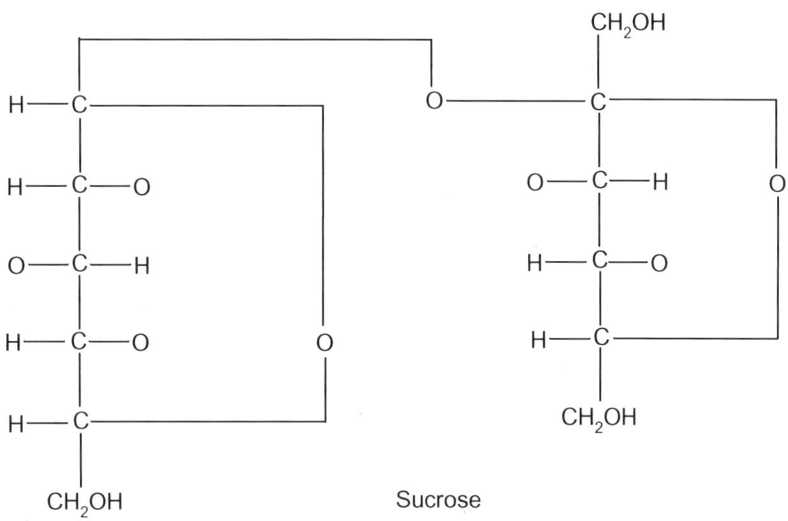

Sucrose

Polysaccharides

Polysaccharides on hydrolysis give many monosaccharides. Chemically polysaccharides are condensation products of monosaccharides. According to the type of monosaccharides presents they can be classified into homopolysaccharides and heteropolysaccharides. If the monosaccharide units are same, can be termed as homopolysaccharides,if they are different can be termed as hetero poly saccharides. Examples for homopolysaccharides include cellulose, inulin and starch. Examples for heteropolysaccharides include α heparin and hyaluronic acid.

Starch

Starch mainly composed of two types of molecules namely amylose and amylopectin. In amylose, glucose molecules are arranged in linear manner and in amylopectin glucose molecules are arranged in highly branched form.

Amylose forms inner portion of the starch grain and is soluble in water. Amylopectin forms outer convering of the starch grain and is insoluble in water. Glucose units of amylose are linked at 1-4 carbon atoms of the successive glucopyranose units. In amylopectin glucose units are linked in 1-4 &1-6 carbon atoms.

Starch is hydrolysed by the enzyme amylase, and is present in saliva as ptyalin, in pancreatic juice as pancreatic amylase. Amylase hydrolyse starch into dextrin and maltose. Intestinal enzyme called oligo -1-, 6 glucosidase acts at 1-6 branching and disintegrates starch completely. Hydrolysis of starch can be briefly outlined as follows;

Starch

↓

Soluble Starch (Gives blue colour with iodine.)

↓

1 maltose + Amylodextrin (Gives Violet colour with iodine.)

↓

2 maltose + Erythrocdextrin (Gives red colour with iodine.)

↓

3 maltose + Achrodextrin (No colour with iodine.)

↓

3 maltose + maltose

Cellulose

Cellulose is the chief constituent of cell wall of all plants. Structurally cellulose is long unbranched chains of β-D glucopyranose units, joined to one another by 1-4 glucosidic linkage. It is insoluble in water. It is soluble in ammoniacal cupric hydroxide solution (schweizer's reagent).

GLYCOSIDES

Glycosides are organic compounds from plants or animal sources which on enzymatic or acid hydrolysis give one or more sugar moieties along with non sugar moiety. Sugar component is called glycone and non-sugar component is known as aglycone. Glycosides are chemically acetals in which hydroxyl group of sugar is condensed with a hydroxyl group of non-sugar component and the secondary hydroxyl group is condensed with the sugar molecule itself to form an oxide ring. So the glycosides can be consider as sugar ethers.

The linkage between glycone and aglycone is called glycosidic linkage, on this basis stereochemically alpha and beta glycosides are possible. But plants contain only beta glycosides. Simply both forms can be synthesized from union of methyl alcohol and glucose. ie alpha- methyl glycoside and beta- methyl glycoside.

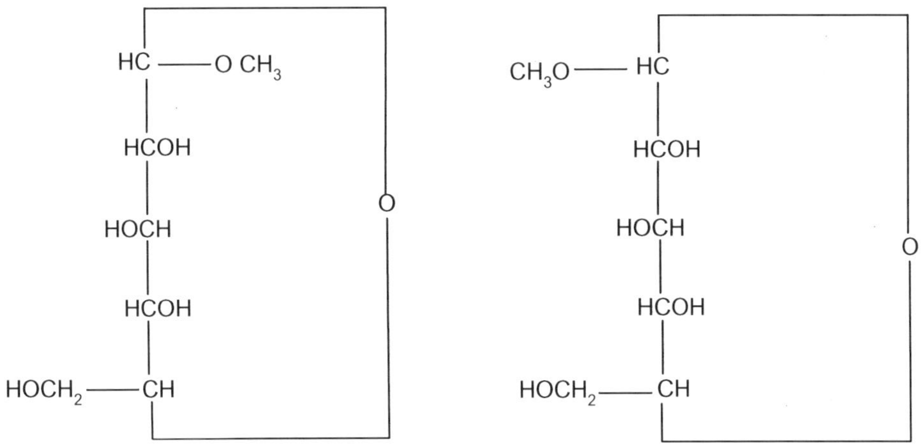

α - Methyl Glycoside β - Methyl Glycoside

Glycosides can be classified according to chemical natrure of aglycone or based on glycosidic linkage exists.

According to chemical nature of aglycone, Glycosides are classified as follows;

1. Anthraquinone or anthracene glycosides.
   eg: Sennosides, Barbaloin, Cascarosides, Hypericin, rhein.
2. Sterol or cardiac glycosides.
   eg: Digitoxin, Digoxin, lanatasides, scillaren, Ouabain, oleandrin.
3. Saponin glycosides.
   eg: Diosgenin, Hecogenin, Glycy rrhizin, shatavarin, Ginsenosides.
4. Cyanogenetic or cyanophoric glycosides.
   eg: Amygdalin, prunasin.
5. Isothiocyanate glycosides.
   eg: Sinigrin.
6. Flavonol glycosides.
   eg: Silybin, Gingkolide, Rutin, Hesperidin.

7. Coumarin and Furanocoumarin glycosides.
   eg: Coumarin, Xanthotoxin, Psoralen, Cantharidin.
8. Aldehyde glycosides.
   eg: Vanillin.
9. Phenol glycosides.
   eg: Arbutin.
10. Steroidal glyco-alkaloids.
    eg: Solasodine.
11. Glycosidal bitters.
    eg: Gentiopicrin, Quassin, Andrographolide.
12. Alcohol glycosides.
    eg: Salicin.

According to glycosidic linkage occured by interaction of OH group of glycone and hydrogen coming through any of the radicals like CH-OH, -SH and -NH present on a glycone part. So they are classified as follows;

1. C- glycosides.

They are formed by

$$\text{Glycone- O}\boxed{\text{H + H}}\text{C - aglycone - Glycone - C- aglycone + } H_2O$$

eg: Aloin, Carminic acid, Cascarosides.

2. O- glycosides.

They are formed by

$$\text{Glycone - O}\boxed{\text{H + H}}\text{O - aglycone - O-aglycone +}H_2O$$

eg: Sennosides.

3. S- glycosides.

They are formed by

$$\text{Glycone - O}\boxed{\text{H + H}}\text{S - aglycone- Glycone -S- aglycone + } H_2O$$

eg: Sinigrin.

4. N= glycosides.

They are formed by

$$\text{Glycone - O}\boxed{\text{H + H}}\text{N - Glycone - Glycone - N - aglycone + } H_2O.$$

eg: Nucleo sides.

Now will see structures of some important glycosides.

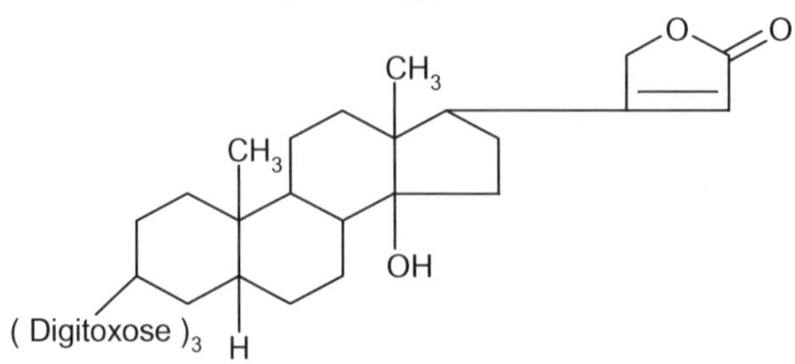

Digitoxin

Digitoxin and Digoxin mainly obtaining from Digitalis purpurea. These are mainly used for cardiac disease.

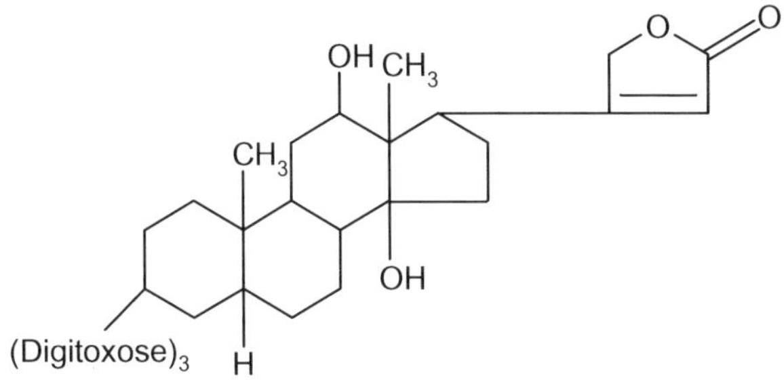

Digoxin

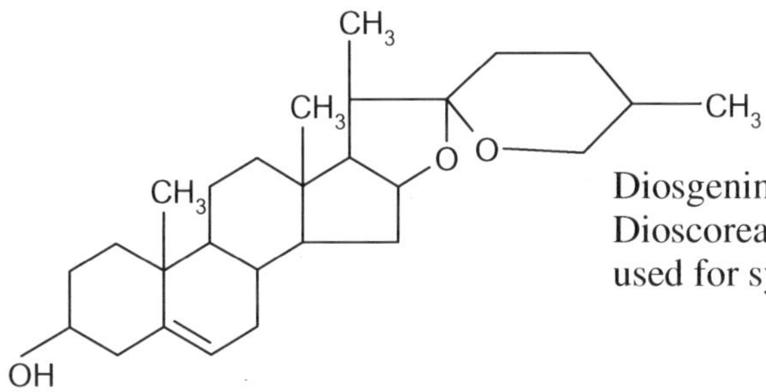

Diosgenin: It is obtained from Dioscorea (yam) It is mainly used for synthesis of medicinal steroids.

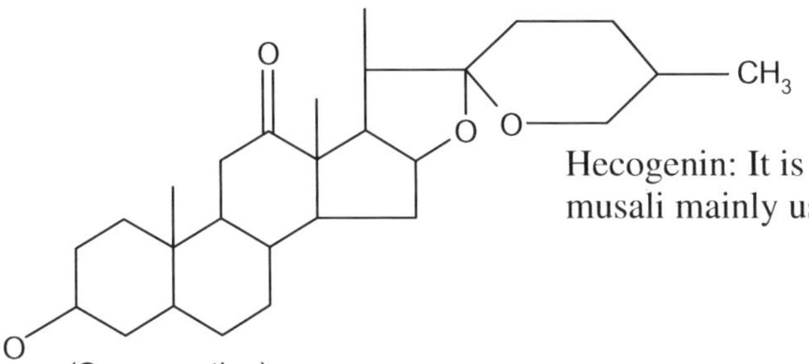

Hecogenin: It is obtained from safed musali mainly used as general tonic.

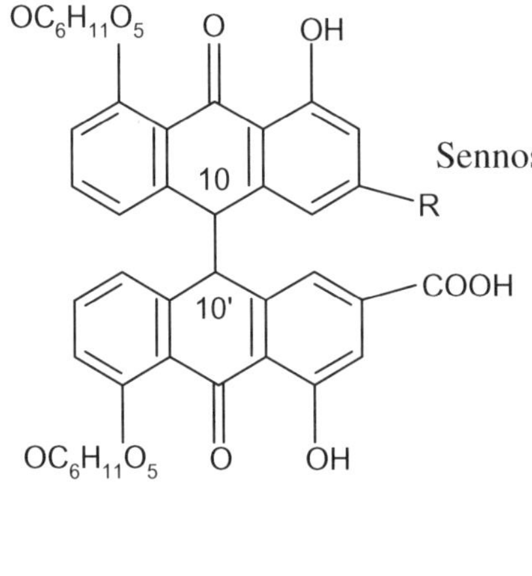

Sennoside (A, B, C and D see below)

R	10, 10`	Sennoside
COOH	trans	A
COOH	trans	B
CH_2OH	trans	C
CH_2OH	trans	D

Sennosides are cbtaining from senna. Sennosides are mainly used as purgatives.

Lanatosides contain Lanatoside A, B, C and D. Lanatosides are obtaining from Digitalis lanata. These are mainly used as Cardio tonic.

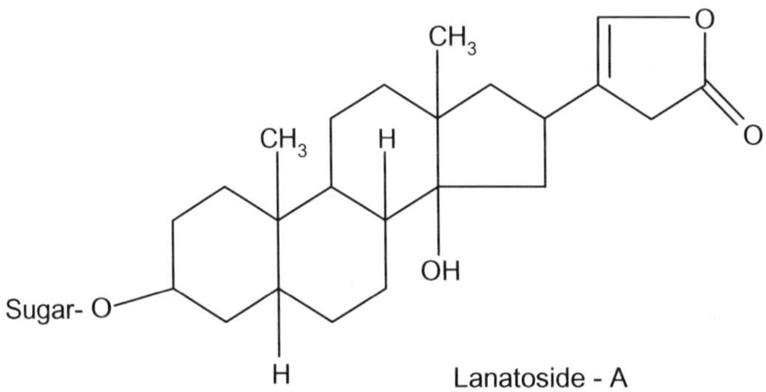

Lanatoside - A

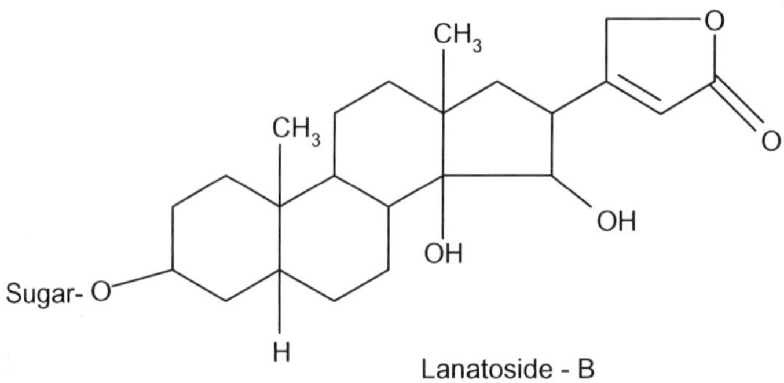

Lanatoside - B

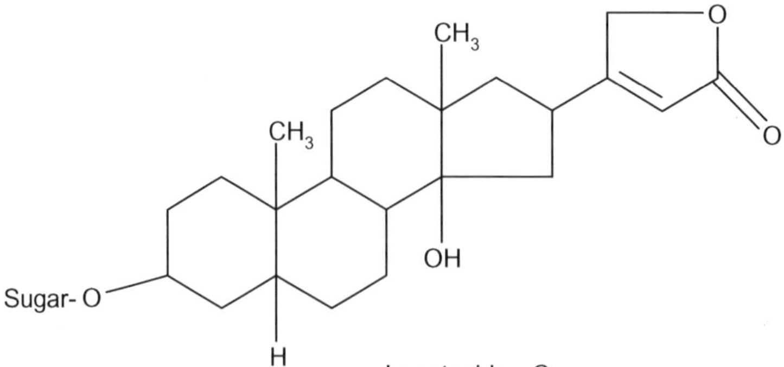

Lanatoside - C

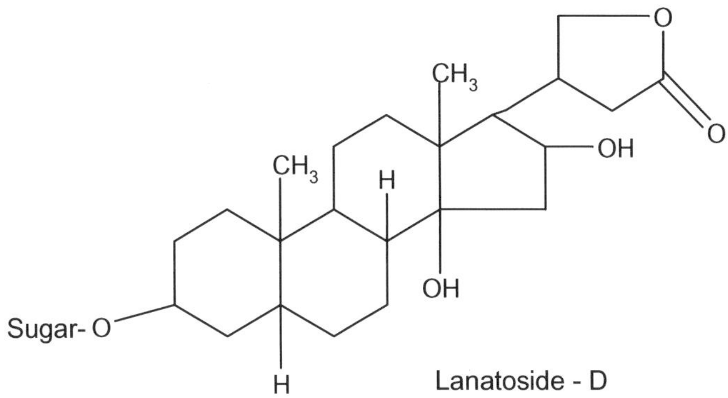

Lanatoside - D

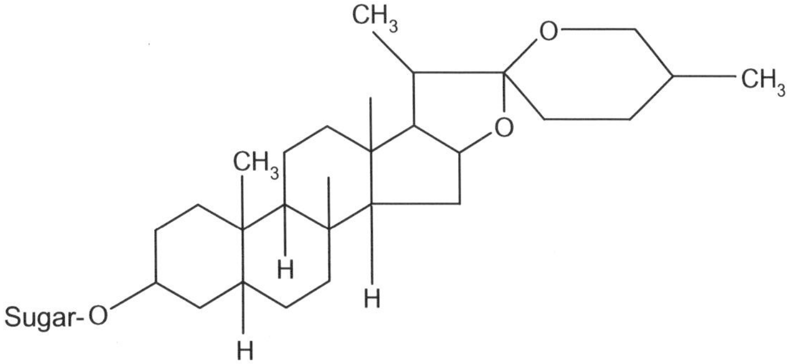

Sarasapogenin: It is obtaining from smilax. It is used as precursors for synthesis of other steroids.

In the above examples, basic nucleus present is steroid, except in sennosides where anthracene is the basic nucleus. Steroids are any compound contains a cylopentano perhydrophenanthrene nucleus. Chemical nomenclature of steroids is based on this fundamental carbocyle with adjacent side-chain carbon atoms. Steroids are numbered and rings are lettered by taking structural formula of cholesterol as the basis. Orientation of steroid substituents can be drawn as follows;

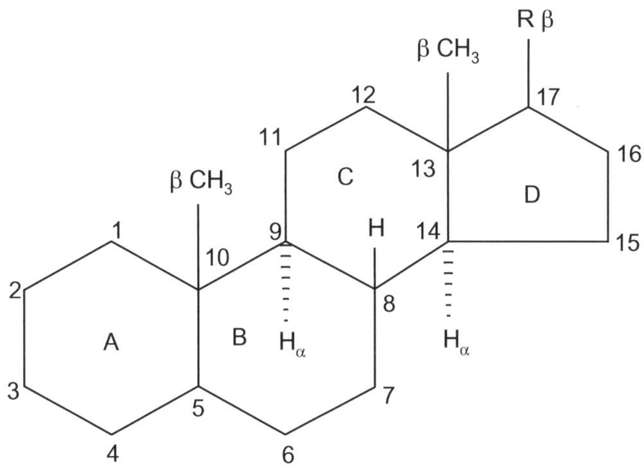

When the rings of a steroid are denoted as projections onto the plane of paper, an atom or group attached to a ring is termed α if it lies below the plane of paper or as β if it lies above the plane of paper.

In the structure, bonds to atoms or groups attached in an α configuration are shown as broken lines, and solid lines as that of β-configuration. In this rings B and C as well as rings C and D are fused trans. Where as rings A and B may be fused either cis or trans.

In the steroid nucleus eight C dissimilar chiral centres (C-3, C-5, C- 8, C-9, C-10, C-13, C-14, C-17) are there.Therefore 2^n ie. 2^8=256 optical isomers are possible. Thus stereo isomerism of steroids can be dealt in two ways, ie the way in which rings are fused together and the configuration of substiuent groups.

Particularly at C-3 and C-17. When a steroid compound is named with "nor" which indicates there is no methylene or methyl group in steroidal nucleus. In one case of cardiac glycosides, steroid aglycones or genins are of two types a cardenolide or bufadienolide. Cardenolides are C_{23} steroids that have 17 β side chain as α-βunsaturated 5- membered lactone ring. Bufadienolides are C_{24} cardenolides with 6-membered lactone ring at 17th position.

AMINO ACIDS AND PROTEINS

Amino Acids are compounds having one or more amino groups and one or more carboxyl groups in the same molecule. Avoiding to relative position the of those two functional groups, they are named in to α, β and γ

Classification of Amino Acids

According to the nature of their occurance, amino Acids are classified into a) Dispensable or Non-essential amino acids (which are synthesized in the body). b) Indispensable or essential amino acids (which are to be furnished through diet). According to Chemical characterestics amino acids are classified into Aliphatic, Aromatic and Heterocyclic amino acids. Aliphatic amino acids are again classified into Neutral, Acidic, Basic and Sulphur containing amino acids.

Neutral Amino Acids

Glycine

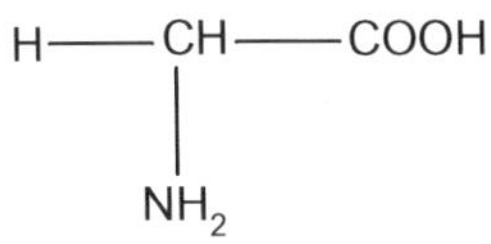

Alanine

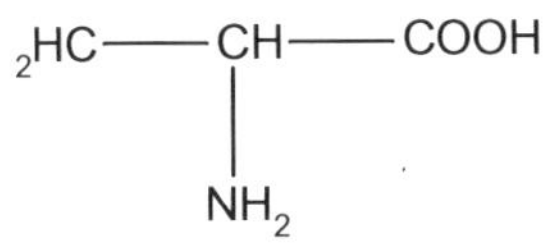

Serine

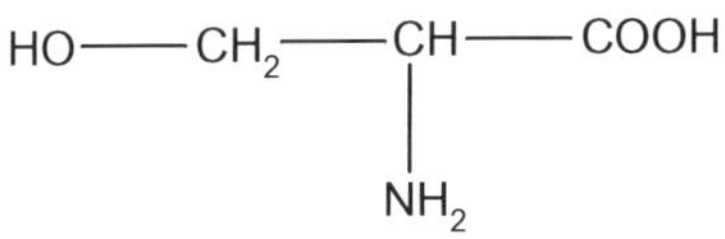

Threonine

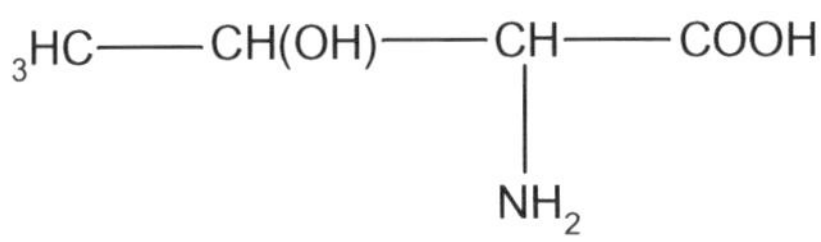

Valine

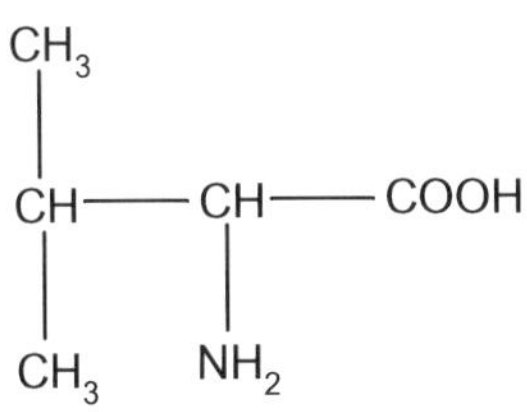

Leucine

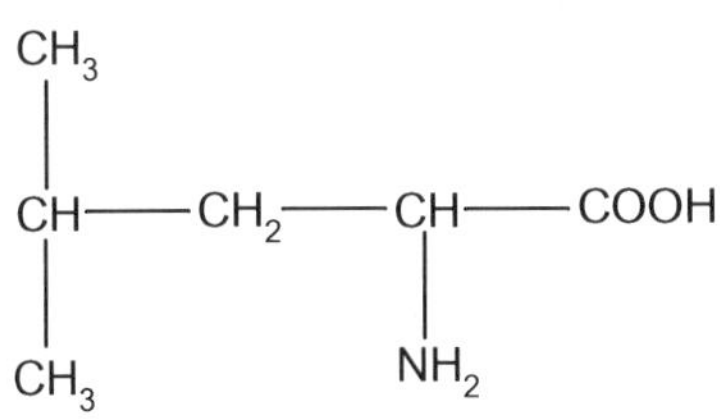

Isoleucine 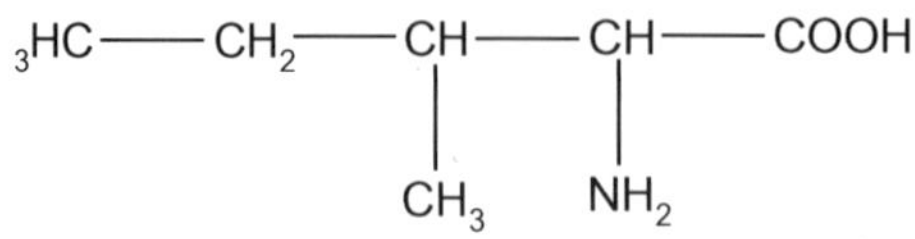

Acidic Amino Acids

Aspartic Acid 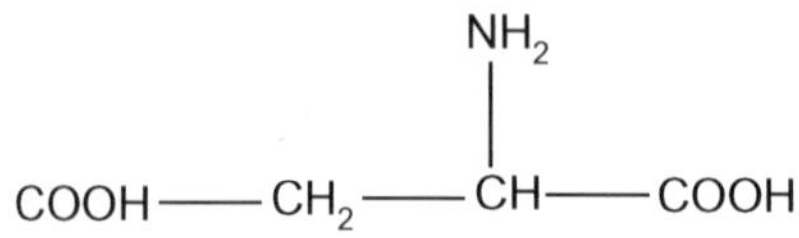

Asparagine 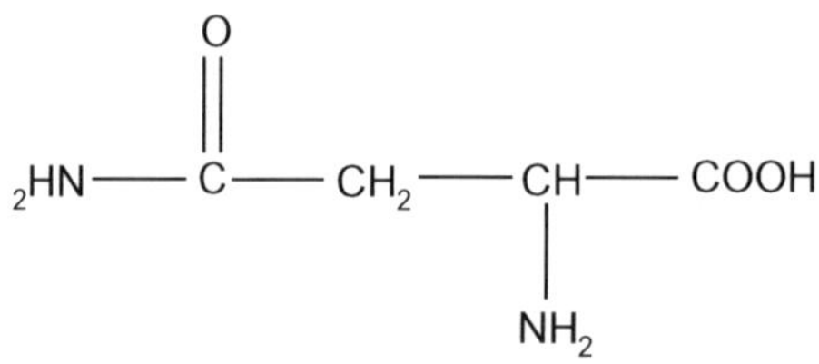

Glutamic Acid 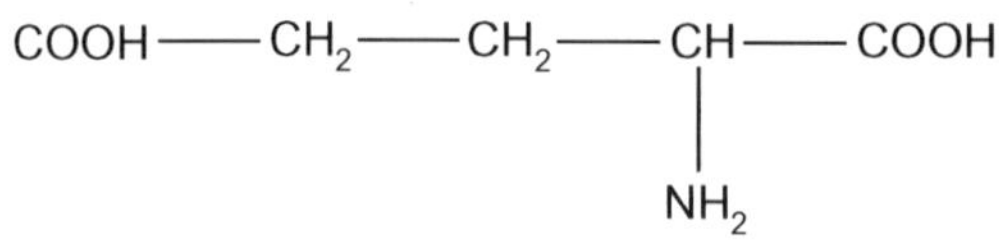

Glutamine 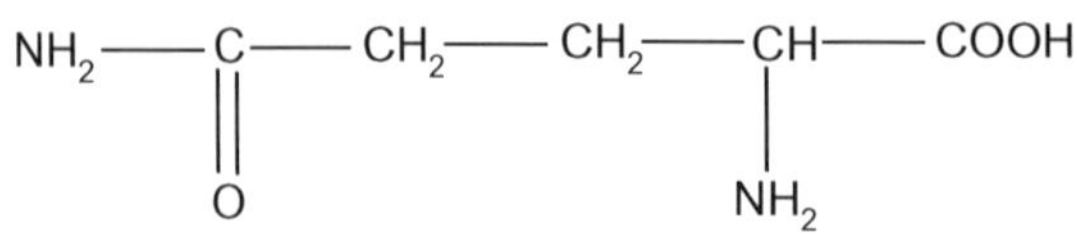

Basic Amino Acids

Arginine 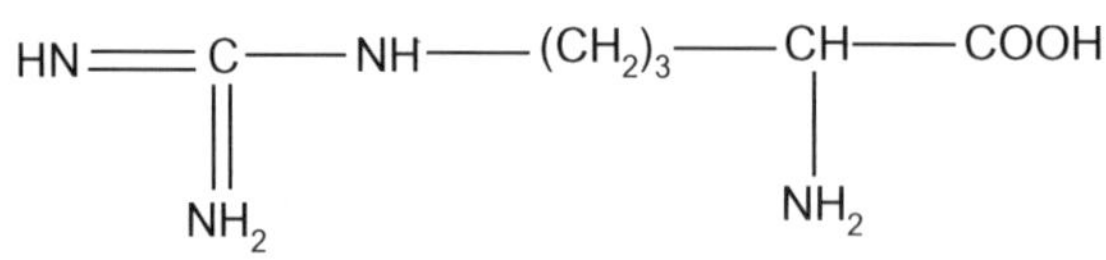

Lysine 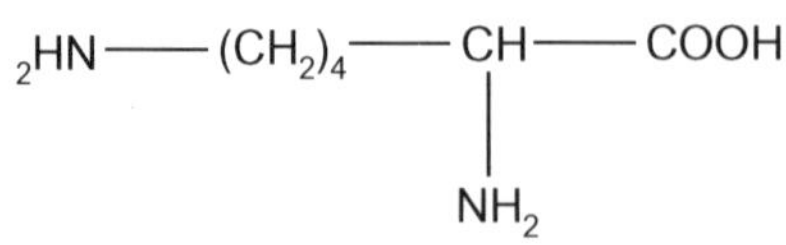

Ornithine 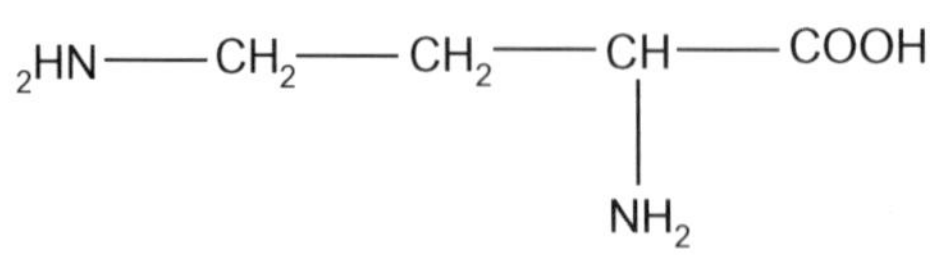

Sulphur Containing Amino Acids

Cysteine

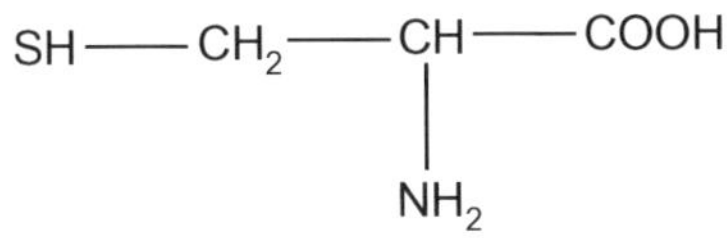

Cystine

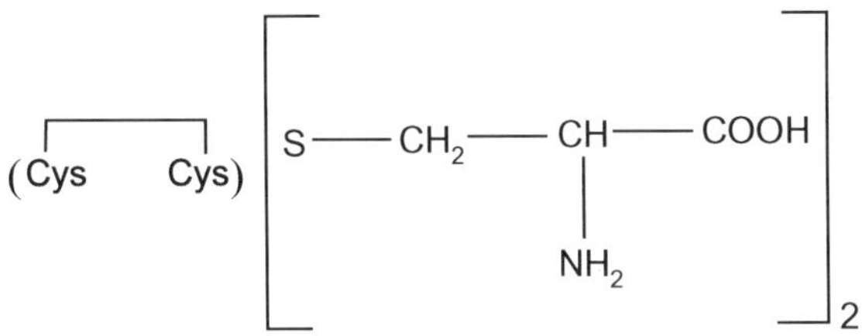

Methionine

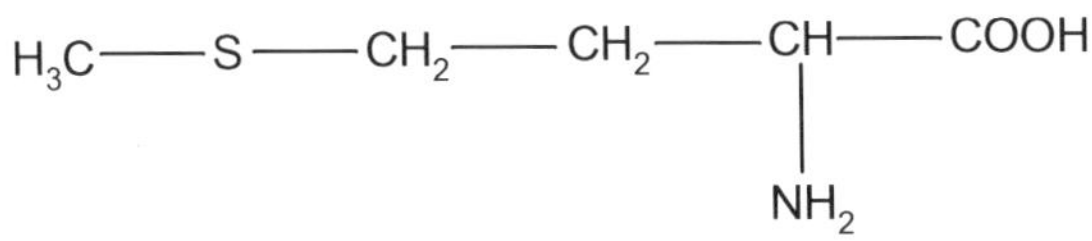

Aromatic Amino Acids

Phenyl alanine

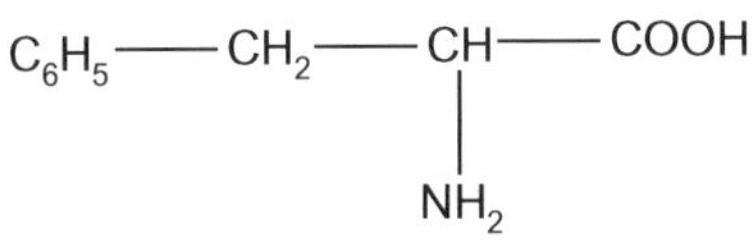

Tyrosine

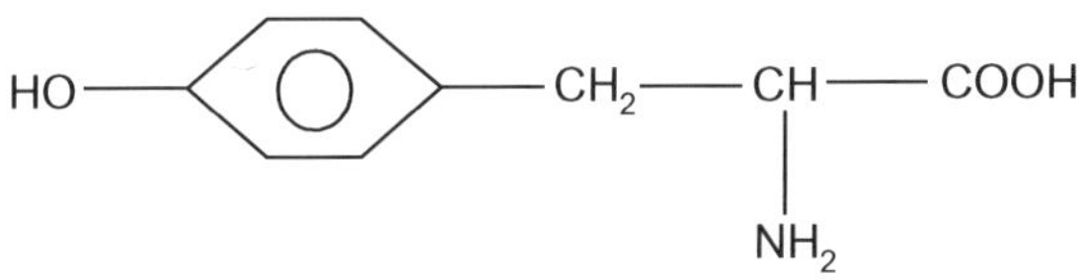

Thyroxine

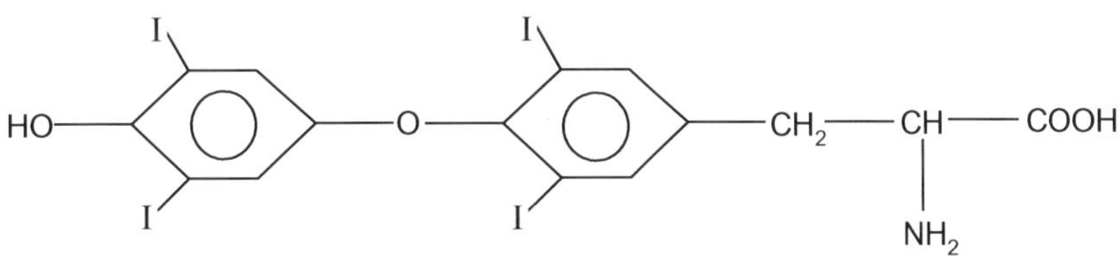

Heterocyclic Amino Acids

Proline

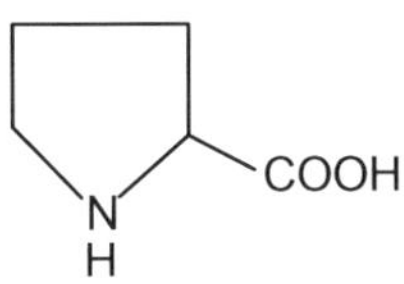

Hydroxy Proline 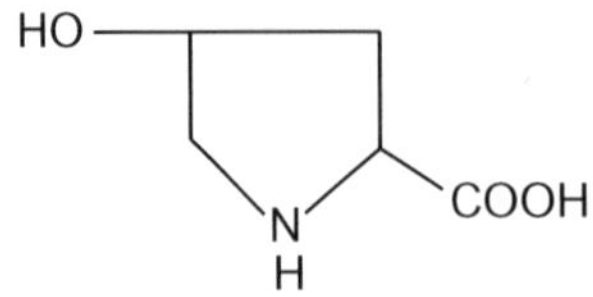

Tryptophan 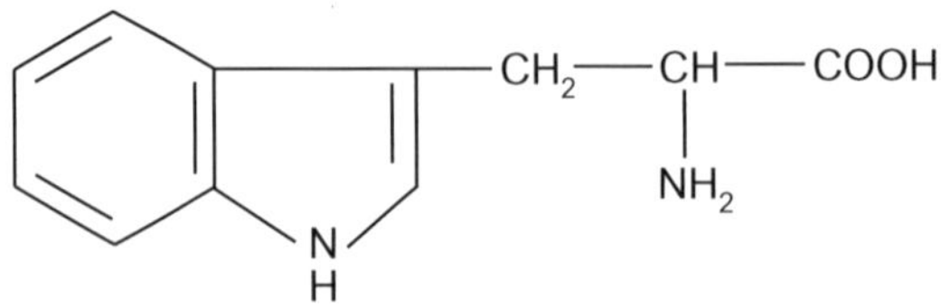

Histidine 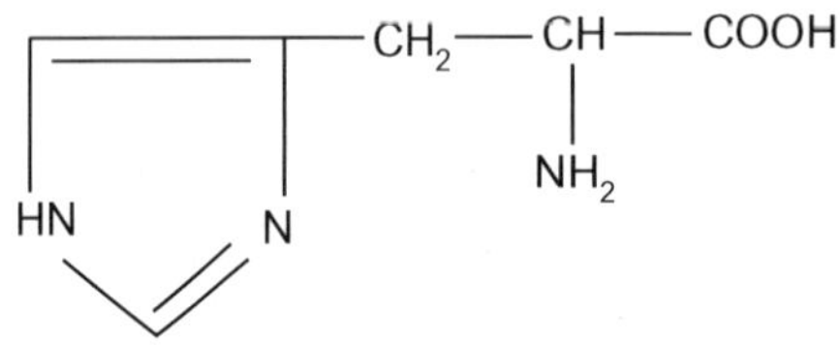

Threonine, Valine, Leucine, Isoleucine, Arginine, Lysine, Methionine, Phenyl alanine, Tryptophan and Histidine are essential amino acids.

General Properties of Amino Acids

Amino acids are colourless crystalline compounds which are generally soluble in water, but sparingly soluble in organic solvents. All amino acids contain atleast one chiral centre except glycine.

I. R Spectra

Most of the Amino acids exhibit absorption bands near 1400 and 1600 $c.m^{-1}$, characterestics of carboxylate ion. Also exhibits characterestic absorption of NH_3^+.

Stereo isomerism of α-Amino acids

Except Glycine, all other amino acids exhibits inversional isomerism.

Absolute configuration

Since all amino acids contain, at least one chiral centre, except Glycine, exhibits optical activity. Natural (-) Serine was chosen as the arbitrary standard for correlating the configuration of amino acids. By optical rotatory dispersion method, proved that all L-amino acids show +ve cotton effects and D-amino acids show -ve cotton effect. Some naturally occuring amino acids have more than one asymmetric centre and can exists in more than two stereo-isomeric forms. Apart from L & D forms, two allo modifications are known which have opposite configuration only at one asymmetric carbon atom relative to former two molecules. Compounds which bear such a relation to each other are referred as diastereomers. They differ in physical properties and in quantitative chemical behaviour such as reaction rate.

Eg: Threonine have L & D and allomodifications.

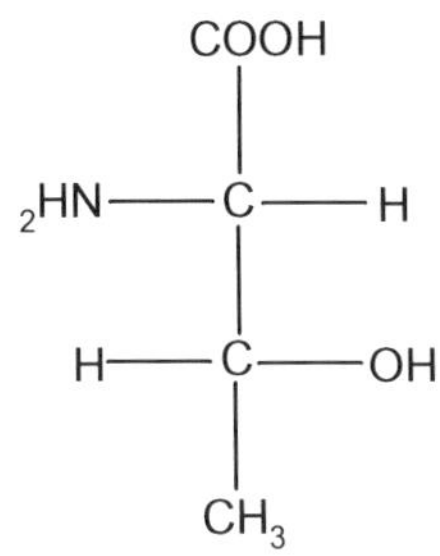
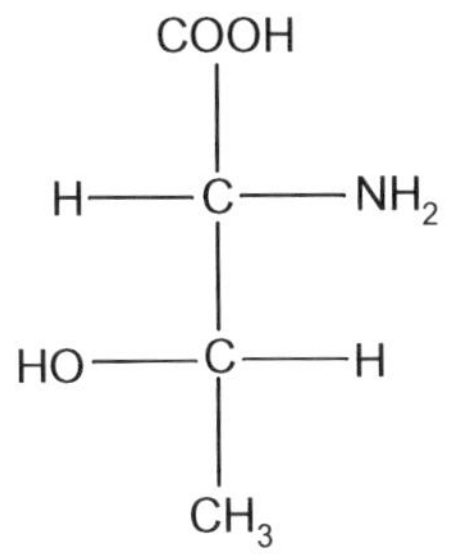
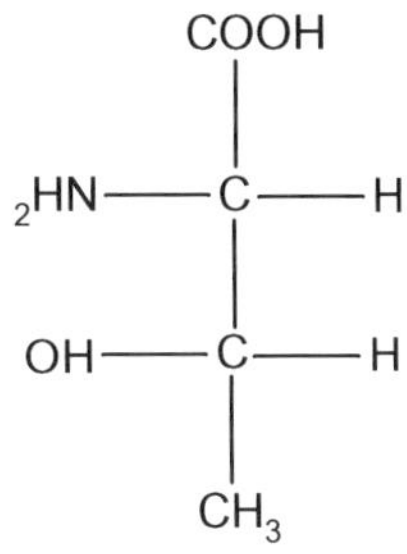
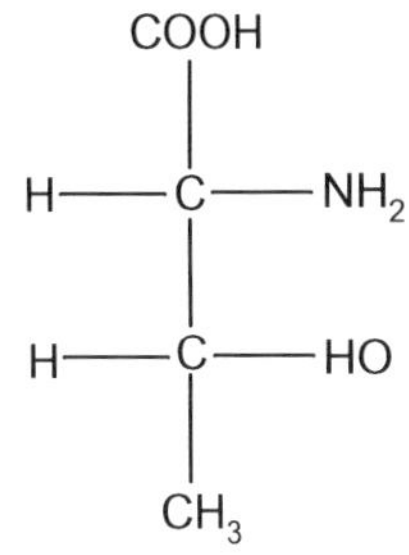

L (-)Threonine | D (+) Threonine | L - allothreonine | D - allothreonine

The symbols 'D' and 'L' are used for the configuration of α-carbon atom and symbols (+) and (-) are used to indicate direction of the rotation.

Reactions due to Amino Group

(i) With strong inorganic acids

Due to the presence of a lone pair of electrons on nitrogen, amino acids form salts with strong inorganic acids.

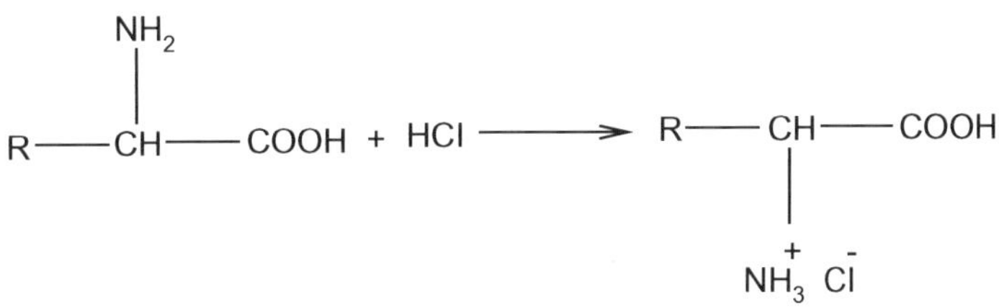

These salts are usually sparingly soluble in water, and the free acids may be liberated by means of a strong organic base. eg: Pyridine.

(ii) Alkylation

In basic solution, the amino group of an amino acid is nucleophilic and can displace the halogen of alkyl halides.

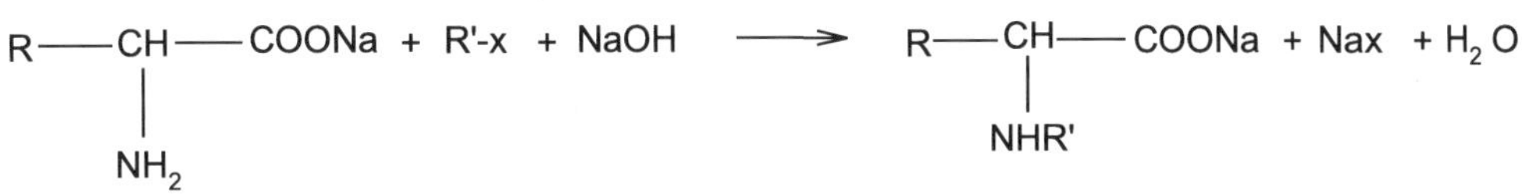

(iii) Arylation

In basic solution, the amino group of an amino acid is nucleophilic and can displace the halogen of any aryl halides.

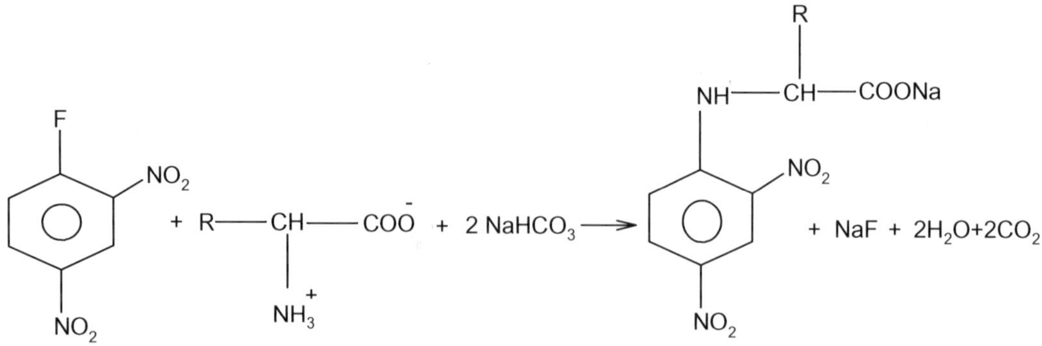

2,4 Dinitro fluorobenzene

(iv) Acylation and Benzoylation

With acetyl chloride or acetic anhydride, amino acid can be acetylated.

$$R-CH(NH_3^+)-COO^- + (CH_3CO)_2O \longrightarrow R-CH(NHCOCH_3)COOH + CH_3COOH$$

Acetic anhydride

Benzoylation can be done with benzoyl chloride.

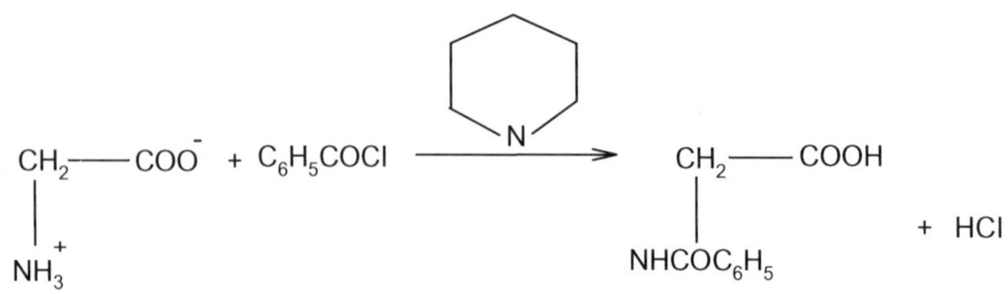

Hippuric Acid

(v) Reaction with Nitrous Acid

Nitrous acid liberates nitrogen from amino acids. The evolved nitrogen can be measured, which forms the basis of van slyke method for analysing mixtures of amino acids.

$$R-CH(NH_3^+)-COO^- + HNO_2 \longrightarrow R-CH(OH)-COOH + N_2 + H_2O$$

(vi) Reaction with nitrosyl chloride or bromide

Amino acids react with these regents, form chloro or bromo products.

$$RCH(NH_2)COOH + NOCl \xrightarrow{HI} RCHClCOOH + N_2 + H_2O$$

$$RCH(NH_2)COOH + NOBr \longrightarrow RCHBrCOOH + N_2 + H_2O$$

(vii) Reaction with Hydriodic Acid

When amino acids heated with hydriodic acid at 200°C, the amino group is eliminated with the formation of fatty acid.

$$RCH(NH_2)COOH \xrightarrow[200^\circ C]{HI} RCH_2COOH + N + H_2O$$

(viii) Reaction with oxidising agents

Oxidising agents attack free amino group and initially either an α-imino acid formed, which hydrolysed to α-keto acid and ammonia. Sometimes oxidation accompanied by decarboxylation and resulted in lower aldehyde and ammonia.

Reactions due to Carboxyl Group

(i) Amino acids react with alkali to form salts.

Eg:

$$\overset{+}{N}H_3—CH_2—COO^- + NaOH \longrightarrow NH_2—CH_2COONa + H_2O$$

(ii) Amino acids with salts of heavy metals.

Amino acid forms chelate compounds with salts of heavy metals.

Eg: Reaction of Glycine with Copper.

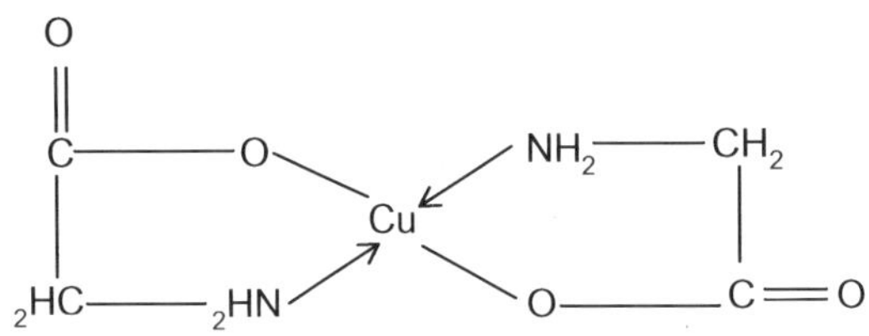

(iii) Amino acids reacts with alcohol to form ester

Carboxyl group of amino acids react with alcohol group forms an ester.

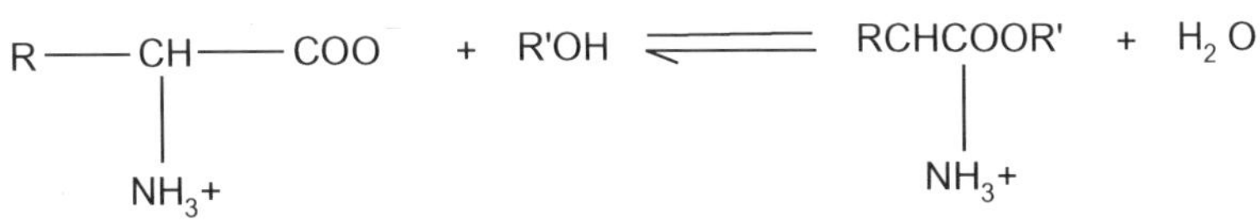

(iv) Reduction of acid group

Amino acids reduced to amino alcohol by metal hydride.

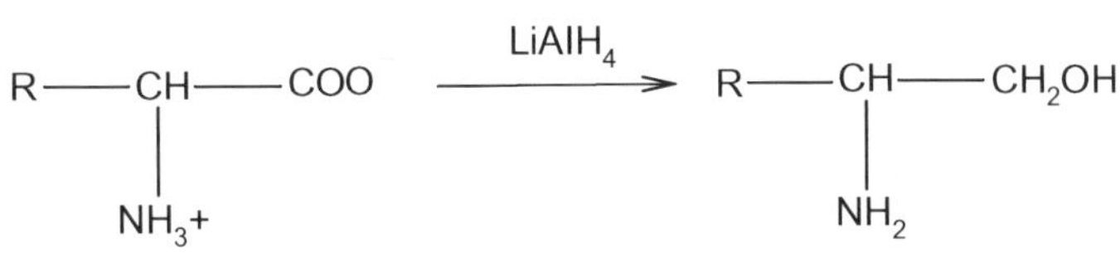

(v) Formation of Acid chlorides

In this reaction, amino group is protected by treating with acetic anhydride. Then acetylated amino acid converted to acetylated amino acid chloride with PCl_5.

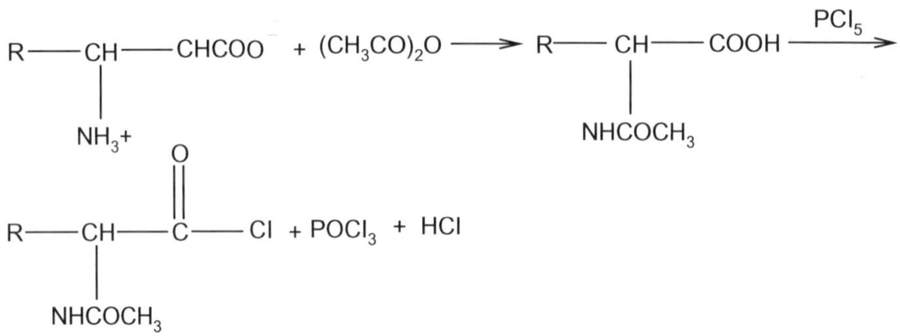

(vi) Dakin-west reaction

When amino acid heated with acetic anhydride in pyridine solution, amino acid converted into methyl α-acetamidoketones. This reaction is known as Dakin west reaction.

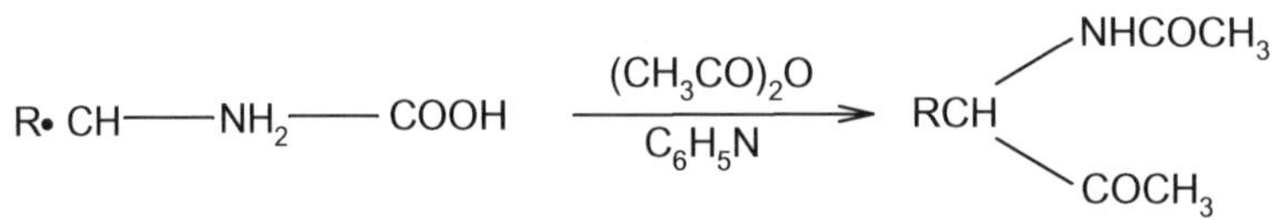

(vii) Decarboxylation

Amino acids on heating with barium oxide ,decarboxylates to amines.

$$R\,CH—NH_2—COOH \xrightarrow{\triangle} RCH_2—NH_2 + CO_2\uparrow$$

Reaction due to both Amino and Carboxyl Groups

(i) Dipolar ions

Amino acids have large dipolemoment in aqueous solution due to their existence as inner salts. Such a double charged ion is known as zwitter ion or ampholyte or dipolar ion. The dipolar ion structure accounts for the absence of acidic and basic properties of amino acids. In neutral solution, amino acids can exists as three species, which are in equilibrium.

$$\underset{\text{Conjugate Acid}}{RCH\overset{+}{N}H_3COOH} \underset{+H^+}{\overset{-H^+}{\rightleftharpoons}} \underset{\text{Dipolar ion}}{RCH\overset{+}{N}H_3CO\overline{O}} \underset{+H^+}{\overset{-H^+}{\rightleftharpoons}} \underset{\text{Conjugate base}}{RCHNH_2CO\overline{O}}$$

(ii) Iso electric point

pH at which amino acids exhibit minimum migration in an electric field is called isoelectric point. For each aminoacids, there is a particular p^H at which concentration of anion and cation in solution will be equal and concentration of dipolar ion in solution will be at maximum. Therefore dipolar ions has a net charge of zero, the migration of ions under the influence of an electric field will be minimum at that p^H.

(iii) Titration of amino acids with alkali

pk_a of amino acid can be determined by titrating with alkali. To do the titration amino group is masked by the addition of formalin. Eg: When formalin added to glycine, methylene glycine and dimethyloglycine is formed.

$$NH_2—CH_2—COOH + HCHO \longrightarrow CH_2{=}NCH_2—COOH + (CH_2OH)_2NCH_2COOH + H_2O$$

This method of masking amino group by formalin and thereafter titration with alkali is known as Sorensen formol titration.

(iv) Action of heat

When amino acids are heated, 2,5 diketopiperazines are obtained.

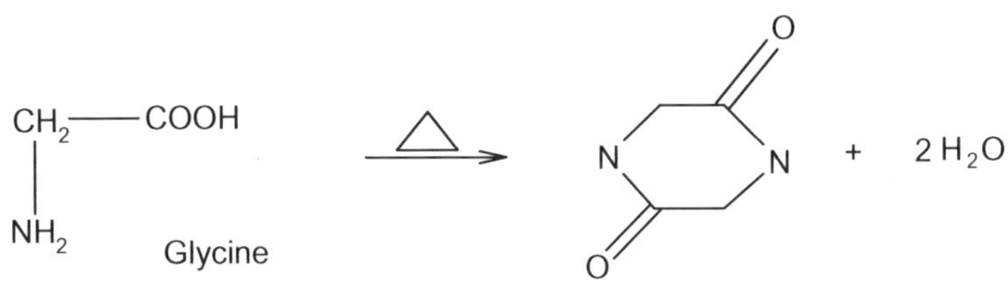

(v) Action of Nitrous acid

With nitrous acid, N-alkyl or arylamino acid yield N-nitroso derivatives which upon dehydration with acetic anhydride yield sydnones.

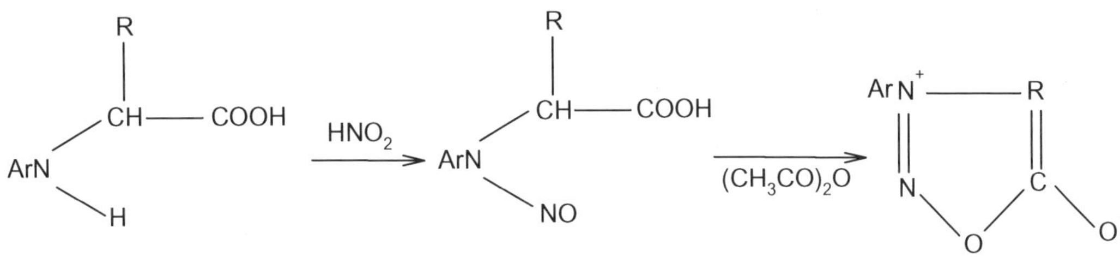

(vi) Formation of Betaines

Amino acid on heating with methyl iodide in methanolic solution give betaines which exists as dipolar ions.

$$\overset{+}{N}H_3CH_2CO\bar{O} + 3\,CH_3I \longrightarrow (CH_3)_3\,\overset{+}{N}CH_2CO\bar{O} + 3\,HI$$

(vii) Action of Phenyl isocyanate

α-amino acids react with phenyl isocyanates to form phenyl-hydantoic acid, which on heating in the presence of acid cyclises to hydantoins which are useful synthetic reagents.

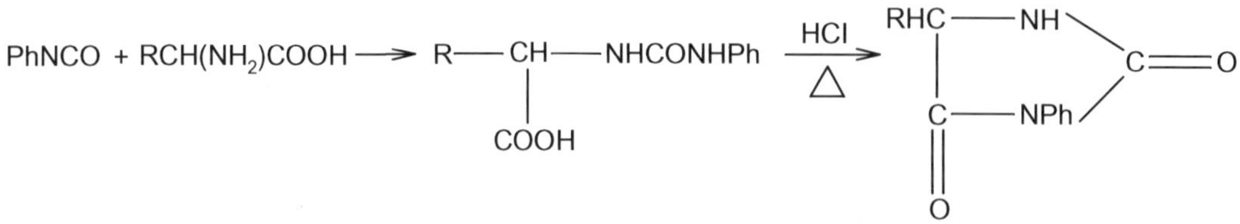

Preparation of Amino Acids

Many methods are there to prepare amino acids. Some important ones are discussed here.

1. Amination of α-halogenated acid

(a) By the action of ammonia

α-chloro and β-bromo acid obtained by direct halogenation of Carboxylic acid or by bromination of corresponding malonic acid can be aminated by alcoholic, aqueous or liquid ammonia.

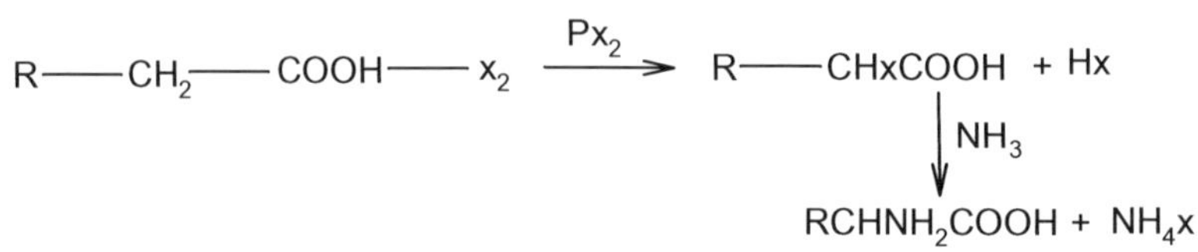

(b) Gabriel's phthalimide synthesis

α-halogenated acid ester is treated with potassium phthalimide yield substituted phthalimide ester which again reacts with hydrazine or 4 N alkali followed by acid hydrolysis give amino acid.

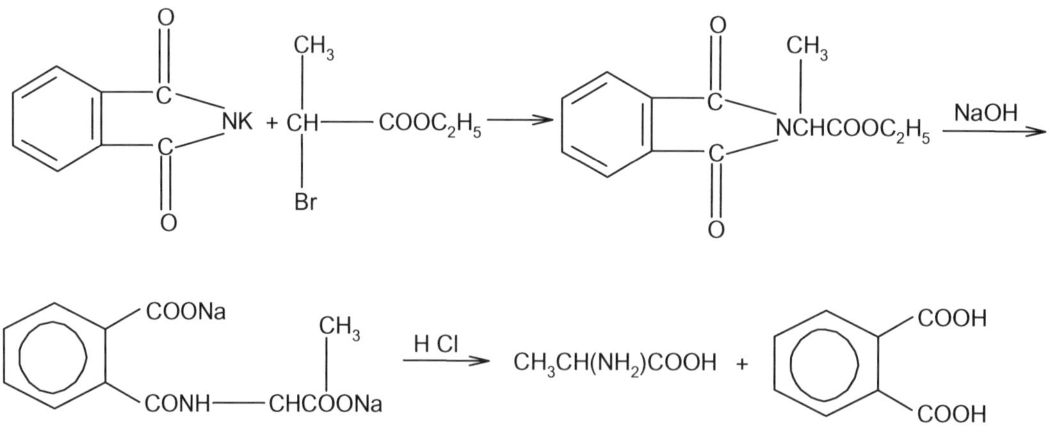

2. Strecker's Synthesis

In this an aldehyde is converted into amino-nitrile by the action of hydrogen cyanide and ammonia. Then amino nitrile is hydrolysed with an acid to get amino acid.

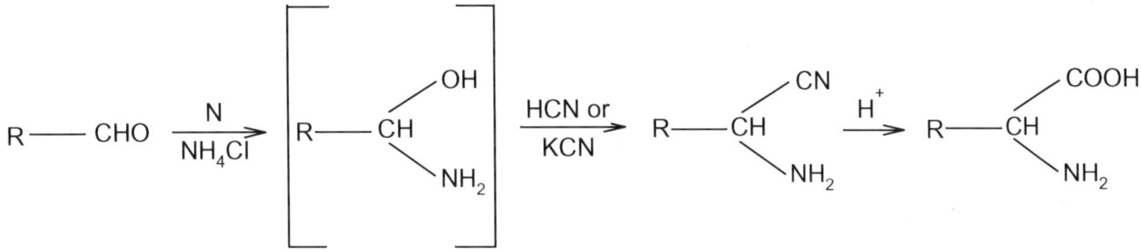

3. Malonic Ester Synthesis

α-halogeno-acid can be prepared by this method.

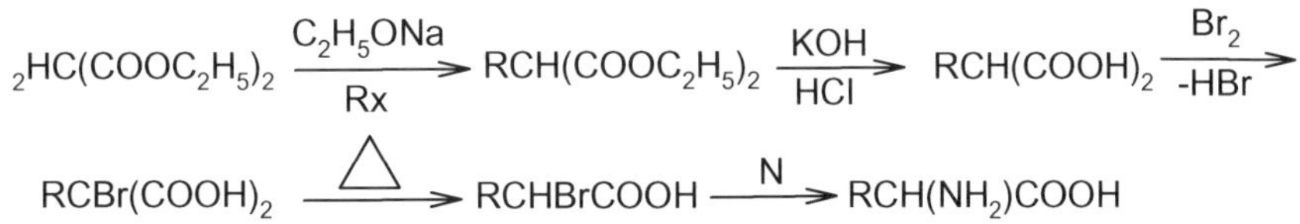

4. Curtius reaction

Malonic or Cyanoacetic ester can be converted into some amino acids.

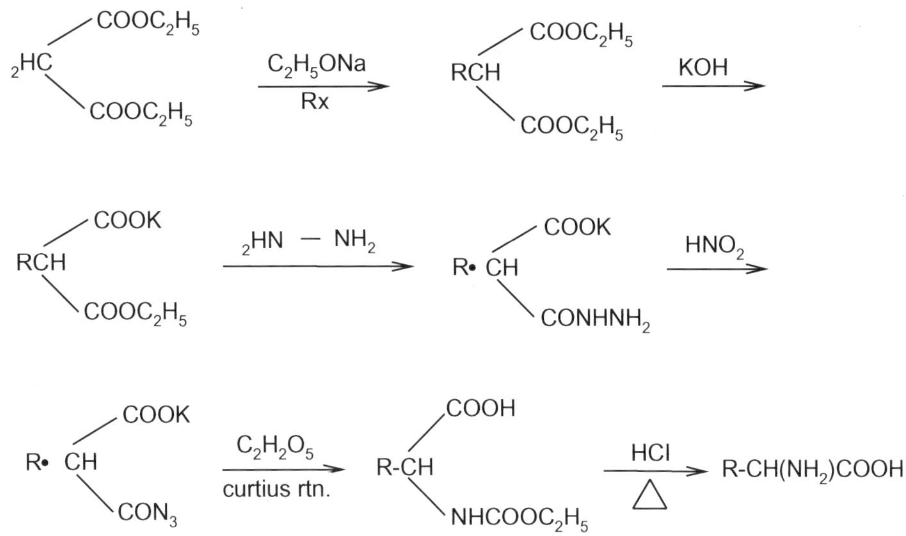

5. Hofmann degradation

Amino acid can be prepared by Hofmann degradation of malonic ester amide.

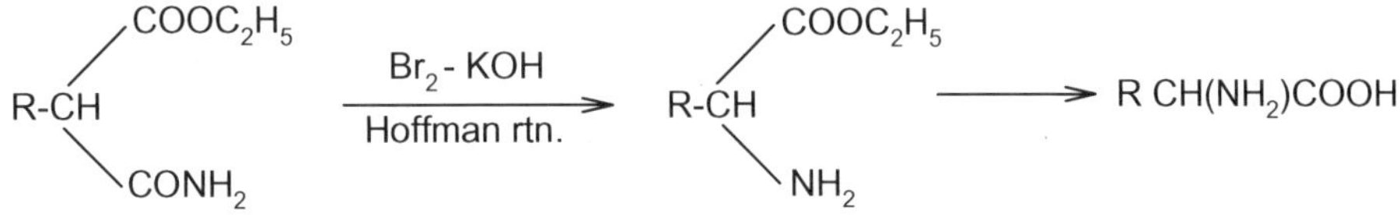

6. Darapsky Synthesis

Amino acids can be prepared by the condensation and simultaneous reduction of an aldehyde and cyanoacetic ester.

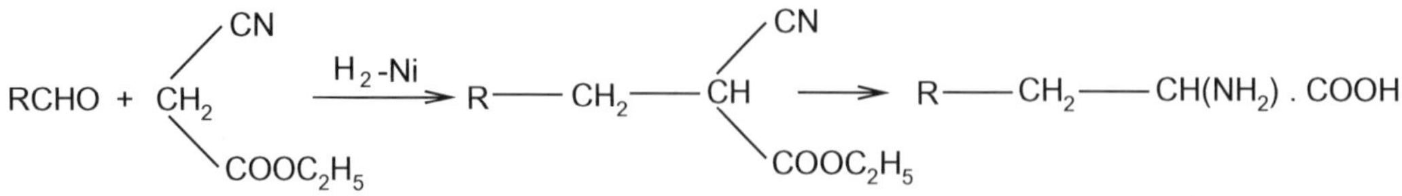

7. Schmidt reaction

Alkylacetoacetic ester can be converted to α-amino acid also by Schmidt reaction.

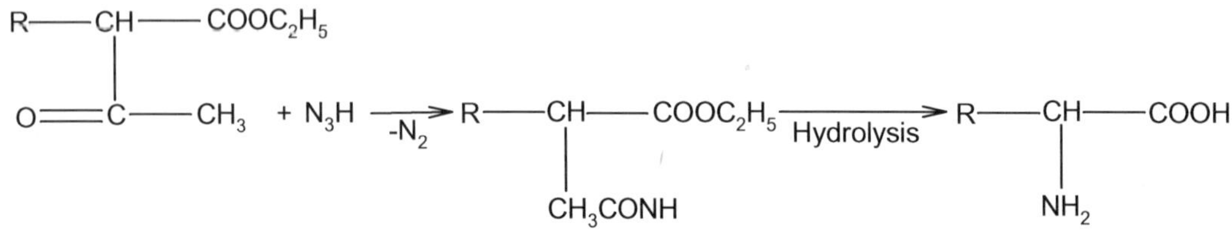

8. Erlenmeyer azlactone synthesis

Aromatic amino acids can be prepared by this method. It includes heating of aromatic aldehyde with hippuric acid (benzoyl glycine) in presence of acetic anhydride and sodium acetate to form azlactone which on warming with 1% alkali followed by reduction with sodium amalgam and hydrolysis with acid give α-amino acid.

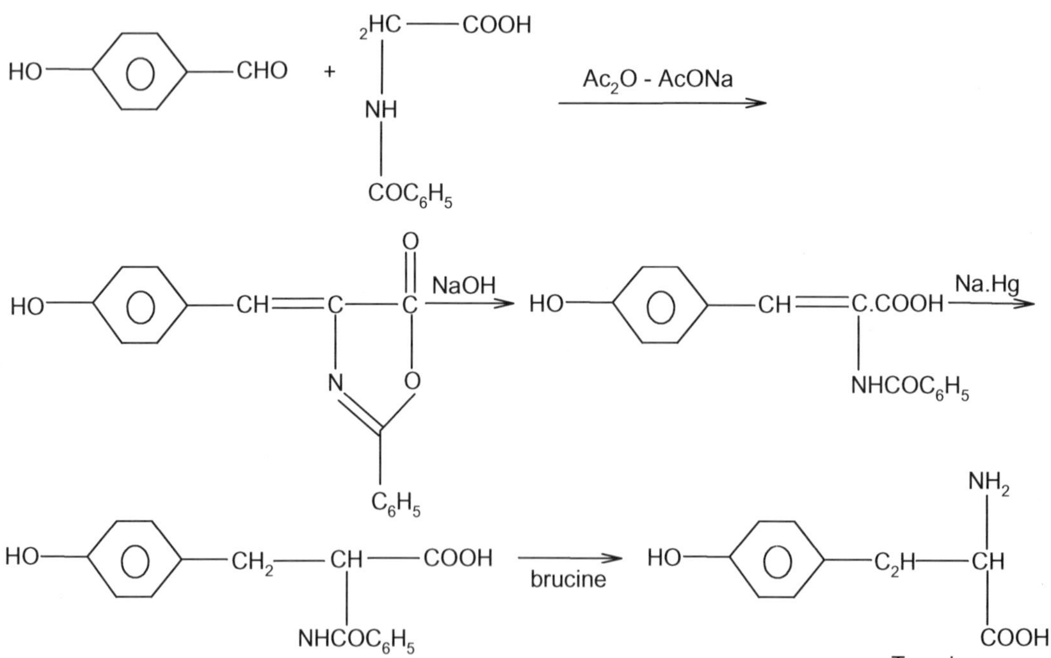

Tyrosine

9. Bucherer's Hydantoin Synthesis

In this method an oxo compound is converted into 5-substituted hydantoin by means of ammonium carbonate and sodium cyanide in aqueous ethanolic solution. Then N-substituted hydantoin on hydrolysis yields amino acid.

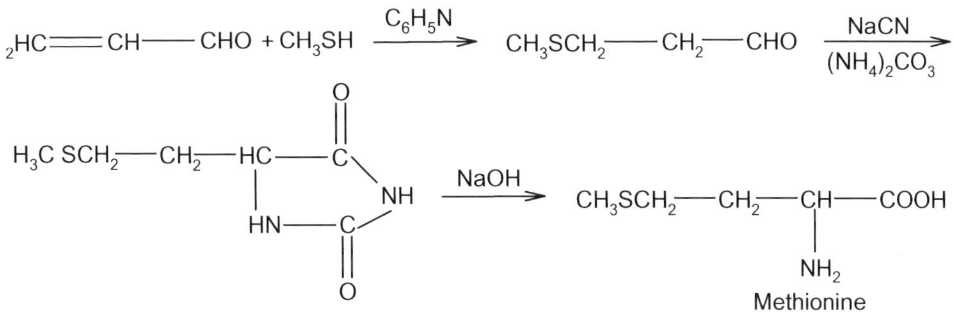

10. Synthesis by Diketopiperazine

Aromatic aldehydes when condensed with diketopiperazine yield substituted products, which upon heating with red Phosphorus and Hydrogen iodide produce α-amino acids.

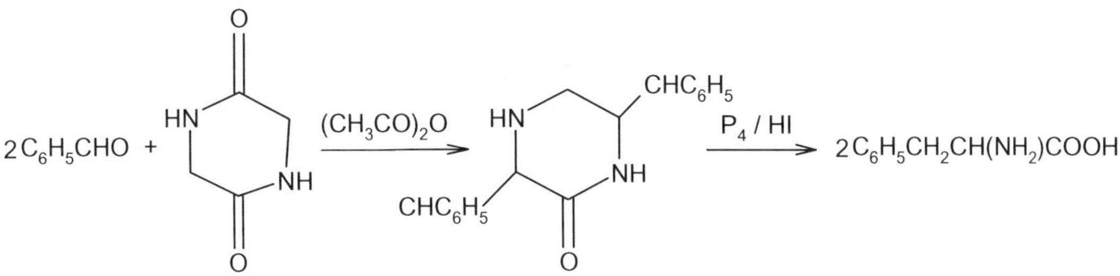

PROTEINS

Proteins are highly complex, nitrogenous compounds occuring in the protoplasm of all animals and plants cell. Proteins are the molecules having molecular weight above 10,000 and polypeptides have less molecular weight. Proteins are amphoteric in nature. At isoelectric point proteins have least solubility, and will have minimum osmotic pressure and viscosity.

According to complexity of structure proteins are divided into Simple proteins, Cojugated proteins and Derived proteins.

Simple proteins

These proteins give only amino acids or their derivatives on hydrolysis. Eg Albumins, Globulins, Prolamines, Glutelins, Albuminoids (Sclero proteins), Histones, Protamines.

Conjugated proteins

Conjugated proteins are proteins which contain a non-protein group (i.e., a compound not containing amino-acid residues) attached to the protein part.

Eg: Glycoproteins, Phosphoproteins, Lipoproteins, Nucleoproteins, Chromoproteins and Metalloproteins.

Derived proteins

These are degradation products obtained by the action of acids,alkalis or enzymes on proteins.

Eg: Denatured proteins, Meta proteins, Polypeptides, Simple peptides.

According to molecular structure and solubility proteins are classified into fibrous proteins and Globular proteins.

Fibrous proteins

These are soluble in concentrated acid or alkali and are long linear protein chains.

Eg: Collagen

Globular proteins

These are soluble in water, dilute acid, dilute alkali and are highly branched, cross linked proteins.

Eg: Casein of milk.

GENERAL CHARACTERESTICS OF PROTEINS

Molecular Weight

Proteins are macromolecules constructed by repetition of one or more structural units called monomers which constitute amino acids. Molecular weight can be determined by Svedberg method which is measurement of sedimentation rates as determined in ultracentrifuge. Other methods are also available to determine the molecular weight like osmotic pressure measurements, X-ray diffraction, light scattering effects,gel filtration and by Chemical analysis. Chemical analysis based on the estimation of amino acids present. Eg: molecular weight of ribonuclease is 13,700, Haemoglobin-68,000.

Denaturation

All proteins are coagulated and precipitated from aqueous solution by heating/by standing in acid/alkaline solution/by treatment with organic solvents such as ethanol or acetone,by high concenteration of urea, by detergents and by physical means such as X-ray, light and shaking. Proteins in this precipitated state are said to be denaturated and process of reaching this state is called denaturation. It mainly occurs at isoelectric point of corresponding protein. Denaturation occurs due to unfolding of proteins. Under careful controlled conditions, renaturation occurs. If denaturation occured by heat, by successive cooling refolding occurs and process is known as annealing.

Salting in and out of Proteins

Solubility of many proteins increases in the presence of small concentration of various neutral salts and is referred as salting in of proteins. When concenteration of neutral salt is increased, the solubility increases to maximum and then decreases, finally protein is precipitated and is referred as salting out.

CHARACTERESTIC COLOUR REACTIONS OF PROTEINS

Biuret Test

When an alkaline solution of protein is warmed with dilute copper sulphate, a red violet colour developed, due to peptide linkage (CONH) At least two peptide linkages needed to respond this reaction.

Xanthoproteic Test

Proteins when warmed with concentrated nitric acid give yellow colour, when it make alkaline produces orange colour. This is due to the nitration of benzene ring.

Millons Test

Addition of millons reagent (mercuric nitrate in nitric acid containing a trace of nitrous acid) to a protien gives a white precipitate which on heating turns to red. This is due to the phenolic group eg: Tyrosin which is a phenolic amino acid.

PEPTIDES

A peptide is composed of two or more amino acids joined through peptide linkage Atoms in the group --CONH--, are planar and the O and H are trans C-N bond length is -O=C-NH-- is 1.32A° which is shorter than the usual C-N bond length(1.47A°).When many amino acids are joined together,the compound is called polypeptide.Below a molecular weight of 10,000, the compound is considered to be polypeptide, above 10,000 is considered to be protein.

GENERAL PRINCIPLES OF POLYPEPTIDE SYNTHESIS

Mainly four steps are there to synthesise polypeptides.

1. Protection of Amino group
2. protection of Carboxyl group
3. Activation of Carboxyl group
4. Coupling

Protection of Amino Group

Active amino group should protected for the regiospecific control. Different types of protecting groups are there. Eg: Benzyloxy Carbonyl (Carbobenzyloxy), t-butyloxy Carbonyl, trityl (triphenyl methyl), Phthaloyl and tosyl (p-toluene sulphonyl) group.

Bergmann's Method

In this method, Benzyloxy Carbonyl Chloride is taken as amino protecting group. It is prepared by the action of Carbonyl Chloride on benzyl alcohol in toluene solution

$$C_6H_5CH_2OH + COCl_2 \longrightarrow C_6H_5CH_2OCOCl + HCl$$

Benzyloxy Carbonyl Chloride reacts with amino acid forms N-benzyloxy Carbonyl peptide. Protecting group removed by hydrogenolysis which is carried out by bubbling hydrogen through a suspension of Palladium Catalyst to peptide.

$$C_6H_5CH_2OCOCl + R\ CH\ (NH_2)\ COOH \xrightarrow[-HCl]{OH-} C_6H_5CH_2OCONHCHR_1COOH \xrightarrow{PCl_5}$$

$$C_6H_5CH_2OCONHCHR_1COCl \xrightarrow[NaOH]{R_2\ (CH)NH_2COOH} C_6H_5CH_2OCONHCHR_1CONHCHR_2COOH \xrightarrow[Pd]{H_2}$$

$$NH_2CHR_1CONHC_2HR_2COOH + C_6H_5CH_3 + CO_2$$

Sulphur containing amino acids cannot be done like this due to unfavourable reaction between Sulphur and Palladium.

Sheehan's Method

Here phthaloyl group is used as protecting group. Amino acid can be converted to N-phthaloyl derivatives by fusion with phthalic anhydride.Protecting group can be removed by treatment with hydrazine hydrate under reflux.

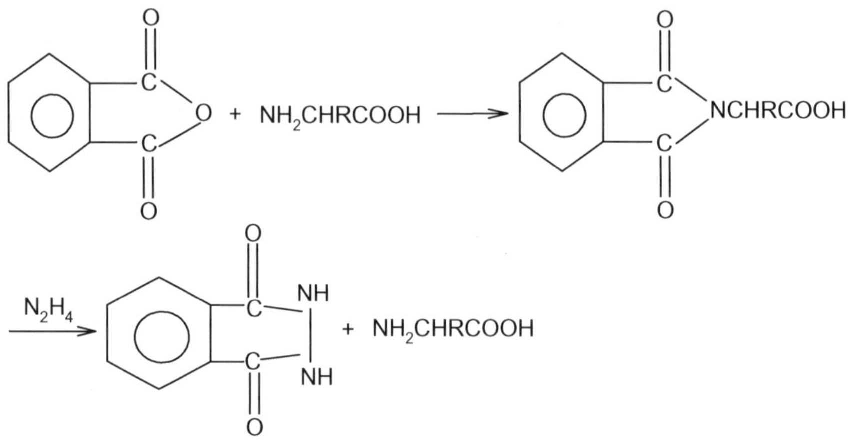

t-butyloxy Carbonyl Group

It is used as its p-nitrophenyl ester.Protecting group removed by acid catalysed cleavage of alkyl-Oxygen bond by trifluoro acetic acid or 2NHCl

$$(CH_3)_3COCOOC_6H_4NO_2 + NH_2CHRCOOH \longrightarrow$$

$$(CH_3)_3CO—CONH—CH—R—COOH + HOC_6H_4NO_2$$

$$\downarrow \text{ClH or } CF_3COOH$$

$$\bar{Cl}\ \overset{+}{N}H_3\ CHRCOOH + (CH_3)_3CCl + CO_2$$

Tosyl Group

P-toluene Sulphonyl Chloride is the protecting group. P-toluene Sulphonyl Chloride reacts with amino acid in the presence of alkali. Protecting group is removed by Sodium in Liquid ammonia.

$$CH_3C_6H_4SO_2Cl + NH_2CHR_1COOH \xrightarrow{NaOH}$$

$$CH_3C_6H_4SO_2NHCHR_1COONa \xrightarrow{CH_3COOH} CH_3C_6H_4SO_2NHCHR_1COOH \xrightarrow[Liq.NH_3]{Na} Na_2CHR_1COOH$$

Protection of Carbonyl Group

Usual method of protecting carboxylic group is esterification. Common esters being methyl, ethyl, benzyl, t-butyl and nitrobenzyl. Methyl or ethyl group is removed by saponification using aqueous alkali-organic solvent mixtures at room temperature.

$$RCH(NH_2)COOH + R'OH(excess) \xrightarrow{H^+} R\ CH(NH_2)COOR' + H_2O$$

Activation of Carboxyl Group

Carboxyl group needs activation which can be done by converting -OH group into a better leaving group.

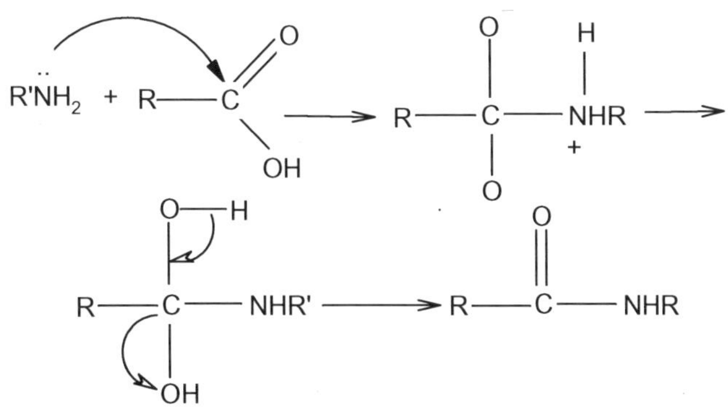

Activating groups include Acid Chlorides, Esters and Acid azides

Acid Chlorides

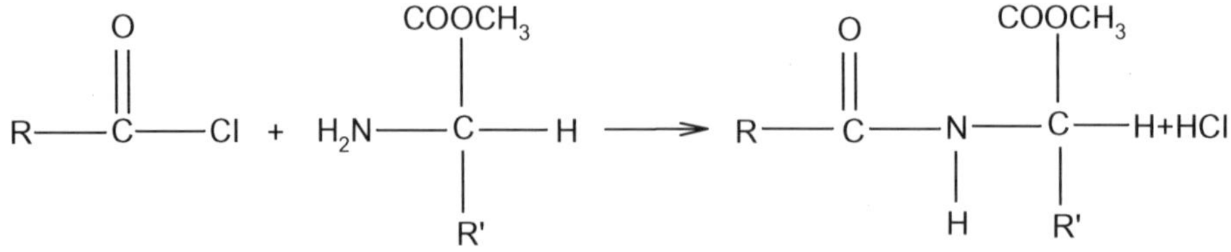

Esters

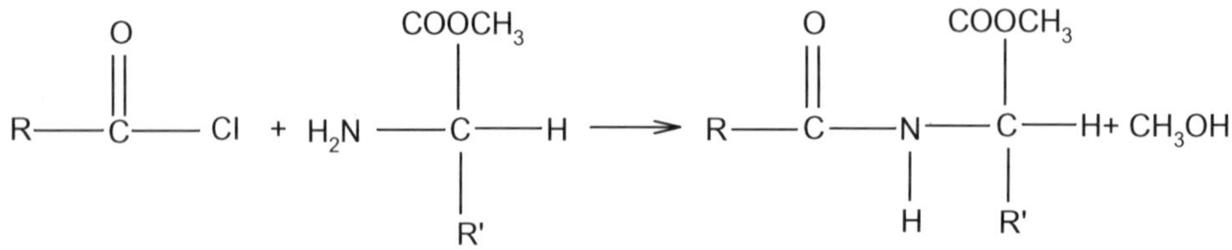

Acid azides

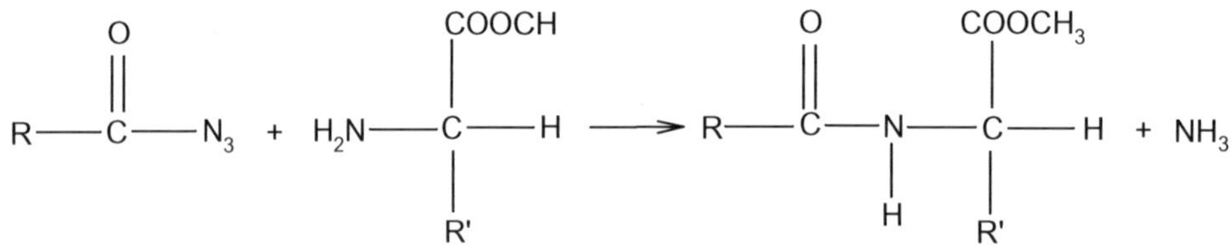

Coupling Step

In coupling step, free amino group and free hydroxyl group joined to give peptide bond. Peptide linkage is formed by nucleophilic attack of free amino group of an amino acid ester or peptide ester on activated Carboxyl end of N-protected amino acid.

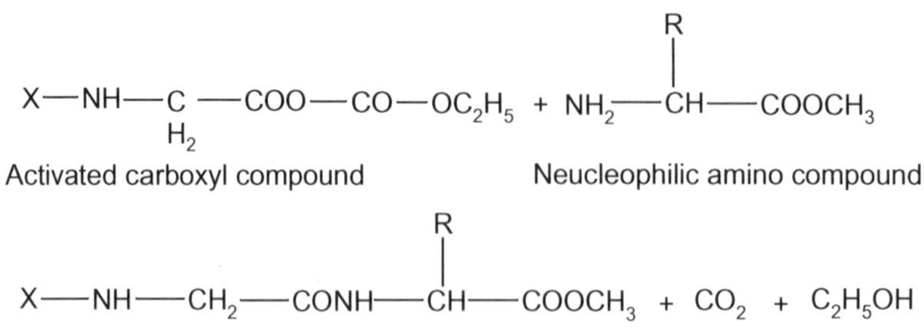

x = Protecting group

SYNTHESIS OF POLYPEPTIDES

Fischer's second method

In this method, ethyl Chloroformate is used to protect the amino group. Fischer prepared a polypeptide by condensation of amino acid, whose amino group protected by means of ethyl Chloroformate with an amino acid ester.

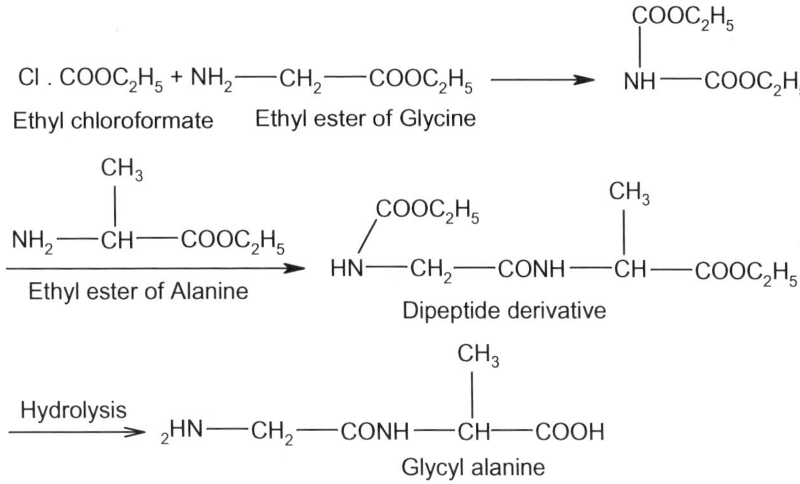

Fischer's third method

In this method tosyl group is used as protecting group. Hydrogen iodide is used to remove tosyl group.

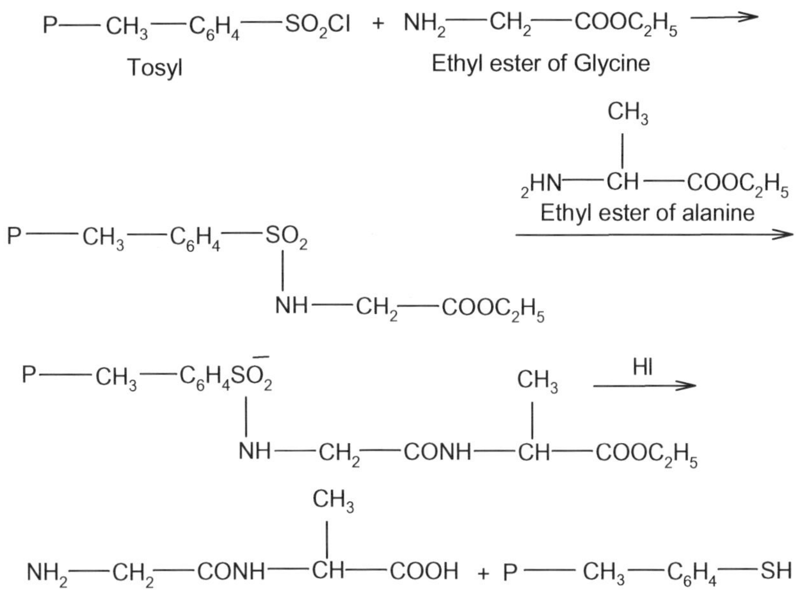

Halpern's method

In this method amino group is protected by means of Dimedone and protective group is removed by mild bromination.

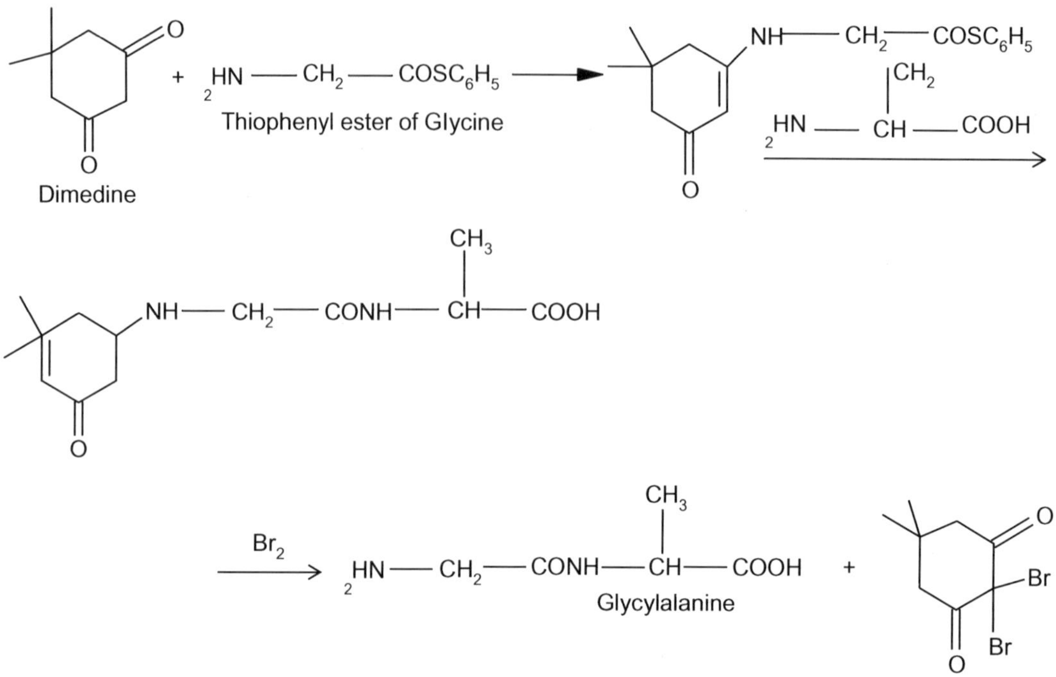

Azlactone Synthesis

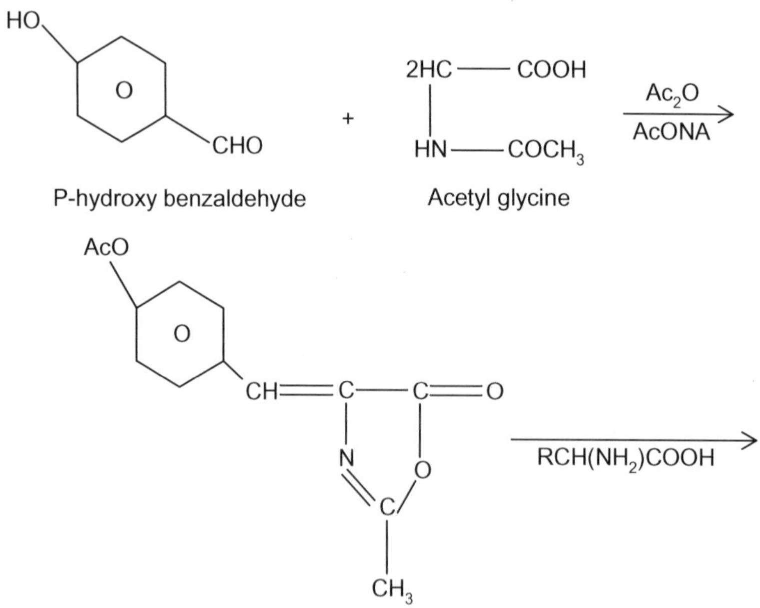

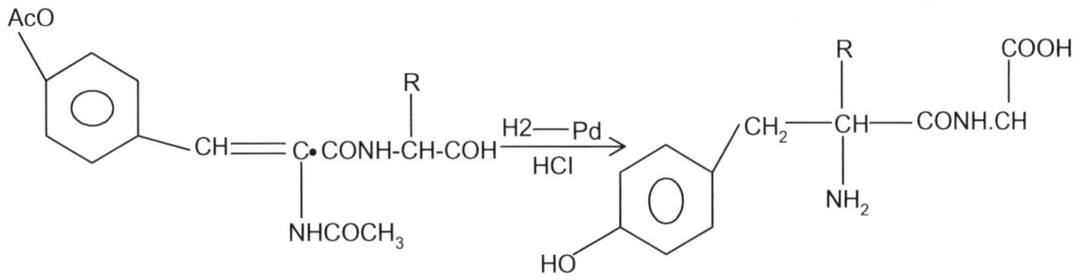

Curtius method

This method consists of condensation of benzoylated amino acid azide with a molecule of amino acid ester.

$$\underset{\text{Glycine}}{2HN-CH_2-COOH} \xrightarrow{C_6H_5COCl} \underset{\text{Benzoylated glycine}}{C_6H_5CO-NH-CH_2-COOH} \xrightarrow{C_2H_5OH}$$

$$C_6H_5CO-NH-CH_2-COOC_2H_5 \xrightarrow{NH_2-N}$$

$$C_6H_5CO-NH-CH_2-CO-NH-NH_2$$

$$\xrightarrow[O^{O}C]{HNO_2} C_6H_5CO-NH-CH_2-CO-N{=}N{\equiv}N$$

$$_2HN-CH(CH_3)-COOC_2H_5$$

$$\xrightarrow[-N_3H]{}$$

$$C_6H_5CO-NH-CH_2-CONH-CH(CH_3)-COOC_2H_5$$

$$\xrightarrow{\text{Hydrolysis}} \underset{\text{Glycine alanine}}{NH_2-CH_2-CONH-CH(CH_3)-COOH} + C_6H_5COOH + C_2H_5OH$$

Mixed anhydride method

It involves conversion of amino acid into anhydrides, which when dissolved in an organic solvent and then treated with water, undergo polymerisation.

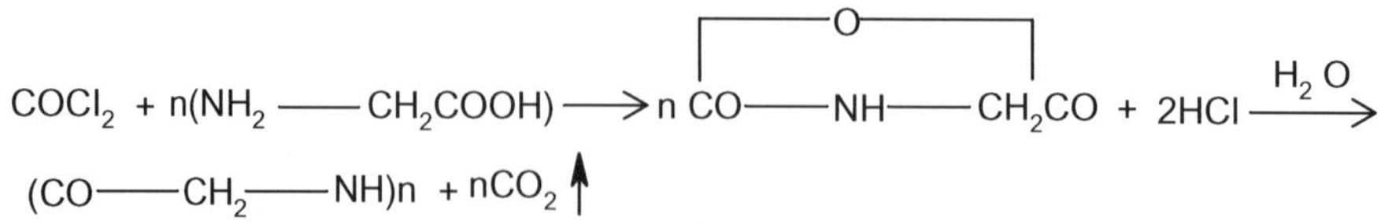

For Berger and Sheehans method refer the protection of amino group.

Structure of Proteins

Proteins are polymers containing large number of amino acids joined to each other by peptide bonds.Structure of proteins can be studied under four heads.

Primary structure

Primary structure deals with a) nature of amino acid b) number of each particular amino acid present in one molecule of protein c) the sequence in which different amino acids are arranged in molecule

To determine the structure of proteins, the peptide or protein must be isolated in pure state,then have to ascertain whether the protein consists of a single peptide chain or whether it is composed of number of subunits.Then each peptide is completely hydrolysed into its constituent amino acids and their nature and amounts are determined.Molecular weight is determined by physical methods.End group analysis is carried out to determine the nature of N- and -C- terminal groups. Then sequence of amino acids determined.

Secondary structure

It deals with shape of the peptide chain that is whether it is linear, cyclic, branched or arranged in the form of helix.

Tertiary structure

It mainly deals forces with which, the peptide chains are held together and the way in which individual peptide chains are arranged in definite manner to a macromolecule of an individual shape. (folded/refolded).

Quaternary structure

It deals with the number of peptide chains and their arrangement in natural proteins.

Now we will see the each structures elaborately.

Primary structure

(a) Purification

In the case of soluble proteins, crude sample of proteins precipitated out near its isoelectric point. The sample is made free from salts by dialysis or gel filtration and then fractionated by chromatographic methods. Purified sample isolated by freeze drying.

(b) Determination of amino acid composition

Protein to be investigated is hydrolysed by means of 6 N hydro Chloric acid at 110° or by peptidase enzyme.Seperated amino acid can be estimated by different methods like ion exchange chromatography, P^H dependent precipitation and electrophoresis.

Ion exchange Chromatography

Chromatographic columns are packed with sulphonated polystyrene divinyl resin which has highly polar-SO_3H group. Solution containing amino acid mixture is placed on column of resin. By protein transfer, amino acid converted into ammonium ion and resin into sulphonate anions. Ammonium ions of different amino acids are then adsorbed on the surface of sulphonic acid resin. Elution of the column with a buffer solution, results in separation of amino acids which can be isolated and weighed. Estimation can be done by reacting with Ninhydrin and measured spectrophotometrically.

P^H dependent precipitation

Since each amino acid have different isoelectric point, can be precipitated by changing the pH.

(c) End group determination (N-terminal and C-terminal)

Amino end degradation

Sanger's method

This method involves treating a polypeptide with Sanger's reagent (1 fluoro 2,4 dinitro benzene-FDNB) in presence of Sodium hydrogen carbonate solution at room temperature to form 2,4 dinitrophenyl (DNP) derivative of polypeptide. Product hydrolysed by acid cleave peptide bond connecting N-terminal amino acid to rest of polypeptide molecule. DNP derivative identified by thin layer chromatography.

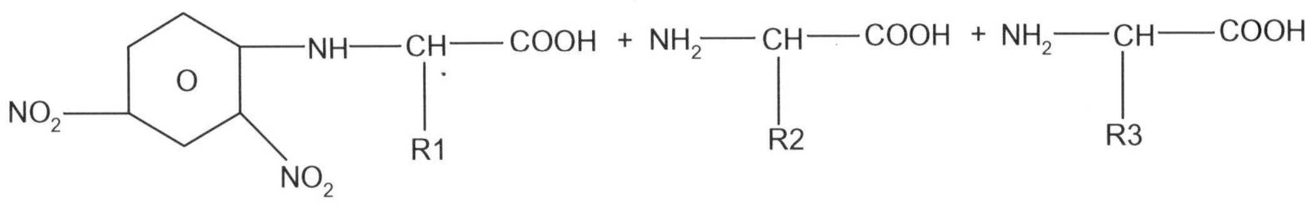

2,4 DNP derivative

Dansyl method

Dansyl reagent (1-dimethylamino naphthalene 5-Sulphonyl-Chloride) is used to make derivative.

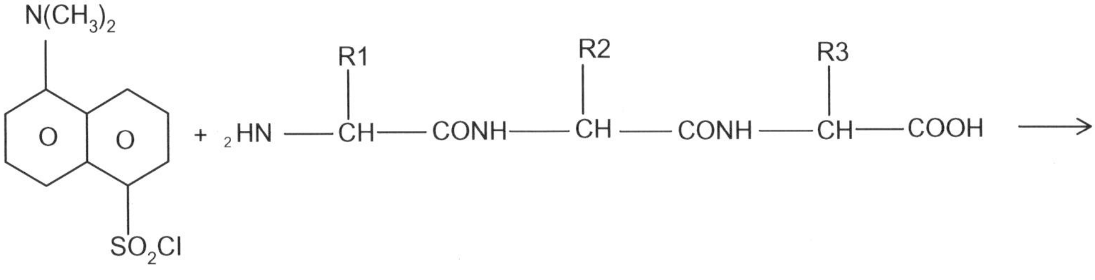

Dansyl Chloride

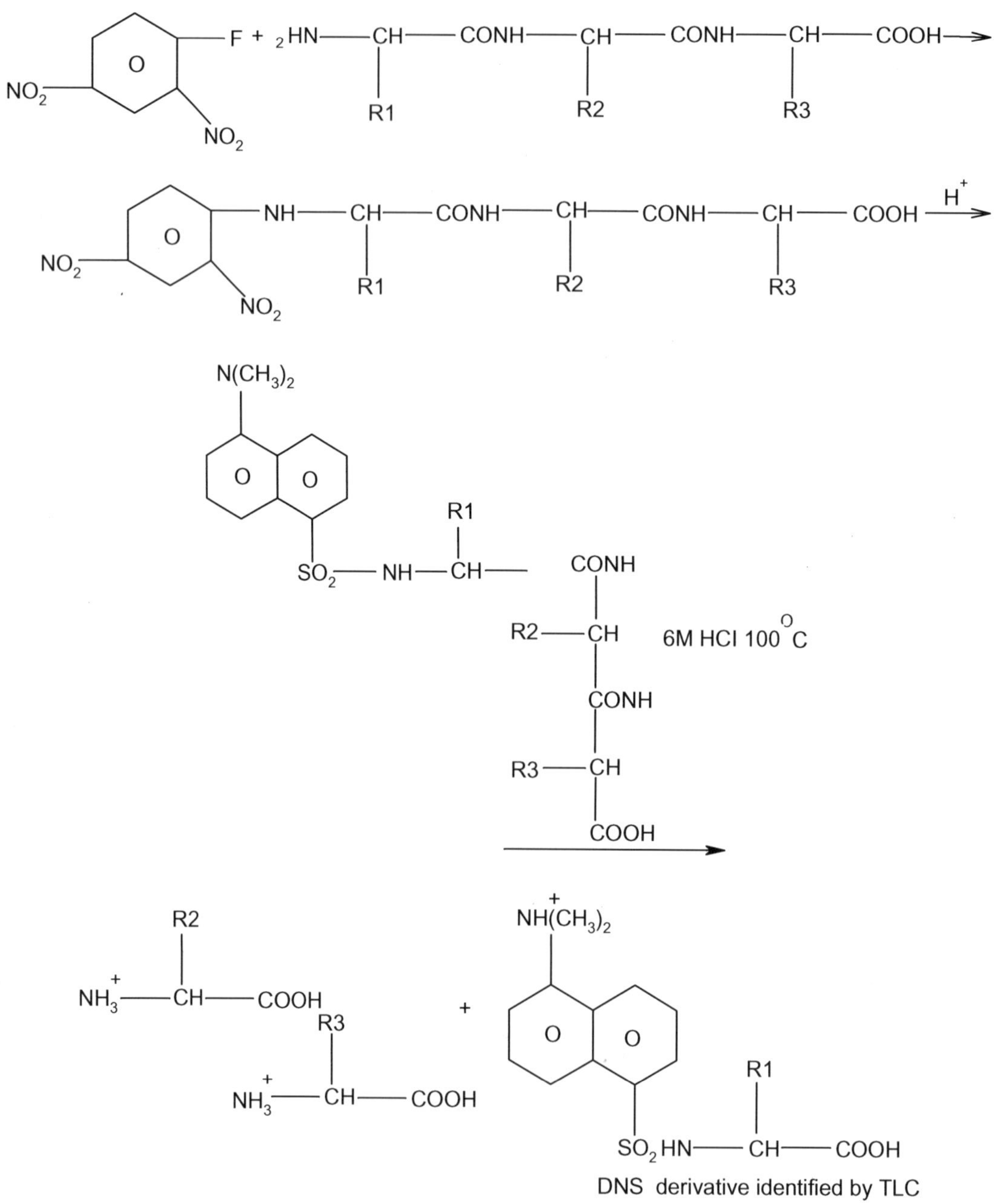

Enzymatic method

Enzyme leucine aminopeptidase attacks peptides only at the end which contains free amino group. When the terminal amino acid released, new terminal will be exposed to enzyme and the reaction continues.

Edman's method

Terminal acid residue having free -NH_2 group picked by Edman reagent (Phenyl isothiocynate) in presence of dilute alkali produce Phenyl thiohydantoin (PTH) derivative which seperated and identified by paper chromatography.

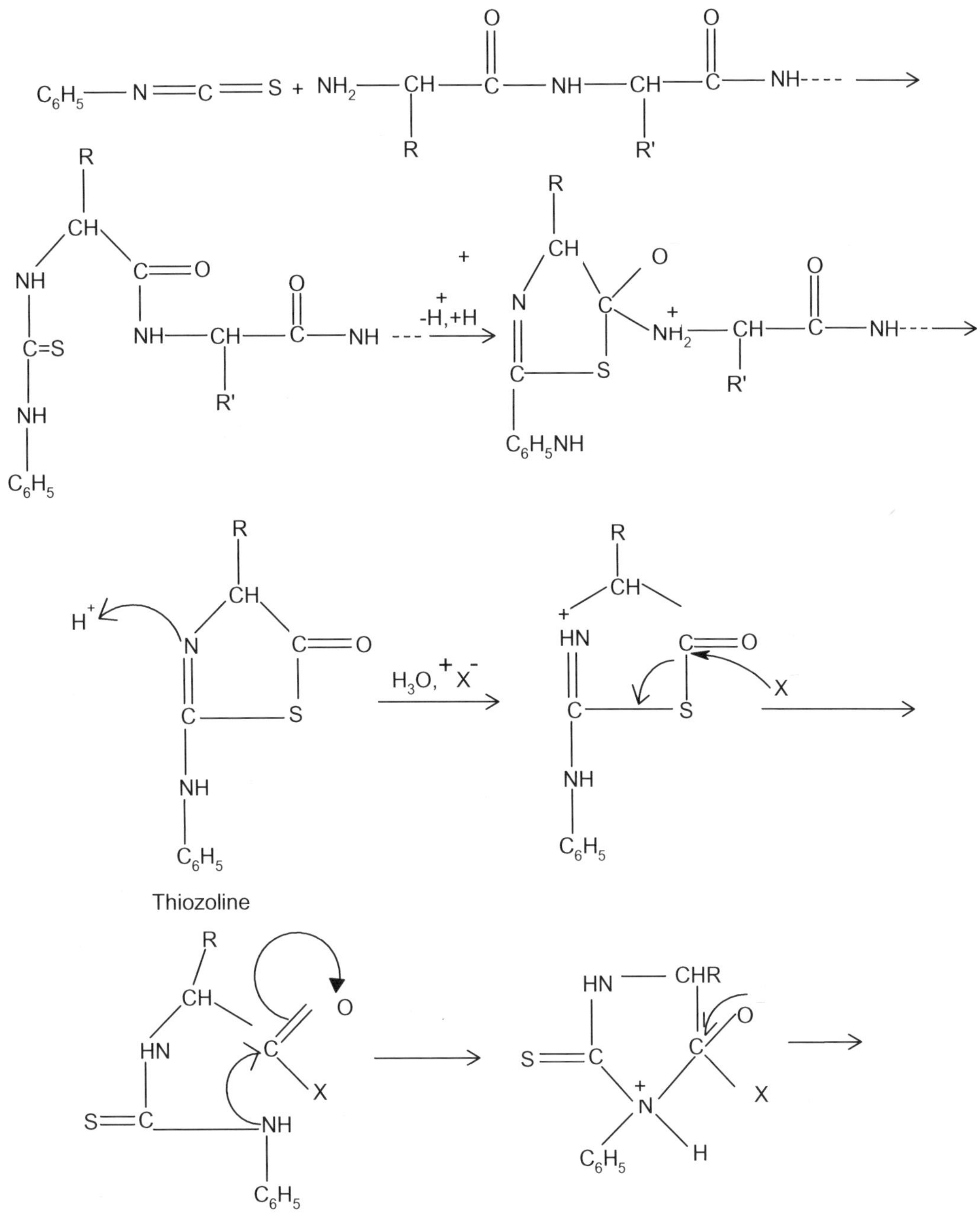

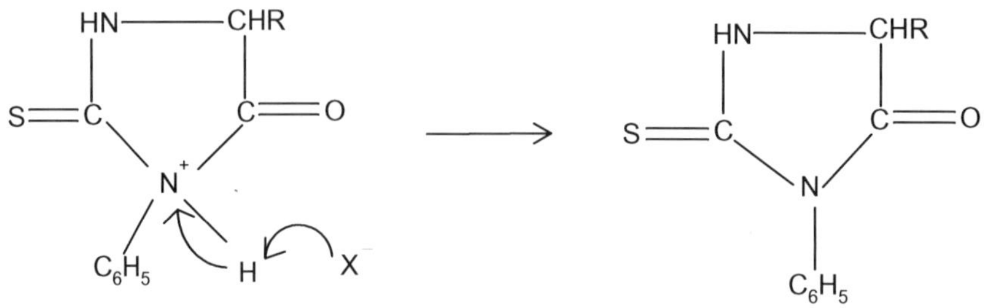

Carboxyl end Degradation

Schlack and Kumpf method

In this method amino group first protected by benzoylation and then C-terminal amino acid converted into thiohydantoin which is hydrolysed ultimately to amino acid just like Edman's method.

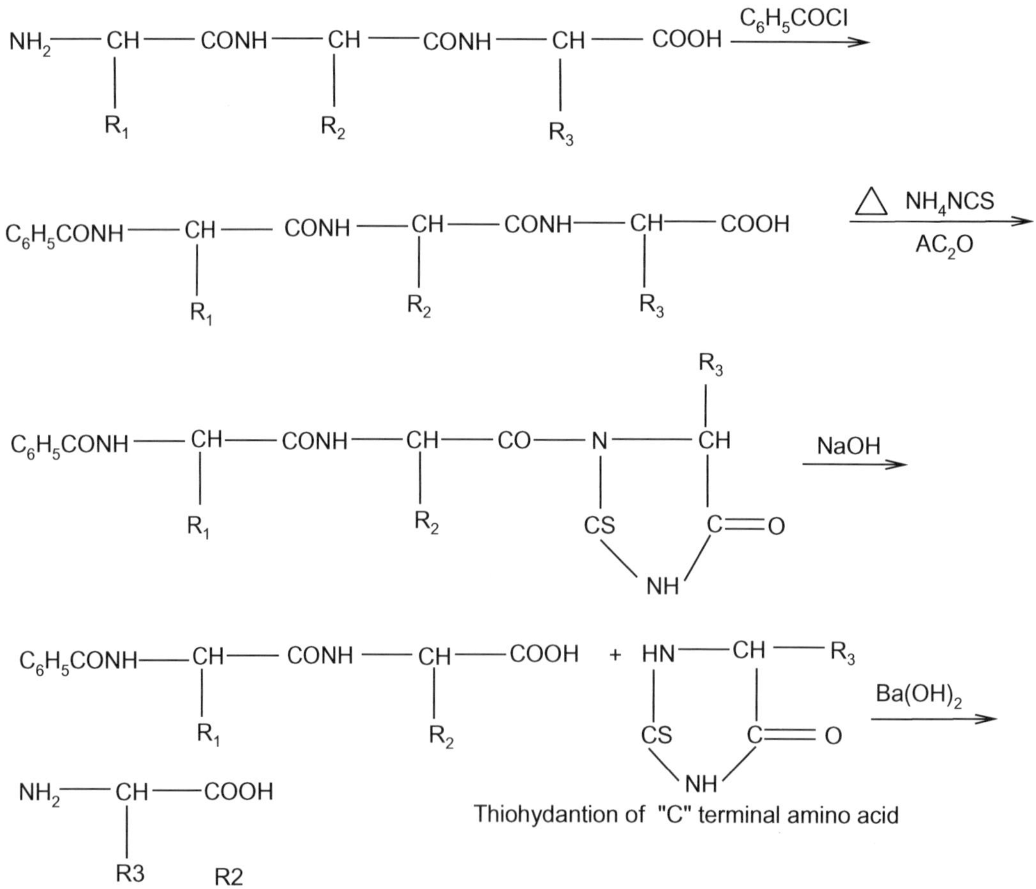

Thiohydantion of "C" terminal amino acid

Reductive method

In this method metal hydride reduces free terminal Carboxyl group of peptide to primary alcoholic group and product on hydrolysis gives amino alcohol (from C-terminal amino acid) along with mixture of amino acids.

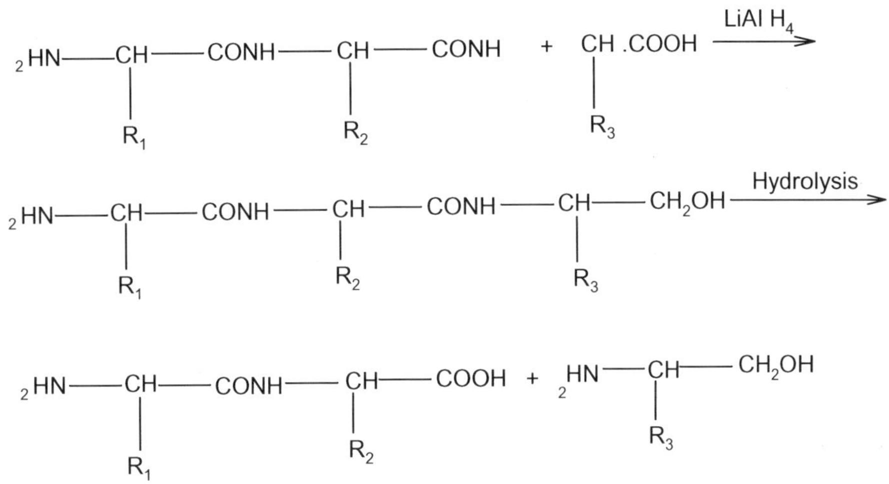

Amino alcohol is separated and identified by paper chromatography.

Hydrazinolysis

In this method, protein is heated with anhydrous hydrazine at 100°, which converts all amino acids except Carbonyl terminal one into amino acid hydrazides. In chromatograph basic hydrazides retained, free amino acid eluted and identified.

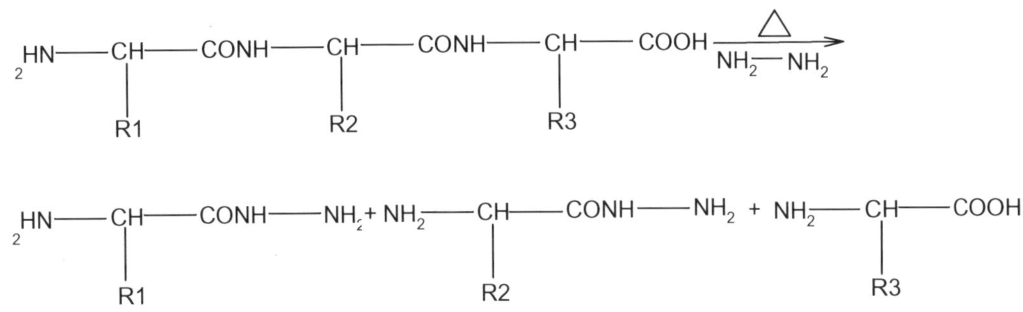

Enzymatic method

The enzyme Carboxyl peptidase attacks peptides only at the end which contains free α-Carboxyl group.

The above mentioned ones are some important methods to determine the terminal end. Next step is cleavage of disulphide bond.

(d) Disulphide bond cleavage

Disulphide bond can be cleaved either by reduction with Sodium borohydride or by oxidation with performic acid.

(e) Determination of Sequence of amino acids

Polypeptide chains obtained after disulphide bond cleavage are seperated and characterised by end group determination. Sequence of amino acids is then determined by Edman procedure in which amino acids are seperated in a stepwise manner.

Enzymatic method is also applied. Eg: Trypsin cleaves CONH involving -CO- part of lysine or arginine molecule. Similarly chymotrypsin splits CONH in which carbonyl group is a part of phenyla lanine, tyrosine or tryptophan residue.

Importance of primary structure

In normal condition Hb of R.B.C have specific sequence of amino acids. In sickle cell anaemic conditions, Hb will have different sequence of amino acids. In normal R.B.C HbA have sequence His-Val-Leu-Leu-Thr-Pro-Glu-Glu-Lys. In sickle cell HbS have sequence His-Val-Leu-Leu-Thr-Pro-Val-Glu-Lys.

So there by studying the primary structure of proteins some genetic diseases can be diagonised.

Secondary Structure

Secondary structure deals with conformation of peptide chain present in protein molecule.Two different conformations existing are α-helix and β conformation. α helix proove peptide group is planar. α helical structure due to resonance in peptide linkage and hydrogen bonding between -H- and C═O group. Hydrogen bonding stabilises the conformation and strength of this bond is a maximum when the atoms concerned (C=O-H-N) are collinear. α-helix is rigid due to the presence of hydrogen bond, which presents free rotation.

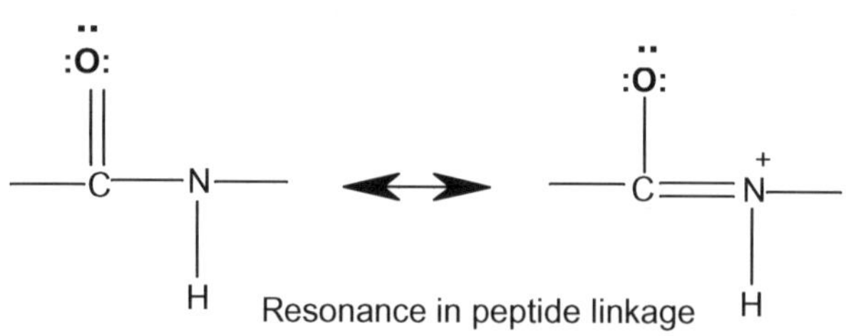

Resonance in peptide linkage

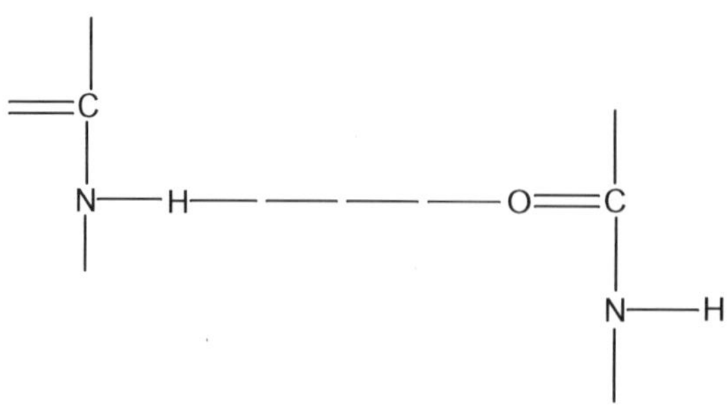

Hydrogen bonding between -NH and -C=O group

α-helix may be left or right handed. Right handed is more stable than left handed helix. Diameter of α-helix found to be 10 A^0.

In β-conformation or pleated sheet, polypeptide chain is extended and chains are held together by inter-molecular hydrogen bonds.Two types of pleated sheets are known-parallel and anti-parallel. In parallel pleated sheet, all polypeptide chains run in same direction. Eg: Keratin. In anti-parallel polypeptide chains run alternatively in opposite directions. Eg: Fibroin.

Tertiary Structure

Tertiary structure refers to its 3-dimensional structure. Here entire molecule is folded. Tertiary structure involves hydrogen bonding,ionic, chemical and hydrophobic bonds. Protein assumes tertiary structure under normal conditions of temperature and pH will be most stable arrangement and is referred as native conformation of that protein. Two major molecular shapes possible are fibrous and globular. Fibrous proteins have a large helical content and are essentially rigid molecules of rod-like shape, where as globular proteins are spherical in shape. Tertiary structure of proteins have been elucidated by X-ray analysis, viscosity measurements, diffusion, light-scattering, ultra-centrifuge method and electron microscopy.

Quarternary structure

Proteins exists as an association of several polypeptide chains and protein is known as oligomeric and individual chains are known as protomers or sub units. These protomers can be separated, even by dissolving in water containing urea. Mycoglobin consists of only one polypeptide chain which contains eight α-helices which are folded in an irregular manner at random coil sections. But Haemoglobin is made up of four sub units-two identical α-chain and two identical β-chain held together by Van der waals forces giving the molecule a quaternary structure.

LIPIDS

INTRODUCTION

Lipids are greasy materials, widely distributed in nature having similar solubility properties. They are insoluble in water, but soluble in polar solvents such as acetone, ether, Chloroform, benzene.....etc. Depending upon the nature of hydrolysis products, lipids are mainly divided into simple, compound and derived lipids.

CLASSIFICATION

1. Simple Lipids

Simple lipids are esters of fatty acids and alcohol. They are further divided into two groups a) fats and oils b) Waxes.

2. Compound Lipids

These are also esters of fatty acids and alcohol but contain some other compounds also. They are further divided into four groups namely;

(a) Phospholipids

These contain fatty acid, glycerol, phosphoric acid and a nitrogenous compound. eg: Lecithin, Cephalin, Sphingomyelin.

(b) Glycolipids

These contain Carbohydrate and Nitrogen.

(c) Sulpholipids

These lipids contain Sulphate group.

(d) Lipoproteins

These lipids are attached to proteins.

3. Derived Lipids

These lipids do not have ester linkage, but derived from simple and compound lipids. They include fatty acids, Glycosides and bases like Choline, Sphingosine, Ethanolamine and serine.

FATS AND OILS

Fats and oils are predominantly glyceryl esters of various higher fatty acids, mainly palmitic, stearic, Oleic, Linoleic & linolenic. Fats are solid or semisolid and oils are liquids at ordinary temperature.Animal as well as plant originated fats and oils are there. eg: Lard (pig fat), tallow (beef and mutton fat), Olive oil, Cottonseed oil, Linseed oil, Coconut oil, Groundnut oil, soyabean oil, Castor oil and Sesame oil.

IMPORTANT PROPERTIES OF FATS

Hydrolysis

Ester linkage of fats are cleaved by aqueous alcoholic alkali yield glycerol and sodium salts of long chain fatty acids. (Soaps.)

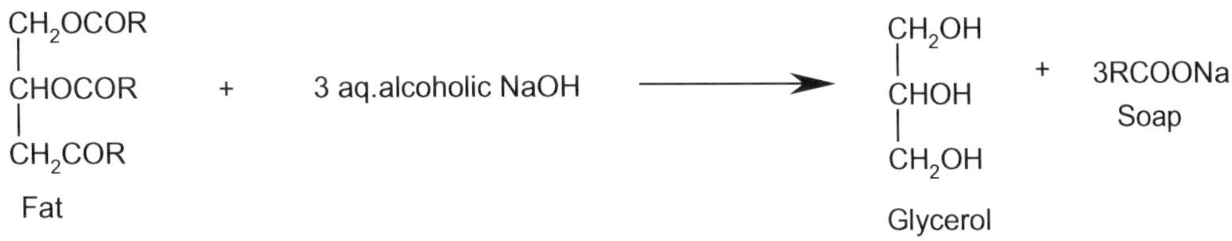

The enzyme lipase splits fat into glycerol and fatty acid.
Eg: Pancreatic lipase or steapsin.

Rancidity

On exposure to moisture and aerobic bacteria, fats are oxidised or hydrolysed into aldehydes, ketones or acids is known as Rancidity. Two types of rancidity are there; Hydrolytic as well as oxidative. Example fo hydrolytic randicity is occuring in butter-which become unpalatable and small amount of butyric acid is produced by the hydrolysis of glyceryl butyrate.

Oxidative rancidity takes place in presence of oxygen, by light, heat, moisture and traces of certain metals like copper. The unsaturated fatty acids oxidised at the double bonds to form peroxides, which then decomposed to aldehydes and ketones of objectionable odour and taste.

Rancidity can be prevented by the addition of traces of organic compounds like phenols, gallic acid, Vitamin C and Vitamin E. This type of substances are called antioxidants. Synthetic derivatives like nordihydro guaiaretic acid (NDGA), 3-tertiary butyl-4-hydroxy anisole,

Dilaurylthiodipropionate also function as anti-Oxidants.

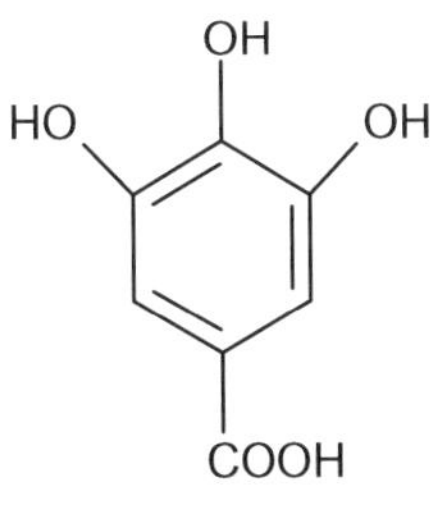

Galic acid

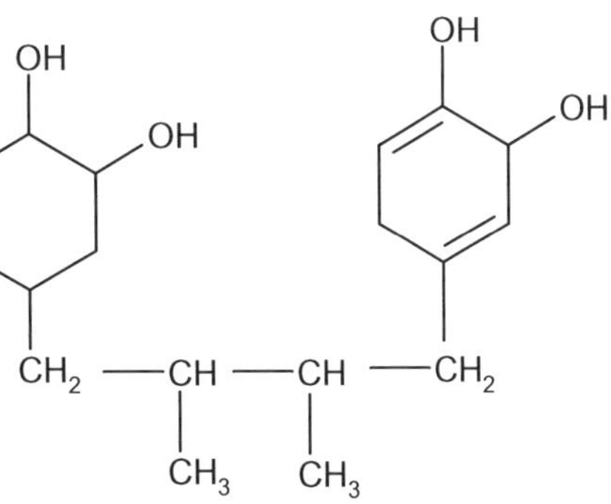

Nordihydro guaiaretic acid (NDGA)

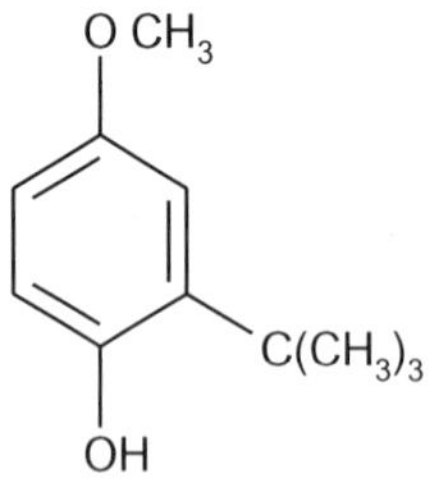

Tertiary butyl-$_4$-hydroxyanisole

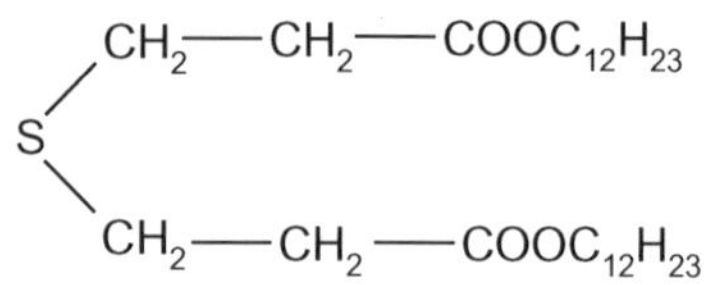

Dilauryl thio dipropionate

Kreis test is used to detect Oxidative rancidity. In this test fat is treated with ether, phloroglusi nol and Hydrochloric acid. Positive test is indicated by the development of red colour, which is due to the presence of epihydrine aldehyde, which is one of the oxidation product.

Drying

Certain Oils, when exposed to air, become thick and harden to resin like solid substance, and the process is known as Drying. Oils are divided into drying, semi-drying and non-drying, according to their behaviour on exposure to light. Drying oils mainly contain Glycerides of Linoleic and Linolenic acids. Eg: Linseed oil, Tung oil, Hempseed oil. A good drying oil on exposure to light and air, dries within 4-5 hours. eg: Linseed oil oxidised and polymerised to thick, brownish, elastic substance known as linoxyn, which is used in the manufacture of linoleum, lincrust and oil-cloth. Linseed oil is used as laxative in veternary purpose.

Semi-drying oil possess low content of linolenic acid than that of drying oils, but linoleic acid content is more than that of non-drying oils.

Eg: Sunflower, Sesame oil, Soyabean oil, cotton seed oil.

Non-drying oils mainly contain triolein. Eg: palm oil, Coconut oil, Olive oil and almond oil. On exposure to light and air, they become rancid. Rancidity developed by the influence of micro-organism which decompose oil into glycerol, saturated and unsaturated fatty acids. The saturated acids decompose to Ketones which causes unpleasant rancid odour. The unsaturated acids oxidised into aldehydes and acids with fewer carbon atoms in their molecule.

Hydrogenation

Certain Oils, especially drying and semi-drying oils adds on hydrogen atoms to the unsaturated linkage of the glycerides, under the influence of suitable catalysts such as finally divided nickel, platinum and copper at high temperature and become more saturated for eg. oleic acid which is an unsaturated fatty acid can be saturated by the addition of 2 H atoms (hydrogenation) to give stearic acid.

$$\underset{\text{Oleic acid}}{CH_3\,(CH_2)_{14}\,CH = CHOOH} \xrightarrow{+2H} \underset{\text{Stearic acid}}{CH_3\,(\,CH_2\,)_{16}\,COOH}$$

In this way, solid edible fats which are saturated can be made from cheap and comparatively inedible oils like cottonseed oils and fish oils. Eg. Margarine & Vanaspathi.

Analysis of Fats

Specific use of fat depends upon degree of unsaturation. Analysis of fats and oils deals with determination of certain constants known as fat constants, they can be either physical constants or Chemical constants.

Physical constants mainly include specific gravity, refractive index, Viscosity and melting point.

Chemical constants include Total fat, Acid value, saponification value. Ester value, Acetyl number, Iodine value, unsaponifiable matter, Reichert Meissl value & polenski value.

Total Fat

Sample containing fat extracted with ether, then ether extract evaporated, fat obtained is measured.

Acid Value

Acid value is defined as the number of milligrams of potassium hydroxide required to neutralise the free fatty acids in one gram of the oil or fat. It is determined by dissolving a weighed amount of fat in alcohol and titrate the solution against standard alkali using phenolphthalein as an indicator.

Saponification Value

Saponification value is defined as the number of milligrams of potassium hydroxide required to saponify entire one gram of oil or fat. It is determined by refluxing a known amount of the sample with excess of standard alcoholic potash solution, & then titrate the unused alkali against a standard acid solution. Since each molecule of fat requires three molecules of KOH to saponify it, so the saponification number readily indicates the number of fat molecules per gram of fat.

Ester Value

Ester value is defined as the number of milligrams of KOH necessary to combine with the fatty acids which are in combination with glycerol in 1 gm. of fat. It is determined by subtracting acid number from the saponification number.

Acetyl Number

Acetyl number is defined as the number of milligrams of KOH required to neutralize the acetic acid obtained by saponifying one gram of acetylated fat. Acetyl number is the measure of number of OH groups present in fat or oil.

Iodine Value

Iodine value is defined as the number of grams of iodine that combine with 100 gms. of an oil or fat. It is determined by treating a known amount of fat or oil dissolved in carbon tetrachloride solution with a known excess of Wij's solution (solution of iodine monochloride in glacial acetic acid) and titrating the unused iodine with a standard hypo solution as usual. The iodine value is a measure of the degree of unsaturation of a fat or oil.

Unsaponifiable Matter

Unsaponifiable matter is the part of fat or oil which is insoluble in water or incapable of forming a soluble soap with alkalies. To get unsaponifiable matter, the given fat is saponified and then warm water is added to it, then unsaponifiable matter appears as oil drops or as a milkiness which is then separated by extraction with petroleum ether.

Reichert Meissl Value

Reichert Meissl value is a measure of the volatile, water soluble acid constituents of the fat. It is defined as the number of millilitres of N/10 potassium hydroxide solution required to neutralise the volatile water-soluble fatty acids obtained by five grams of fat. To determine this, sample is heated with a solution of potassium hydroxide in glycerol until completely saponified. The mixture is then acidified with sulphuric acid, & distilled. The distillate is filtered and water-soluble acids in the filtrate are neutralised with N/10 potassium hydroxide solution.

Polenski Value

It is the measure of steam-distillable, water insoluble acid constituents of the fat. It is defined as the number of millitres of N/10 potassium hydroxide required to neutralize the water insoluble, steam-distillable acids liberated by the hydrolysis of 5 gm of the fat.

Important fatty acids obtaining from fats hydrolysates can be classified into saturated, unsaturated and Hydroxy fatty acids

Eg. for Saturated fatty acids

Butyric acid - $CH_3\ (CH_2)_2COOH$

Caproic acid - $CH_3\ (CH_2)_4COOH$

Caprylic acid - $CH_3\ (CH_2)_6COOH$

Capric acid - $CH_3\ (CH_2)_8COOH$

Lauric acid - $CH_3\ (CH_2)_{10}\ COOH$

Myristic acid - $CH_3\ (CH_2)_{12}\ COOH$

Palmitic acid - $CH_3\ (CH_2)_{14}COOH$

Stearic acid - $CH_3\ (CH_2)_{16}COOH$

Arachidic acid - $CH_3\ (CH_2)_{18}\ COOH$

Eg. for unsaturated fatty acids

Oleic acid - Cis - $CH_3\ (CH_2)_7\ CH = CH\ (CH_2)_7.COOH$

Linoleic acid - Cis,cis $CH_3(CH_2)_4.CH = CH.CH_2.CH = CH.(CH_2)_7.COOH$

Linolenic acid - Cis,cis,cis

$-CH_3CH_2CH = CH.CH_2.CH = CH.CH_2.CH =CH.(CH_2)_7.COOH$

Arachidonic acid - $CH_3\ (CH_2)_3.(CH_2.CH = CH_4.(CH_2)_3.COOH$

Eg. for Hydroxy fatty acids

Ricin oleic acid - $CH_3\ (CH_2)_5\ CHOH.CH_2.CH = CH\ (CH_2)_7COOH$

Cerebronic acid - $C_{23}H_{46}.(OH)COOH$

Eg. for Cyclic fatty acids.

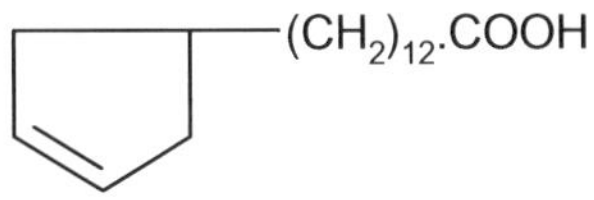

Chaulmoogric acid

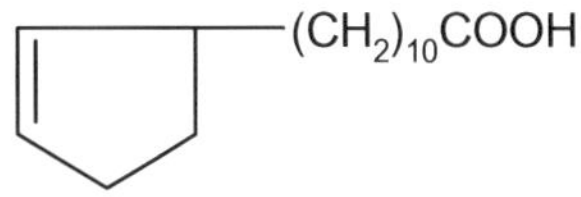

Hydrocarpic acid

Physiological Importance of Fats and Oils

Fats and oils are acts as storage of energy in plants as well as animals. Fats give 21/4 times as much energy as carbohydrates or proteins. Fat is a poor conductor of heat, thus fatty layer prevent loss of heat from the body. Some unsaturated fatty acids are indispensable constituents in diet and their deficiency leads to certain diseases

Waxes

Waxes are esters of long chain fatty acids and long - chain alcohols or sterol. Important acids in waxes are Myristic acid, palmitic acid, Cerotic acid, Melissic acid. Important alcohols constitute Lauryl alcohol, Cetyl alcohol, Octodecyl alcohol, carnaubyl alcohol ceryl alcohol, myricyl alcohol Cocceryl alcohol. Cholesterol. Some examples of common waxes are given below.

Name of Wax	**Important ingradient present**
Spermaceti	Cetyl palmitate
Beeswax	Myricyl palmitate

Waxes are acting as protective coatings in plants and animals.

VITAMINS

Vitamins are organic compounds, required in small quantities, but difficiency causes symptomatic disease. They are mainly classified as either fat soluble-Vitamin A, D, E and K or Water soluble Vitamin B complex and C.

VITAMIN A

Vitamin A is otherwise known as Retinol. It is enriched in fish liver oil. It's dificiency causes Night blindness, severe deficiency leads to xerophthalmia (hardness of Cornea.)

Chemistry of Vitamin A

Vitamin A_2 is dehydrogenated form of Vitamin A_1. Dehydrogenation is takes place in Vivo.

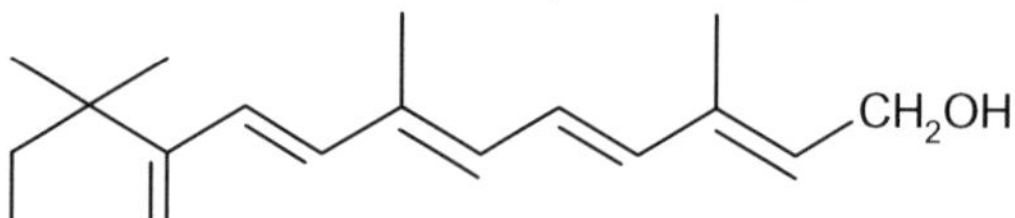

Vitamin A_1

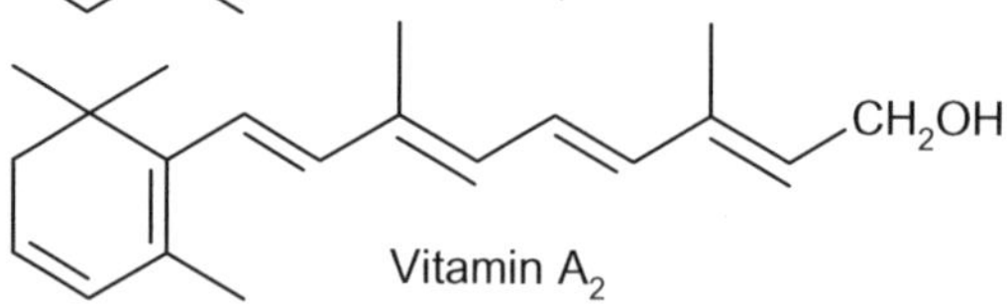

Vitamin A_2

1. **Molecular composition of Vitamin A_1 is $C_{20}H_{30}O$**
2. **Presence and nature of oxygen**

   Formation of ester indicate oxygen is present as alcoholic Vitamin A undergo oxidation to yield an aldehyde indicating the presence of primary Alcohol.
3. **Presence of Ring**

   On catalytic reduction of Vitamin A, absorbs 5 molecules of hydrogen and forms perhydroretinol ($C_{20}H_{40}O$). So the molecular formula of parent compound will be $C_{20}H_{40}$ which corresponds to the general formula C_nH_{2n} for the compounds having one ring.
4. **Presence of Conjugated system of double bonds**

   Vitamin A_1 forms an adduct with maleic anhydride indicating the presence of conjugated system of double bonds.
5. **Presence of β-Ionone**

   Ozonolysis of one molecule of Vitamin A_1, produces one molecule of geronic acid indicating the presence of One β-Ionone nucleus.

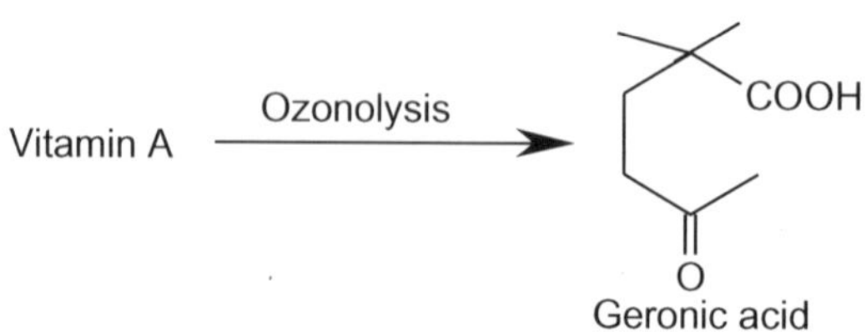

6. Presence of -C (CH_3) groups in side chain

One molecule of Vitamin A undergoes, permanganate oxidation to give two molecules of acetic acid , indicating the presence of -C (CH_3) groups in side chain.

7. Position of C- Methyl Groups

Most of the carotenoids found to have isoprene units.

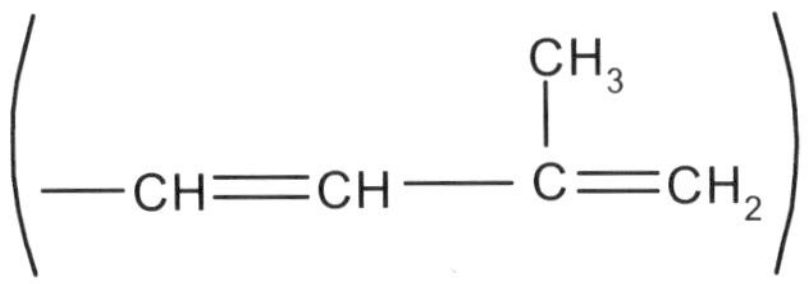

8. Number of Isoprene units

Permanganate oxidation of Vitamin A gives two molecules of acetic acid indicating the presence of two isoprene units. Along with CH_3COOH, other products like 2-2-dimethyl glutaric acid, 2,2-dimethyl succinic acid and dimethyl malonic acid are also formed. Formation of 1,6-Dimethyl naphthalene also explains the presence of two isoprene units.

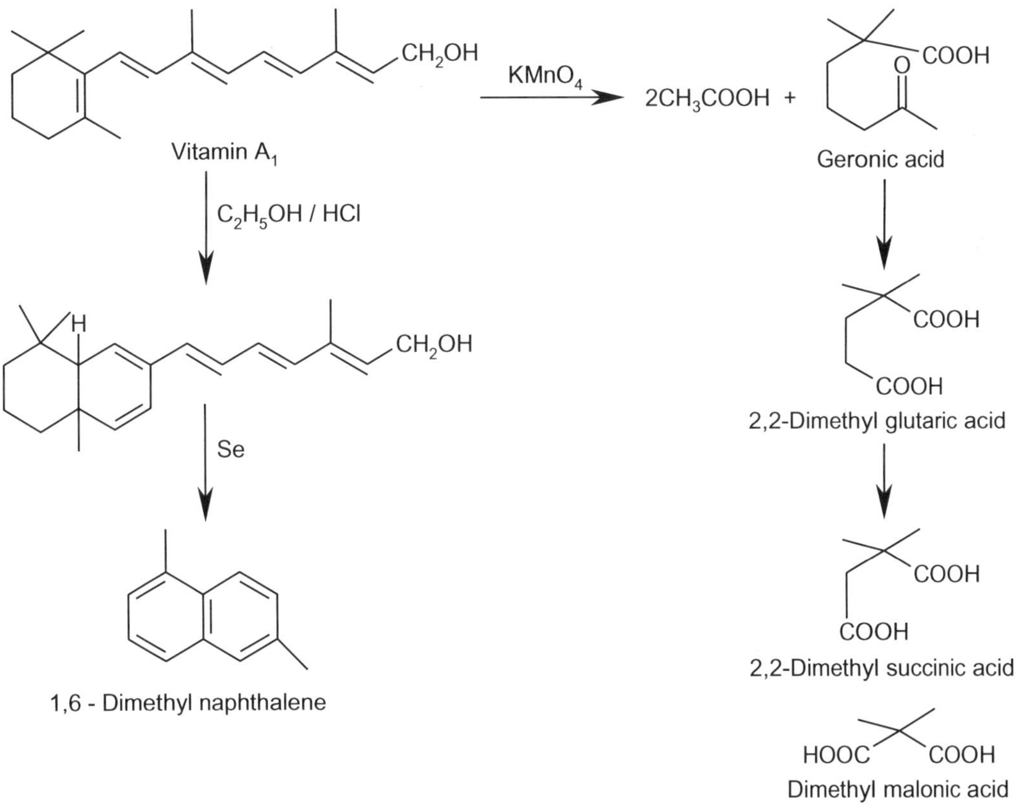

Finally the structure of Vitamin A_1 can be confirmed by its synthesis.

Synthesis of Vitanin A_1

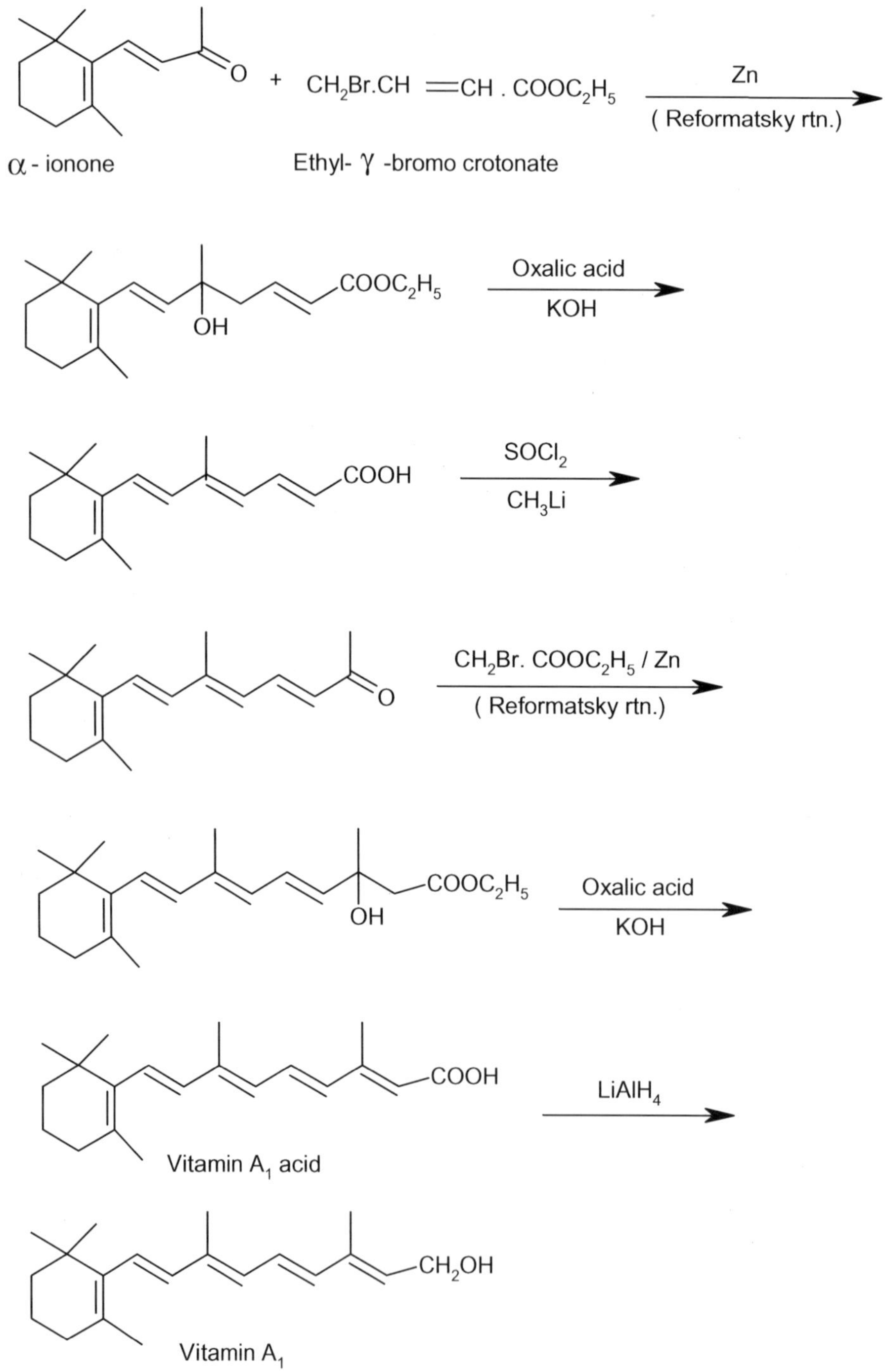

Conversion of Vitamin A_1 in to Vitamin A_2.

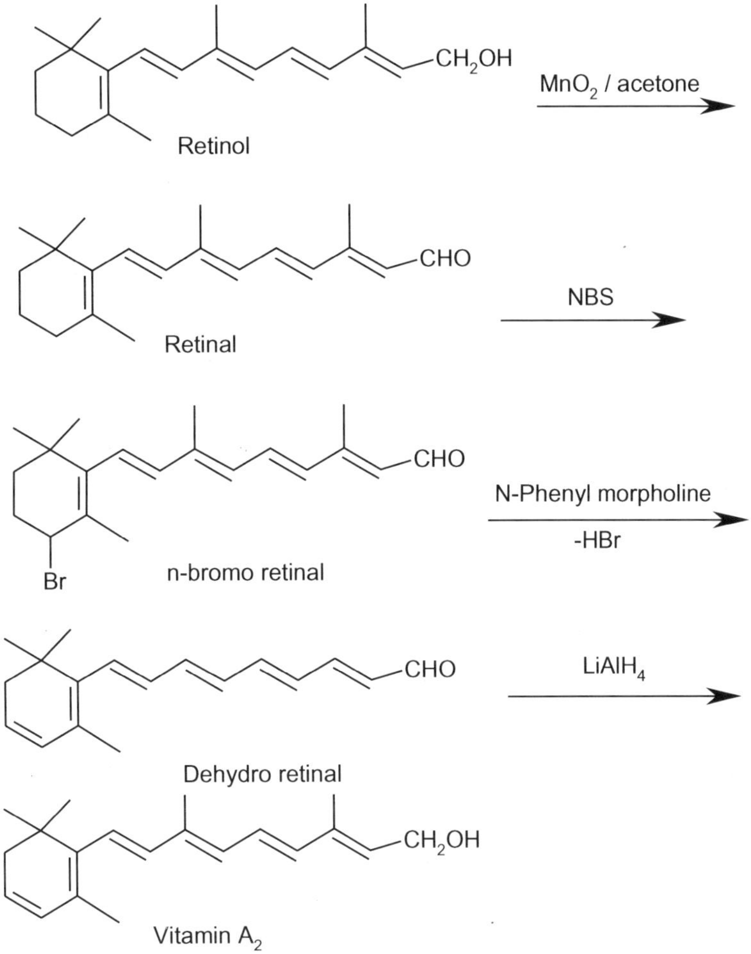

VITAMIN D

Vitamin D enriched in Cod-liver oil. So far five different Vitamins like D_1, D_2, D_3, D_4 & D_5 have been isolated. All vitamins of this group are formed by irradiation of specific sterols which are known as pro-Vitamins.

Provitamin	Vitamin
Ergosterol	Vitamin D_2 (Calciferol) (Ergocalciferol)
7-Dehydro - Cholesterol	Vitamin D_3 (Cholecalciferol)
22, 23 - Dihydroergosterol	Vitamin D_4
7 - Dehydro - Sitosterol	Vitamin D_5

Deficiency of Vitamin D leads to a disease called rickets.

Chemistry of Vitamin D_2 (Calciferol or Ergocalciferol)

Vitamin D_2 is formed from Ergosterol. Both are isomers having similarity in their molecular formulae.

1. Molecular formula is $C_{28}H_{44}O$

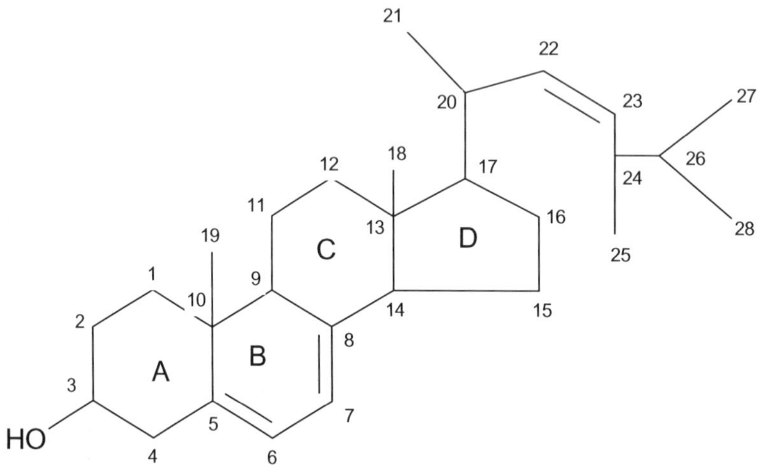

2. Presence and nature of hydroxyl group

On acetylation it forms monoacetate and on benzoylation it forms monobenzoate,indicating the presence of one hydroxyl group. Vitamin on oxidation gives a ketone indicating hydroxyl group is secondary in nature.

3. Nature of double bonds

Four molecules of hydrogen is added to Vitamin D_2 to give octahydro compound $C_{28}H_{52}O$. So the parent hydrocarbon will be $C_{28}H_{52}$, it belongs to the general formula C_nH_{2n-4} indicating the presence of tricyclic compound. Eventhough formation of octahydro derivative indicate the presence of four double bonds, three of the double bonds are in the nucleus, one must be in side chain to explain formation of aldehyde. Conjugated triene system confirmed by reaction with maleic anhydride to form adduct.

5. Confirmation of Tricyclic system

Presence of tricyclic system already explained in previous point. On selenium distillation Vitamin D does not give Diel's hydrocarbon indicate one of the rings of ergosterol is opened during irradiation to form Vitamin D_2

6. Nature of the rings C and D

Ergosterol acetate on reaction with maleic anhydride forms an adduct (I) which on saponification gives a dicarboxylic acid (II), which on treatment with diazomethane gives a diester (III), which is reduced catalytically to a dihydro compound (IV) which on ozonolysis gives a saturated ketone. (V)

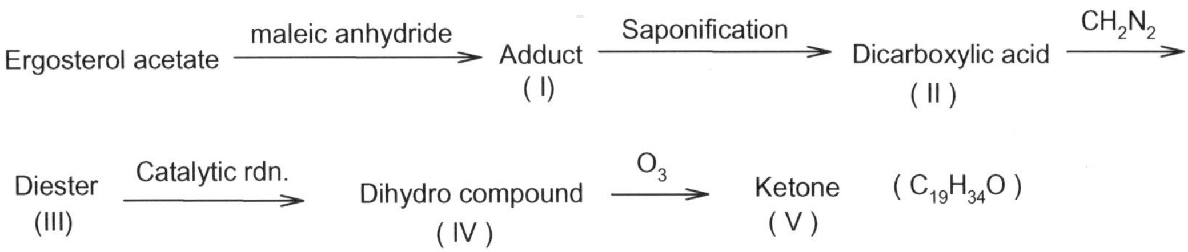

Since molecular formula for parent hydrocarbon (V) is $C_{19}H_{36}$, it is suppose to have two rings. Higher number of hydrogen atoms (34) of ketone indicates, presence of side chain with angular methyl group. Due to this side chain, rings present must be C and D.

Formation of ketone from Dihydro compound suggests ring C linked to ring B by means of a double bond. The double bond must be between C_7 and C_8. The ring B is opened between C_9 and C_{10}. So the structure of Ketone can be drawn as follows,

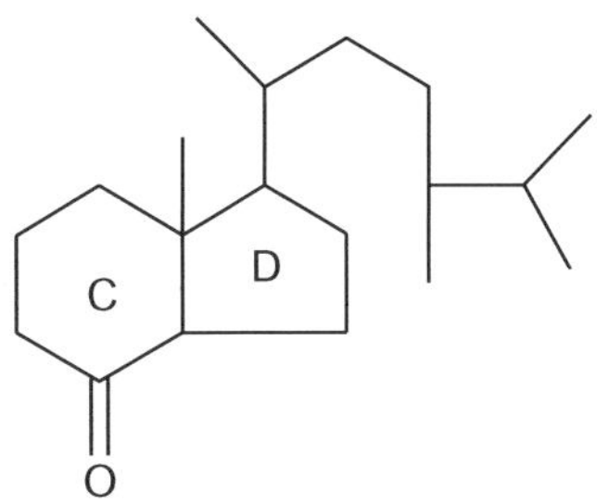

Saturated Ketone (V)

7. Nature of Ring A

The dicarboxylic acid (Compound II) formed in above reaction undergo catalytic dehydrogenation to form naphthalene (VI) and β-naphthoic acid (VII)

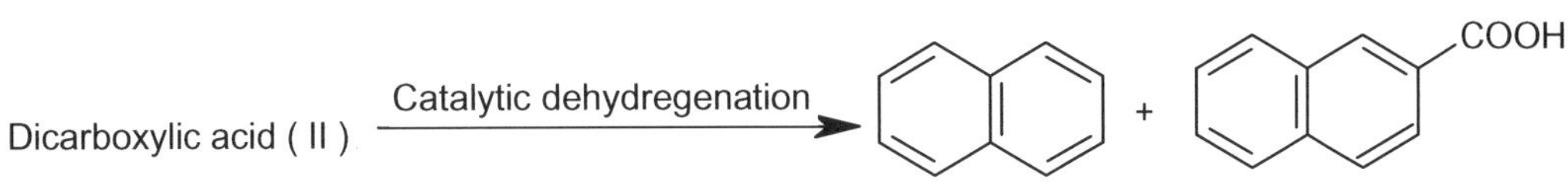

naphthalene beta-naphthoic acid (VII)

Diester formed above undergo selenium dehydrogenation to form 2,3- Dimethyl naphthalene.

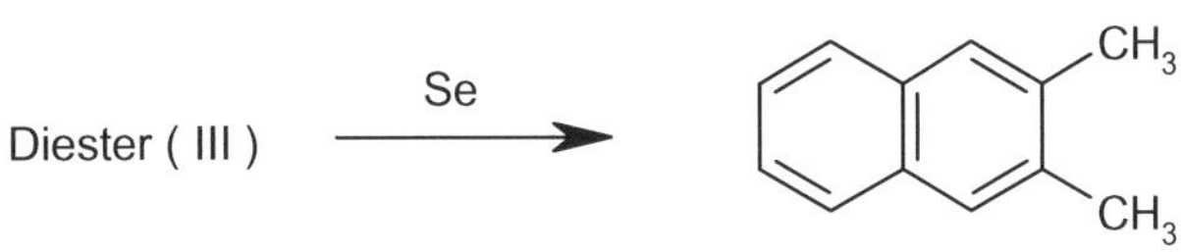

2,3-Dimethyl naphthalene

Dimethyl groups of 2,3-Dimethyl naphthalene indicate position of two COOH in Dicarboxylic acid II and $COOCH_3$ in Diester. Formation of naphthalene and β-naphthoic acid confirm the presence of hydronaphthalene in Dicarboxylic acid compound. From all above, the structure of ergocalciferol can be proposes as follows,

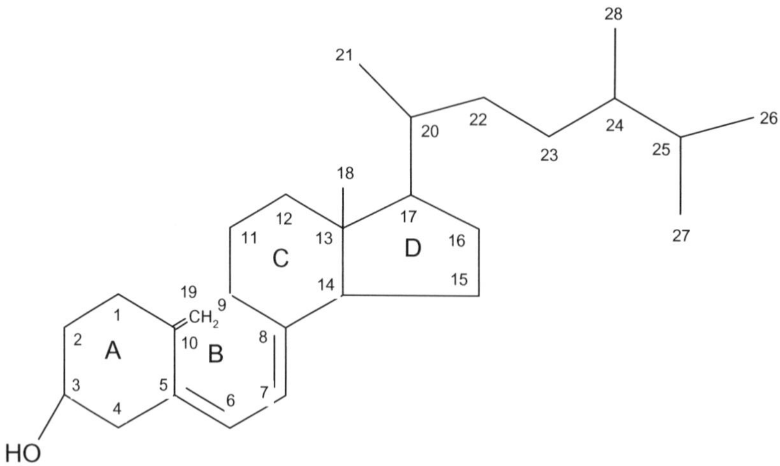

Formation of Vitamin D_3, D_4 & D_5 from their provitamins.

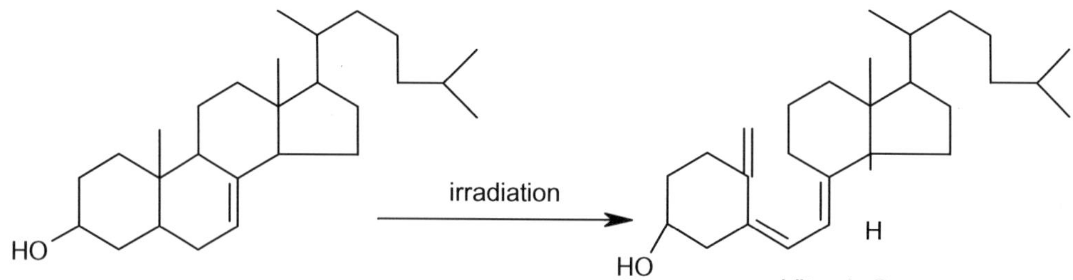

7-Dehydrocholesterol

Vitamin D_3

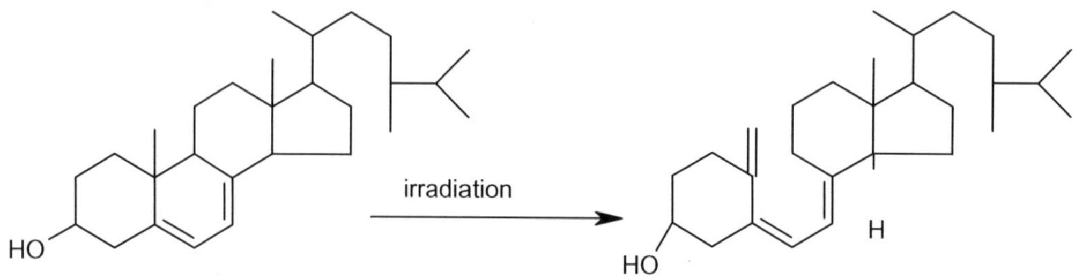

22,23-Dihydro ergosterol

Vitamin D_4

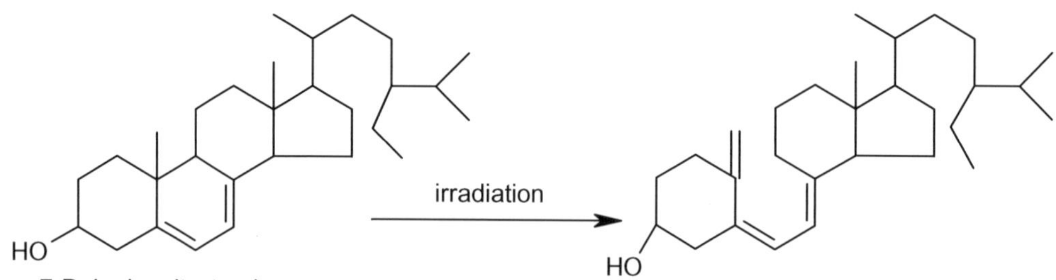

7-Dehydro sitosterol

Vitamin D_5

VITAMIN E

Vitamin E is otherwise known as tocopherol. It is also called antisterility factor, since it causes sterility in animals. It is enriched in wheat germ oil.

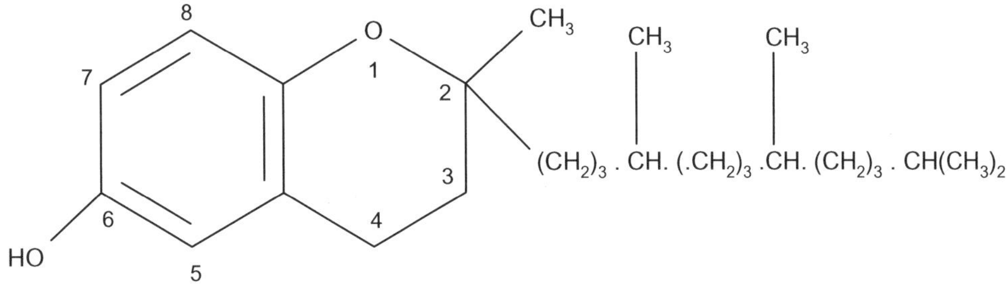

Chemistry of Tocopherol

1. **Molecular composition is $C_{29}H_{50}O_2$**
2. **Presence and nature of Hydroxyl group**

   On acetylation and esterification α-Tocopherol forms mono-acetate and mono ester indicating the presence of one hydroxyl group. By chemical tests this 'OH' is found to be Phenolic in nature.
3. **Nature of 2nd Oxygen atom**

   Second oxygen atom found to involved in cyclic ether.
4. **Presence of Benzenoid nucleus**

   Pyrolysis of α-tocopherol at 350°C gives duroquinol indicating the presence of benzenoid nucleus.

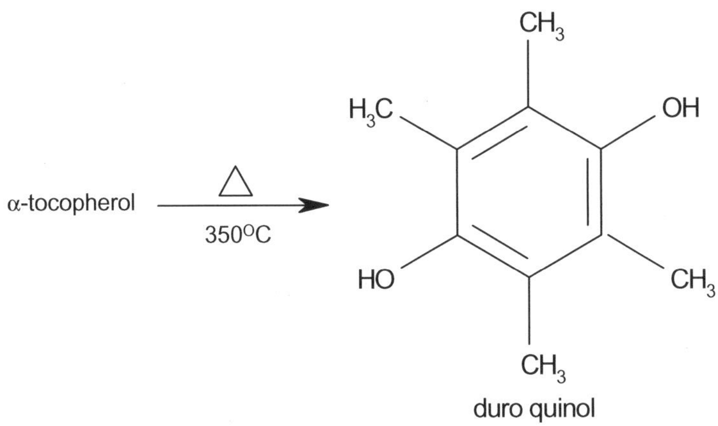

5. **Degree of hydroxyl group**

   α-tocopherol under mild oxidation with chromic acid yield dimethylmaleic anhydride and lactone whose precursor is Hydroxy acid. Since lactonisation is very rapid, indicating that hydroxy acid as well as lactone is γ-one.

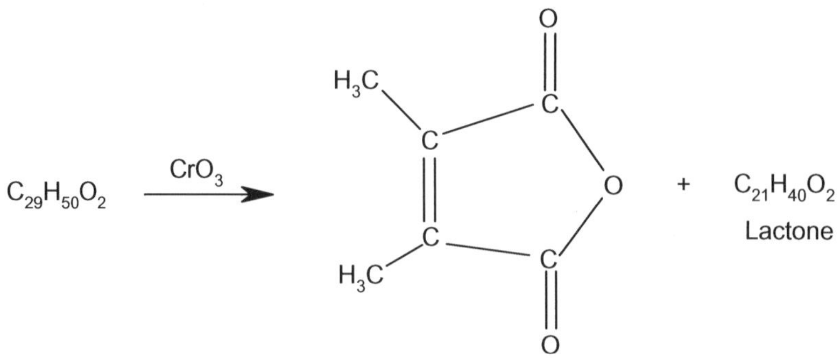

Resistance to oxidation and difficulty in esterification of Methyl ester of hydroxy acid indicate hydroxyl group is tertiary one.

6. Structure of γ-Lactone

$C_{21}H_{40}O_2$ (γ-Lactone) undergo vigorous oxidation with chromic acid produce an acid $C_{16}H_{32}O_2$ and a ketone $C_{16}H_{33}.CO.CH_3$. Acid shown to have three -C- CH_3 group by Kuhn - Roth method and most of the natural compounds may have isoprene unit, so the structure of acid can be assigned as,

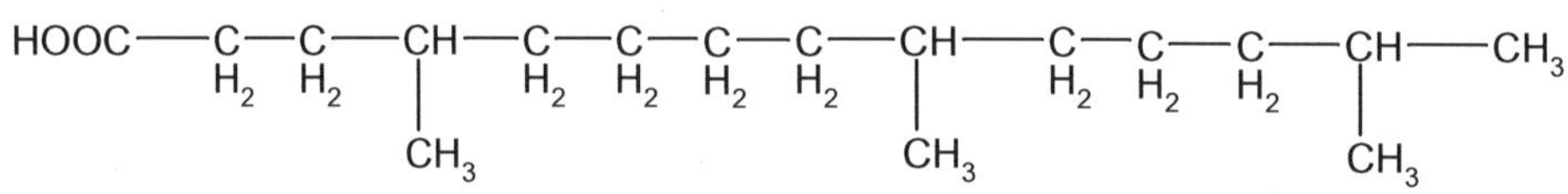

This acid is considered as one of the degradation product of γ-Lactone. Therefore the structure of γ-Lactone can be drawn as,

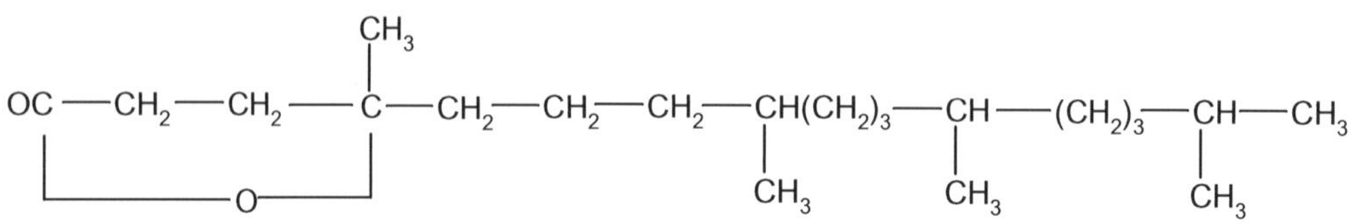

γ-Lactone

Finally the structure of α-Tocopherol can be proved by its synthesis.

Synthesis of α-Tocopherol

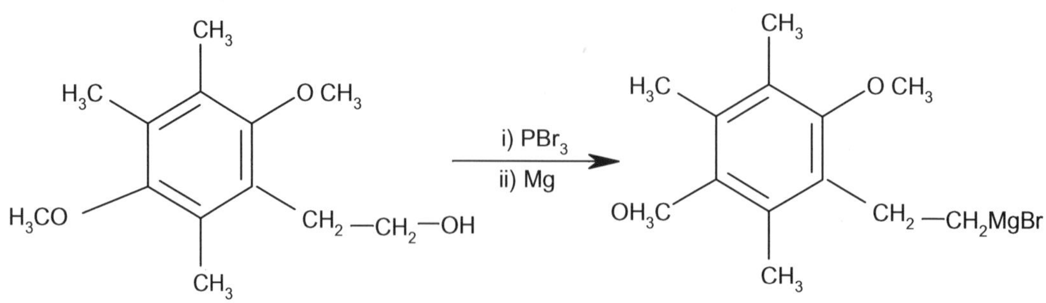

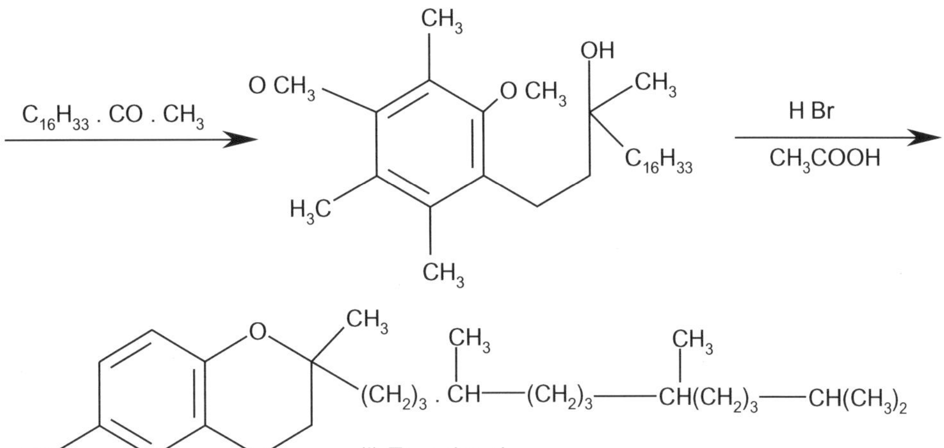

(I)-Tocopherol

VITAMIN K

Vitamin K is enriched in cereals and leafy tissues. It is essential for blood clotting. Two important vitamins of K called K_1 and K_2 are isolated. It is also known as anti-haemorrhagic Vitamin.

Constitution of Vitamin K_1

1. **Molecular composition is $C_{31}H_{46}O_2$**
2. **Presence of Naphthaquinone**

   λ-max of Vitamin K_1 is similar to that of 2,3-disubstituted 1,4-naphthaquinone. So probably 2,3-disubstituted 1,4-naphthaquinone may present in Vitamin K_1.
3. **Nature of Quinone**

   Vitamin K_1 is yellow in colour and can be reduced to a colourless octahydro derivative by absorbing four molecules of hydrogen.

   $$\text{Vitamin } K_1\text{(yellow)} \xrightarrow{4H_2} C_{31}H_{54}O_2 \text{ (Colourless).}$$

   It indicates, Quinone must be 1,4 because 1,2-quinone are usually red.
4. **Confirmation of Methylated 1,4-naphthaquinone**

   Vitamin K_1 undergoes oxidation with Chromic acid gives phthalic acid and 2-methyl-1,4-naphthaquinone-3-acetic acid.

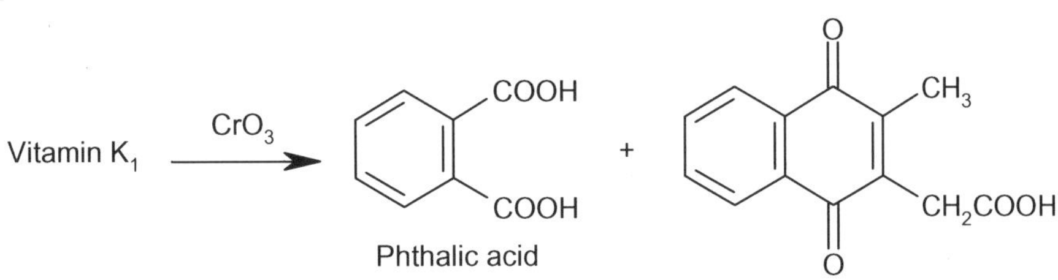

Formation of phthalic acid indicate benzene ring is unsubstituted formation of another acid indicate, vitamin have 1,4-naphathquinone skeleton methylated at second position and another substituent is at third position. So the partial structure of Vitamin K_1 can be written as;

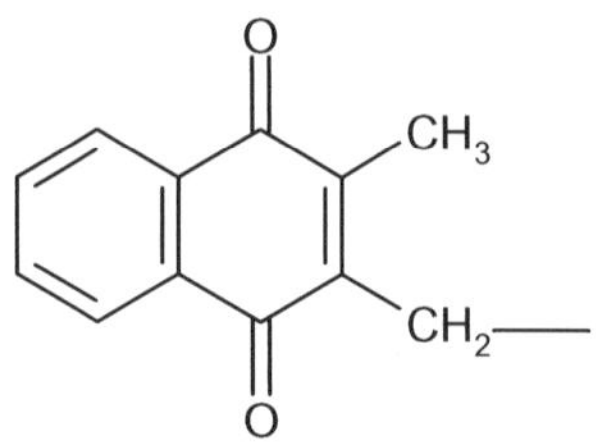

5. Presence of double bond in side chain

When 1,4-naphthaquinone which is obtained as a product during reduction, as we seen in third point, subjected to reduction utilizes 6 hydrogen atoms therefore, one double bond must be present in the side chain to account for the utilization of eight hydrogen atoms by Vitamin K_1.

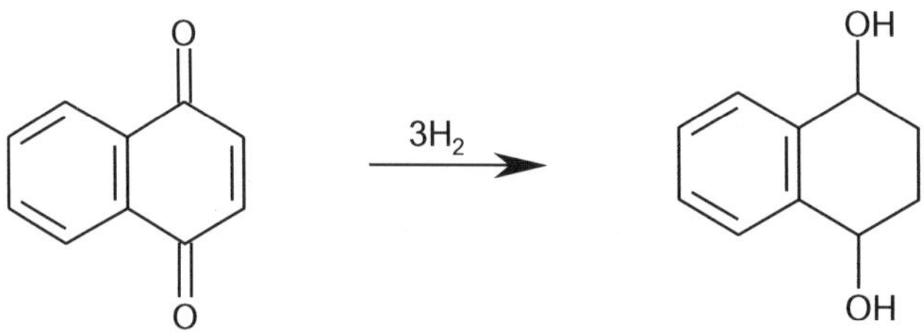

6. Structure of side chain

Reductive acetylation of Vitamin K_1 gives a diacetyl derivative which on ozonolysis gives an acid and a ketone. The ketone obtained here have structural similarity with that of ketones obtained by oxidation of phytol. So the side chain can be written as;

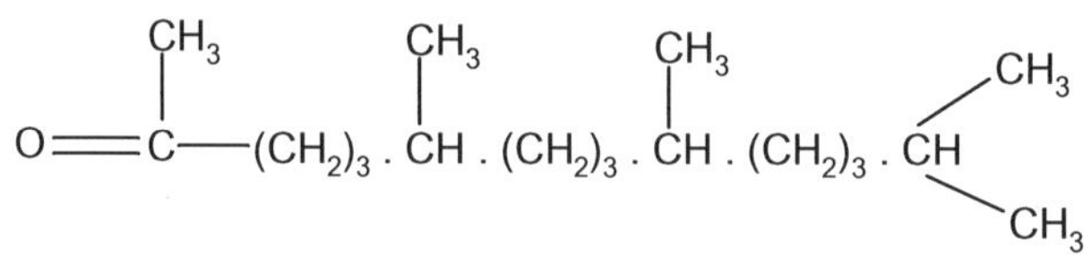

On the above basis, the structure of Vitamin K_1 can be written as,

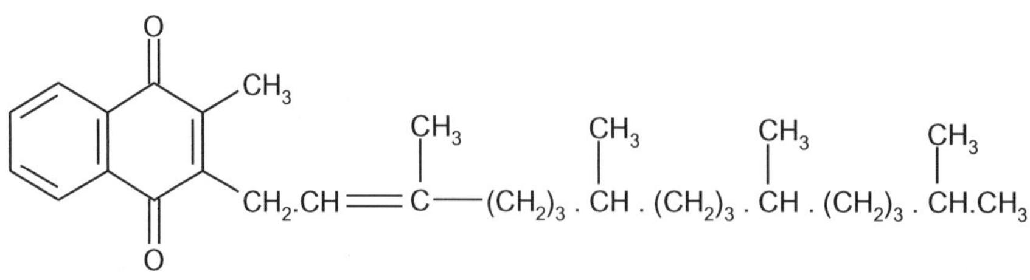

Finally structure of Vitamin K_1 can be confirmed by its synthesis.

Synthesis of Vitamin K_1

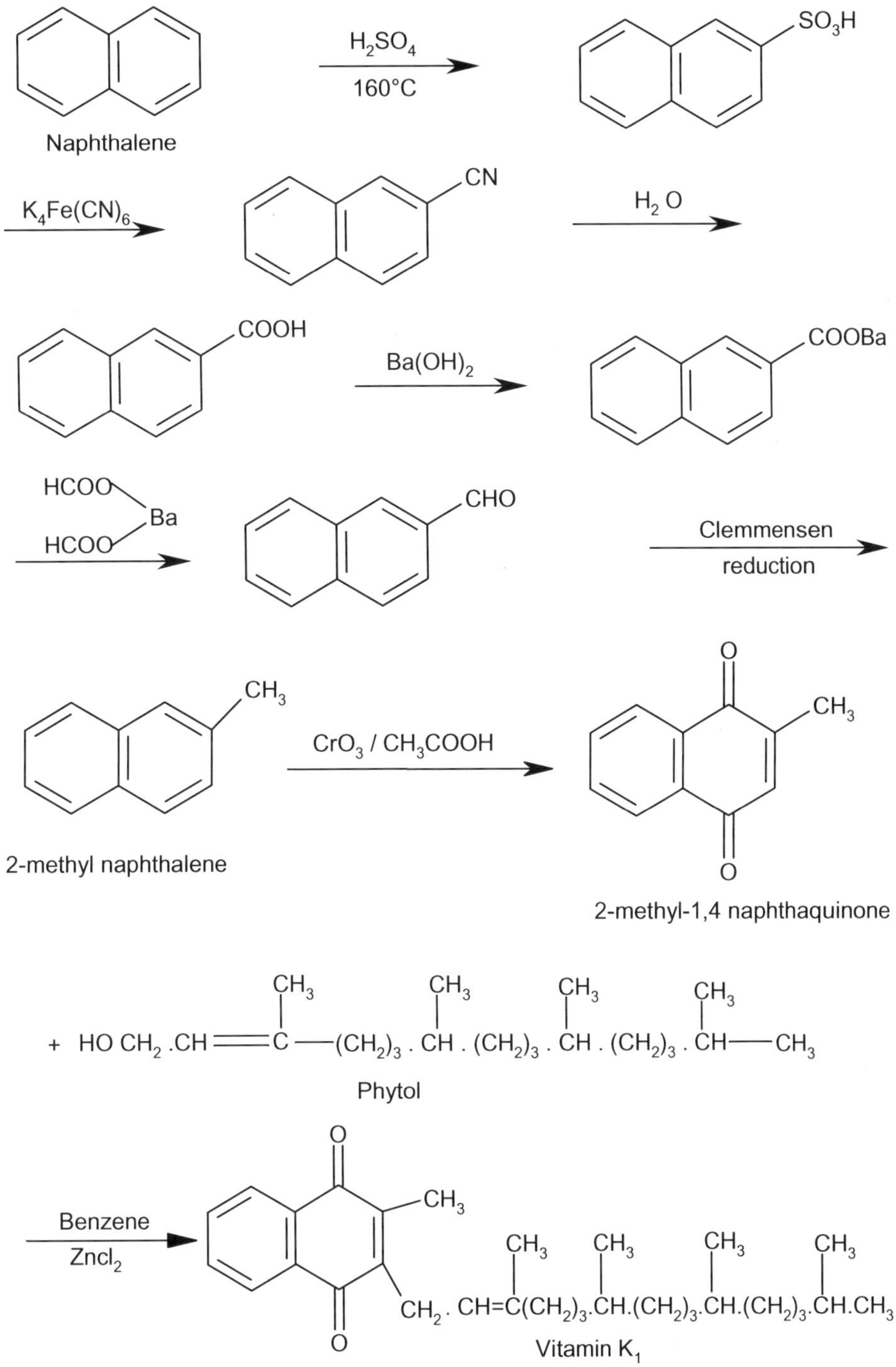

VITAMIN B_1 (Thiamine or Aneurine)

It is water soluble Vitamin, enriched in rice polishing and yeast. It's deficiency causes Beriberi. Thiamine is obtained in it's salt form as Thiamine hydrochloride

Chemistry of Thiamine hydrochloride

1. **Molecular composition of thiamine hydrocloride is $C_{12}H_{18}C_{12}N_4OS$ Cleavage of vitamin by sodium sulphite**

Thiamine on treatment with a solution of sodium sulphite saturated with SO_2 at room temperature broken into compound A and compound B. So we shall discuss each compound to draw the entire structure of Thiamine

Constitution of Compound A

(i) Molecular composition is C_6H_9NOS

(ii) Nature of Nitrogen

It shows to be basic in nature, but dosen't have reaction with nitrous acid, indicating that nitrogen is tertiary

(iii) Functional nature of oxygen

Oxygen is shown to be as alcoholic when this compound is treated with hydrochloric acid, a hydroxyl group is replaced by chlorine atom. UV spectrum of chloro compound is same as that of hydroxyl compound suggest hydroxyl group is in side chain.

(iv) Position of sulphur

U.V spectrum as well as unreactivity of sulphur indicates, sulphur is present in a thiazole ring.

(v) Structure of compound A

Compound A as well as Thiamine on oxidation with nitric acid give same compound $C_5H_5NO_2S$. It is found to be identical with 4-methyl thiazole-5-carboxylic acid.

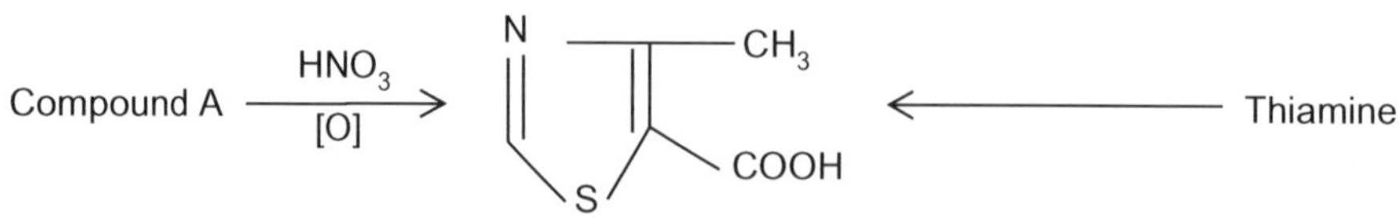

4-methyl thiazole-5-carboxylic acid

Since the presence of alcoholic group in side chain have been confirmed, the side chain could be either -CH_2-CH_2-OH or -$CHOHCH_3$ But since Compound A is not optically active and does not give iodoform test indicate side chain will be CH_2-CH_2-OH only. So the structure for compound A can be stated as

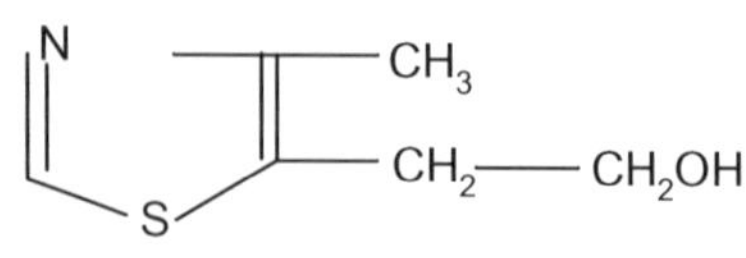

It is confirmed by its synthesis. Synthesis of compound A from 2-methyl furan

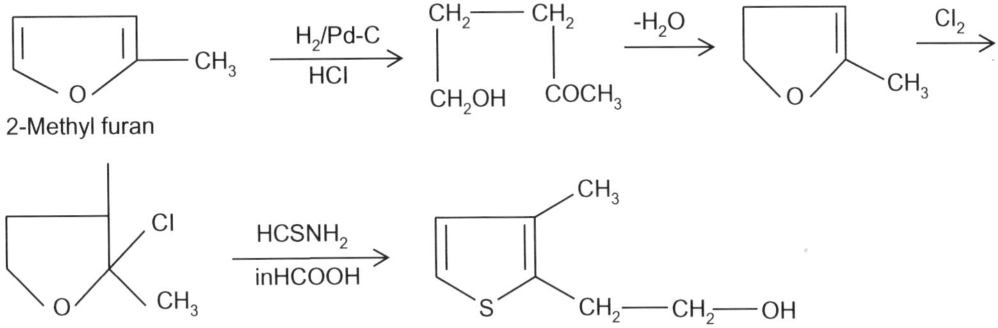

Compound A

Constitution of Compound B

1. **Molecular composition is found to be $C_6H_9N_3O_3S$**
2. **Nature as sulphonic acid**

   Compound B on heating with water under pressure at 200°C gives sulphuric acid. On treatment with sodium hydroxide forms sodium sulphite
3. **Presence and nature of Nitrogen**

   Nitrogen evolved on treatment with nitrous acid. Since evolution of nitrogen was slow, and reaction with benzoyl chloride was slow, indicate nitrogen is present in amidine functional group Compound B on heating with hydrochloric acid at 150°C under pressure produced a compound C and ammonia.

$$C_6H_9N_3O_3S \quad + \quad H_2O \longrightarrow C_6H_8N_2O_4S \quad + \quad NH_3$$

Formation of ammonia indicates replacement of an amino group by a hydroxyl group. It is characterestic of 2 and 4-aminopyrimidines. UV spectrum of compound (c) is similar to that of synthetic 4-hydroxypyrimidines. Therefore compound B probably a 4-aminopyrimidine derivative.

4. **Presence of methylated amino derivative**

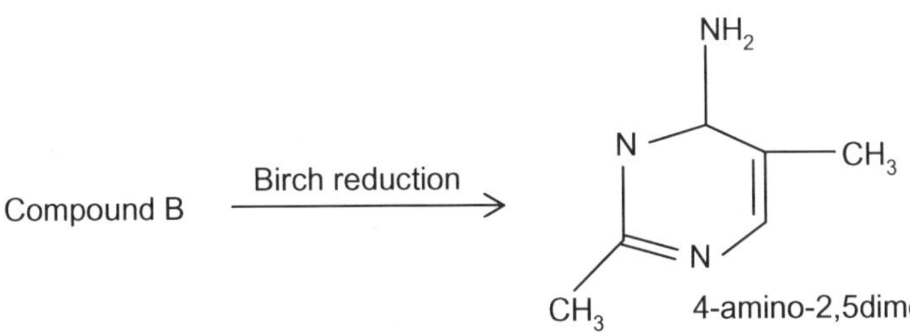

4-amino-2,5dimethylpyrimidine

It's structure is confirmed by its synthesis.

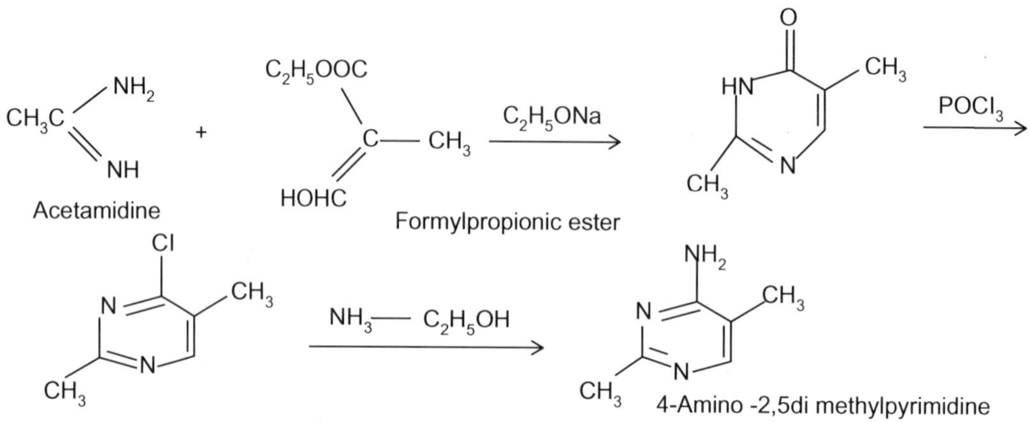

5. position of linkage of sulphuric acid with methyl group

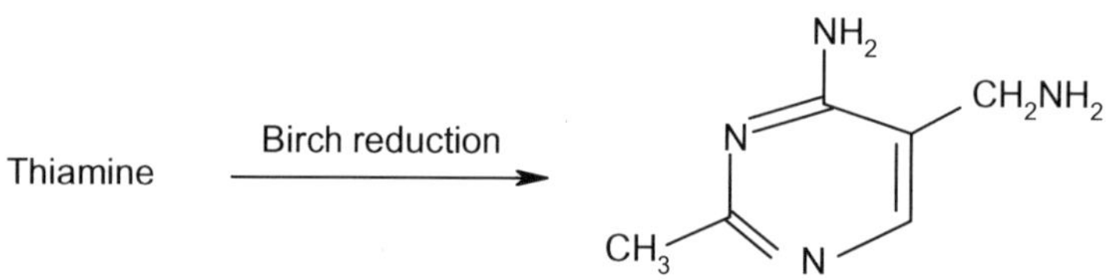

Compound D (4-amino-5-amino methyl 2-methyl pyrimidine)

So in compound D, one amino group is present instead of sulphuric acid. Therefore it is confirmed that sulphuric acid group in compound B is joined to methyl group at 5th position. It is confirmed by the reaction of 5-ethoxy methyl-4-hydroxy -2- methyl pyrimidine with sodium sulphite produced 4-hydroxy -2- methyl pyrimidyl -5- methane Sulphonic acid. It is found to be identical with compound C

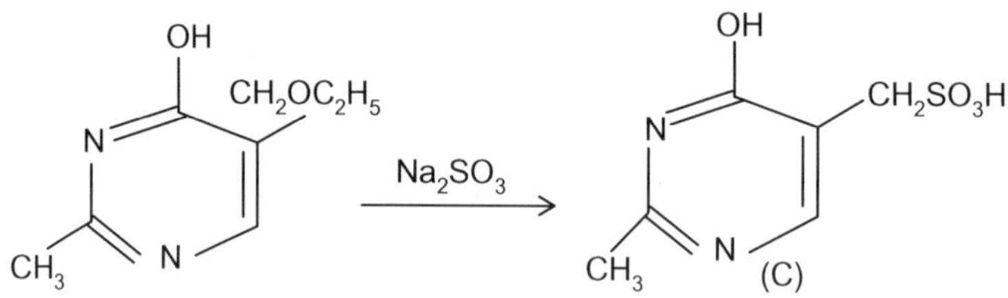

So the structure of (B) can be proposed as;

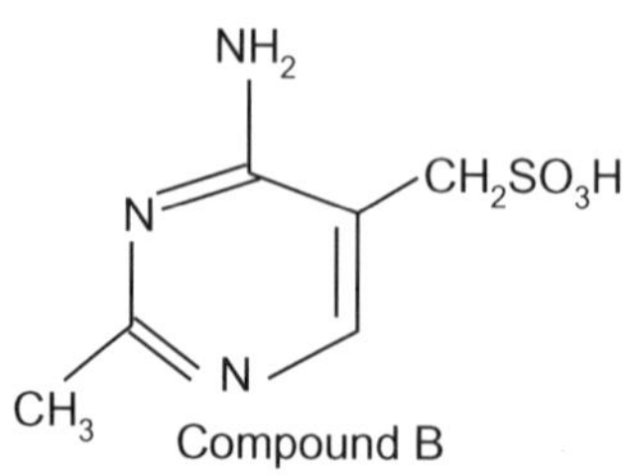

Compound B

Finally it's structure is confirmed by it's synthesis.

Synthesis of Compound (B)

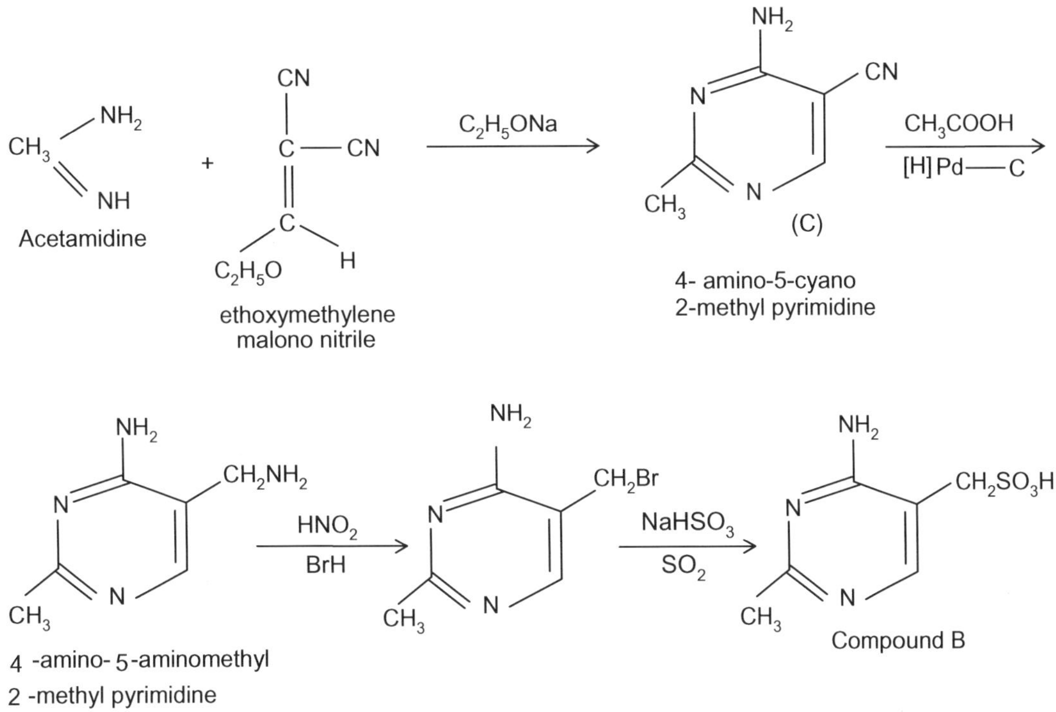

Point of Linkage between Compound A and Compound B

Sulphonic acid group in compound B is introduced during the fission of thiamine with sodium sulphite. Thus compound B is attached at CH_2 group at 5th position. Formation of compound D can be explained, if the compound B is attached to nitrogen of compound A by means of methylene bridge. It is again confirmed by the resemblance of thiamine to quaternary ammonium salts. So the complete structure of thiamine can be drawn as;

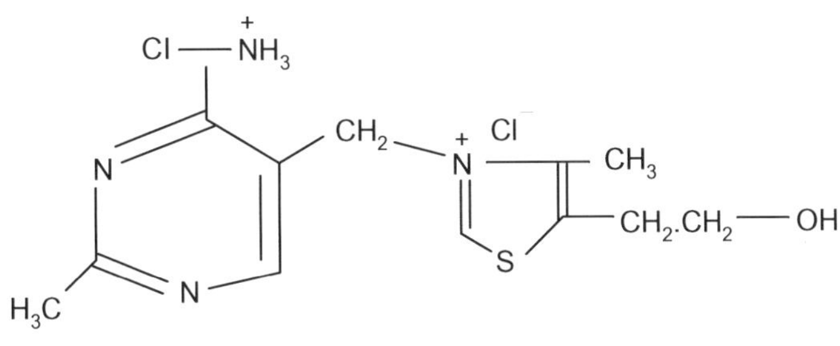

The structure of thiamine has been confirmed by its synthesis which involve two steps.

Step I Synthesis of pyrimidine moiety

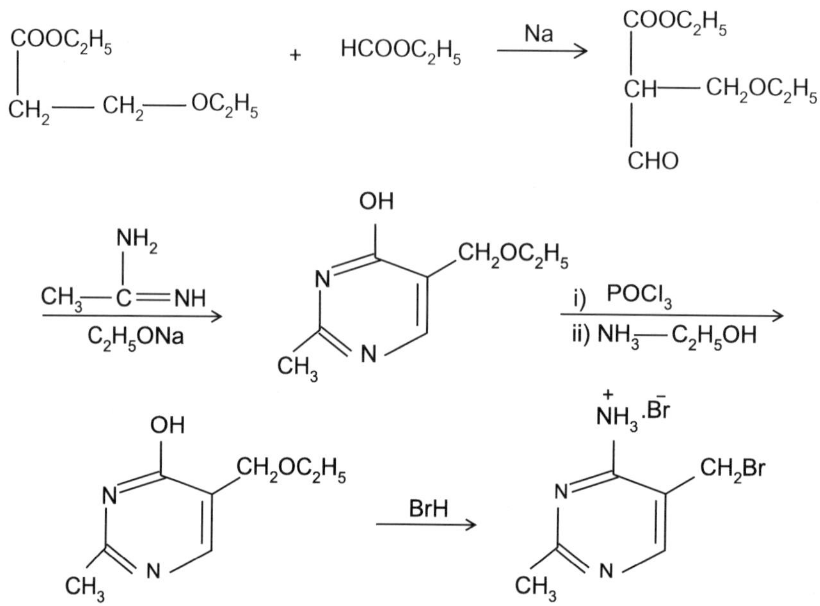

Step II Condensation of pyrimidine and thiazole moieties

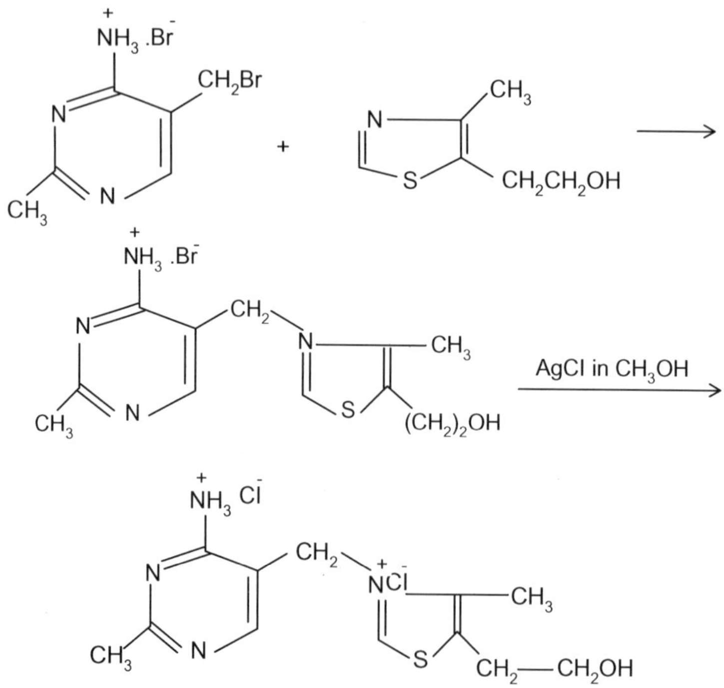

Thiamine chloride hydrochloride

VITAMIN B_2 (Riboflavin) (Lacto Flavin)

Riboflavin is a yellow crystalline, water soluble, heat stable soild, enriched in yeast, green vegetables, liver and wheat germ. It's deficiency causes cheilosis and corneal opacity.

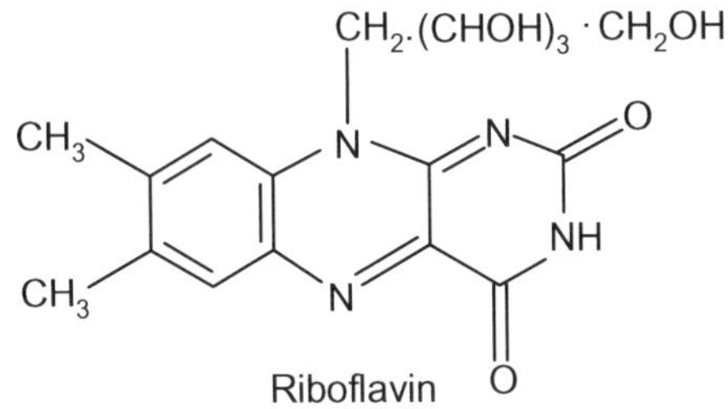

Riboflavin

Chemistry of Riboflavin

1. **Molecular composition is $C_{17}H_{20}N_4O_6$**
2. **Presence of four hydroxyl groups**

   On acetylation silver salt of riboflavin gives a tetraacetate, indicating the presence of four hydroxyl groups.
3. **Presence of primary alcoholic group**

   Oxidation of riboflavin with lead tetra-acetate produce formaldehyde, indicating the presence of primary alcoholic group.
4. Phtolysis of Riboflavin in alkaline medium yield lumiflavin or photoflavin, in acidic medium give Lumichrome. So the structure of Riboflavin can be deduce from Lumiflavin and Lumichrome.

Structure of Lumiflavin

(i) Molecular composition of Lumiflavin is $C_{13}H_{12}N$.

(ii) Nature of side chain

Lumiflavin can neither be acetylated nor oxidised by lead tetra acetate showing that C4 fragment is tetra hydroxy butyl side chain, (R-CHOH-CHOH-CHOH-CH_2OH).

(iii) Presence of methylimino group (>N-CH_3).

Lumiflavin shown to have methylimino group, but was not present in riboflavin . It indicates side chain in riboflavin attached at the position occupied by methyl imino group in lumiflavin.

(iv) Presence of ring system

Alkaline hydrolysis of lumiflavin yields urea and amino carboxylic acid (compound A). This reaction needed two molecules of water, so the urea must come from a ring system.

$$C_{13}H_{12}N_4O_2 + 2H_2O \xrightarrow{Ba(OH)_2} \underset{\text{Compound A}}{C_{12}H_{12}N_2O_3} + \underset{\text{Urea}}{CH_4N_2O}$$

(v) Nature of compound A

Compound A is found to be a β-keto carboxylic acid, since it easily eliminates CO_2 molecule to give a substance B

$$\underset{\text{Compound A}}{C_{12}H_{12}N_2O_3} \xrightarrow{-CO_2} \underset{\text{Compound B}}{C_{11}H_{12}N_2O_2}$$

(vi) Nature of compound B

Compound B shows the properties of lactam and on boiling with NaOH solution gives Glyoxalic acid and compound C

$$\underset{\text{Compound B}}{C_{11}H_{12}N_2O} \xrightarrow{NaOH} \underset{\text{Glyoxalic acid}}{CHO.COOH} + \underset{\text{Compound C}}{C_9H_{14}N_2}$$

(vii) Compound C is found to be an aromatic diamino derivative by usual tests. It give a blue precipitate with ferric chloride, indicate that compound C must have N-methyl-O-phenylenediamine nucleus.

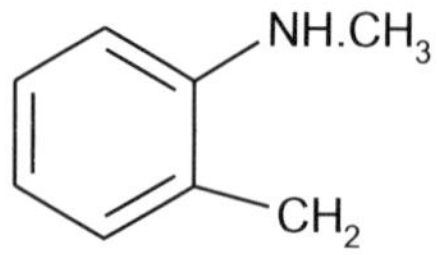

By a series of synthetic reactions, presence of two methyl groups, as well as its's structural identity have been proved as N-methyl-4, 5-diamino O-xylene

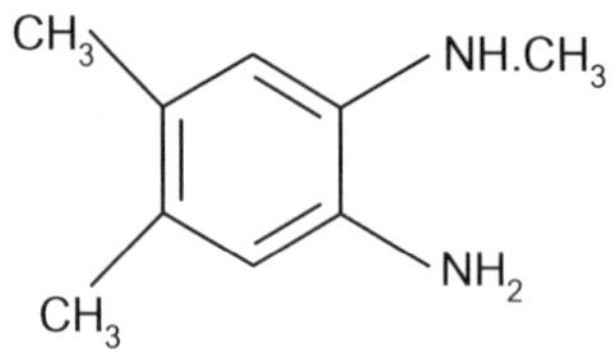

Compound C

Structure of compound C has been proved by it's synthesis.

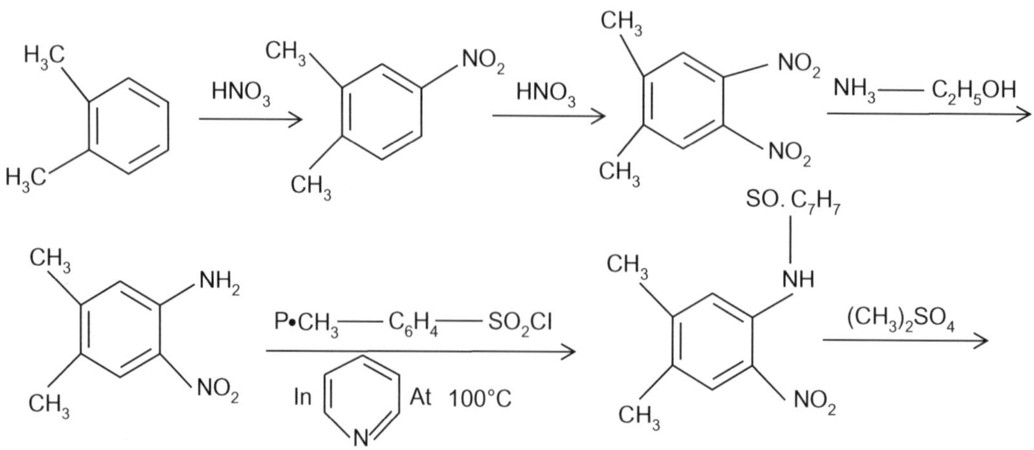

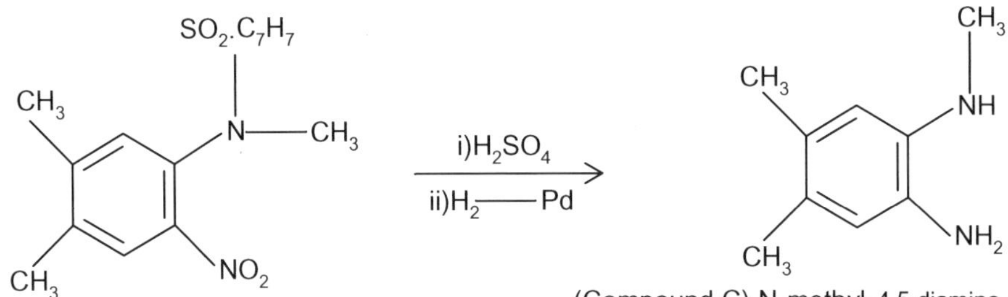

(Compound C) N-methyl-4,5-diamino - Oxylene

From the above points structure of lumiflavin can be represented as follows;

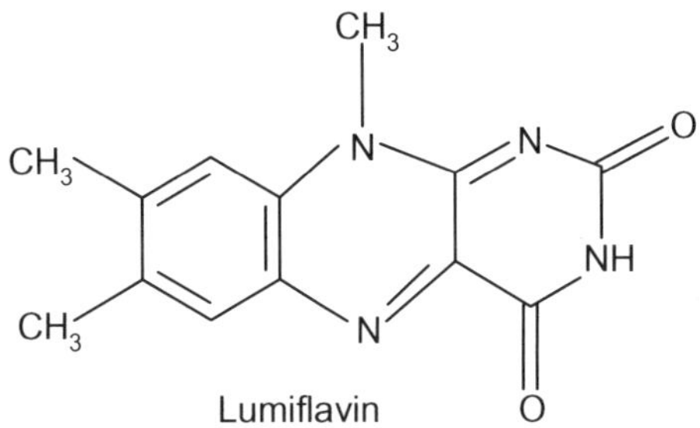

Lumiflavin

Finally structure of Lumiflavin can be confirmed by synthesis.

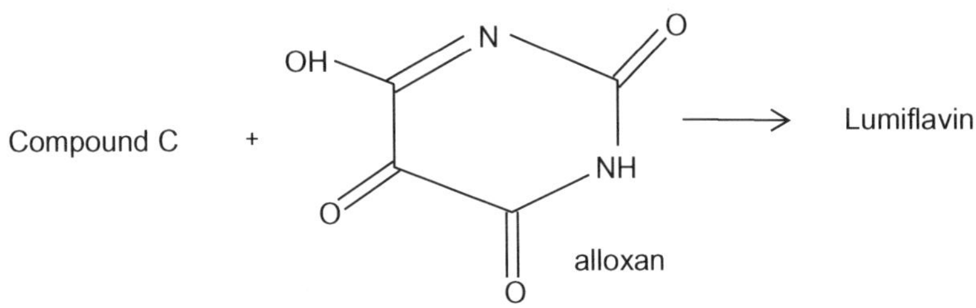

Structure of Lumichrome

Analytical work shows structure of Lumichrome is 6,7-dimethyl alloxazine ie. lumichrome is lumiflavin with a hydrogen atom instead of methyl group at 9th place. It also suggests lactoflavin contains a side chain attached to Na.

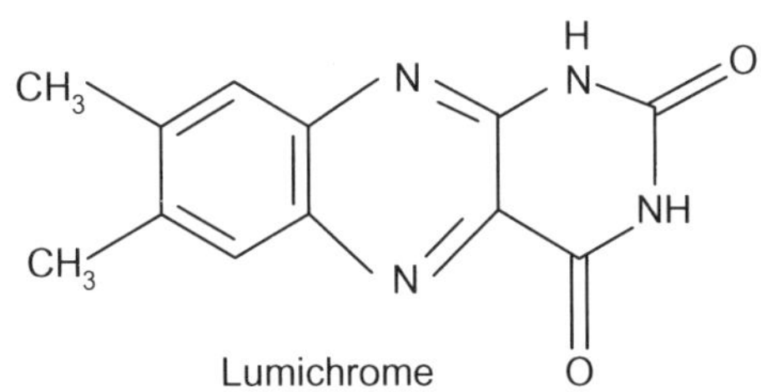

Lumichrome

Side Chain of Ribo-flavin

(i) Presence of Sugar

Reaction mixture from which lumichrome isolated gave positive test for pentose sugar.

(ii) Presence of five active hydrogen atom

Ribo flavin is found to have five active hydrogen atoms by Zerewitnoffs method. Since one active hydrogen atom present on N_3 of lumiflavin, rest four active hydrogen is present as four hydroxyl groups in side chain.

(iii) Riboflavin undergo oxidation with lead tetra acetate gives formaldehyde, one -OH should be in terminal CH_2OH. From the above points, side chain of riboflavin is found to be

$$—CH_2—CHOH—CH—OH—CHOH—CH_2OH$$

So the entire structure of Riboflavin can be represented as follows,

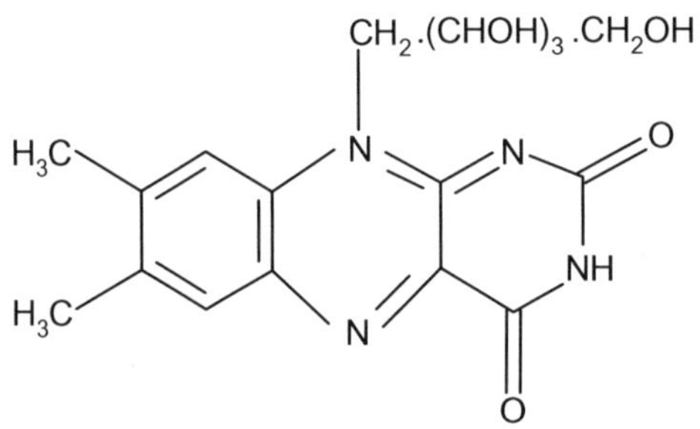

Fianally structure of Riboflavin confirmed by synthesis.

Kuhn Synthesis of Riboflavin

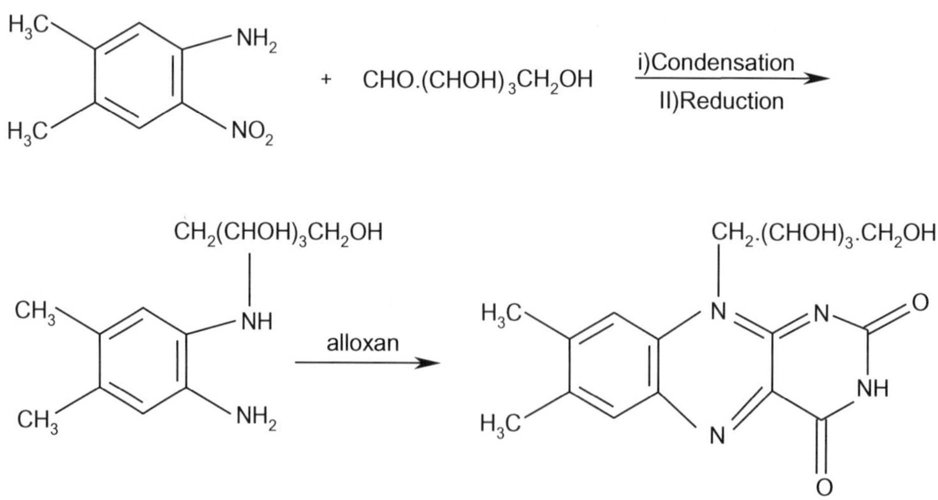

Riboflavin

VITAMIN B_6 (Pyridoxine) (Adermin)

Pyridoxine is enriched in rice bran and yeast. It is used to cure dermatitis in rats.

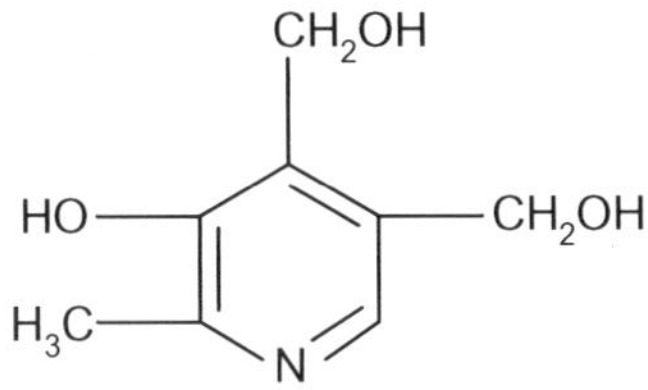

Chemistry of Pyridoxine

1. **Molecular composition is $C_8H_{11}NO_3$**
2. **Presence of active hydrogen atoms.**

   Presence of three active hydrogen atoms have been confirmed by Zerewitnoff method.
3. **Presence of Phenolic Hydroxyl group.**

   Formation of Mono-Methyl ether with diazomethane and deep red color with $FeCl_3$ indicate the presence of one phenolic hydroxyl group.
4. **Presence of alcoholic hydroxyl group.**

   Since Mono-methyl ether of pyridoxine does not give colour reaction with $FeCl_3$ and forms diacetate with acetic anhydride and a hydrobromide of a dibromide with HBr, indicate remaining two hydroxyl groups are alcoholic in nature.
5. **Presence of pyridine neucleus**

   UV Spectrum of pyridoxine shows similarity to 3-hydroxy pyridine indicating the presence of pyridine nucleus,with phenolic group in 3rd position group
6. **Position of two alcoholic groups on adjacent carbon atoms.**

   Lead tetraacetate has no action on monomethyl ether of pyridoxine indicate, two alcoholic groups are not on adjacent carbon atoms in side chain.
7. **Presence of -C-CH_3 group**

   Oxidation by chromic anhydride (kuhn-Roth method) indicate the presence of one -C-CH_3 group.
8. **Structure of pyridoxine**

   Monomethyl ether of pyridoxine on careful oxidation with potassium permanganate, gives methoxy pyridine tricarboxylic acid and gives blood-red colour with ferrous sulphate which is a characterestic reaction of pyridine -2- carboxylic acid indicating one of the COOH in tricarboxylic acid must be in 2nd position. When methyl ether of pyridoxine oxidised with alkaline permanganate under ordinary conditions, CO_2 and anhydride of dicarboxylic acid is obtained. It indicates carboxyl groups are in ortho position. Anhydride on hydrolysis gives corresponding acid which didn't give red colour with ferrous sulphate, indicating no carboxyl group in 2nd position. So it assumes, on decarboxylation tricarboxylic acid eliminates 2-carboxyl group to form an anhyride. Thus tricarboxylic acid can be either of the following structures:

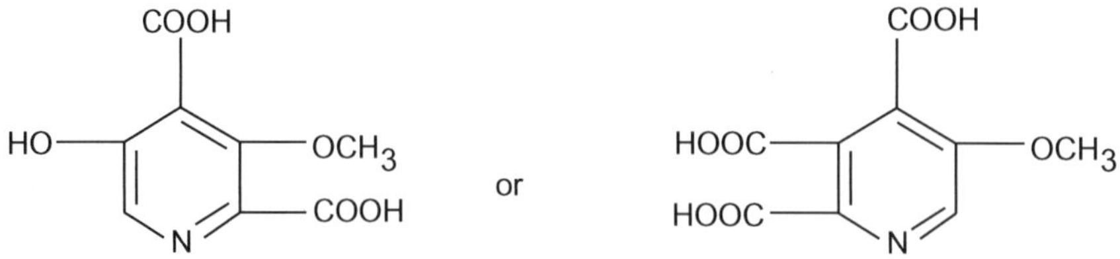

Since pyridoxine methyl ether contains three oxygen atoms (one as methoxyl and other two alcoholic) it is possible that two carboxyl groups in tricarboxylic acid may arise from two CH_2OH group and third COOH may from methyl group. So the pyridoxine may be either of the following.

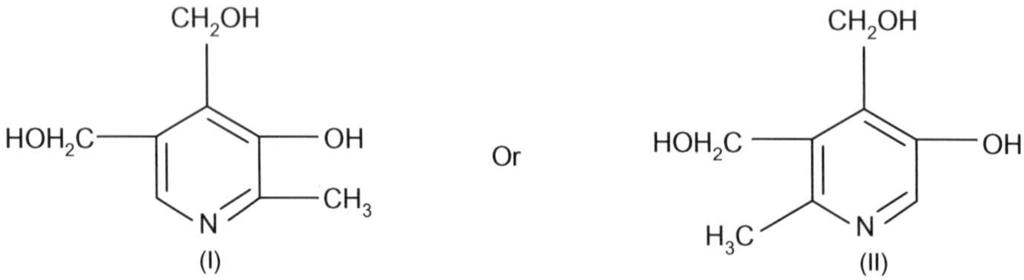

Now Pyridoxine is I or II?

When pyridoxine methyl ether was oxidised with barium permanganate a dicarboxylic acid given which form an anhydride and give a dye namely phthalein on fusion with resorcinol, so the two carboxyl groups must be in ortho position. Analysis of both dicarboxylic acid and its anhydride showed the presence of a methyl group. So the structure of dicarboxylic acid can be either of the following;

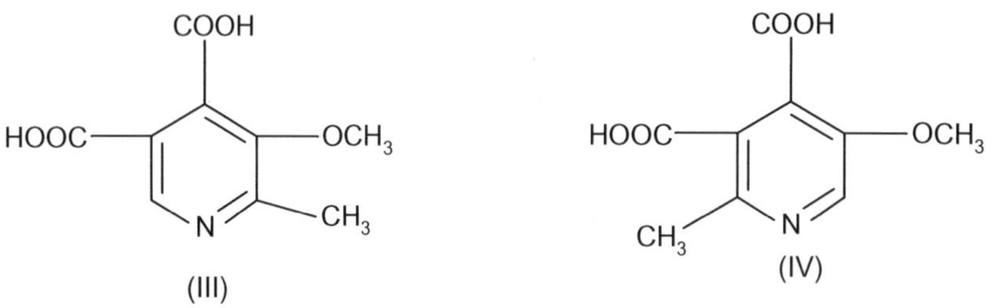

anhydride from III is similar to that of obtaining from 4-methoxy 3-methyl isoquinoline. From these points structure of pyridoxine is as I

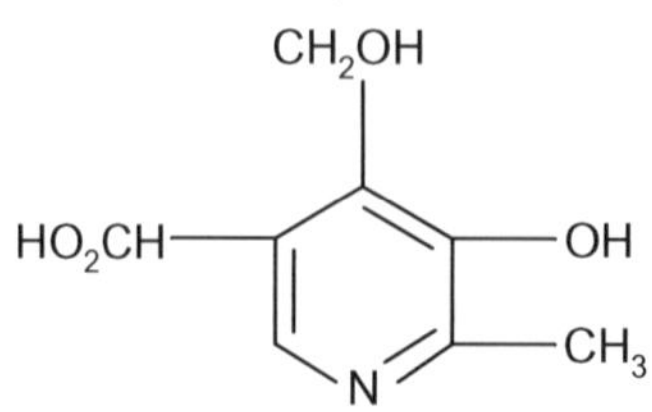

Pyridoxine

Synthesis of Pyridoxine

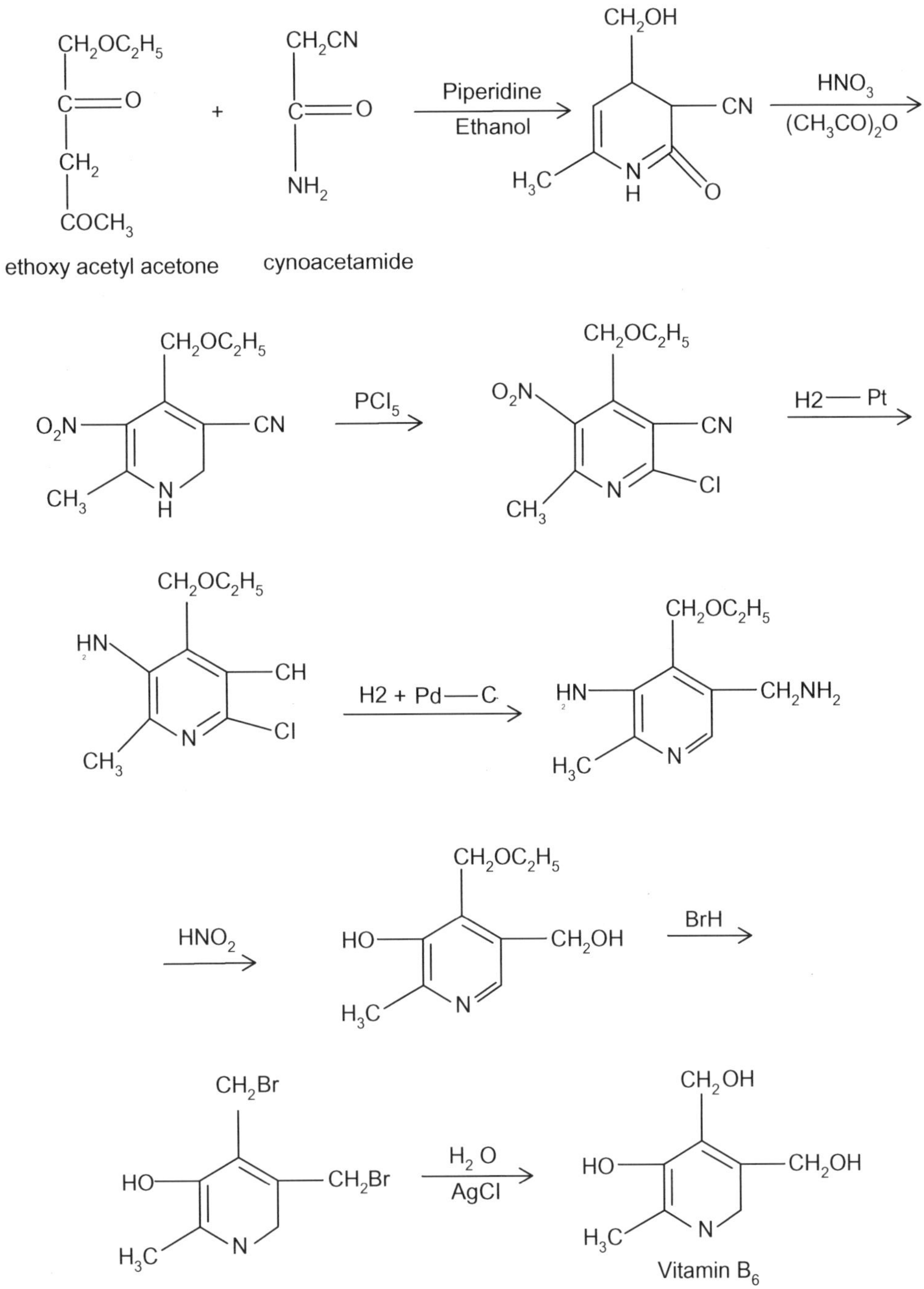

VITAMIN B_{12}

Vitamin B_{12} is otherwise known as Cyanocobalamin and is enriched in liver.

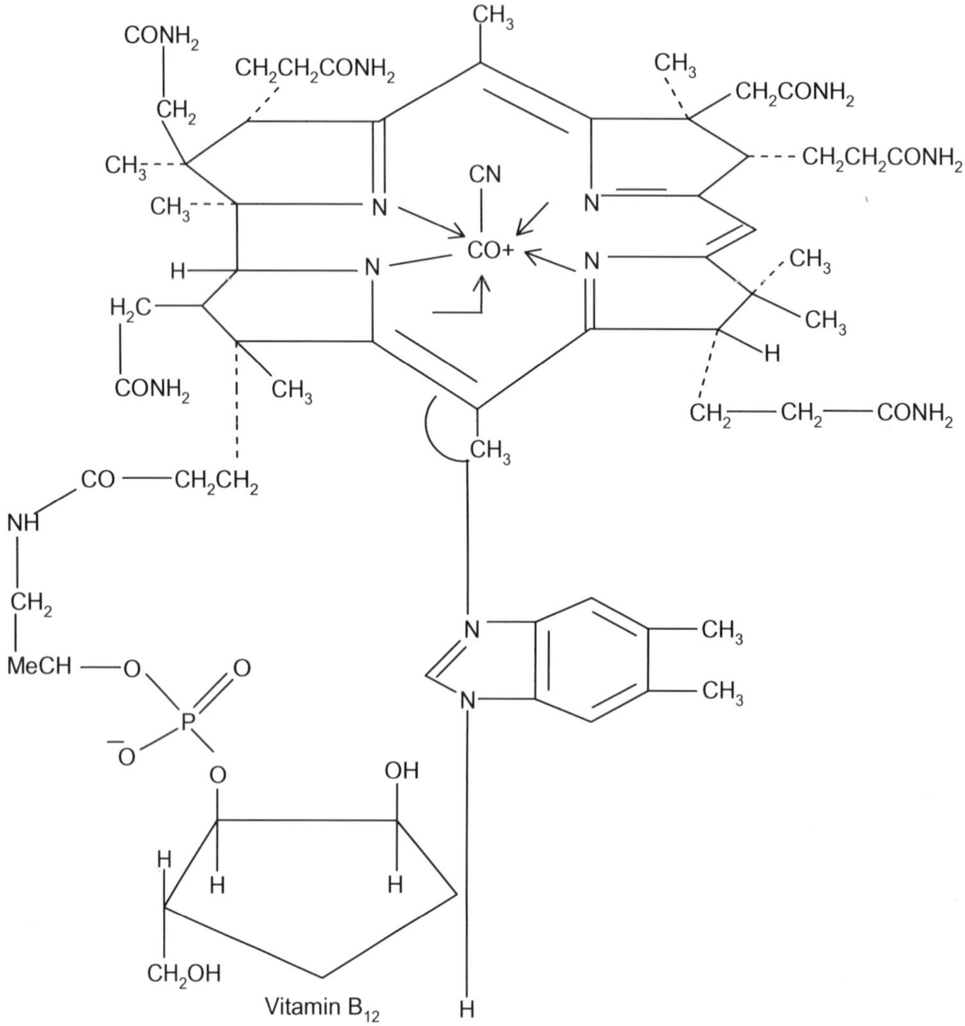

Vitamin B_{12}

Chemistry of Vitamin B_{12}

1. **Most accepted molecular formula of vitamin B_{12} is $C_{66}H_{88}N_{14}O_{14}PC$**
2. **Nature of Cobalt atom**

   Magnetic susceptibility measurements indicate cobalt atom is in trivalent state.
3. **Presence of Cyanide group**

   I.R indiacte the presence of Cyano group and Cyanide group is directly linked to Cobalt atom.

4. Acid hydrolysis of Vitamin B_{12}

Acid hydrolysis of Vitamin B_{12} produces ammonia, compound I namely 1-amino-propan-2-Ol, Compound II namely 5-6, dimethyl benzimidazole, Compound III namely 5,6-dimethyl-benzimidazole-1-α-D-ribofuranoside.

Structure of compound I

Molecular composition of Compound I is C_3H_9NO. It is found to have one aliphatic $-NH_2$ group. Compound I undergoes oxidation with periodic acid, yields acetaldehyde and formaldehyde, indicate compound I is as 1-amino-2-propanol. It is confirmed by its synthesis.

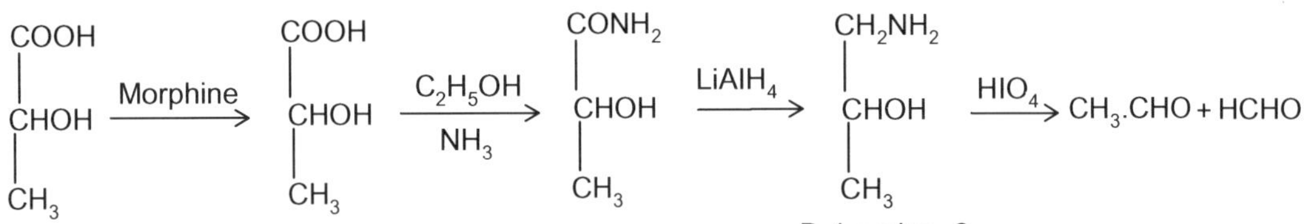

DL-lactic acid D-lactic acid D-1-amino-2-propanol (compound I)

Structure of compound II

Compound II on reaction with benzoyl chloride gives one compound identified as 4,5- dibenzamido. -1,2-dimethyl-benzene. Therefore the compound II should be 5,6-dimethyl benzimidazole.

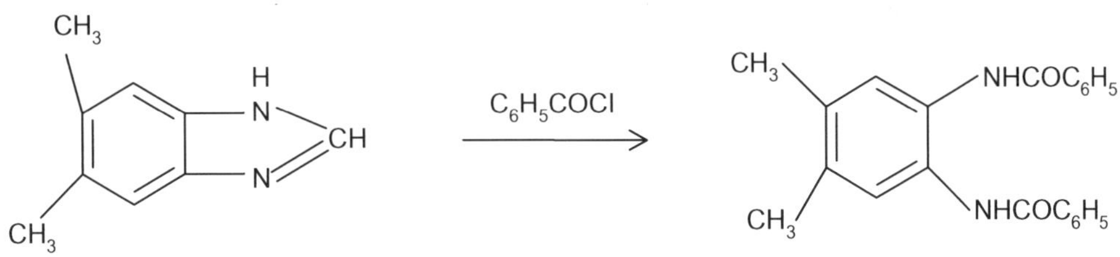

5,6-dimethyl benzimidazole (compound II) 4,5-dibenzamido-1,2 dimethyl benzene

Structure of compound II confirmed by synthesis.

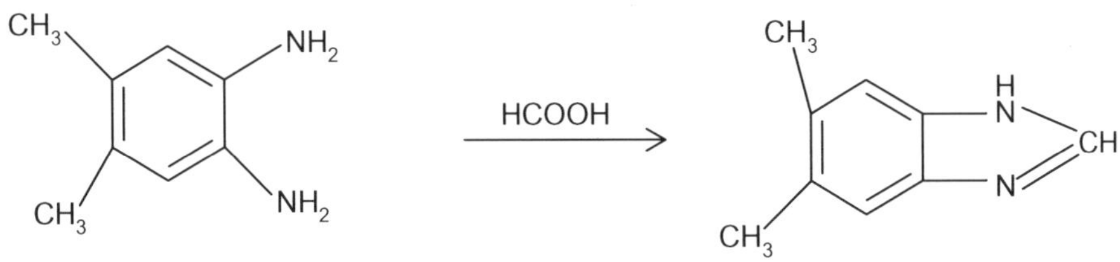

4,5 - diamino - 1,2 - dimethyl benzene (Compound II)

Structure of Compound III and Compound IV

Hydrolysis of Vitamin B_{12} in 6NHCl at 100°C for eight hours yield two bases. One of them is isolated as picrate and gave positive test of carbohydrates which was found to be pentose. It consume one molecule of HIO_4 indicate pentose is in furanose form. Thus compound III is 5,6- dimethylbenzimidazole -1-ribofuranoside-which is confirmed by its synthesis.

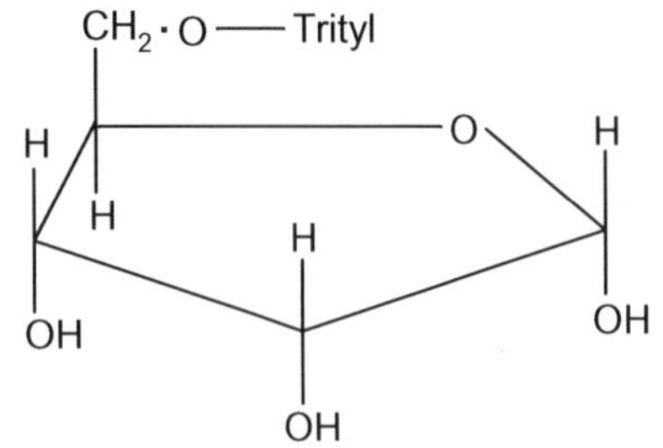

5, - trityl - d- ribofuranose

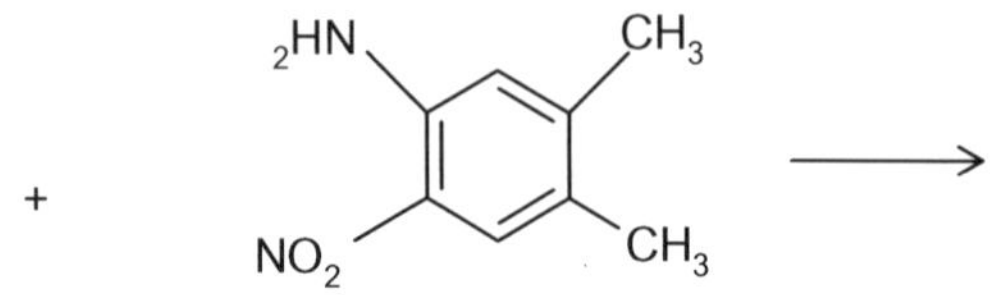

4,5 - dimethyl-2-nitroniline

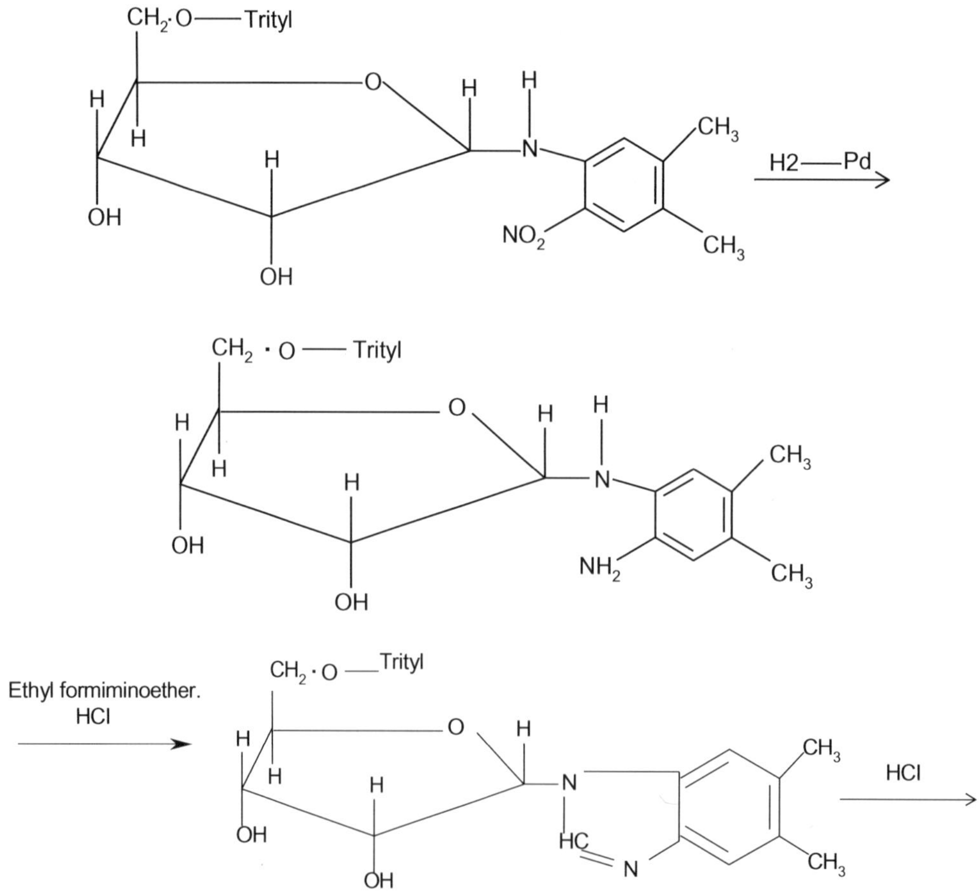

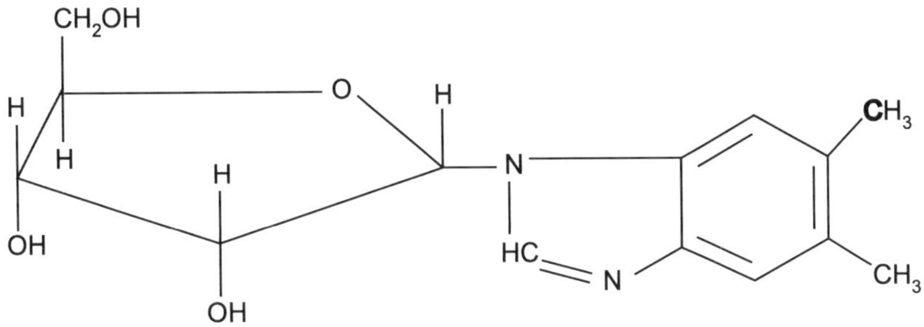

1-α-D- ribofuranosyl -5,6 - dimethyl benzimidazole

5. Vitamin B_{12} reacts with cyanide ion to produce a purple complex containing two cynide groups. U.V spectrum indicate nitrogen of benzimidazole at 3rd position co-ordinately attached to cobalt atom.

6. Involvement of propyl amine part in the linkage of nucleotide to cobalt containing part of Vitamin hydrolysis of Vitamin B_{12} with Conc.H_2SO_4 removes nuecleotide but propylamino and amide group remain attached. It indicate that propyl amine part involved in linkage of nucleotide to cobalt containing part of Vitamin.

7. Amide linkage between propanol and cobalt containing fragment propanol is linked to cobalt containing fragment by amide group have been prooved.

8. Presence of six primary amide group

Vitamin B_{12} undergo hydrolysis with nitrous acid yield hexacarboxylic acid. Showed the presence of six primary amide groups.

9. Presence of pyrrolidine ring

Oxidation of Vitamin B_{12} with sodium chromite in acetic acid givesubstituted succinimides which indicate the presence of pyrrolidine ring.

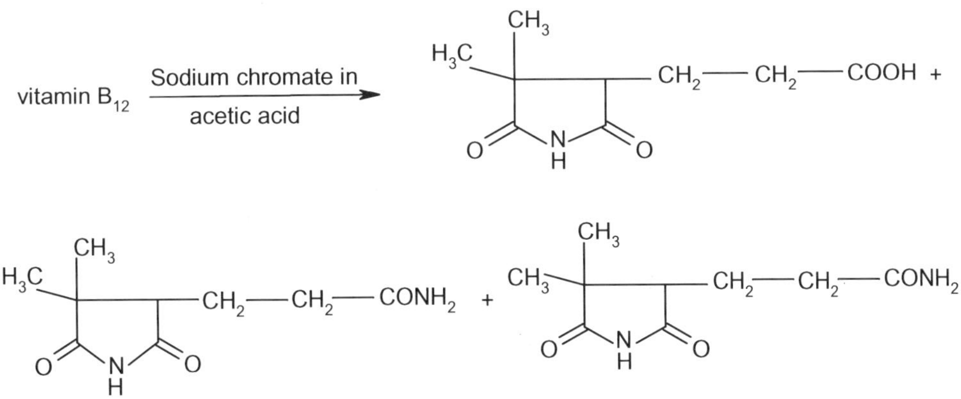

Based on these facts and physico-chemical studies, structure of Vitamin B_{12} can be drawn as given earlier.

FOLIC ACID

Folic acid is otherwise known as pteroylglutamic acid which has been isolated from various sources like yeast, spinach. It's deficiency causes macrocyclic anaemia.

All experiments lead to structure of folic acid has been performed on an yeast namely Lactobacillus Casei. Alkaline hydrolysis of the fermentation Lactobacillus casei factor, in the absence of oxygen, formed two molecules of D-glutamic acid and DL-form of liver Lactobacillus casei factor. Where as alkaline hydrolysis of Lactobacillus casei factor in the presence of air gave compound A and compound B.

Structure of Compound A

1. Molecular composition of compound A is found to be $C_7H_5N_5O_3$ and containing one carboxyl, one amino and one enolic hydroxyl groups.
2. **Presence of 2-aminopyrimidine skeleton**

Compound A on oxidation with chlorine water followed by hydrolysis with HCI, compound A gives guanidine which indicates the presence of 2-aminopyrimidine. So the partial structure of compound can be written as either pteridine derivative or purine derivative. But UV spectrum reveals the presence of pteridine nucleus.

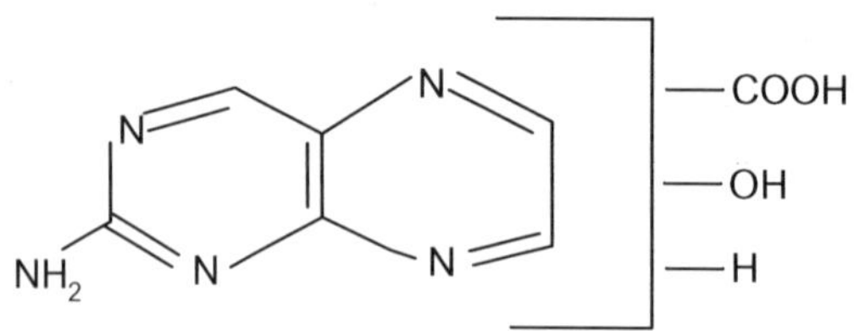

3. **Presence of one carboxylic group**

Compound A on decarboxylation gives a compound identical with 2-amino-4-hydroxypteridine. So the compound A must have one carboxylic group.

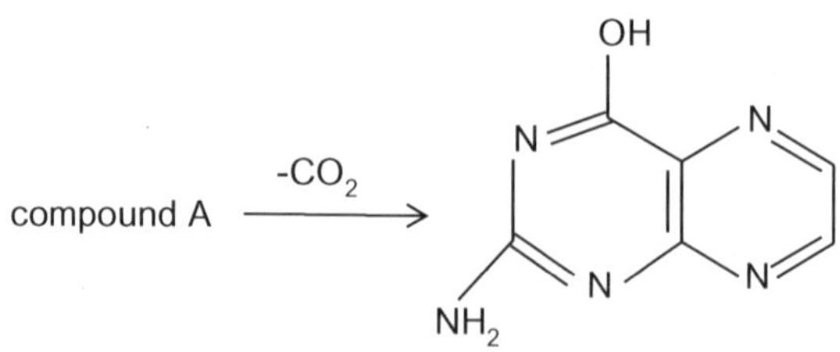

4. **Position of carboxyl group**

Lactobacillus casei factor on treatment with aqueous sulphuric acid gives an aromatic amine and an aldehyde. Aldehyde undergo reaction with aqueous alkali in absence of air gives an acid and an another compound which degraded into 5-amino-2-methyl pyrazine. Thus the structure of compound A can be drawn.

1. Lactobacillus casei factor Aromatic amine+

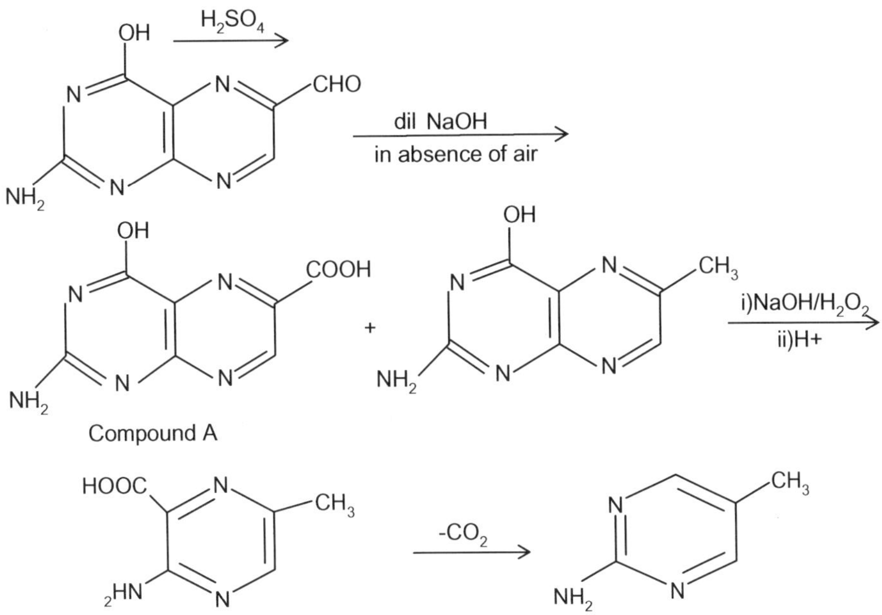

The structure of compound A can be confirmed by its synthesis.

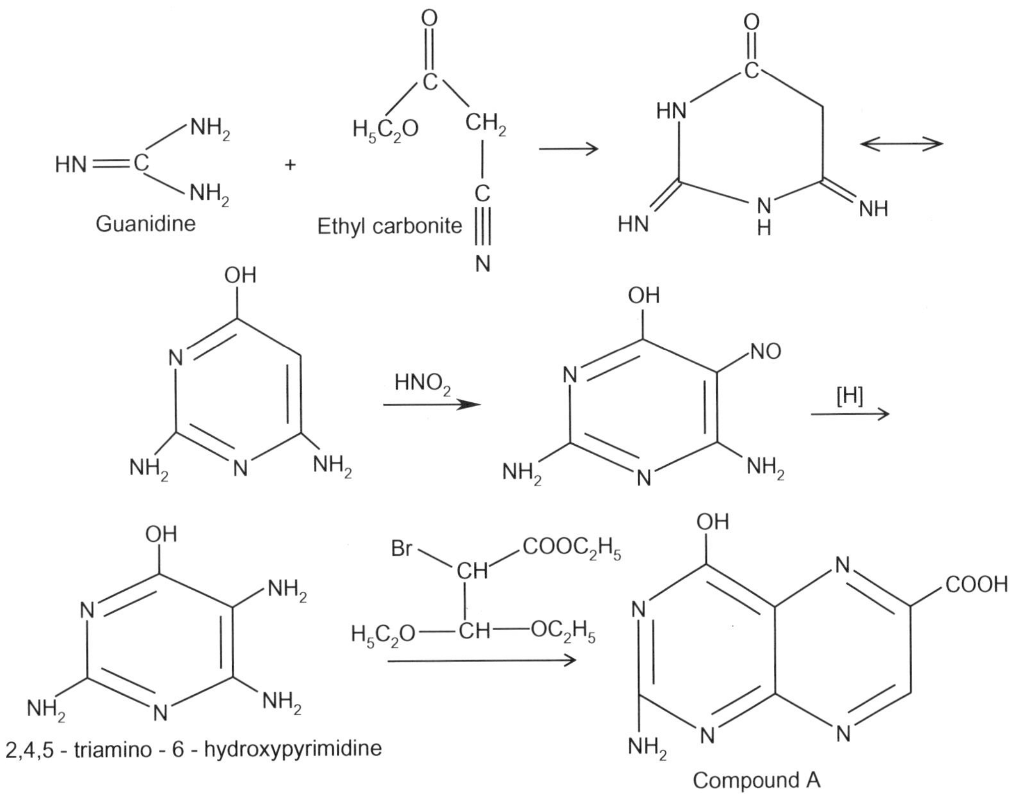

Structure of compound B

1. By usual tests, compound B found to have primary aromatic amino group
2. Peptide nature of compound B

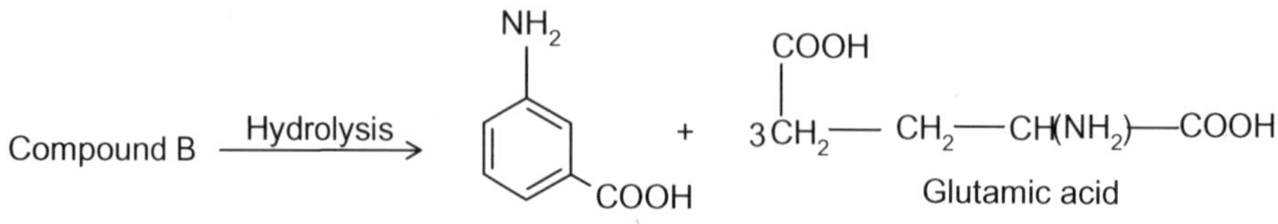

Therefore compound B must be a tripeptide of PABA and glutamic acid.

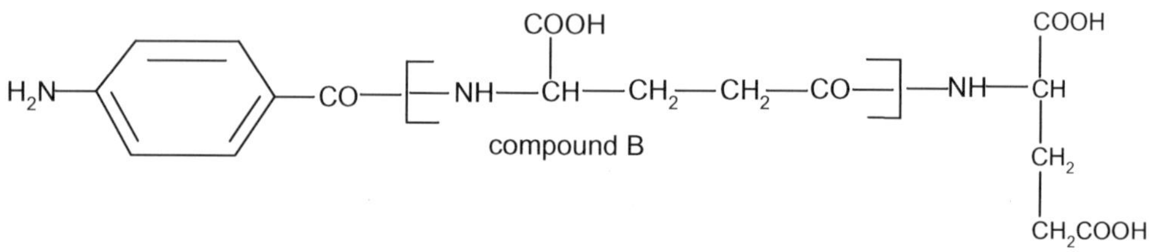

Point of linkage of Compound A and compound B

Compound A and compound B are found to be bridged through methylene group. Finally the structure can be proved by its synthesis. Lactobacillus caseifactore can be synthesised by reacting equimolecular quantities of compound A and 2,3-dibromopropoinaldehyde and p-aminobenzoyl L(+)-glutamic acid in presence of sodium acetate.

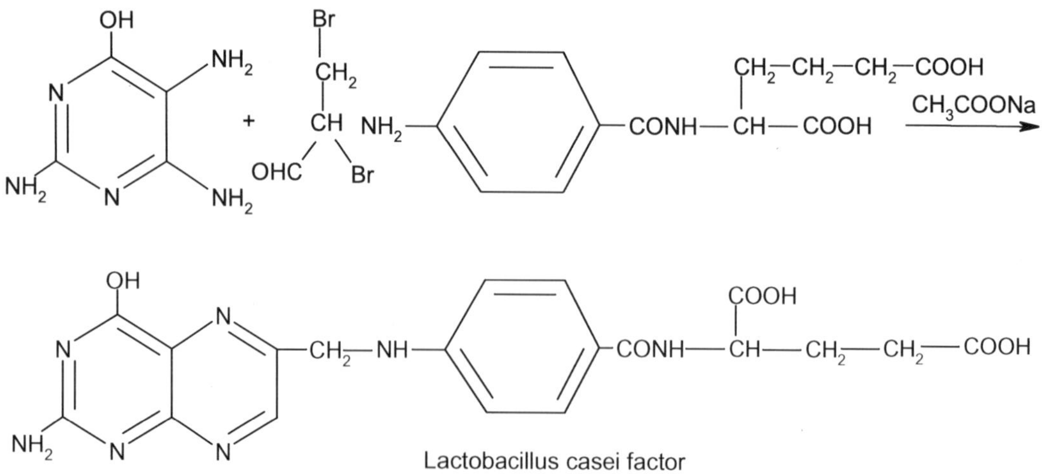

Lactobacillus casei factor

TERPENOIDS

Terpenoids are hydrocarbons of plant origin having the general formula $(C_5H_8)n$ as well as their oxygenated, hydrogenated and dehydrogenated derivatives. Most of the terpenoids are colourless liquids, lighter than water and boil between 150-180°C. Most of them are optically active. On thermal decomposition, most of the terpenoids yield isoprene as one of the products. Isoprene rule states that skeletol structures of all naturally occuring terpenoids are built of isoprene units. They are joined in head to tail fashion.

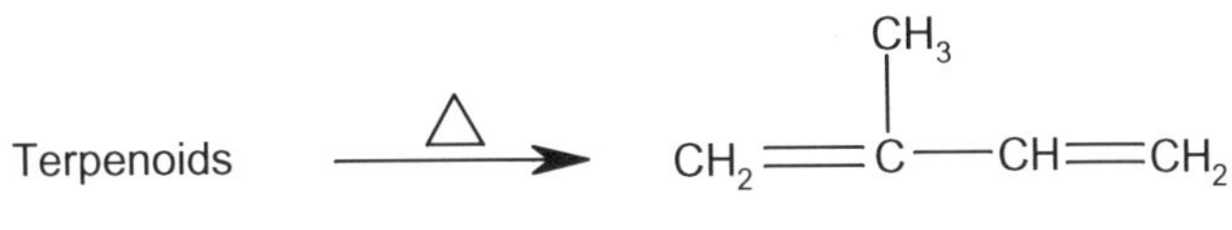

Isoprene

But some exceptions are there in lavandulol and eremophilone the isoprenes are joined tail to tail at their centre. Under experimental conditions isoprene undergoes polymerisation to yield various terpenoids.

$$2C_5H_8 \xrightarrow[280^\circ C]{\triangle} C_{10}H_{16}$$

Dipentene

CLASSIFICATION OF TERPENOIDS

According to number of isoprene units, terpenoids can be classified as follows;

Class	No. of isopren	Molecular formula
Hemiterpene or isoprene	1	C_5H_8
Monoterpene or Terpenes	2	$C_{10}H_{16}$
Sesquiterpenes	3	$C_{15}H_{24}$
Diterpenes	4	$C_{20}H_{32}$
Triterpenes	6	$C_{30}H_{48}$
Tetraterpenes	8	$C_{40}H_{64}$
Polyterpenes	n	$(C_5H_8)_n$

On the basis of number of rings present, terpenoids can be classified into as follows.

Cyclic nature	General formula	Example
Acyclic	CnH_{2n+2}	Citral
Monocyclic	CnH_{2n}	Menthol
Bicyclic	CnH_{2n-2}	Eudesmol
Tricyclic	CnH_{2n-4}	Cedrol
Tetracyclic	CnH_{2n-6}	Cafestol

Generally four methods are applied to extract terpenoids. They are expression, steam distillation, extraction by volatile solvents and adsorption in purified fats. Among these steam distillation is the widely used one.

General Methods of Determining Terpenoid Structure

1. Analytical methods
2. Synthetic methods
3. Physical methods

1. Analytical methods

(a) Molecular formula

After getting the isolated pure specimen, molecular formula is ascertained by usual methods and also by means of mass spectrometry.

(b) Nature of the oxygen atom

Oxygen can be present as hydroxy, aldehyde, keto and carboxylic functional groups. Functional groups like methoxyl, amide, Nitrite ....etc are not yet reported in terpenoids.

(i) Hydroxy group

Hydroxy group can be detected by the formation of acetate, benzoate or urethane esters. Eg.

$$\text{R-OH} + (CH_3CO)_2O \longrightarrow \underset{\text{Acetate}}{ROCOCH_3} + CH_3COOH$$

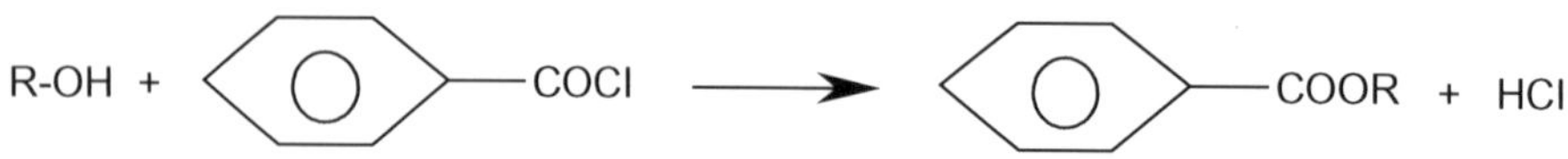

Benzoate

$$\underset{\text{Phenyl isocyanate}}{\text{R-OH} + O{=}C{=}N{-}C_6H_5} \longrightarrow \underset{\text{Substituted methane}}{R{-}O{-}\overset{\overset{O}{\|}}{C}{-}NH{-}C_6H_5}$$

(ii) Carbonyl group

Carbonyl group can be detected by the formation of Bisulphite derivative, oxime and phenylhydrazone.

Sodium bisulphite derivative.

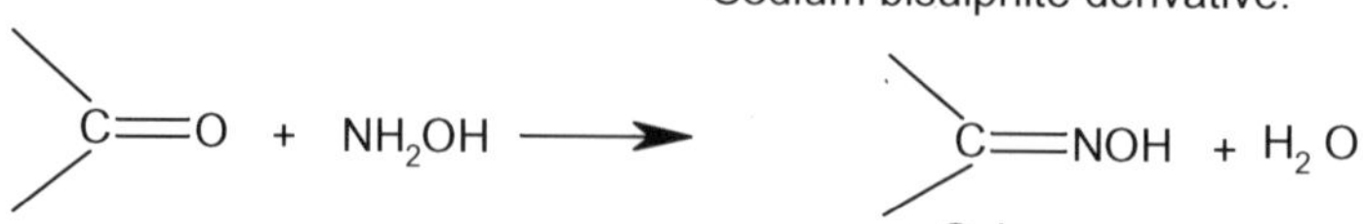

Oxime

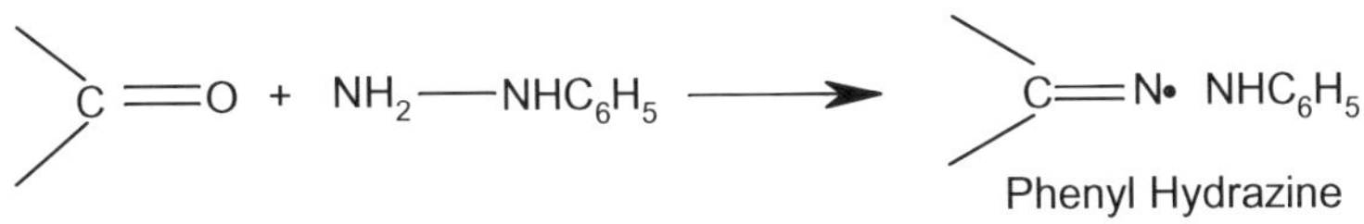

The carbonyl group-aldehyde or Ketone can be ascertained by oxidation. The aldehyde on oxidation yields monocarboxylic acid without loss of carbon atom, whereas ketone on oxidation yields a mixture of compounds having lesser number of carbon atom.

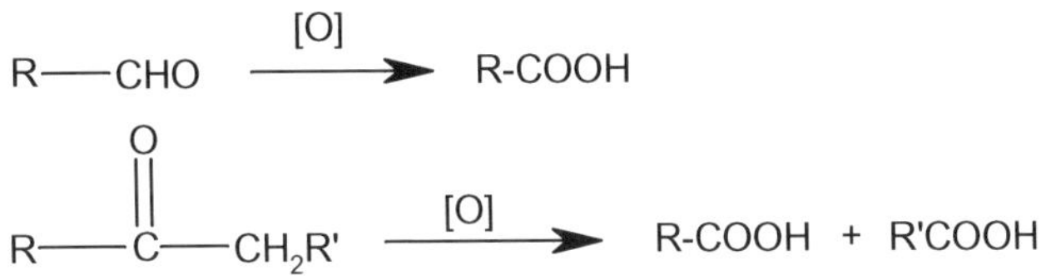

(iii) -CH_2CO- group

-CH_2CO- group forms oximes with nitrous acid in presence of hydrochloric acid.

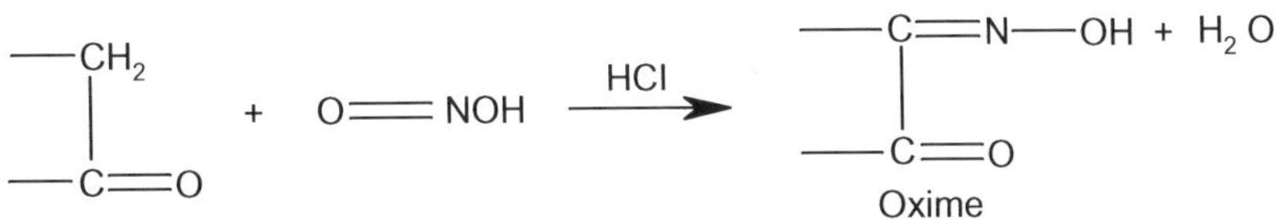

If - CH_2CO- functional group present in the ring which on oxidation yield a dicarboxylic acid without loss of carbon atom.

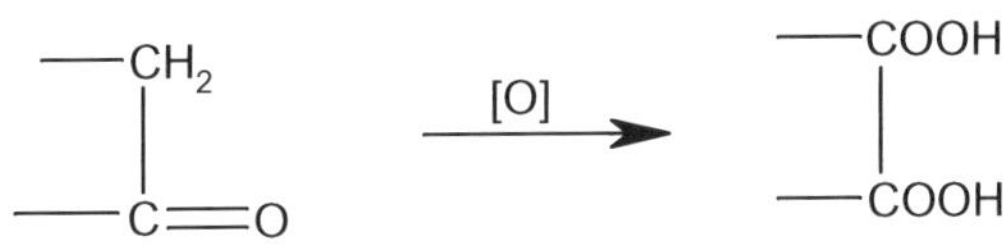

(iv) -$COCH_3$ group

$COCH_3$ group can be detected by Haloform reaction.

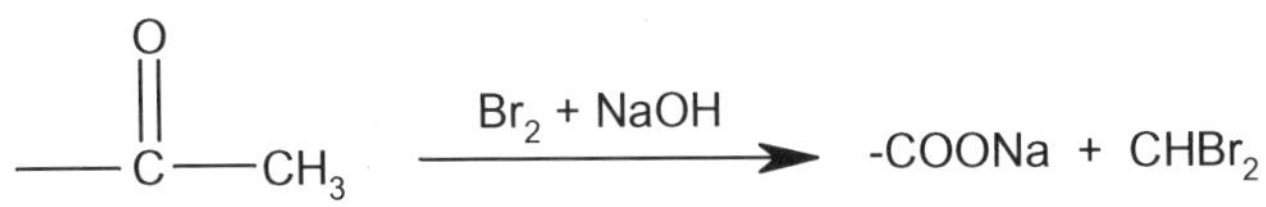

(v) -COOH group

If a compound is soluble in ammonia and gives effervescence with sodiumbicarbonate, indicate the presence of carboxyl group. Acid group can also detected by esterification.

(c) Unsaturation

Presence and number of olefinic double bonds in terpenoids can be detected by the formationof addition products with halogens, halogen acid, hydrogen, peracid and nitrosyl chloride (Tilden reagent). In catalytic hydrogenation, the extent of unsaturation can be calculated from the amount of hydrogen consumed.

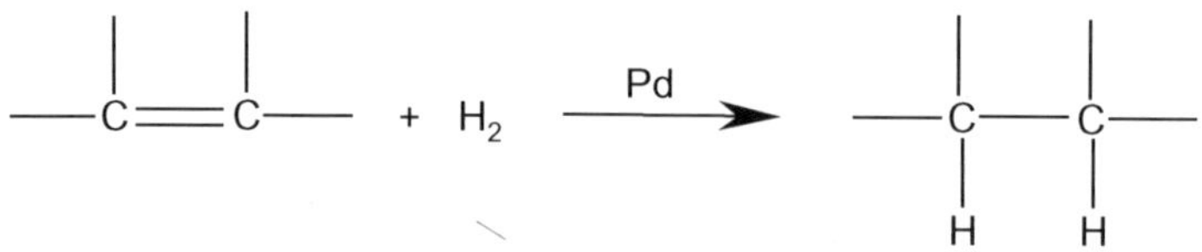

By halogenation reaction, measurement of amount of halogen used gives the amount of unsaturation

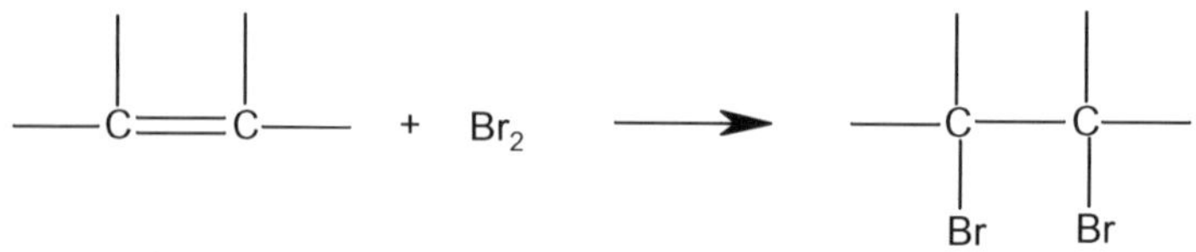

Olefinic bonds form epoxides with peracid

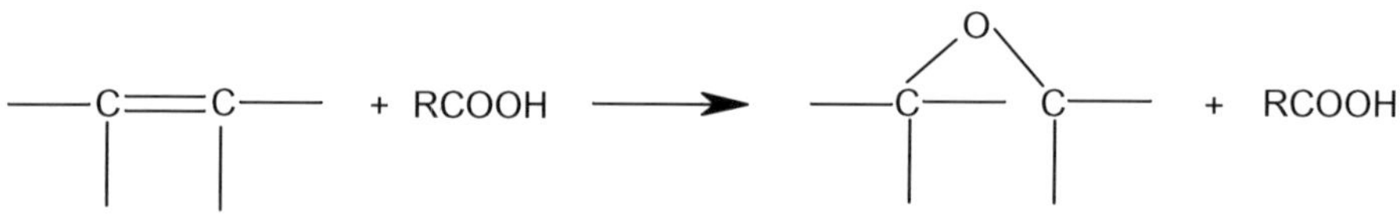

Conjugated system of double bonds canbe detected by Diels Alde reaction (many examples for Diels Alder reaction quoted in the topic-Heterocyclics)

(d) Number of rings

Number of rings can be obtained from isoprene rule. For eg: molecular formula of Citral is $C_{10}H_{16}O$. It contains two double bonds and one oxygen atom as in carbonyl group. Thus molecular formula of parent hydrocarbon would be

$$C_{10}H_{16}O \equiv C_{10}H_{16} + 4H \text{ (for two double bonds)} + 2H \text{ (for Carbonyl oxygen)}$$

$$\equiv C_{10}H_{22} \longrightarrow C_nH_{2n+2} \text{ therefore Citral is acyclic.}$$

(e) Degradation

Terpenoids can be degraded into simple fragments of known structures. Degradation mainly done by oxidation.

(i) With Ozone

Ozone attacks olefinic linkage of the molecule to form ozonide which either by hydrolysis or catalytic reduction yields corresponding carbonyl compounds.

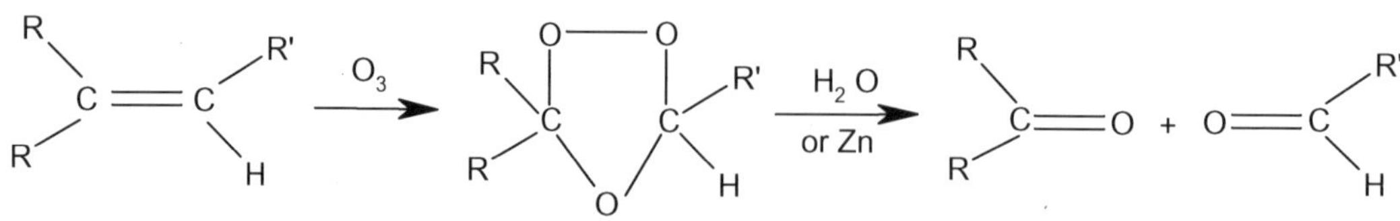

Ozonide

Ozonolysis generally done to locate the position of double bonds in a molecule.

Formation of formaldehyde reveals the presence of terminal double bond.

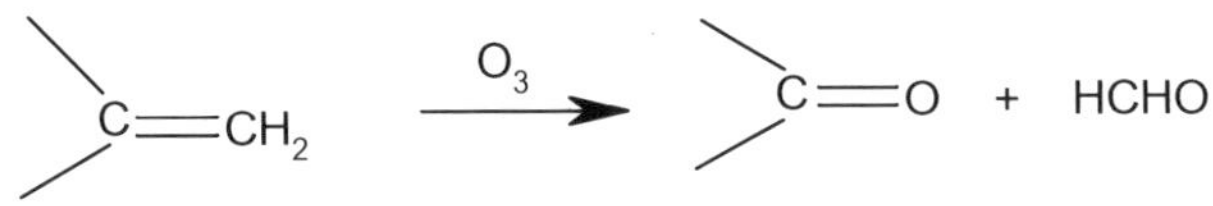

(ii) With Nitric acid

Nitric acid oxidise terpenoid into a mixture of aliphatic and aromatic acids.

(iii) Sodium hypohalite

Sodium hypohalite is used for removal of one carbon atom as bromoform or iodoform from methyl Ketone ($-COCH_3$) The reaction is known as haloform reaction.

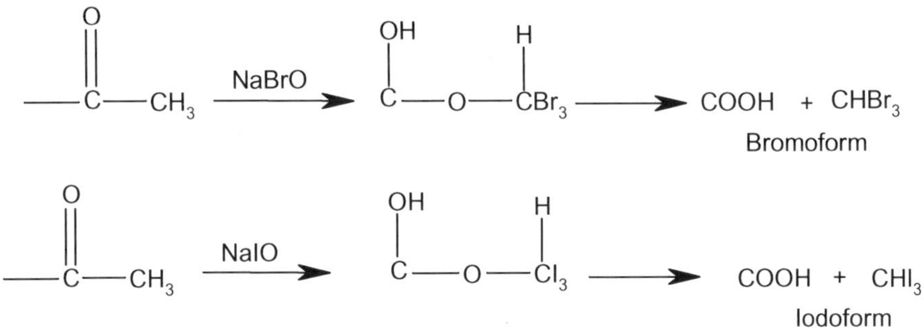

(iv) Oxidizing agents

When hydroxylating agents like lead tetra-acetate in hot acetic acid, peracids, Osmiumtetroxide, Hydrogen peroxide, and potassium permanganate attack olefinic double bonds of terpenoids yield 1,2-glycols.

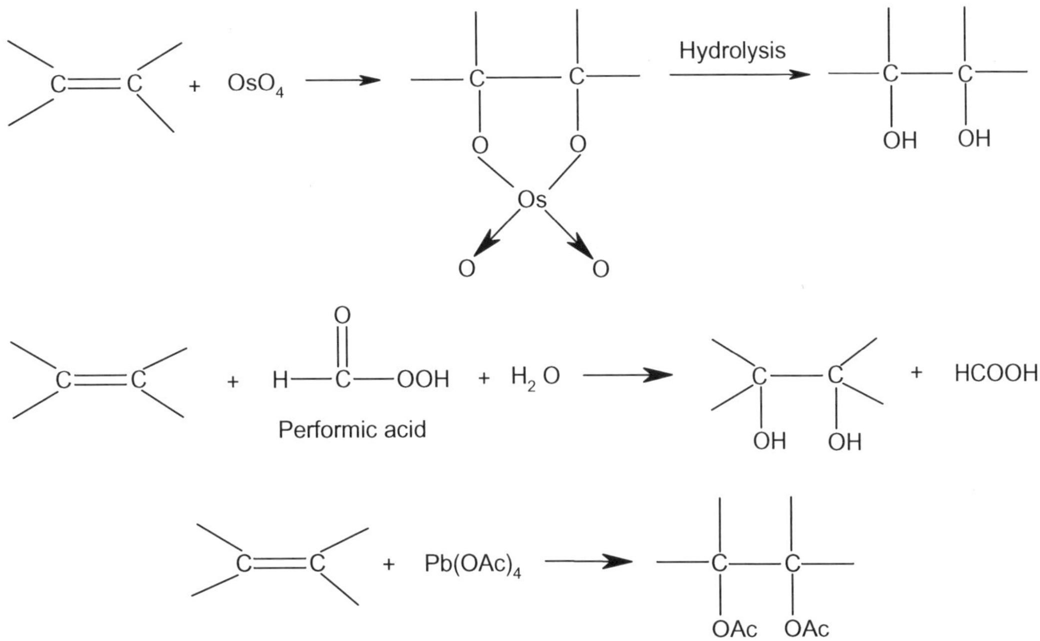

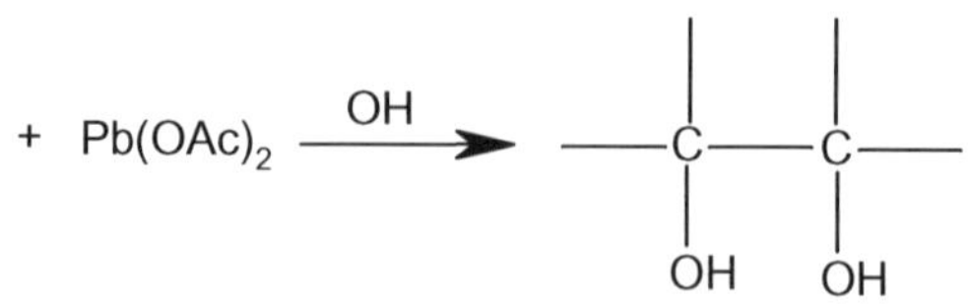

(v) Dehydration

When terpenoids containing alcoholic and ketonic group are heated with dehydrating agents, loose a molecule of water and converted to simple aromatic compounds.

Eg:

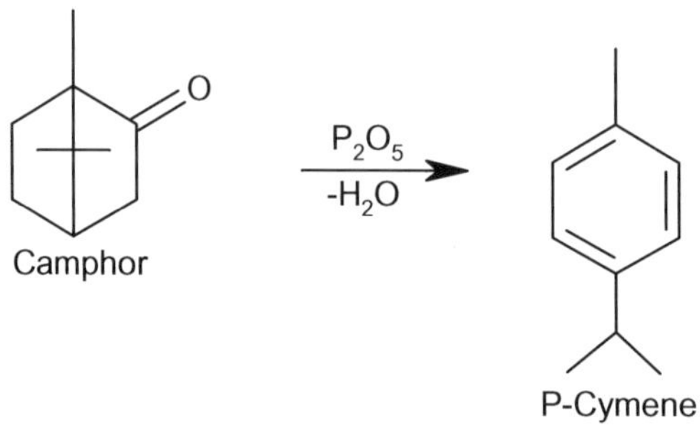

(vi) Dehydrogenation

When terpenoids heated with zinc, Iodine, Bromine sulphur converted to aromatic compounds of known structure

2. Synthetic methods

(a) Catalytic hydrogenation

Thymol can be reduced by Nickel to menthol.

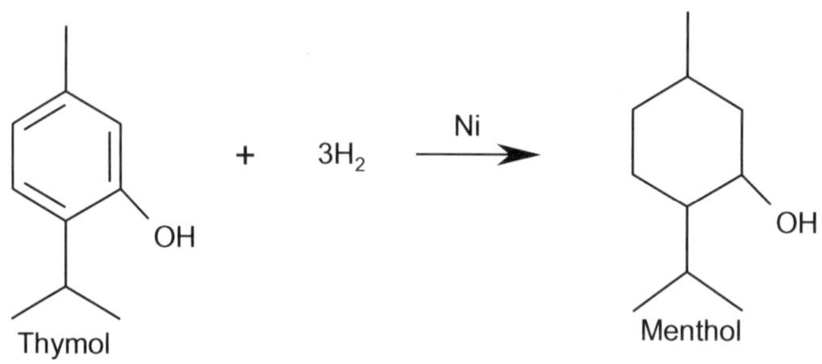

(b) Grignards reaction

By this method methyl or isopropyl groups can be introduced into a compound having carbonyl group.

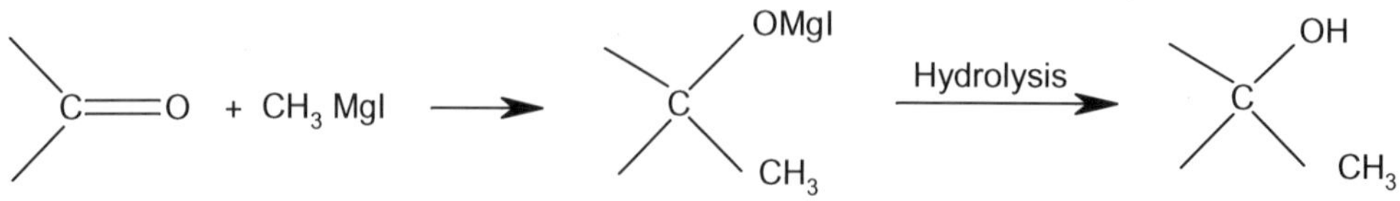

(c) Reformatsky reaction

In this reaction, α-halogen substituted ester is treated with a carbonyl compound (CHO, C= or OCO) in the presence of zinc to form β-hydroxy ester which on treatment with dilute acid yield β-hydroxy acid which converted to unsaturated acid.

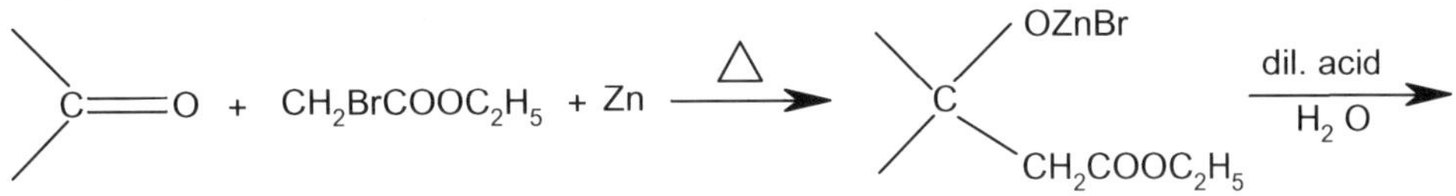

α-bromo ethyl acetate

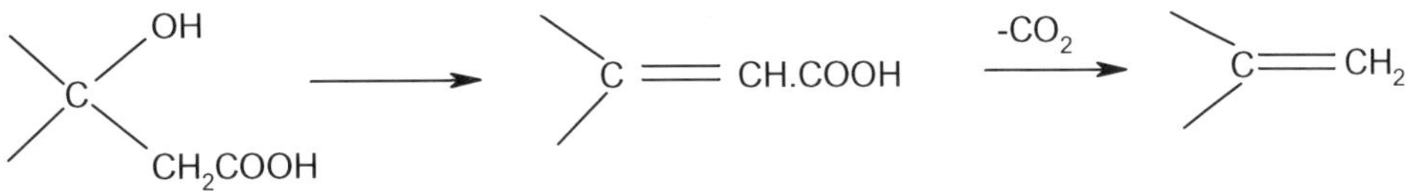

α-hydroxy acid — Unsaturated acid — Hydrocarbon

3. Physical methods

(a) U.V Spectroscopy

It is used in terpenoid chemistry for the detection of configuration according to the presence of double bond, λ-max will be different for different compounds.

For Eg:

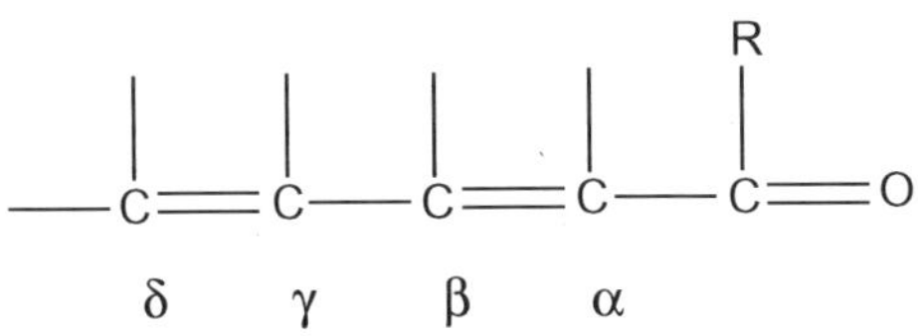

for parent chain given value is 215 n.m

for α substitution = 10 n.m

for β substitution = 12 n.m

for γ substitution = 18 n.m

for exocyclic double bond = 05 n.m

(b) Infra-red Spectroscopy

I.R spectroscopy is useful in detecting the presence of a hydroxyl group, Oxo group and α, β-Unsaturation. It is very useful in detecting isopropenyl group and can distinguish between cis and trans isomers.

(c) NMR Spectroscopy

It is used to identify double bonds and to determine end groups. This method is also used to determine the number of rings present and also to reveal orientation of methyl groups.

(d) Mass spectrometry

This technique is used to elucidate the structre of terpenoids. Molecular weights, Molecular formulae, nature of various functional groups, relative positions of double bonds ... etc can be determined.

(e) Optical rotation

Optical Rotatory Dispersion studies can be used to assign absolute configurations.

(f) X-ray Analysis

X-ray technique can be used even for elucidating the structure and to study the stereo-chemistry of Terpenoids.

After employing all general methods, the structure canbe confirmed by its synthesis.

CITRAL

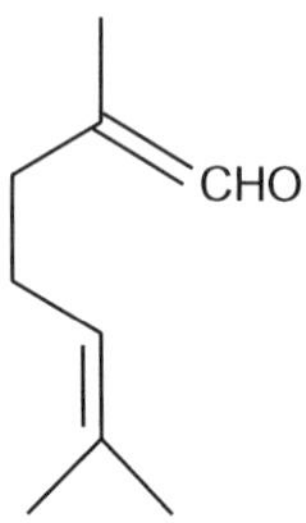

Citral is widely distributed in nature mainly in lemon grass oil. Citral is a liquid having the smell of lemons Citral is acyclic monoterpenoid having the molecular formula $C_{10}H_{16}O$.

1. Presence of two double bonds

Citral adds two moles of bromine - shows citral contains two double bonds.

$$C_{10}H_{16} + 2Br_2 \longrightarrow C_{10}H_{16}OBr_4$$

2. Presence of aldehyde group

(a) Citral forms Oxime with hydroxylamine.

$$>C=O + NH_2OH \longrightarrow >C=NOH + H_2O$$

(b) Citral forms phenyl hydrazone with phenylhydrazine.

$$>C=O + NH_2NHC_6H_5 \longrightarrow >C=N{\bullet}NHC_6H_5 + H_2O$$

(c) Citral on reduction with sodium amalgam gives geraniol.

$$C_{10}H_{16}O \xrightarrow[\text{[H]}]{\text{Na - Hg}} \underset{\text{geraniol}}{C_{10}H_{18}O_4}$$

(d) Citral on Oxidation with silver oxide gives geranic acid.

$$C_{10}H_{16}O \xrightarrow[\text{[O]}]{Ag_2O} \underset{\text{Geranic acid}}{C_{10}H_{18}O_2}$$

Formation of Geraniol and Geranic acid confirms oxo group present in Citral is an adehyde. (There is no reduction in number of carbon atoms in products)

3. Acyclic nature of Citral

Presence of two double bonds and an aldehyde group in Citral leads to a saturated hydrocarbon of molecular formula $C_{10}H_{22}$ which corresponds to general formula CnH_{2n+2} for acyclic compounds indicating that Citral must be an acyclic compound.

4. Skeletal structure of Citral

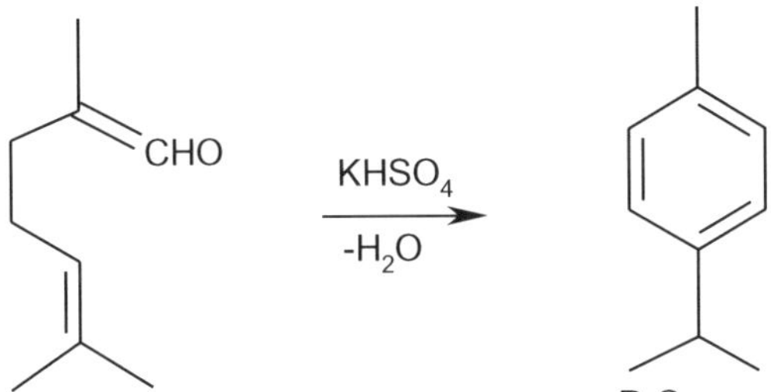

Citral   P-Cymene

Formation of a known cyclic structure of p-cymene indicate citral having the skeletal structure

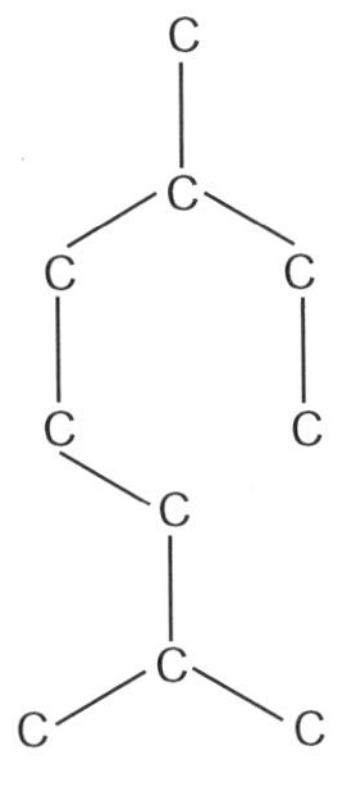

5. Structure of Citral by Ozone degradation

Citral on ozonolysis forms diozonide, which on hydrolysis yields Glyoxal, laevuladehyde and Glyoxal. Formation of these products confirm the structure of citral.

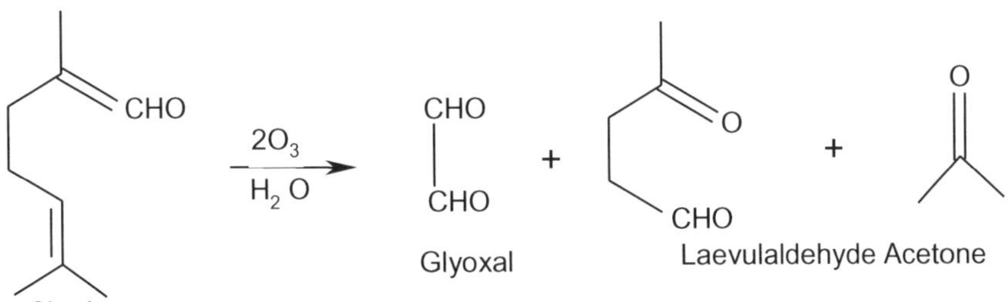

Glyoxal   Laevulaldehyde Acetone

Citral

Finally the structure of Citral confirmed by its synthesis.

Barbier - Bouveault - Tiemanns synthesis for citral

In this synthesis methyl heptenone is converted into Geranic ester by Reformatskys reaction, which is converted into citral by heating a mixture of calcium salts of geranic and formic acids.

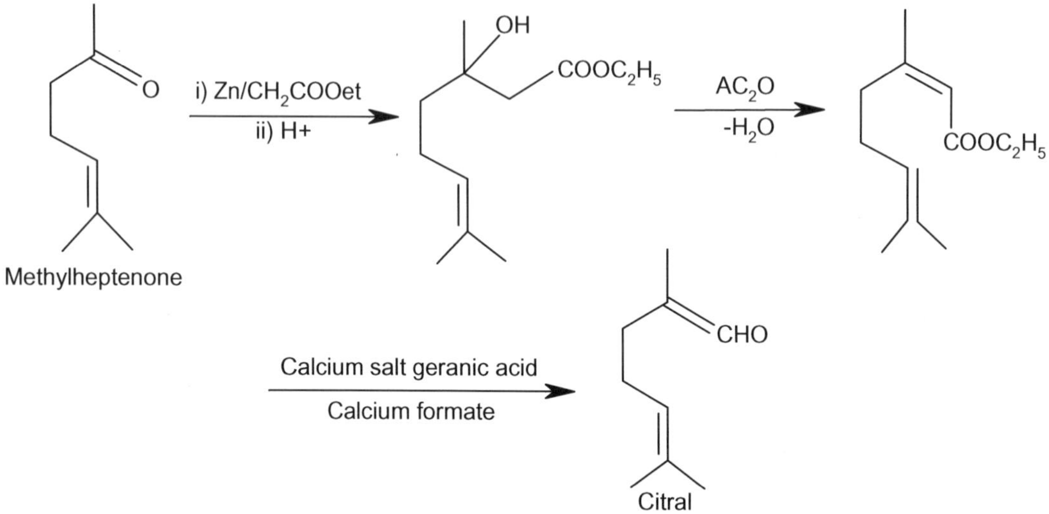

Two geometrical isomers cis and trans forms are possible with respect of aldehyde to methylene Citral is used for synthesis of β-ionone which is used in perfumery.

MENTHOL

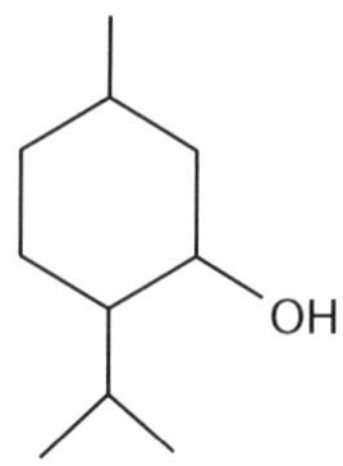

Menthol is optically active and naturally -ve form is occuring mainly in peppermint oil. It have the molecular formula $C_{10}H_{20}O$. It is used as antiseptic and anaesthetic.

1. Presence of alcoholic group

Menthol reacts with an acid to form ester. Menthol on oxidation give menthone which indicates hydroxyl group in menthol is 2° alcohol.

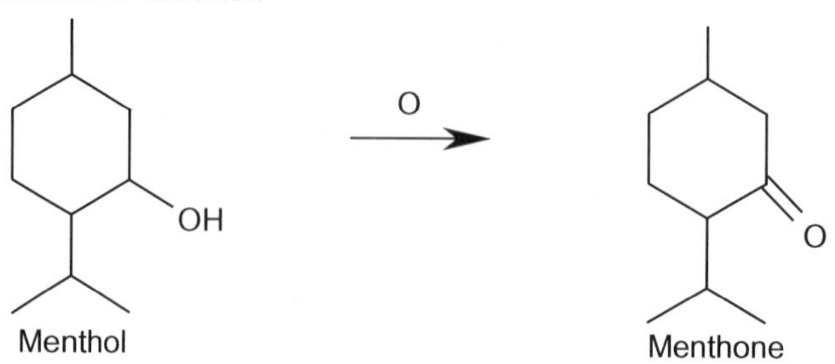

2. Structure of Menthol

Menthol can be obtained from pulegone - whose structure is known. Aromatisation of menthol to thymol again reveals the structure of Thymol.

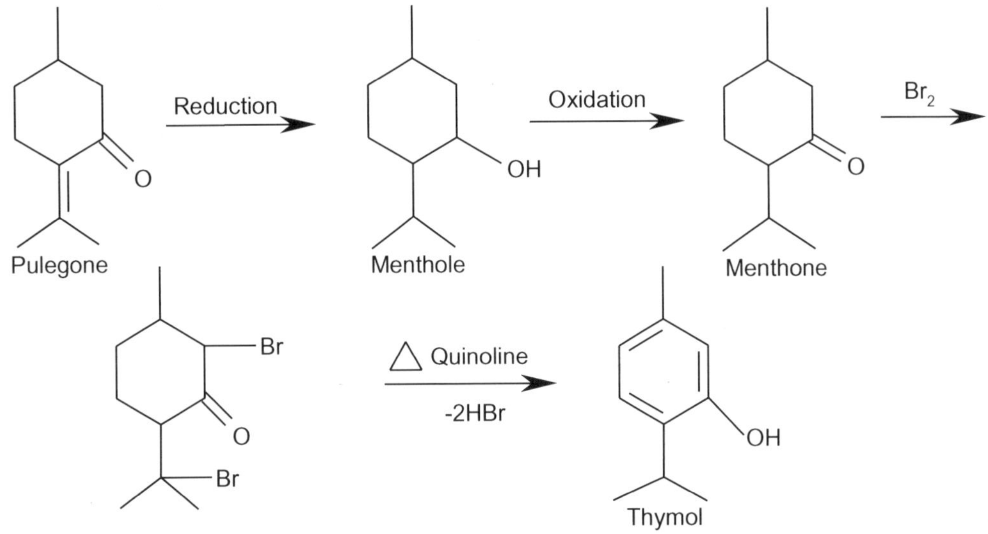

Finally structure of menthol can be confirmed by its synthesis.

3. Synthesis of Menthol

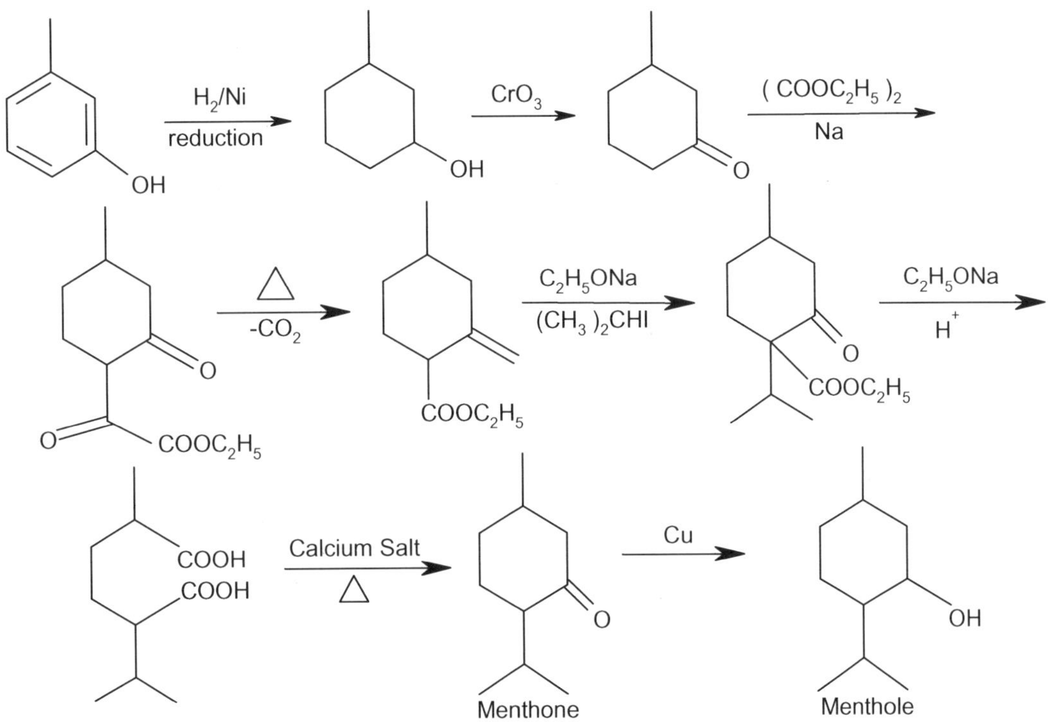

Stereo Chemistry of Menthol

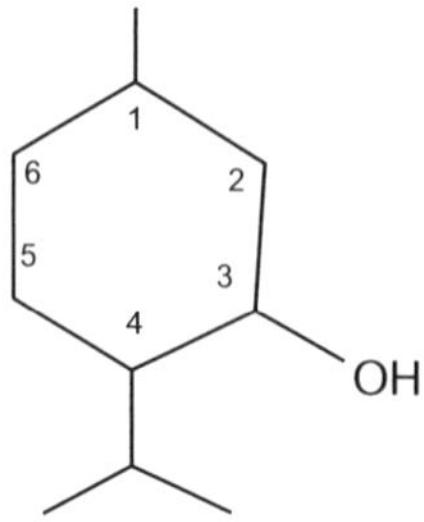

Since menthol molecule has 3 dissimiliar Chiral carbon atoms (1, 3, & 4), it exist in 8 ($2^3 = 8$) optically active forms ie 4-enantiomeric pairs.

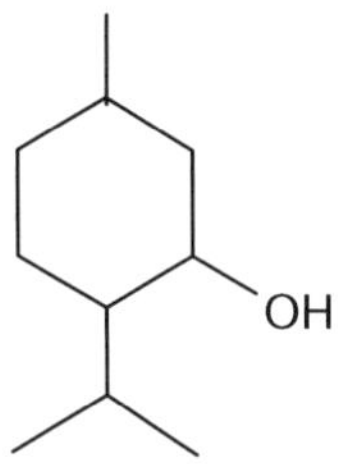

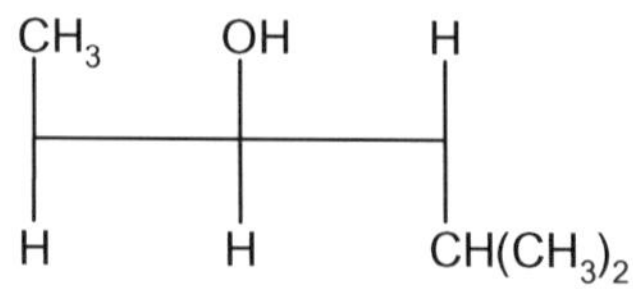

Menthol

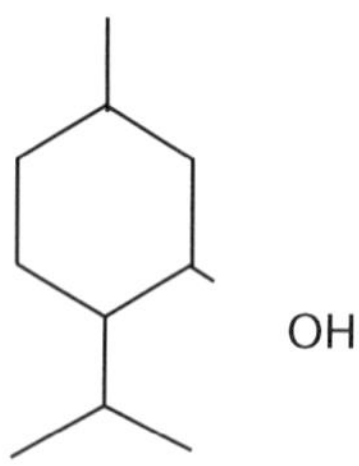

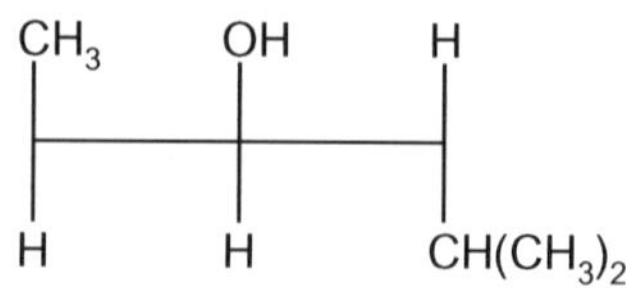

Neomenthol

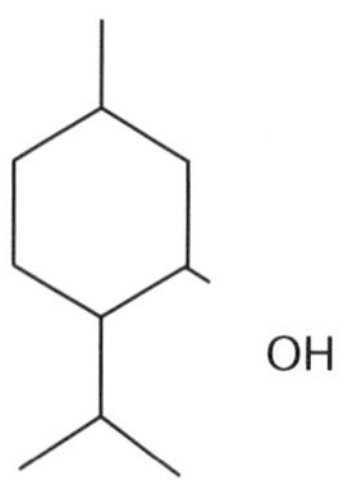

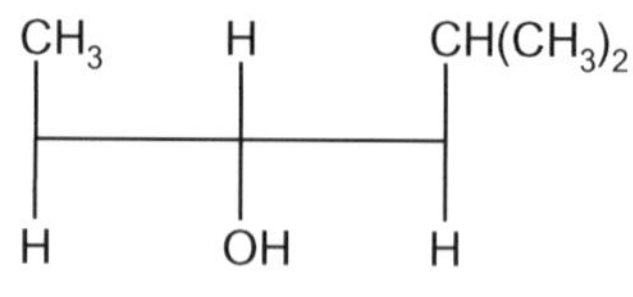

Isomenthol

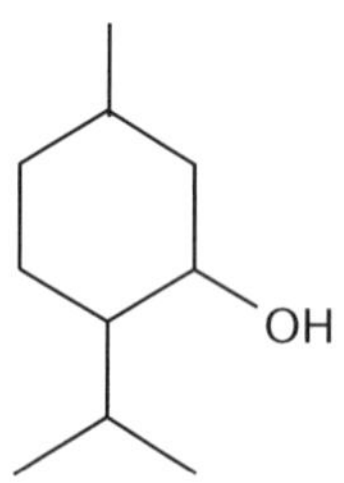

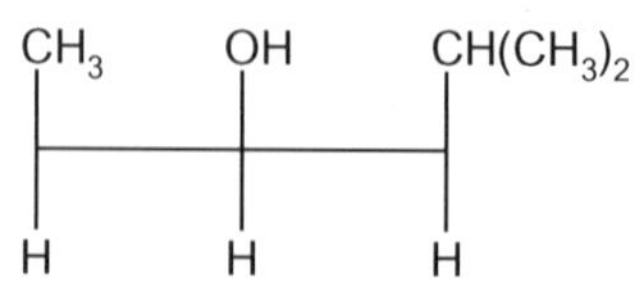

Neoisomenthol

Conformations of the above can be represented as

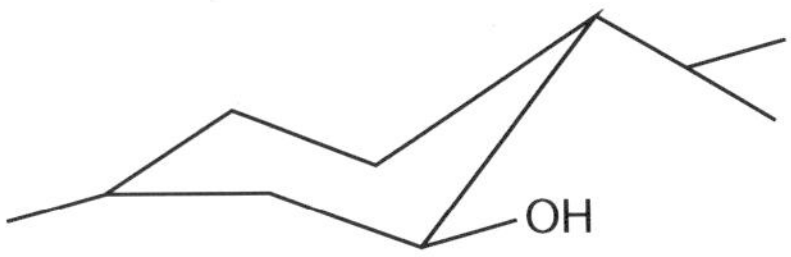

Menthol

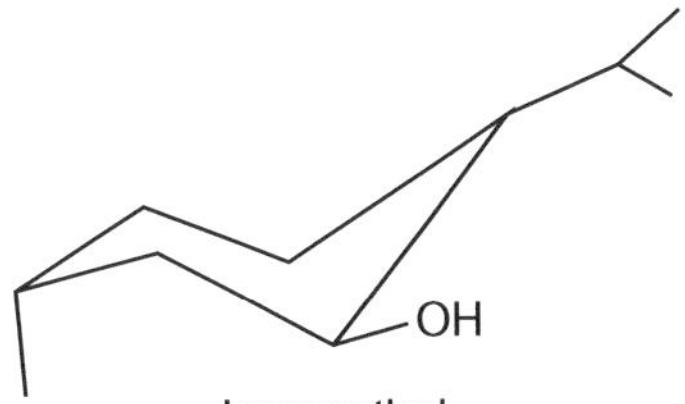

Isomenthol

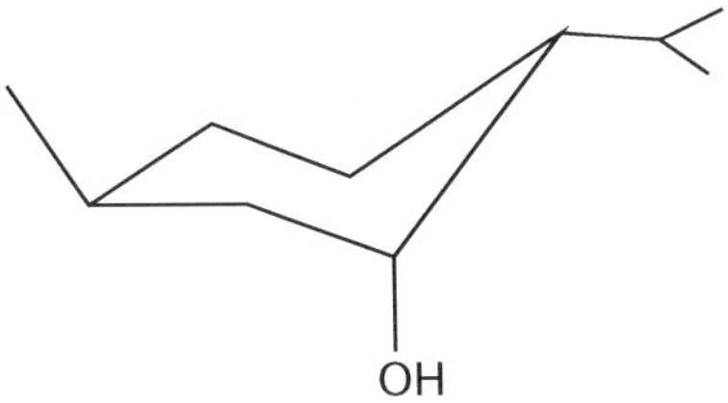

Neomenthol

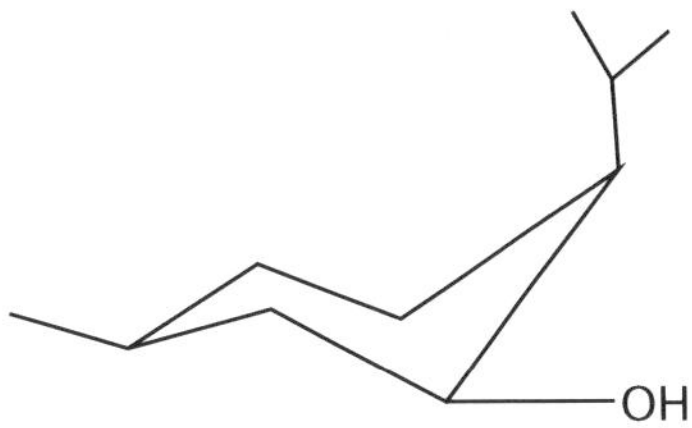

Neoisomenthol

CAMPHOR

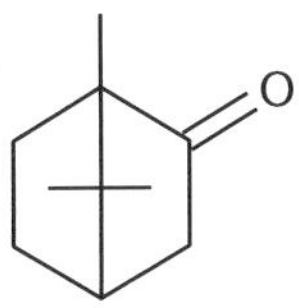

Camphor is an optically active solid, occur in the camphor tree of formosa and Japan. Camphor is used as plasticizer for the manufacture of celluloid and photographic films. It is used as mild disinfectant. It is also used as insect repellent. It is having the molecular formula $C_{10}H_{16}O$. Camphor is a bicyclic monoterpenoid.

1. Nature of Oxygen atom

Camphor on reaction with semicarbazide gives semicarbazone. Camphor on reaction with phenyl hydrazine gives phenyl hydrazone. Camphor on reaction with hydroxylamine gives camphor oxime.

$$\underset{\text{Camphor}}{C_6H_{16}O} + \underset{\text{Hydrxylamine}}{NH_2OH} \longrightarrow \underset{\text{Camphoroxime}}{C_{10}H_{16} \equiv N - OH}$$

Camphor on oxidation with nitric acid gives camphoric acid.

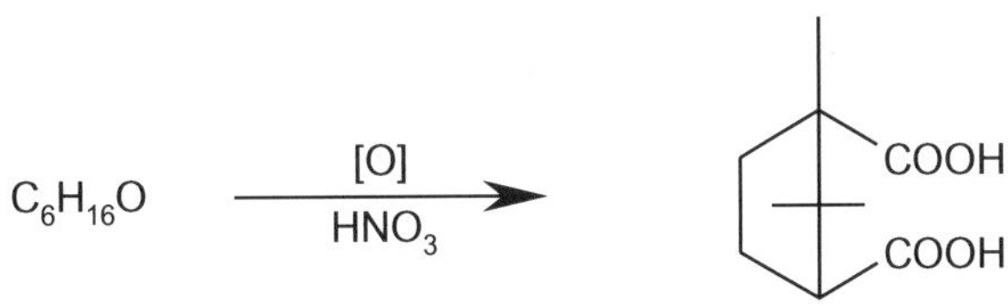

Camphor

Camphoric acid

Camphor on reduction with sodium amalgam gives Borneol which is a secondary alcohol. From the above reactions, camphor is considered to be a cyclic Ketone.

2 Saturated Characterestics

Camphor does not undergo addition reactions with bromine or nitrosyl chloride. Therefore camphor is considered to be a saturated compound.

3. Presence of Bicyclic system

Molecular formula of saturated parent hydrocarbon of camphor is $C_{10}H_8$, which corresponds to general formula CnH_2n-2. It indicate camphor is a bicyclic compound.

4. Presence of -CH_2CO group

Camphor on condensation with benzaldehyde forms monobenzylidene derivative

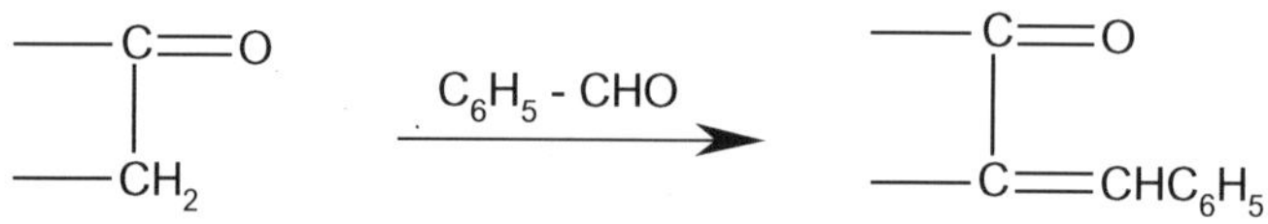

5. Presence of Six membered ring

Camphor on reaction with phosphorous pentoxide or zinc chloride gives P-cymene. It indicates the presence of six membered ring, one, methyl and gemdimethyl group.

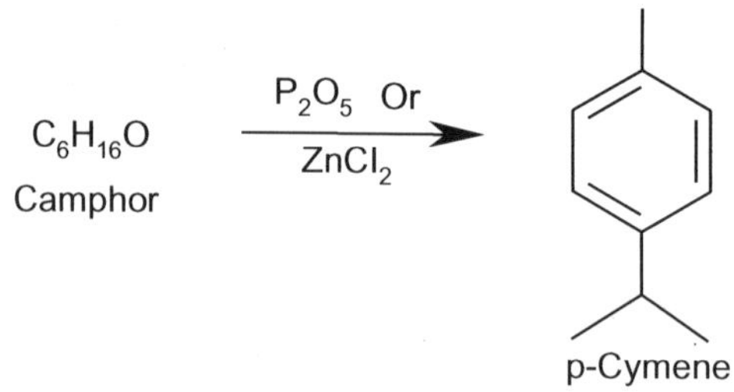

Camphor on oxidation by nitric acid gives camphoric acid, which on further oxidation gives camphoronic acid

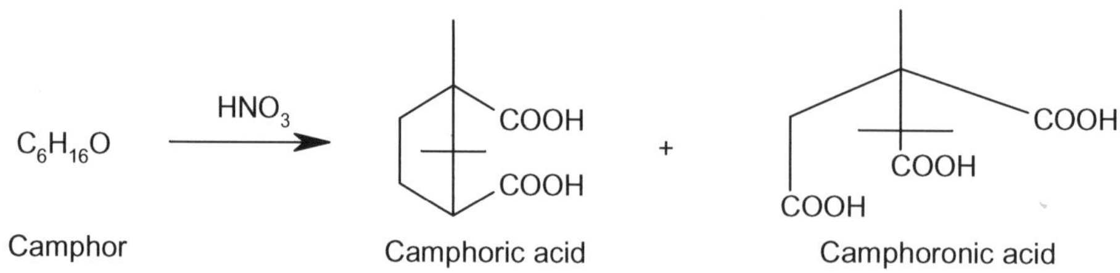

The structure of Camphoronic acid.

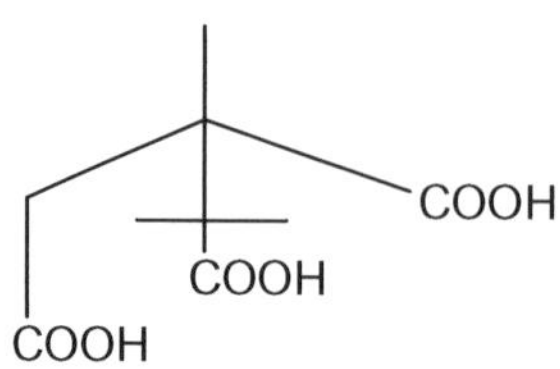

Its molecular formula is $C_9H_{14}O_6$.

Presence of tricarboxylic group in different carbon atoms.

Camphoronic acid does not undergo decarboxylation under ordinary conditions. Therefore carboxyl group should be attached to 3 different carbon atoms.

Presence of α, β-tricarballylic acid

Camphoronic acid on distillation at atmospheric pressure gives isobutyric acid, trimethyl succinic acid and carbondioxide.

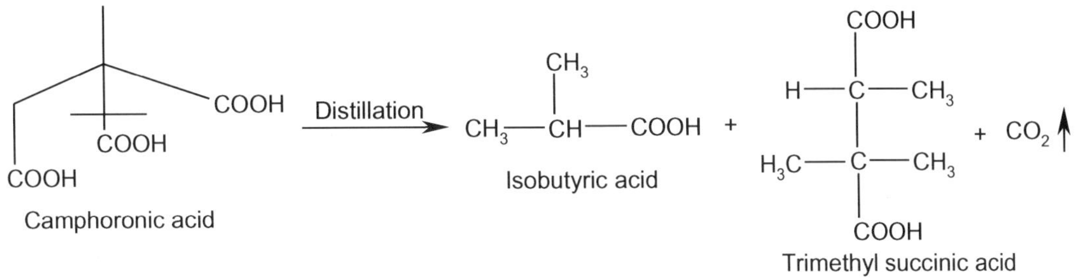

The structure of camphoronic acid can be confirmed by synthesis

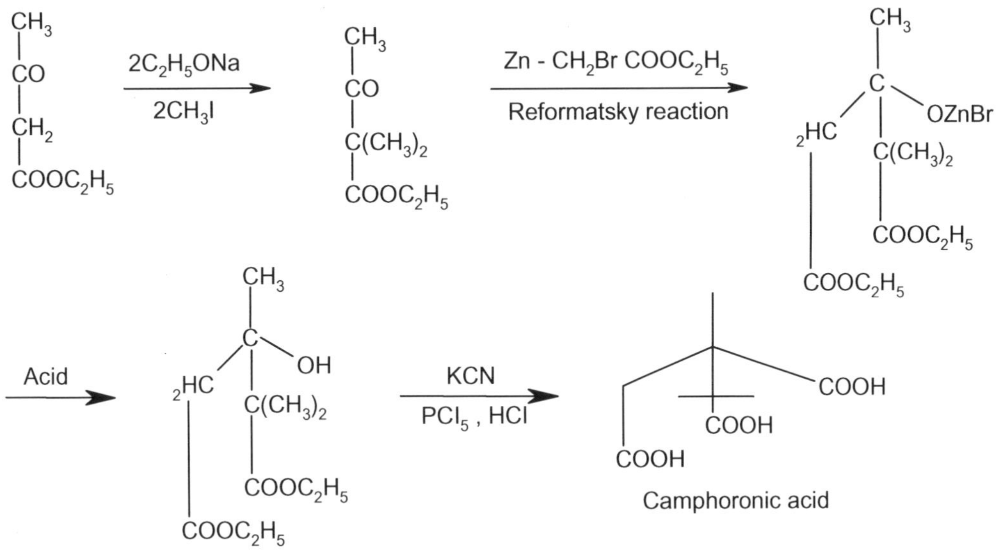

Structure of Camphoric Acid

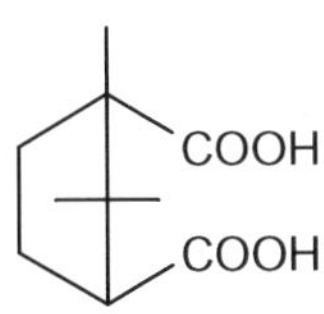

Molecular formula of camphoric acid is $C_{10}H_{16}O_4$. By qualitative Chemical tests, camphoric acid is found to be a saturated dicarboxylic acid.

Nature of carboxylic acid group

Camphoric acid forms monoester easily but diester with some difficulty. So one COOH group may be 1° or 2° and other is 3°. Camphoric acid forms monobromo derivative, which is possible only when one COOH group is 2°.

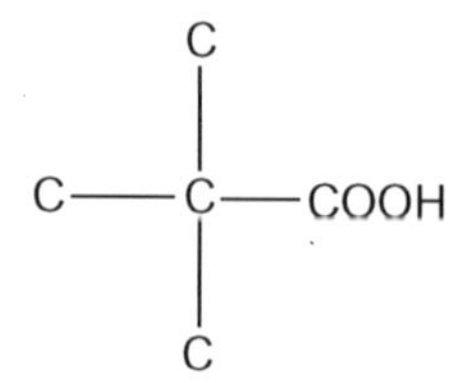

3° Carboxylic group

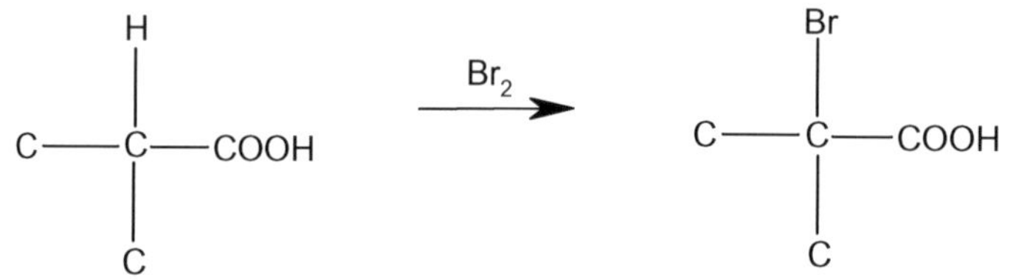

2° Carboxylic group — Monobromo derivative

As Glutaric acid derivative

Camphoric acid is found to be a ring substituted glutaric acid on the basis of Blanc rule which states that on heating with acetic anhydride, glutaric aci give anhydride, adipic acid give cyclopentanones and pimelic acid give cyclohexanones. Since camphoric acid gives an anhydride, it must be a glutaric acid derivative.

Synthesis of Camphoric Acid

Reaction between 3,3-dimethyl glutaric ester and diethylester in presence of sodium ethoxide will lead to the formation of camphoric acid.

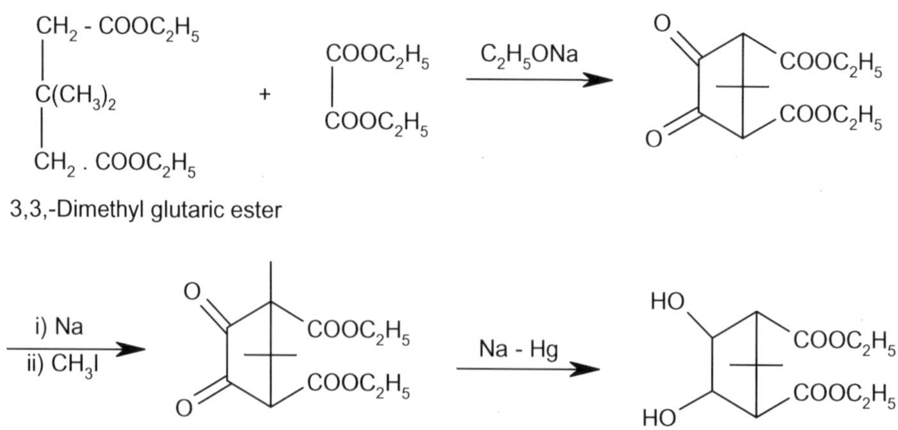

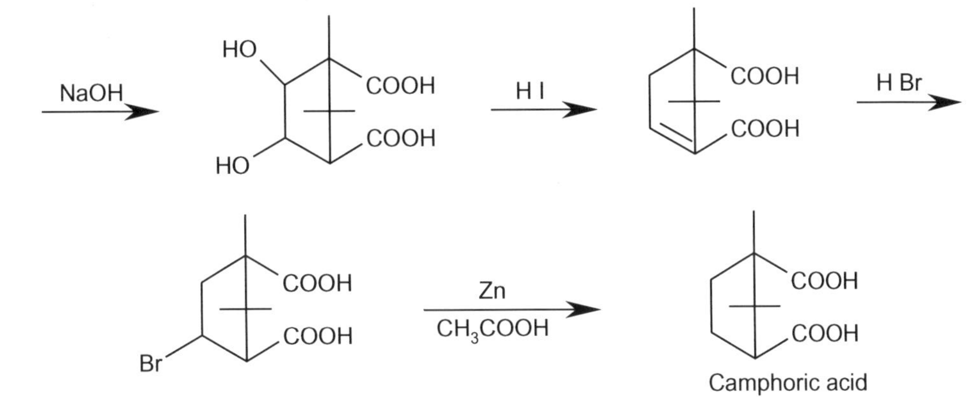

Finally structure of camphor can be confirmed by its synthesis

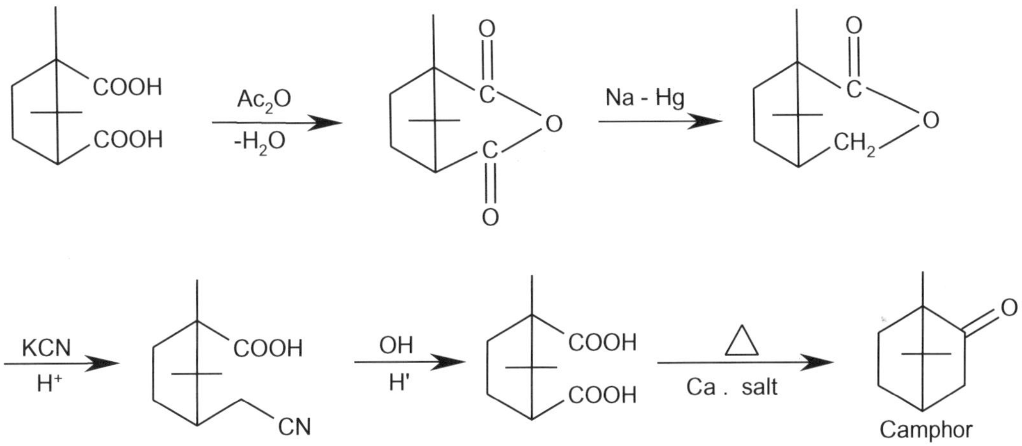

Stereochemistry of Camphor

Eventhough camphor has two dissimilar chiral centres, only one pair of enantiomer is known -ie Cis form. Trans fusion of the gem-dimethylmethylone bridge to the cyclohexane ring is impossible. Due to this, camphor exists in boat conformation.

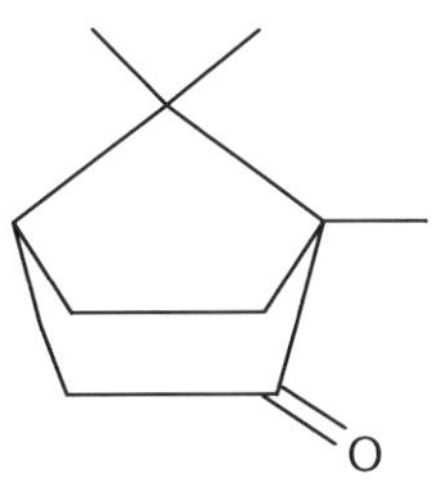

Camphor

α-TERPINEOL

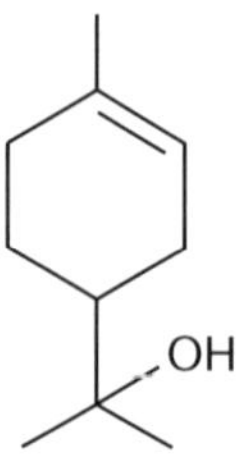

α-Terpineol is a monocyclic monoterpenoid. It is an optically active compound, occurs naturally in (+), (–) and in racemic modification. It can exist in other isomeric forms such as β-Terpineol and γ-Terpineol

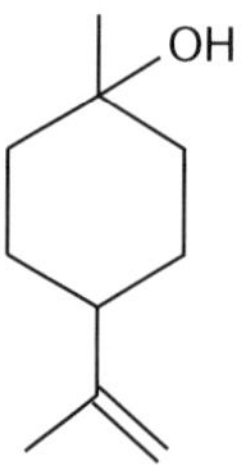

β-Terpineol

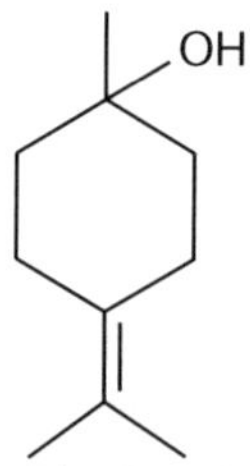

γ-Terpineol

Molecular formula of α-terpineol is $C_{10}H_{18}O$.

Presence of double bond.

α-terpineol adds two bromine atoms to form addition compound. So one double bond is present

$$C_{10}H_{18}O + Br_2 \longrightarrow C_{10}H_{18}OBr_2$$

Presence of Monocycle

Parent (saturated) hydrocarbon of α-terpineol has the molecular formula $C_{10}H_{20}$ which corresponds to general formula of monocyclic compound i.e. CnH_2n.

Skeletol structure

When α-terpineol heated with sulphuric acid, give p-cymene.

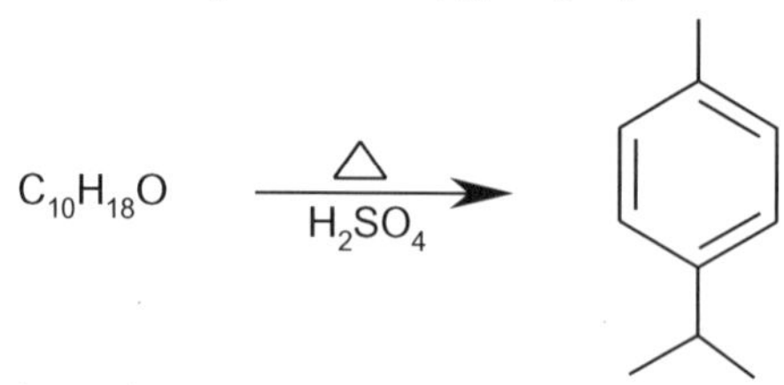

α-terpineol also responds to the tests for 3° alcoholic group.

Presence of double bond in the ring.

α-Terpineol on reaction with 1%. Alkaline $KMnO_4$ give trihydroxy compound, indicate double bond get attacked to give trihydroxy compound. Which on conversion to a keto lactone having the same number of carbon atoms suggests double bond must be inside the ring.

α-terpineol (C10) $\xrightarrow{1\ \%\ KMnO_4}$ Trihydroxy compound $\xrightarrow{CrO_3}$

Ketohydroxy acid (C10) $\xrightarrow{\text{-water}}$ Ketolactone (C10) $\xrightarrow{KMnO_4}$

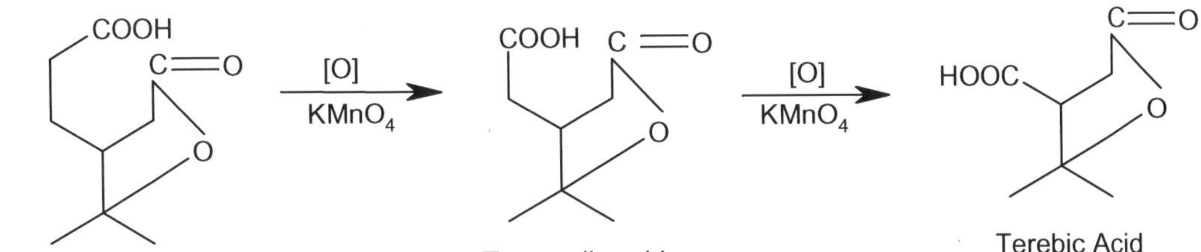

Homoterpenylic acid → Terpenylic acid → Terebic Acid

Finally structure of α-Terpineol can be confirmed by its synthesis.

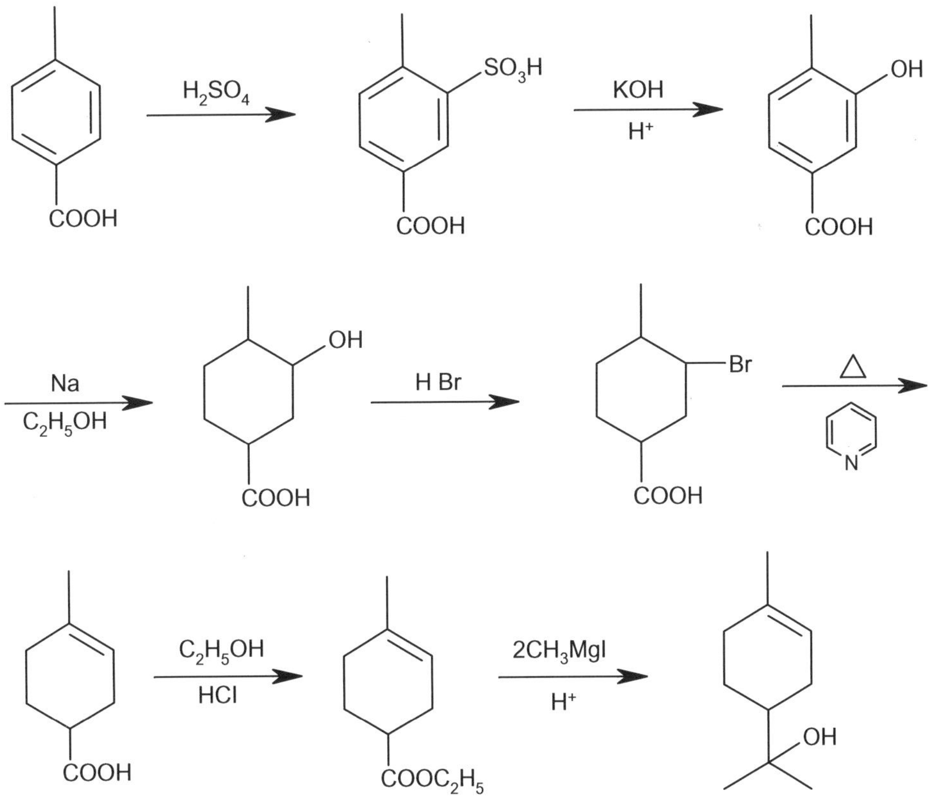

α-terpineol

α-PINENE

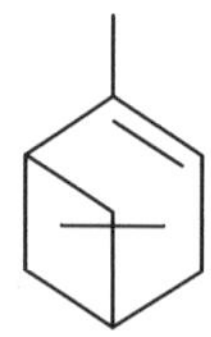

It is a liquid, occurs as both (+) and (–) forms in all turpentine oils. It is having the molecular formula, $C_{10}H_{16}$

Presence of double bond

α-Pinene adds on two, bromine atoms, therefore one double bond must be present.

$$\underset{\alpha\text{-Pinene}}{C_{10}H_{16}} \xrightarrow{Br_2} \underset{\alpha\text{-Pinene dibromide}}{C_{10}H_{16}Br_2}$$

As a bicyclic compound

Molecular formula of parent saturated hydrocarbon is $C_{10}H_{18}$ which corresponds to the general formula CnH_2n-2; therefore α-Pinene is bycyclic.

Presence of a six membered ring

α-Pinene on heating with alcoholic sulphuric acid yields α-terpineol.

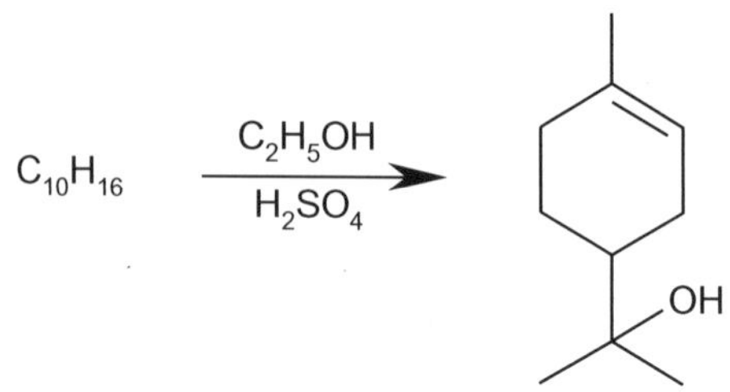

α-terpineol

Formation of α-terpineol suggests in α-Pinene, a six membered ring having a double bond of α-terpineol is present. In α-terpineol hydroxyl group present at C_6, but no hydroxyl group in α-Pinene. Therefore C_6 of Pinene must be involved in one three membered and one four membered/three membered ring. Nature of the second ring whether three on four membered can be confirmed by oxidative degradation of α-Pinene.

Oxidative degradation of α-pinene

$$\underset{C\text{-}10}{\alpha\text{-Pinene}} \xrightarrow{1\,\%.\text{alk.}KMnO_4} \underset{C\text{-}10}{\text{Pinene glycol}} \xrightarrow{\text{alk. }KMnO_4}$$

$$\text{Pinonic acid} \xrightarrow[-CHBr_3]{NaOBr} \underset{C\text{-}9}{\text{Pinic acid}} \xrightarrow[Ba(OH)_2]{Br_2} \text{Cis-norpinic acid}$$

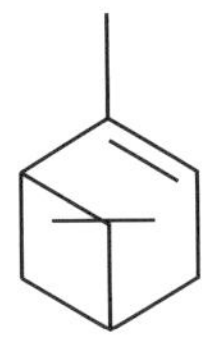

Alpha -Pinene

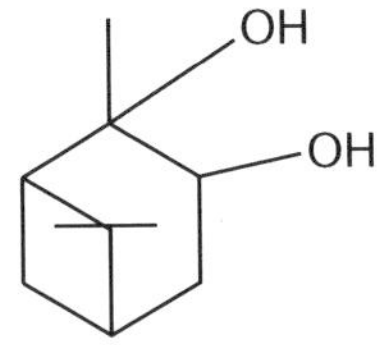

Pinene glycol

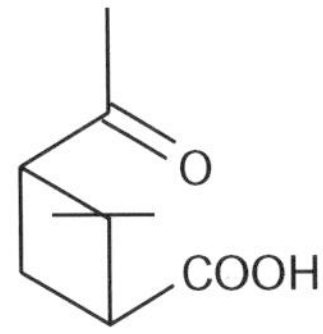

Pinonic acid

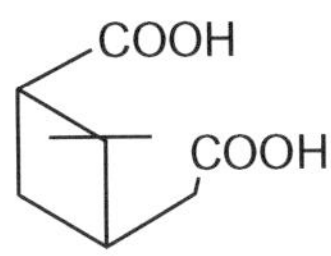

Pinic acid

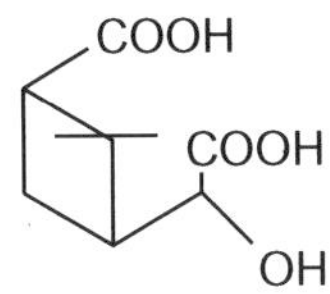

Hydroxypinic acid

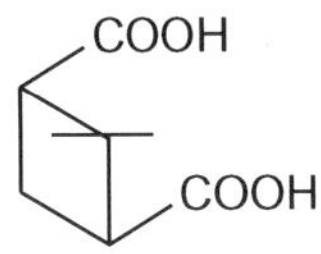

Cis-norpinic acid

Conversion of Pinene glycol to pinonic acid indicates 6-membered ring having glycolic group and double bond is oxidised. Since pinonic acid undergo haloform reaction to form pinic acid suggests pinonic acid have an acetyl group. Structure of nor-pinic acid can be confirmed by its synthesis.

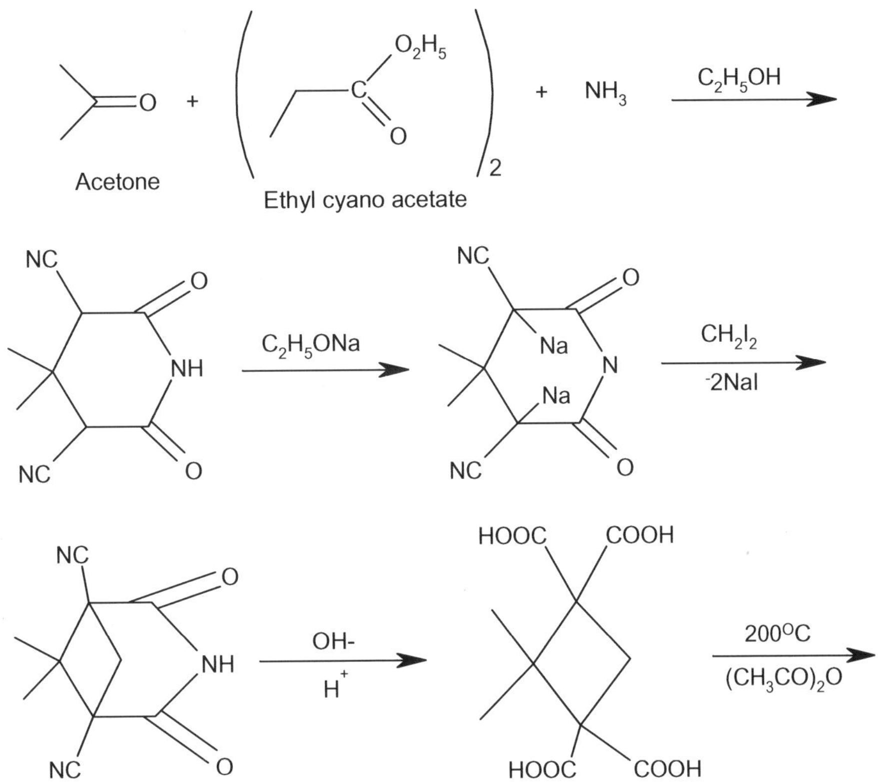

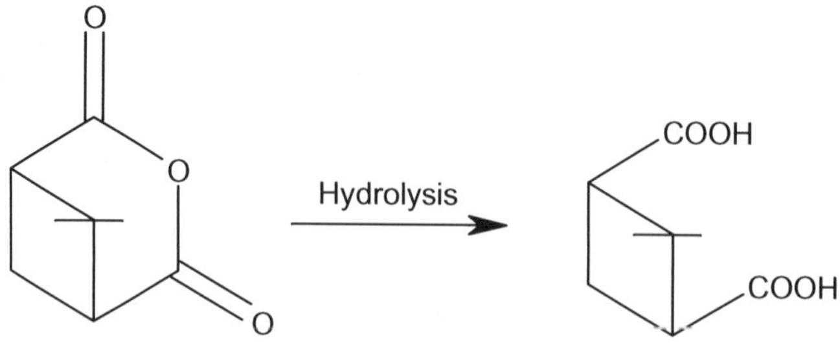

Cis-norpinic anhydride

Cis - norpinic Acid

Finally structure of α-pinene can be confirmed by its synthesis.

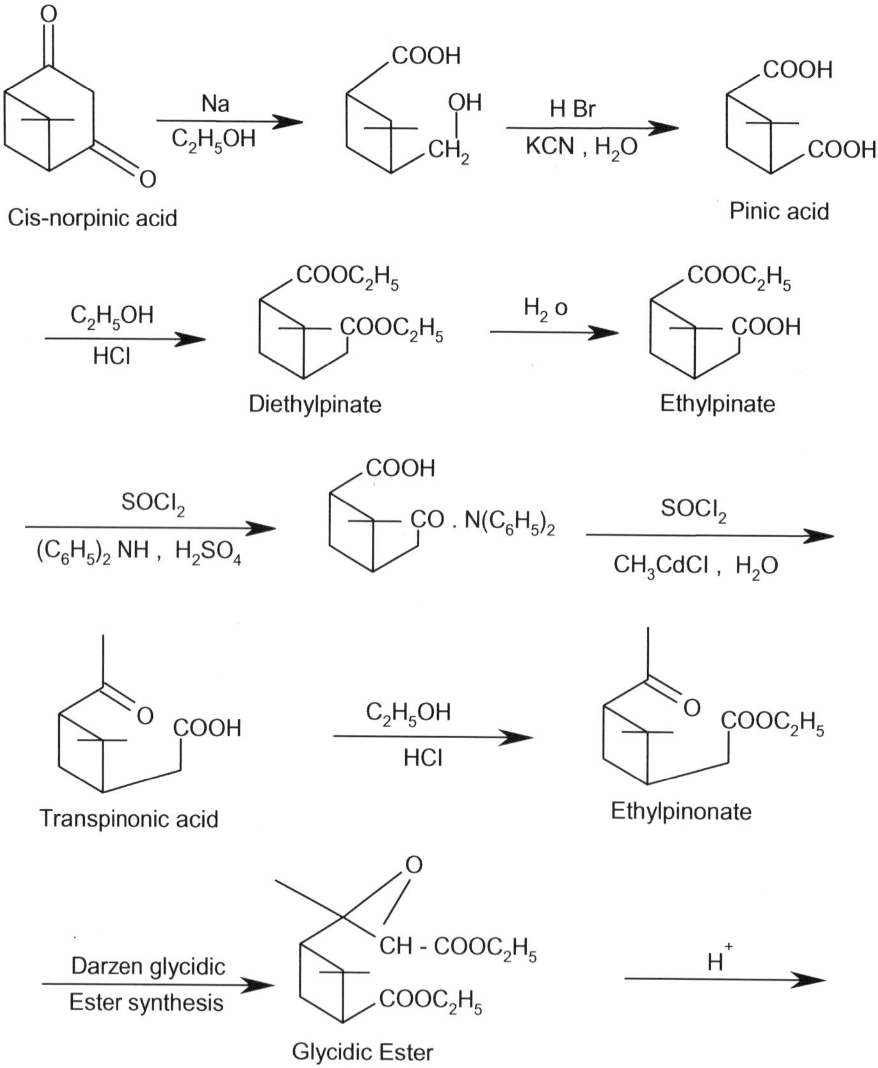

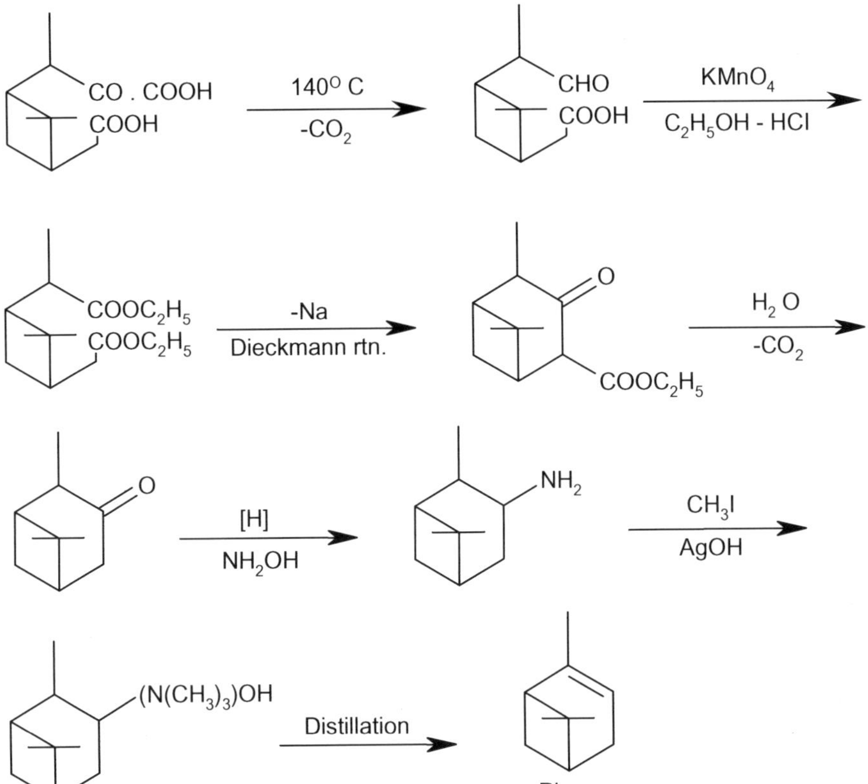

Pinene

Two dissimilar Chiral Centres are present in α-Pinene. Only Cis enantiomer is possible due to the fact that four membered ring can only be fused to Six-membered one in Cis position. Fusion of two rings in trans pattern is impossible.

ALKALOIDS

Alkaloids are physiologically active basic compounds of natural origin, having atleast one nitrogen atom in the basic ring. According to the natutre of nucleus present in the molecule, alkaloids can be classified as;

(a) Phenylethylamine alkaloids Eg: Ephedrine, Adrenaline
(b) Pyrrolidine alkaloids Eg: Hygrine, Stachydrine
(c) Pyridine and piperidine alkaloids Eg: Ricinine, Conine
(d) Pyrrolidine - Pyridine alkaloids Eg: Nicotine
(e) Quinoline alkaloids Eg: Cinchonine, Quinine.
(f) Isoquinoline alkaloids Eg: Papaverine
(g) Phenanthrene alkaloids Eg: Morphine, codeine
(h) Indole alkaloids Eg: Reserpine, Gramine
(i) Tropane alkaloids Eg: Atropine
(j) Tropolone alkaloids Eg: Colchicine

Extraction of Alkaloids

The dried plant material, finely powdered and extracted with methanol. The methanol distilled off and residue treated with inorganic acids, so the bases are extracted as their soluble salts. Sodium carbonate is added to liberate free bases which is extracted with various organic solvents like ether, chloroform... etc. The extract is evaporated to get crude alkaloids.

General Properties

Alkaloids are colourless, (Berberine is yellow coloured is an exemption.) crystalline, non-volatile solids (Conine and Nicotine are liquids which are exemption.) which are soluble in organic solvents. Most of the alkaloids are optically active, nitrogenous substances having bitter taste.

General Methods for Determining Molecular Structure of Alkaloids

Pure substance is subjected to qualitative analysis to know the nature of carbon, hydrogen and nitrogen. Empirical formula obtained from quantitative analysis. Presence of unsaturation ascertained by addition reaction with bromine.

Molecular formula derived from molecular weight.

I. Functional nature of Oxygen

Oxygen atom can be present as phenolic hydroxyl group (=C -OH), alcoholic hydroxyl group (-C-OH), carboxyl group (-COOH), alkoxyl group(-OR), Carbonyl group (>C=O), and ester group (-OCOR)

(a) Phenolic hydroxyl group (=C-OH)

If phenolic hydroxyl group present, alkaloid is made to soluble in sodium hydroxide and reprecipitated by Carbon dioxide colour reaction with ferric chloride indicate the presence of Phenolic group. The number of Phenolic group can be estimated by acetylation.

(b) Alcoholic hydroxyl group (-C-OH)

Alcoholic hydroxyl group is generally indicated by its acylation reaction. Alcoholic group can be further confirmed by dehydration and oxidation. The nature of alcoholic group ie primary, secondary or tertiary can be confirmed by oxidation reactions.

Primary alcohol (-CH_2OH) on oxidation gives first an aldehyde and then acid, both having the same number of carbon atoms as that of parent alcohol.

$$\text{—CH2OH} \longrightarrow \text{—CHO} \longrightarrow \text{—COOH}$$

Secondary alcohol (>CHOH) on oxidation gives first a ketone having the same number of carbon atoms and then acid with fewer number of carbon atoms.

Tertiary alcohol on oxidation gives ketone and acid both having fewer number of carbon atoms. The number of alcoholic hydroxyl group can be estimated by zerewitnoff active hydrogen determination. This method consist of heating the alcohol with methyl magnesium iodide and measures the methane so formed.

Carboxyl group (-COOH)

Solubility of the alkaloid in aqueous sodium carbonate or ammonia indicates the presence of a carboxyl group. Esterification also indicate presence of acid. Acid group can be estimated generally by acid-alkali titration or by silver salt method.

Alkoxyl group (-OR)

Presence of methoxyl groups and their number can be determined by zeisel method. The alkaloid is heated with concentrated hydriodic acid at its boiling point; the methoxyl groups are thereby converted into methyl iodide which is then absorbed by ethanolic silver nitrate and the silver iodide is weighed.

Carbonyl group (>C=O)

Carbonyl groups such as aldehydes or ketones are detected by usual carbonyl reagents like hydroxyl amine, Phenyl hydrazineand 2,4-dinitrophenylhydrazine. Distinction between aldehydic and ketonic group can be made on the basis of reduction and oxidation reactions.

Ester group (-OCOR)

Hydrolysis of the alkaloid with water, dilute acids or alkali and on examination of the products led to information, wheather the compound is an ester, lactone, amide lactam or a betaine. The nature is established by knowing the nature of acid, which is the hydrolysed product. For eg:

$$\underset{\text{Amide}}{-CONH_2} + NaOH \xrightarrow{\text{Heat}} COONa + NH_3$$

$$-COOR' + NaOH \xrightarrow{\text{Heat}} COONa + R'\,OH$$

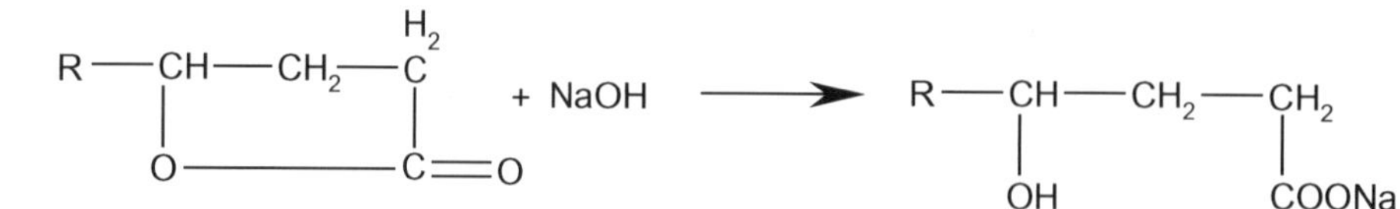

Lactone

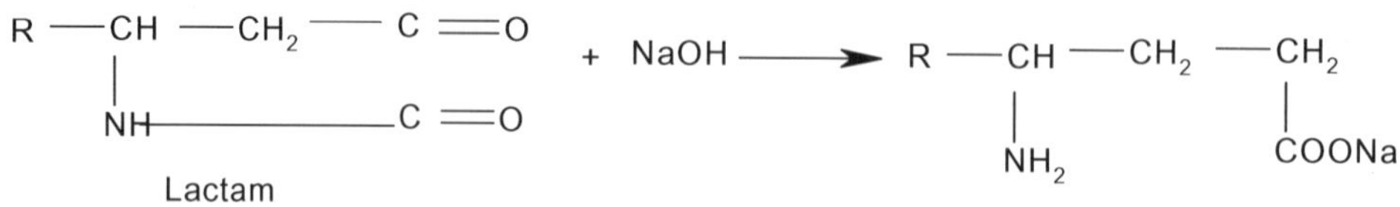

Lactam

Methylenedioxyl group (-OCH_2O-)

Presence of Methylenedioxyl group indicated by the formation of formaldehyde when alkaloid is heated with hydrochloric or sulphuric acid.

II. Functional nature of Nitrogen

(1) The nature of nitrogen can be know from the general reactions of alkaloid with - acetic anhydride, methyl iodide and nitrous acid. If all these reactions are negative then nitrogen atom will be in-tertiary nature. It can be confirmed by reaction with 30% hydrogen peroxide to form amine oxide.

(2) Number of alkyl groups attached to Nitrogen atom when the alkaloid distilled with aqueous potassium hydroxide will form methylamine, dimethylamine or trimethyamine indicate the number of methyl groups attached, one, two or three. If ammonia produces which indicates the presence of amino group. Alkyl groups can be estimated by Herzig Meyer method in which alkaloid is heated with hydriodic acid at 150-300°C, Under pressure, so that alkyl groups are converted into alkyl iodides which are estimated as silver iodide by means of alcoholic silver nitrate eg:

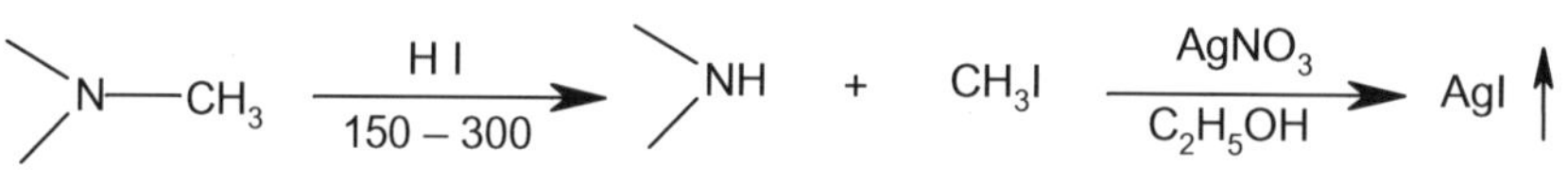

(3) Quantitation of C-methyl groups.

By Kuhn -Roth Oxidation, number of methyl groups attached to carbon atom can be estimated. In this method alkaloid is heated with acidified potassium dichromate to form acetic acid, wich is titrimetrically estimated using a base

(4) Degradation studies on alkaloids.

Degradation of alkaloid into known structures will give infromation about basic structure of alkaloid.

1. Hofmann's exhaustive methylation method

By this method heterocyclic rings are opened with the elimination of nitrogen and the nature of carbon skeleton is thereby obtained. In this method unsaturated heterocyclic ring hydrogenated and converted into quaternary methyl ammonium hydroxide by methylation and hydrolysis, which is heated and decomposes with loss of water formed by hydroxyl group from hydroxide and hydrogen from β-carbon with respect to nitrogen.Carbon -nitrogen linkage cleared to give olefin. For example degradation of pyridine is given here:

Pyridine is catalytically reduced to piperidine which on treament with methyl iodide yield quaternary ammonium iodide. It is treated with moist silver oxide or potassium hrydroxide to form quaternary ammonium hydroxide which on heating water get liberated. The product again moist with silver oxide and then heated. Water again liberated along with trime thylamine and an unsaturated olefin.

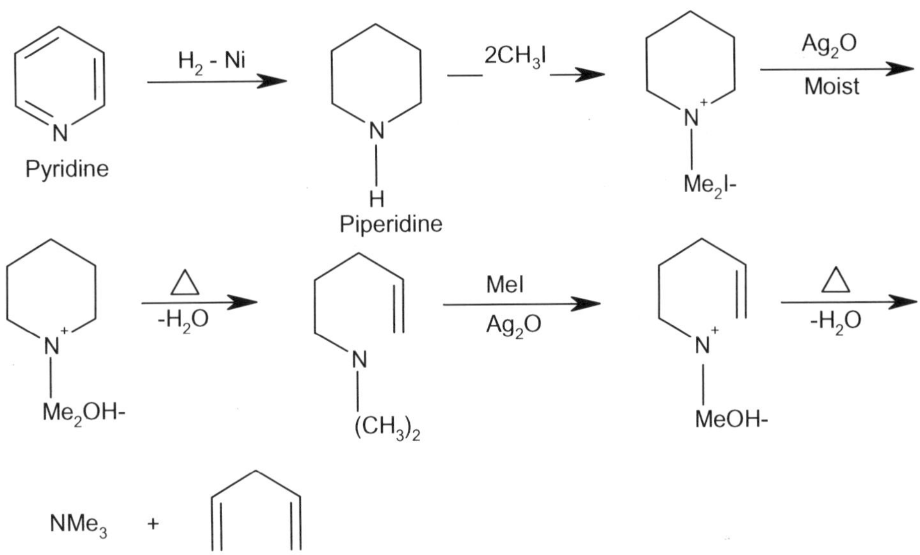

Hofmann's method is applicable only to compound having β-hydrogen atom with respect to nitrogen.

2. Emde modified method

When the base not contain a β-hydrogen atom, Emde modified method applied. Here quaternary ammonium halide reduced with sodium amalgam in aqueous ethanol or with sodium in liquid ammonia or is catalytically hydrogenated.

For example will see degradation of Isoquinoline.

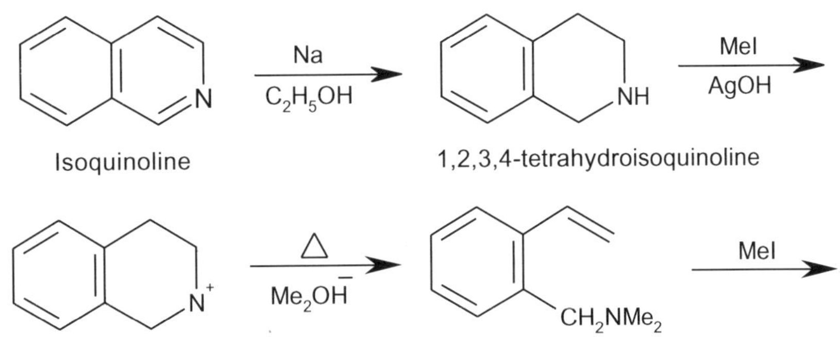

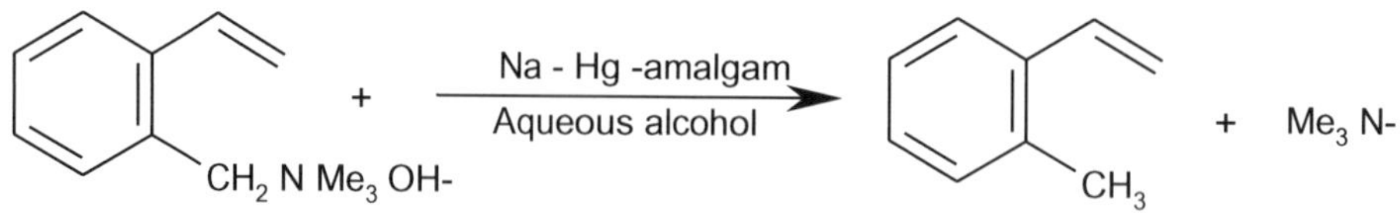

β-hydrogen absent here

3. Von Braun's method for tertiary cyclic amines.

In von Braun's cyanogen method, alkaloid containing tertiary nitrogen atom in the ring is treated with cyanogen bromide, in which bromine attached to carbon atom and cyanogen to nitorgen atom. Brominated cyanamide undergo hydrolysis to a brominated secondary amine.

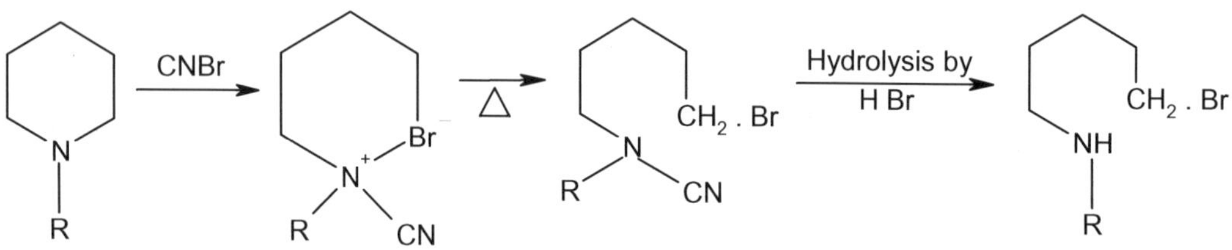

4. Von braun's method for secondary cyclic amines

In this method compound benzoylated and treated with phosphorus halide, then nitrogen atom is eliminated as benzonitrile along with the formation of α, ω dihalo compound.

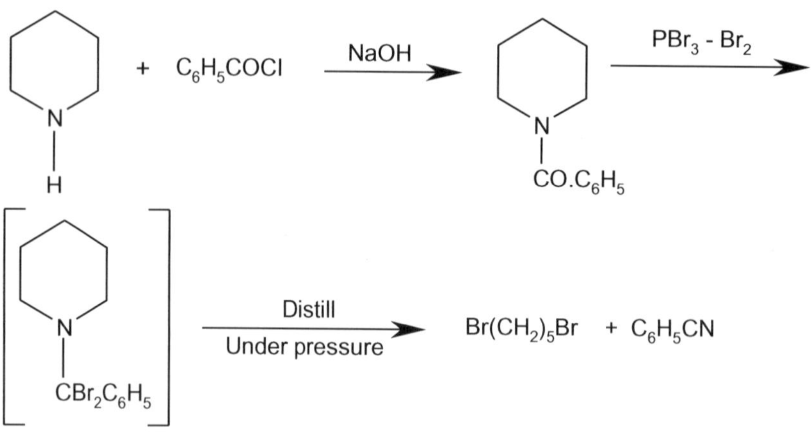

Oxidation

From oxidation produts, nature of some functional groups like C=C, -CHOH ....etc can be obtained. By varying the strength of oxidising agent, it is possible to obtain avariety of products. Mild oxidation is usually effected with hydrogen peroxide, ozone, iodine in ethanolic solution, or alkaline potassium ferricyanide. Moderate oxidation can be carried out by means of acid or alkaline potassium permanganate or chromium trioxide in acetic acid. Vigorous xidation effected by potassium dichromte-sulphuric acid, concentrated nitric acid or a manganese dioxide-sulphuric acid.

6. Fusion with Solid potassium hydroxide

Fusion of an alkaloid with solid pottassium hydroxide produces small fragments, from which nuclei present in the molecule can be detected.

7. Zinc dust distillation

Distillation of alkaloid over hot Zinc dust degrade alkaloid into stable aromatic derivatives. From the derivatives, nature of parent compound can be elucidated.

V. Physical methods

In conjunction with chemical methods, physical methods can also employed. IR spectra reveals functional groups present. U.V spectra indicate the type of structure present. X-ray studies also, reveals even stereochemical nature of compounds. Basic nucleus of compounds can be studied from NMR as well as Mass spectra.

VI. By Synthesis

Finally structure of alkaloid can be confirmed by its synthesis.

ATROPINE

Atropine mainly occurs in Atropa belladonna of solanaceous family.

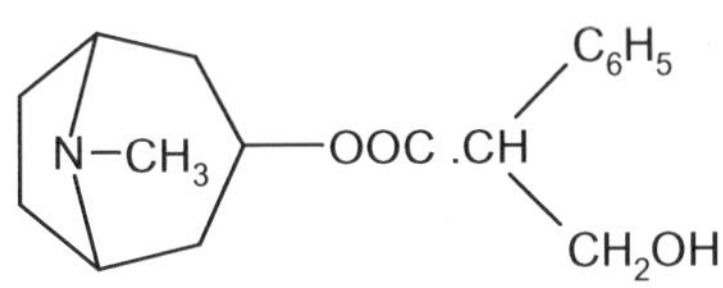

Molecular formula of atropine is $C_{17}H_{23}NO_3$. Atropine on warming with barium hydroxide, hydrolysed to tropic acid and tropine. Therefore atropine is considered as an ester.

Constitution of tropic acid

1. Molecular formula is $C_9H_{10}O_3$

2. Presence of acid

Tropic acid takes one mole of alkali, and does'nt add bromine, so it is a saturated monobasic acid.

3. Presence of OH group

Tropic acid must have one -OH group since it give a monoacetate on acetylation.

4. Presence of benzene ring with one side chain

When heated, tropic acid loses a molecule of water to form atropic acid, -$C_9H_8O_2$. Which on oxidation gives benzoic acid. Thus tropic and atropic acids contain a benzene ring with one side chain.

5. Structure of atropic acid

From the above point, structure of atropic acid can be any one of the following.

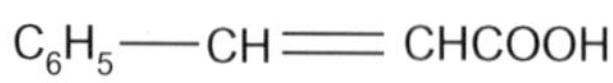

(a)

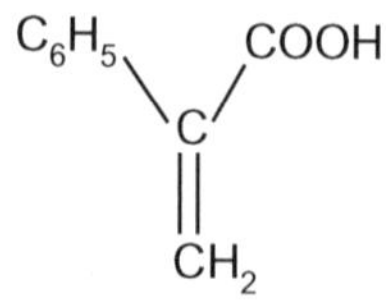

(b)

Since structure (a) is known to be cinnamic acid, (b) must be atropic acid. It is supported by the fact that oxidation of acid by potassium permanganate gives phenyl glyoxylic acid (C_6H_5CO-COOH).

6. Structure of tropic acid

Addition of a molecule of water to atropic acid give tropic acid, which can be either of the following.

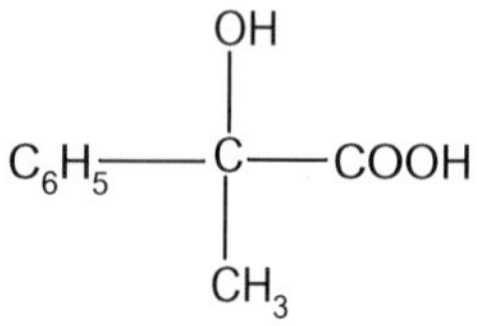

(c)

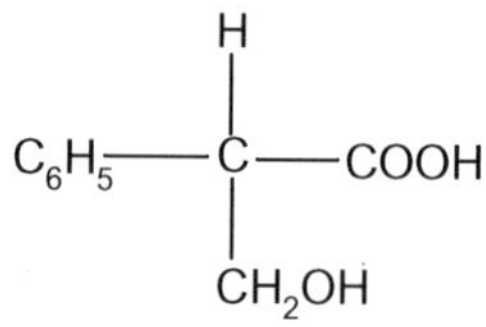

(d)

Finally structure of tropic acid is confirmed as (D) by its synthesis.

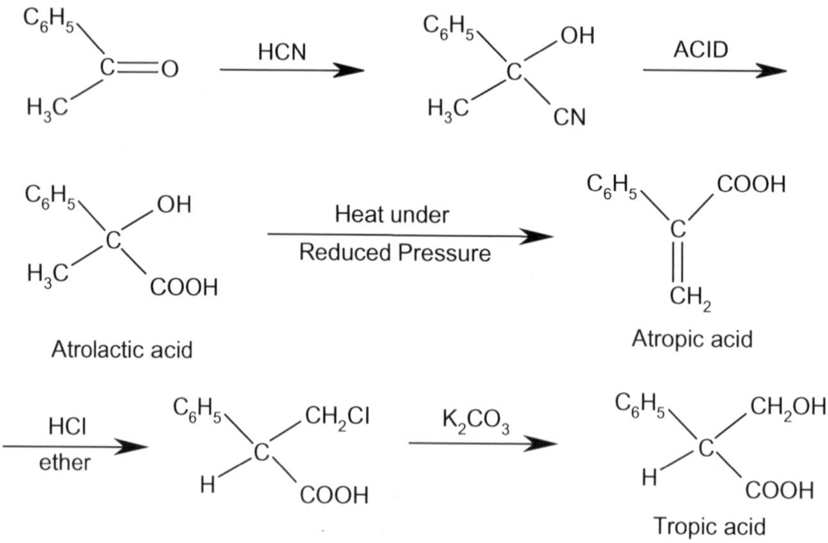

Constitution of Tropine (Tropanol)

1. Molecular formula is C_8H_5NO

2. Presence of tertiary nitrogen atom

Tropine forms quaternary salt with methyl iodide, therefore nitrogen must be tertiary.

3. presence of one hydroxyl group

Since tropine forms monoacetate and mono benzoate, tropine must have one hydroxyl group.

$$C_{18}H_{14}N(OH) \xrightarrow[NaOH]{C_6H_5COCl} C_8H_{14}N\,(OCOC_6H_5)$$

4. Nature of Hydroxyl group

Tropine on oxidation with chromic acid yield tropinone which is a ketone, therefore hydroxyl group must be secondary alcoholic.

$$C_7H_{13}(CHOH) \xrightarrow{[O]} \underset{\text{Tropinone}}{C_7H_{13}N{-}C{=}O} + H_2O$$

5. Presence of reduced pyridine nucleus

Tropine on treatment with hydroiodic acid gives tropineiodide which on reduction with zinc and hydrochloric acid give Dihydrotropidine which on distillation by hydrochloride give Nordihydrotropidine, which undergo zinc dust distillation give 2-Ethyl pyridine.

$$\underset{\text{Tropine (Below 150° C)}}{C_8H_{15}NO} \xrightarrow{HI} \underset{\text{Tropineiodide}}{C_8H_{14}NI} \xrightarrow{[H]} \underset{\text{Dihydrotropdine}}{C_8H_{15}N} \xrightarrow{HCl}$$

$$\underset{\text{Non-dihydrotropidine}}{C_7H_{13}N + CH_3Cl} \xrightarrow[\text{distillation}]{\text{Zn dust}} \underset{\text{2- Ethylpyridine}}{C_7H_9N}$$

On this basis, assumes tropine is a redcued pyridine derivative.

6. Presence of Hydroxyl group in the ring

Tropine on oxidation with chromium trioxide give tropinic acid, which is a dicarboxylic acid, since there is no loss of carbon on its formation, therefore hydroxyl group must be inside the ring.

7. Preesence of CH $_2$COCH$_2$ group

Tropinone (formed by oxidation of Tropine) forms a dibenzylidene derivative with benzaldehyde and a di-oximino derivative when treated with amyl nitrite and hydrochloric acid. It indicates the presence of -CH$_2$.CO.CH$_2$- group.

8. Presence of pyrrolidine ring in tropinone

It can be proved in three ways.

(i) Exhaustive methylation of tropine gives tropilidene (cycloheptatriene)

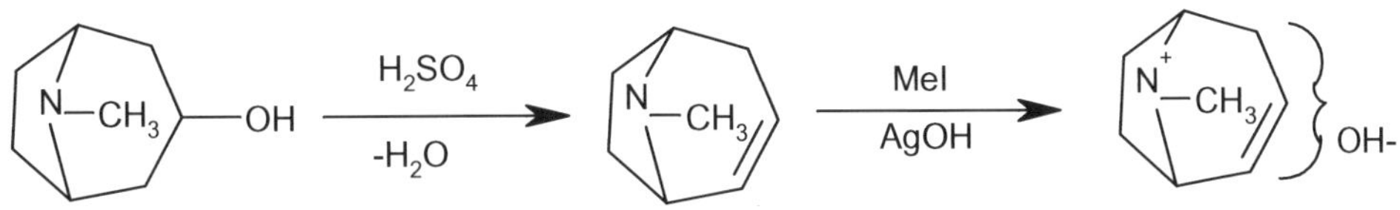

Tropine

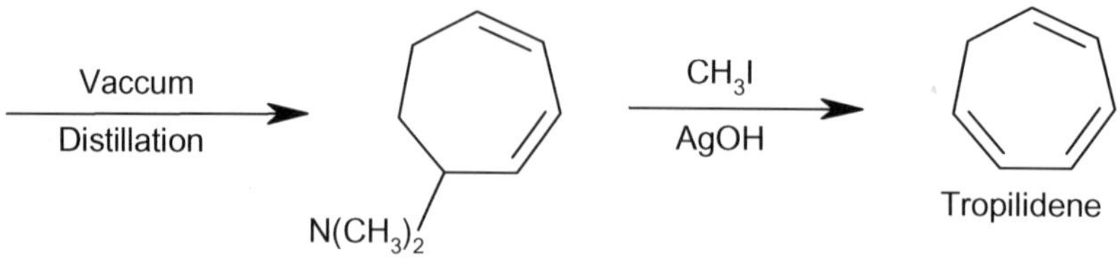

(ii) Exhaustive methylation of tropinic acid gives an unsaturated dicarboxylic acid which on reduction forms pimelic acid.

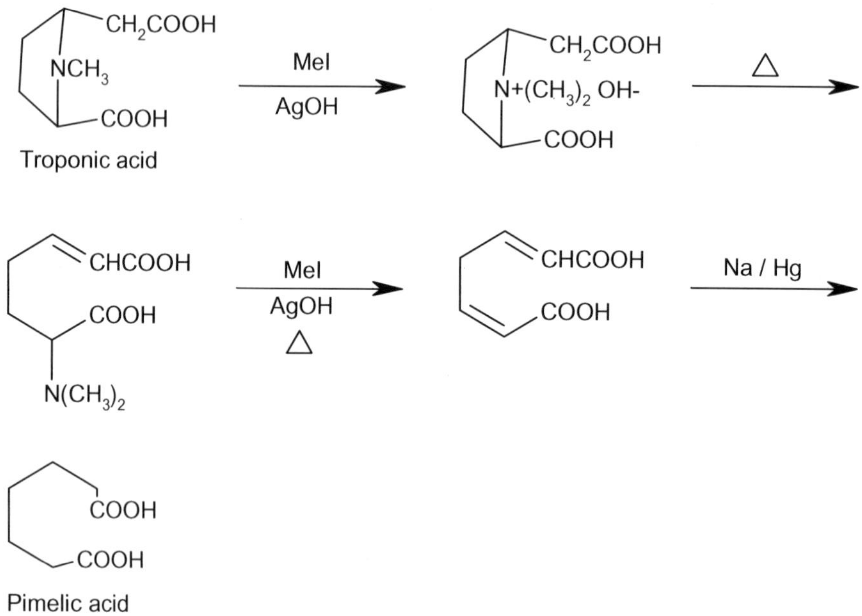

(iii) Tropinone on oxidation with CrO_3-H_2SO_4, gives -N- methyl succinimide.

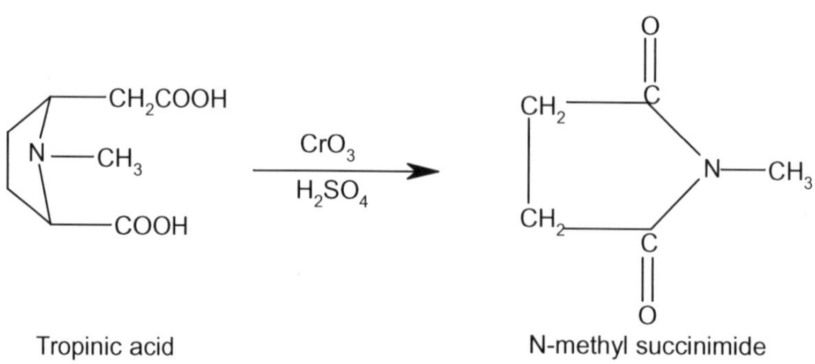

Finally structure of Tropine can be confirmed by its synthesis.

Willstatter's Synthesis for Tropine

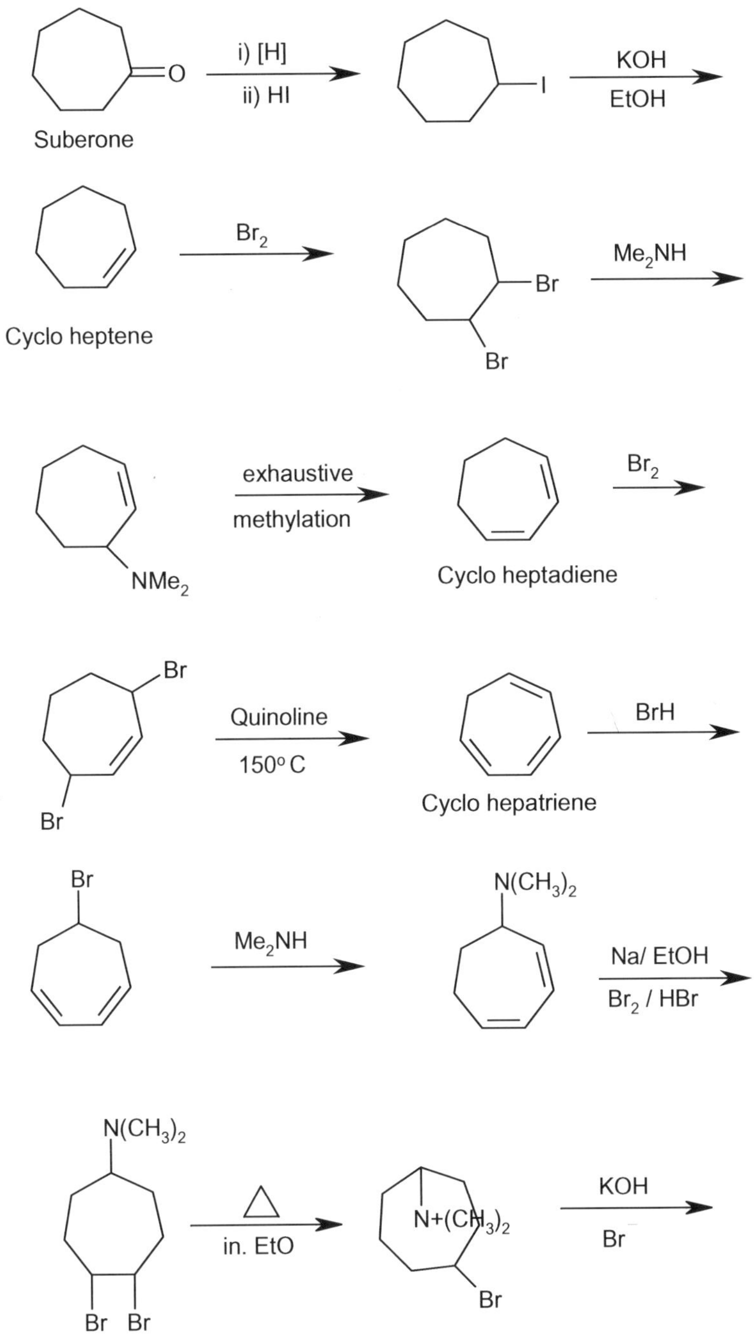

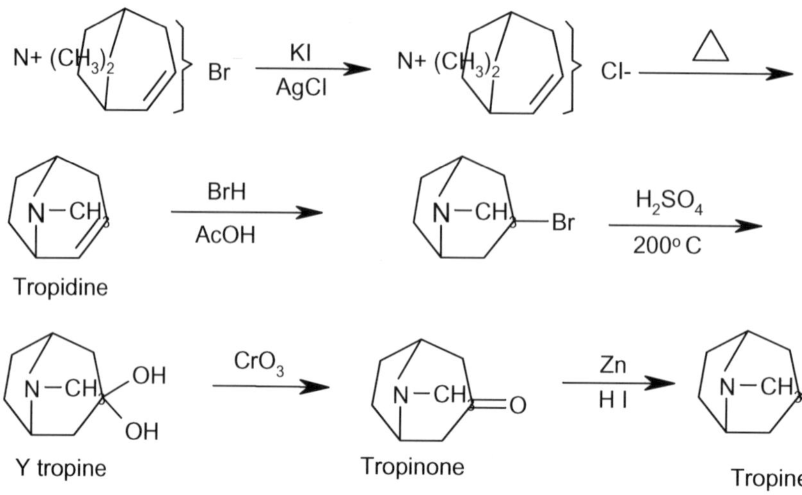

Process of combining Tropine and Tropic acid

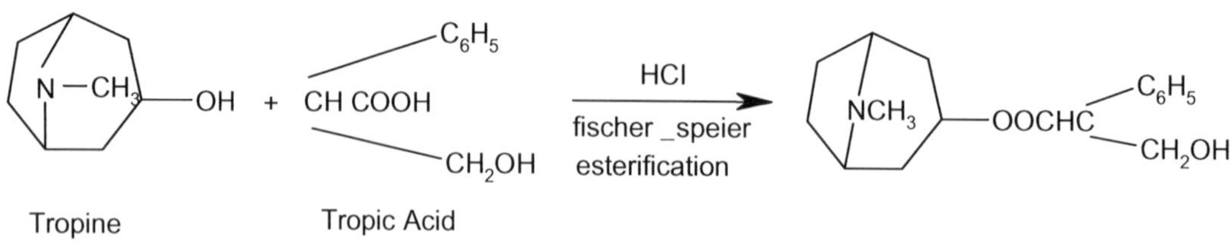

Atropine is optically inactive and it have dialating action on pupils of the eyes. Tropine is racemic modification of hyoscyamine.

QUININE

Quinine is a well known antimalarial drug mainly occurring in cinchona bark.

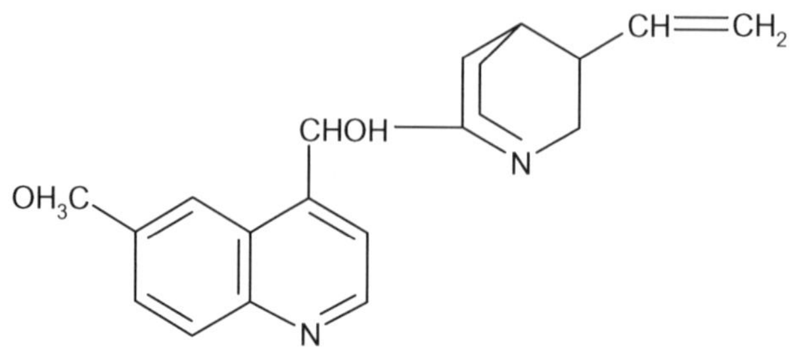

Quinine

Constitution of Quinine

1. **Molecular formula**

From the elemental analysis and molecular weight determination, quinine is having the molecular formula $C_{20}H_{24}N_2O_2$

2. **Presence of ditertiary nitrogen atom**

Quinine adds on two molecules of methyl iodide to form diquaternary salt. It indicates the presence of two nitrogen atoms.

$$C_{20}H_{24}O_2 + 2CH_3I \longrightarrow C_{20}H_{24}N2.2CH_3I$$

3. **Presence of methoxyl group**

When heated with hydrohloric acid, quinine eliminates one carbon atom as methyl chloride, which indicates the presence of one methoxyl group.

4. **Presence of hydroxyl group**

Quinine on benzoylation forms monobenzoate and on acetylation forms monoacetate. It indicate the presence of one hydroxyl group.

5. **Nature of hydroxyl group**

Quinine on oxidation by chromium trioxide produces Quinone a ketone,

$$\underset{\text{Quinine}}{C_{20}H_{24}N_2O_2} \xrightarrow{CrO_3} \underset{\text{Quinone}}{C_{20}H_{22}N_2O_2}$$

There fore hydroxyl group present in Quinine is secondary alcoholic in nature.

6. **Presence of one ethylenic double bond**

Quinine adds on one molecule of bromine indicate the presence of one double bond.

7. **Presence of Quinoline nucleus**

When Quinine is fused with concentrated potassium hydroxide it yields mixture of many Quinoline derivatives like 6- methoxy quinoline and 4-methylquinoline.

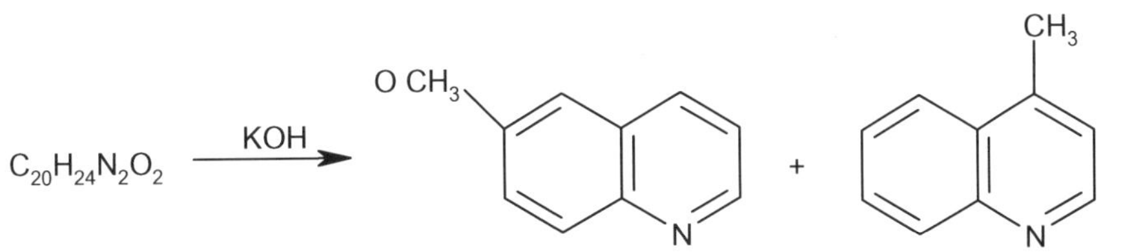

6-methoxy quinoline 4-methyl quinoline

8. **Oxidation of Quinine**

Controlled oxidation of quinine with chromic acid gives quininic acid and meroquinone.

9. **Structure of Quininic acid**

(a) when Quininic acid is heated with sodalime, it undergoes deacarboxylation yielding 6-methoxy quinoline. The 6th position of methoxyl group has been confirmed by the converssion of Quininic acid to 6-hydroxyquinoline by heating with hydrochloric acid.

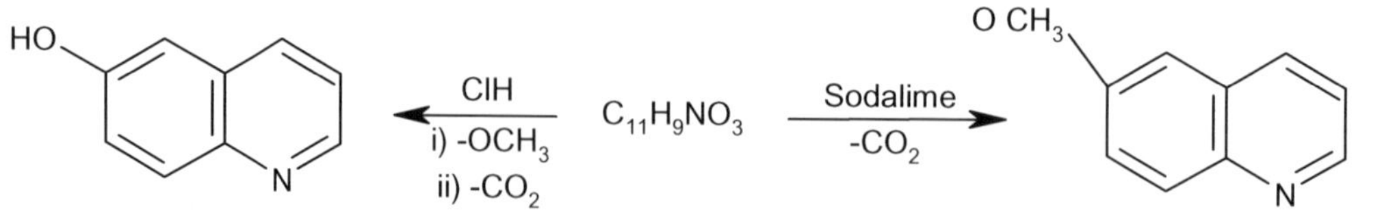

6-methoxy quinoline

(b) When quininic acid is oxidised, by chromic acid yields 2,3,4-tricarboxylic acid, showing that benzenering of the Quininic acid having the methoxyl group which is oxidised and -COOH group is present at 4th position.

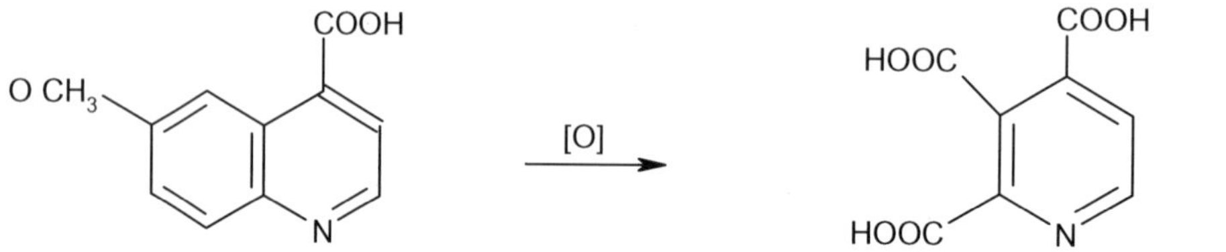

Quininic acid

Pyridine - 2,3,4 - tricarboxylic acid

(c) Finally structure of quininic acid has been confirmed by synthesis.

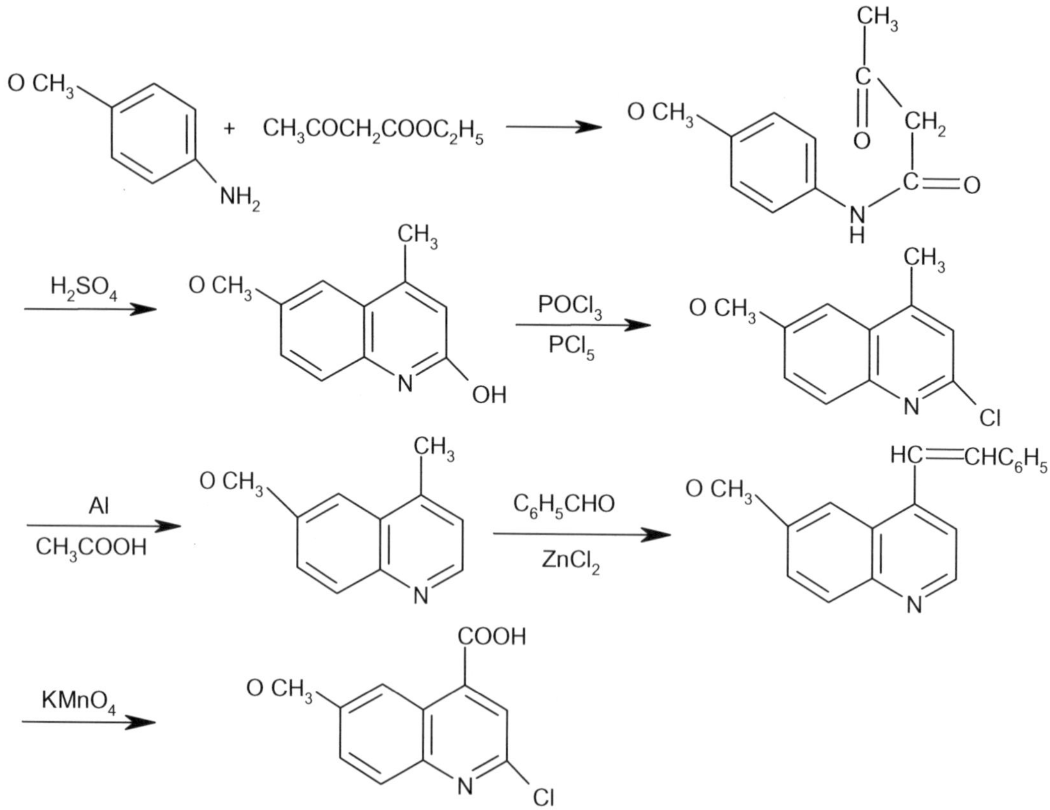

Quninic acid

10. Structure of Meroquinene

(a) It's molecular formula is $C_9H_{15}NO_2$.

(b) It forms an ester indicating the presence of one carboxylic acid group.

(c) When meroquinene undergoes reduction it consumes one hydrogen indicating the presence of one ethylenic double bond (-C.H = C.H $_2$)

(d) When meroquinene oxidised with cold acidified $KMnO_4$ yields Cincholoiponic acid - which is a dicarboxylic acid along with formic acid.

$$C_9H_{15}NO_2 \xrightarrow{[O]} HCOOH + \underset{\text{Cincholoiponic acid}}{C_8H_{13}O_4}$$

(e) When Cincholoiponic acid, oxidised with acid permanganate yield an another dicarboxylic acid called loiponic acid ($C_7H_{11}NO_4$) with the loss of one methylene group. So it assumes Cincholoiponic acid, may have a methylene derivative.

(f) Since Cinchonoloiponic acid have more than one -CH_2- group than loiponic acid, Cincholoiponic acid may have either of the following structure.

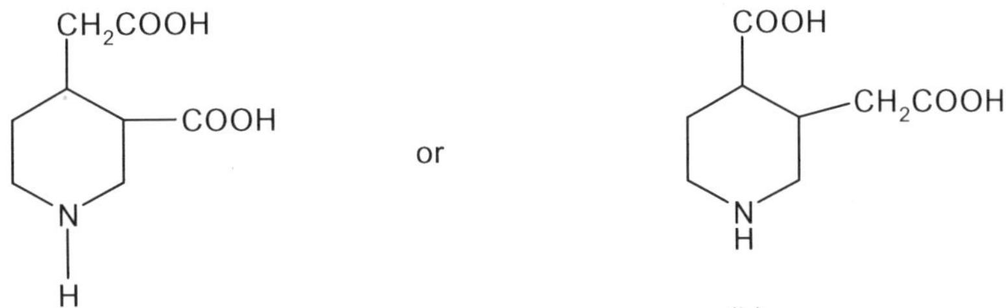

(a) (b)

Since Cincholoiponic acid on heating with conc. H_2SO_4 gives γ-picoline, structure of Cincholoiponic acid is found to be (a).

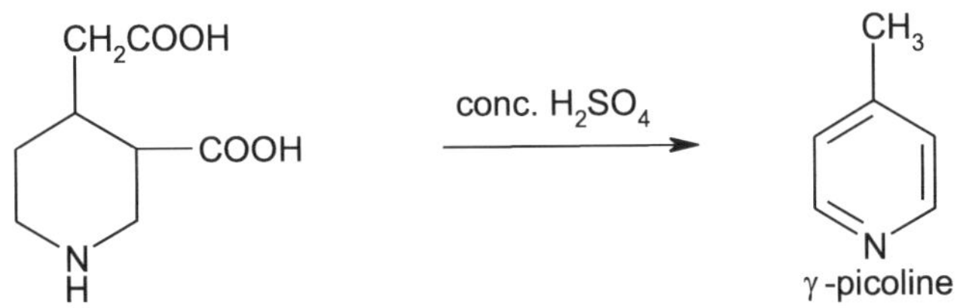

γ-picoline

The structure of Cincholoiponic acid has been proved by its synthesis.

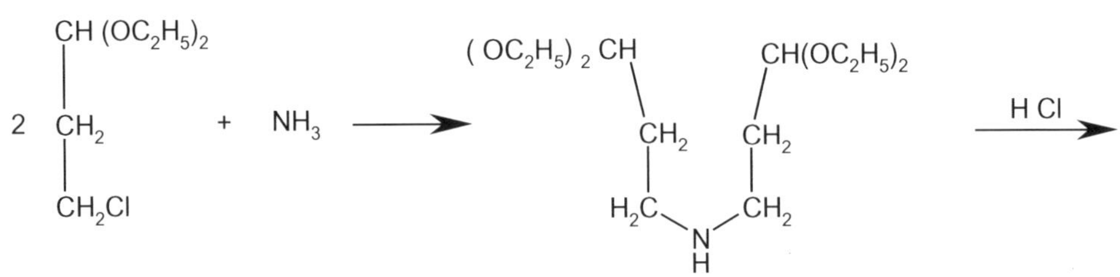

β-chloropropionacetal Iminodipropionacetal

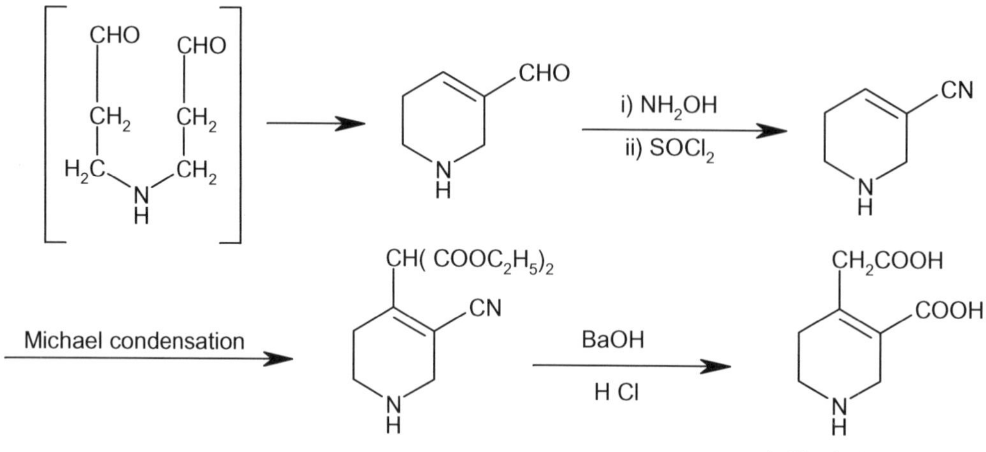

± Cincholoiponic acid

(g) Meroquinene on reduction with zinc and hydroiodic acid yields Cincholoipon ($C_9H_{17}NO_2$) which is having Carboxyl and ethyl group.

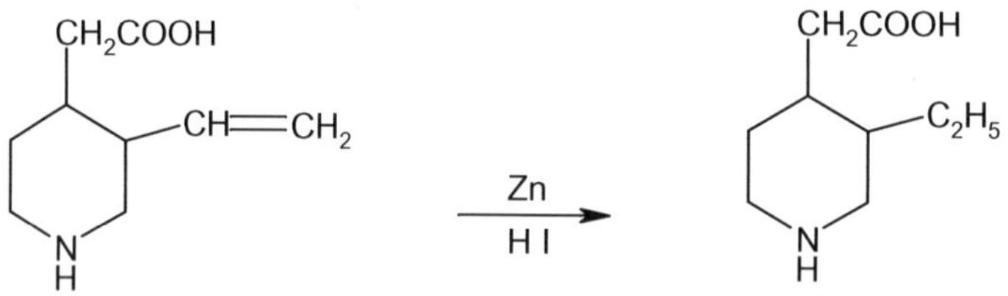

Cincholoipon

(h) Meroquinene on heating with hydrochloric acid at 240°C yields 3-ethyl, 4-methylpyridine.

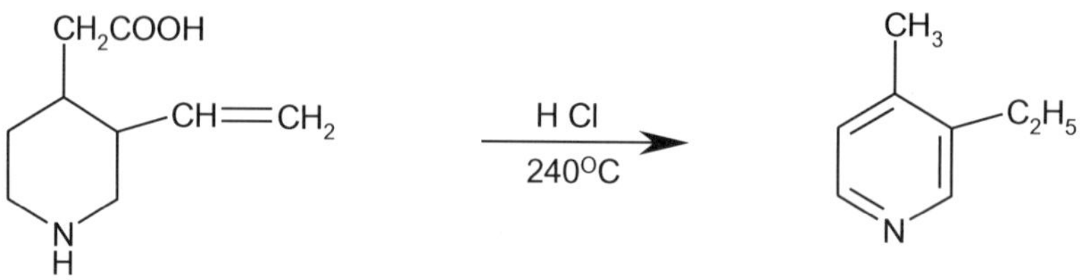

Linking between quininic acid and Meroquinene in Quinine

Carboxylic groups are not present in Quinine molecule. But its oxidation products, Quininic acid and Meroquinene posess free Carboxylic acid groups indicating that both were linked by means of Carboxylic Carbon atoms.

Finally Structure of Quinine can be confirmed by its synthesis.

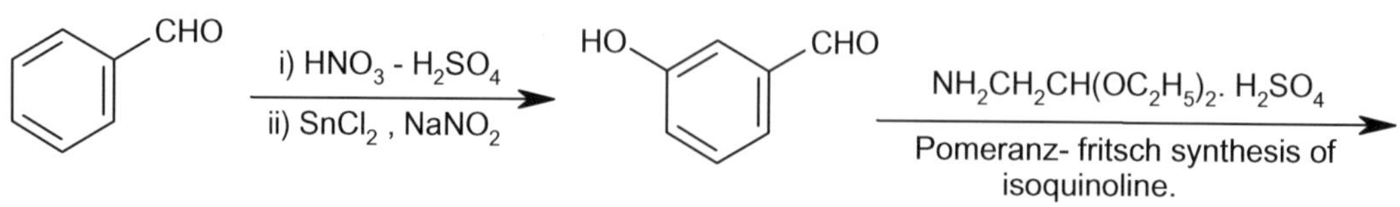

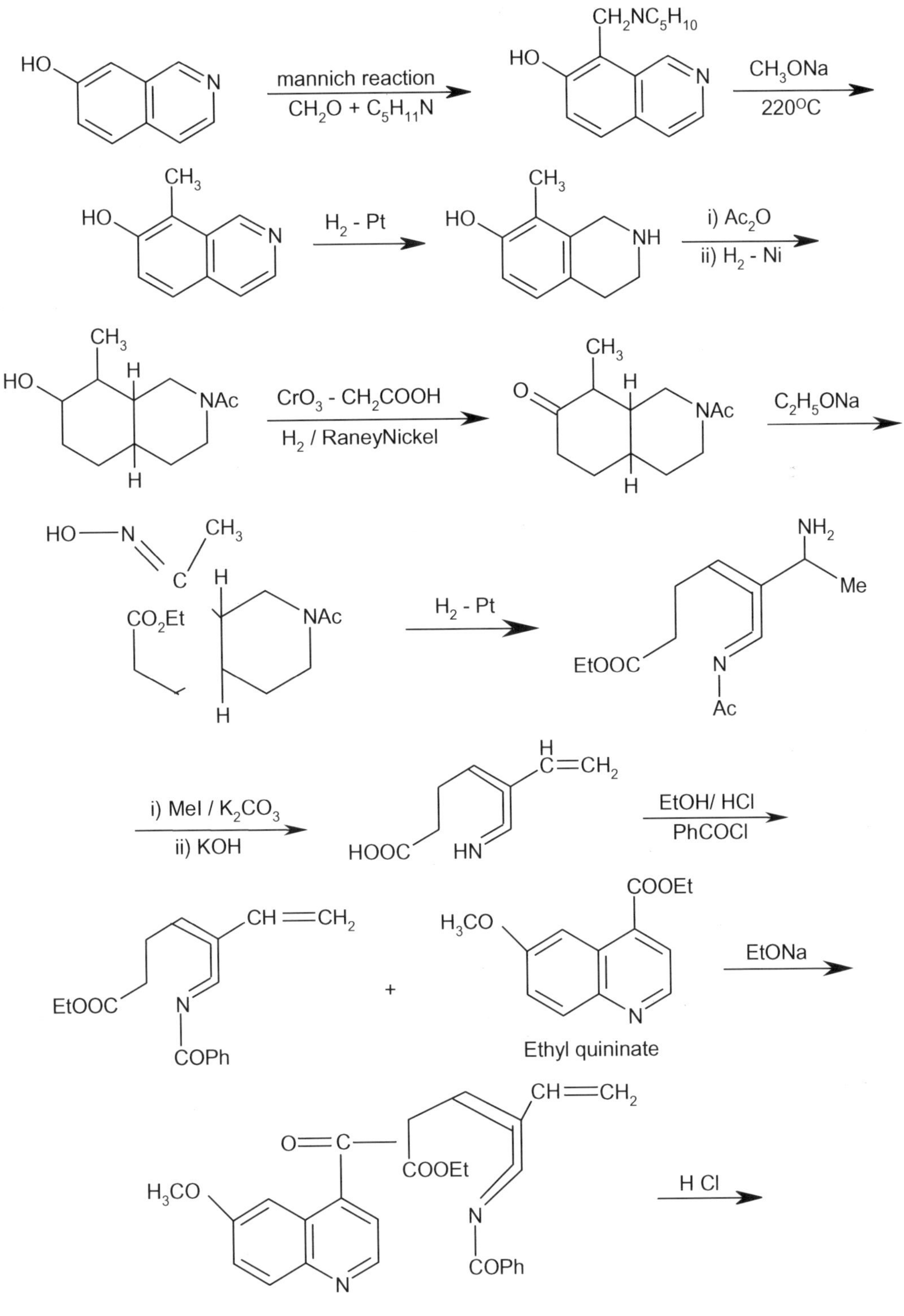
mannich reaction
CH2O + C5H11N
CH2NC5H10
CH3ONa
220°C
H2 - Pt
i) Ac2O
ii) H2 - Ni
CrO3 - CH2COOH
H2 / RaneyNickel
C2H5ONa
H2 - Pt
i) MeI / K2CO3
ii) KOH
EtOH/ HCl
PhCOCl
Ethyl quininate
EtONa
H Cl

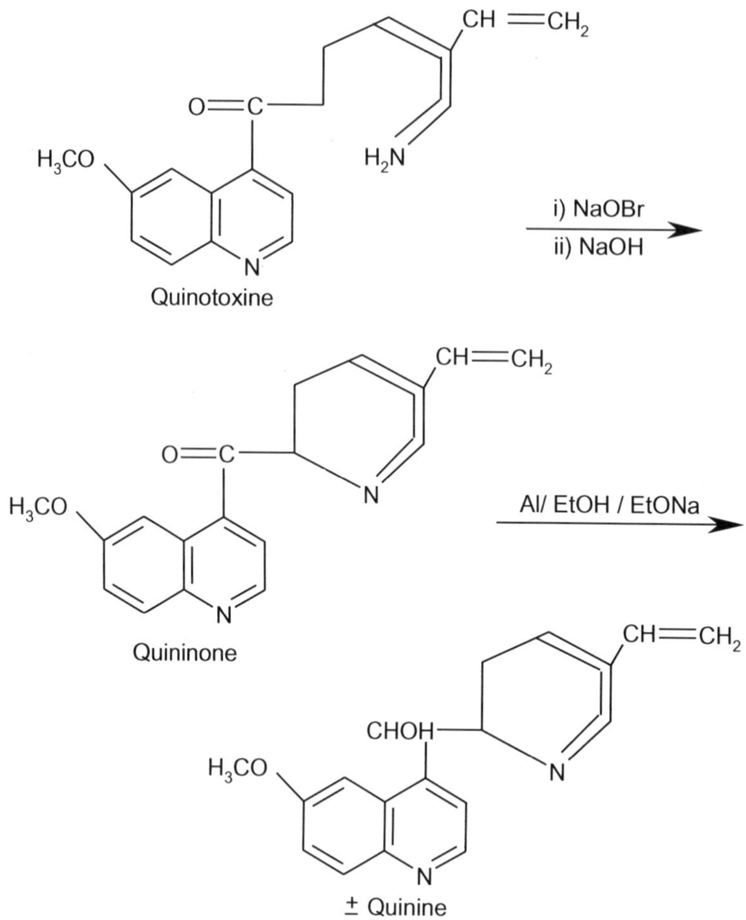

RESERPINE

Reserpine mainly occurs in Rauwolfia Serpentina. It is mainly used as antihypertensive agent. It is also used in epilepsy, insomnia, fever, cholera, dizziness and headaches.

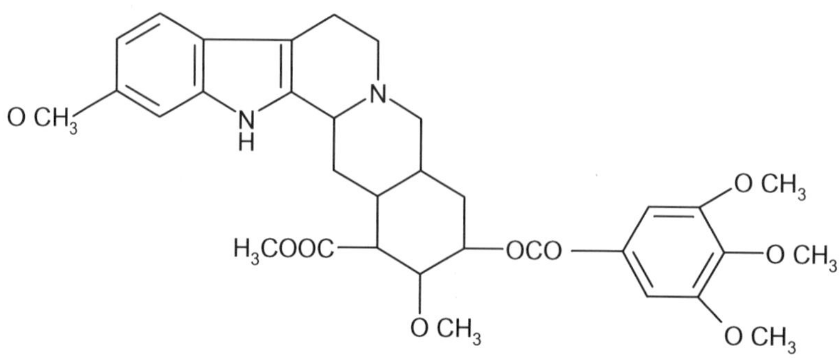

Reserpine

Constitution of Reserpine

1. **Molecular formula of reserpine is $C_{33}H_{40}N_2O_9$**
2. **Presence of five methoxyl group**

   Reserpine on heating with HI gives 5 methoxyl groups (zeisel method)
3. **Presence and nature of Nitrogen**

   Since reserpine is weak base, both nitrogen atoms must be in the ring. Reserpine forms acetyl derivative on acetylation indicating the presence of -NH- group. Since reserpine readily gives a methiodide, second nitrogen atom must be tertiary.
4. **Reserpine as a diester**

   Reserpine on alkaline hydrolysis gives methanol, 3,4,5-trimethoxy benzoic acid and an another acid namely reserpic acid.

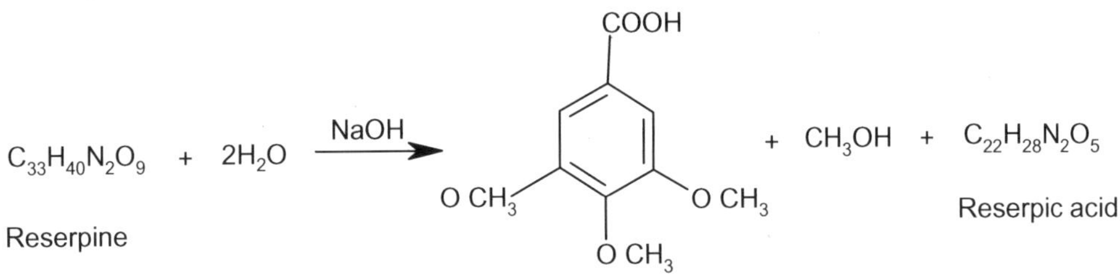

In the hydrolysis products, two -COOH ie one in trimethoxy benzoic acid and reserpic acid and two alcoholic groups one in methanol and other in reserpic acid suggests reserpine is a diester.More over it can be confirmed by metal hydride reduction on reserpine to give reserpic alcohol and 3,4,5-trimethoxy benzyl alcohol.

5. **Structure of Reserpic acid**
   1. Molecular formula of reserpic acid is $C_{22}H_{28}N_2O_5$
   2. Presence of two methoxyl groups, one carboxyl group, one secondary alcoholic group, one >NH and one tertiary nitrogen atom confirmed by usual tests.
   3. Presence of indole nucleus

      Reserpic acid on permanganate oxidation gives 4- methoxy -N- oxalyl anthranilic acid indicate the presence of indole nucleus.

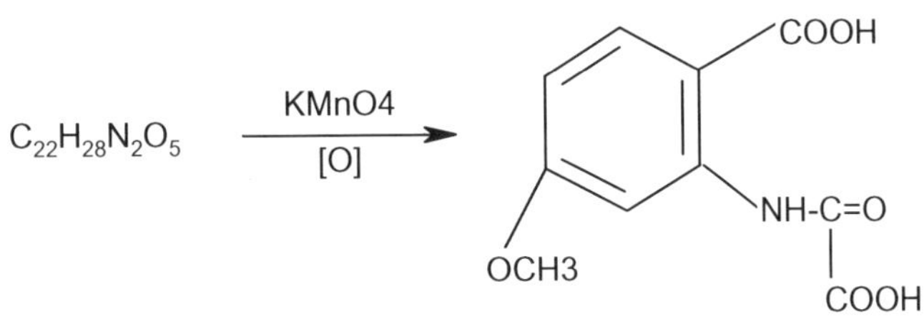

   4. Position of hydroxyl and carboxyl group in reserpic acid. Reserpic acid on alkaline fusion gives 5-hydroxy isophthalic acid. Reserpic acid on treatment with acetic anhydride gives γ-lactone suggesting -OH and -COOH group are meta to each other.

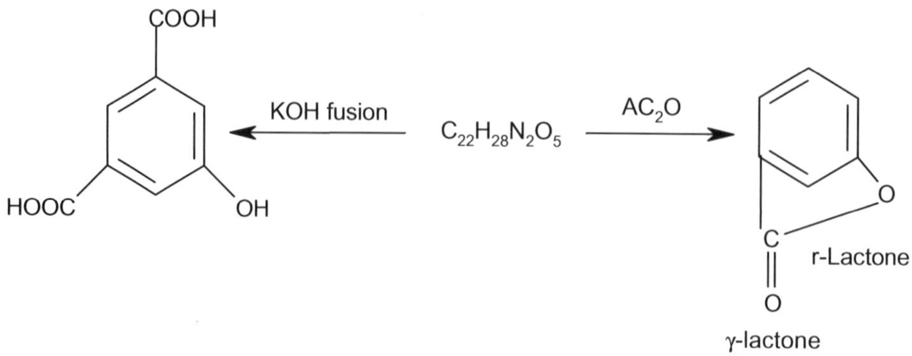

5. Formation of Yobyrine.

   Methyl reserpate on selenium dehydrogenation give Yobyrine by which carbon skeleton of reserpic acid and hence that of reserpine can be traced.

Structure of Yobyrine

(a) Molecular formula of Yobyrine is found to be $C_{19}H_{16}N_2$

(b) Presence of pyridine nucleus.

   Yobyrine condenses with aldehydes suggests the presence of pyridine nucleus with $-CH_2-$ substituent adjacent to nitrogen.

(c) Presence of indole nucleus.

   Yobyrine on zinc dust distillation gives 3-ethylindole and isoquinoline suggests the presence of indole nucleus.

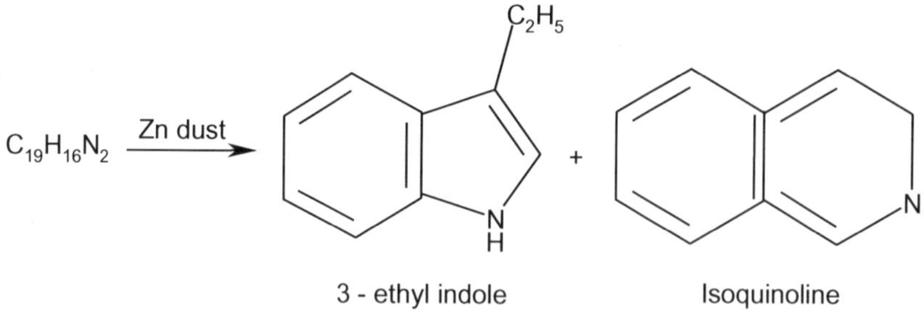

(d) Oxidation of Yobyrine.

   Yobyrine on oxidation by different oxidising agents give different products.

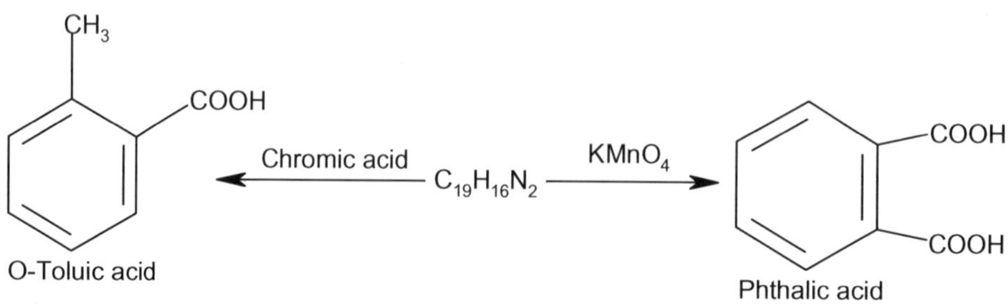

The above facts lead to structure of Yobyrine as follows. Which is also confirmed by its synthesis.

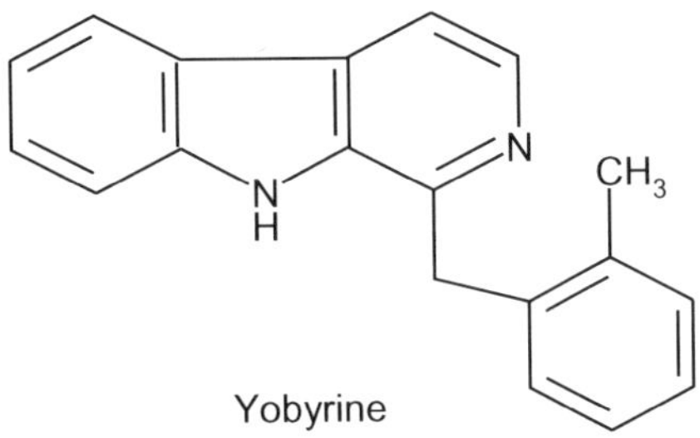

Yobyrine

Formation of yobyrine reveals the carbon skeleton of reserpine as;

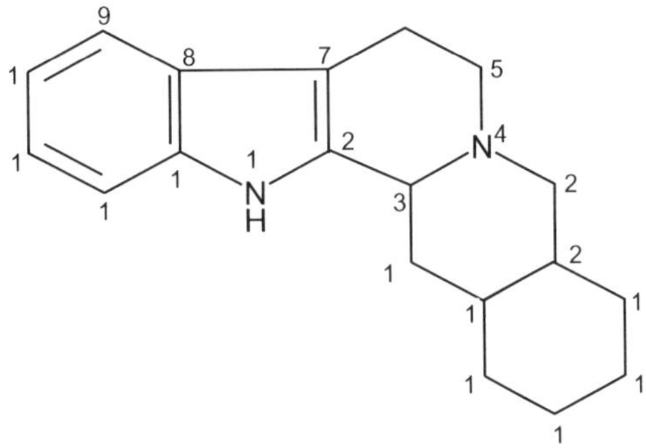

Finally structure of Reserpine proved by its synthesis.

Synthesis of Reserpine

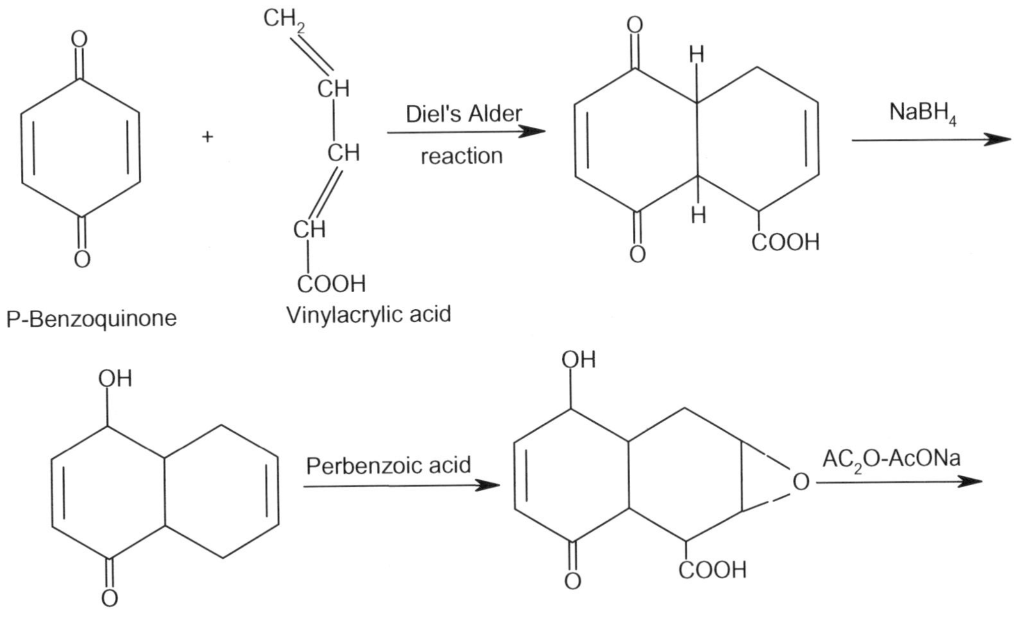

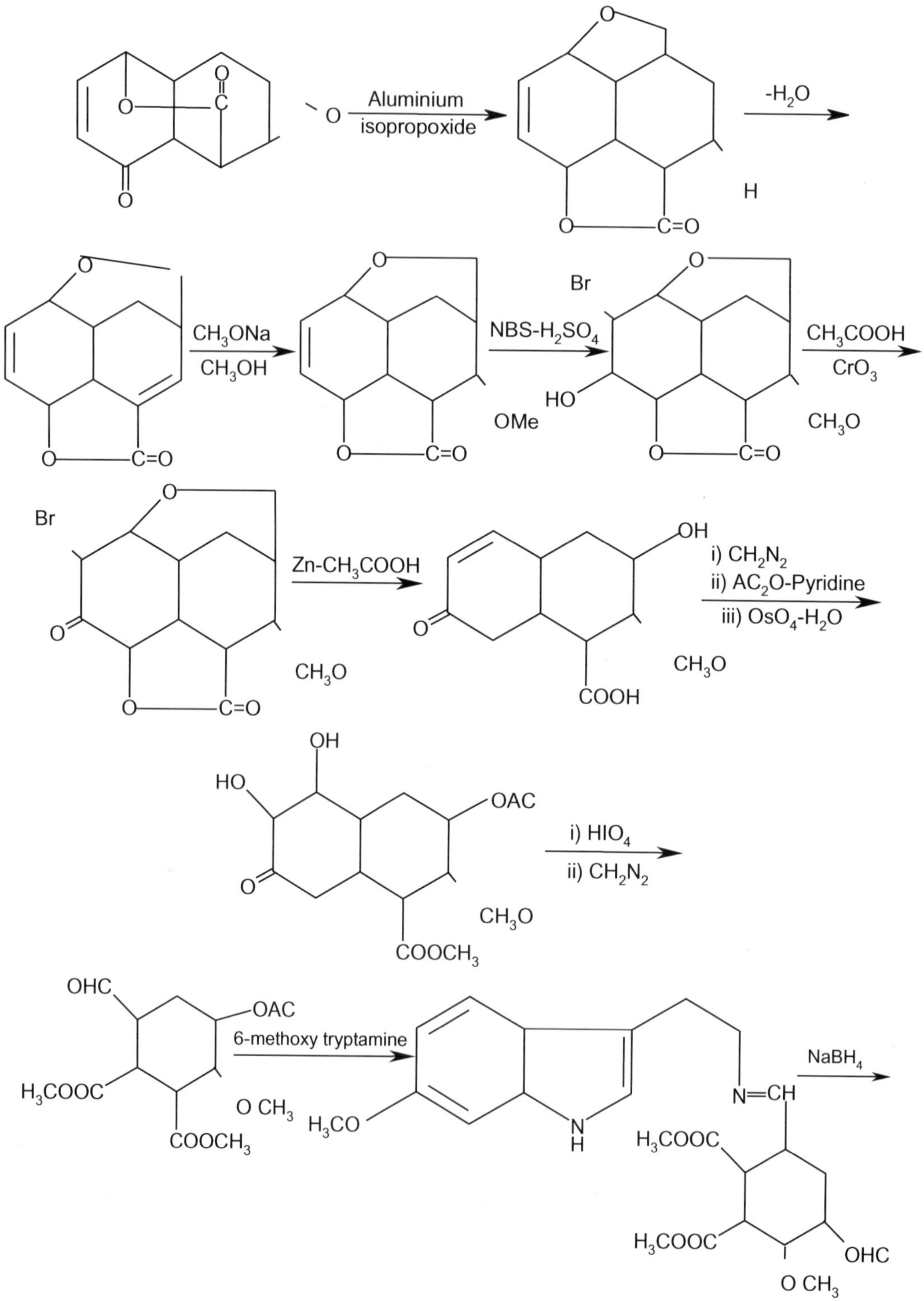

Aluminium isopropoxide
-H_2O
H
CH_3ONa
CH_3OH
OMe
Br
NBS-H_2SO_4
HO
CH_3COOH
CrO_3
CH_3O
Br
Zn-CH_3COOH
CH_3O
OH
COOH
i) CH_2N_2
ii) AC_2O-Pyridine
iii) OsO_4-H_2O
CH_3O
OH
HO
OAC
i) HIO_4
ii) CH_2N_2
CH_3O
$COOCH_3$
OHC
OAC
6-methoxy tryptamine
H_3COOC
O CH_3
$COOCH_3$
H_3CO
N
H
N=CH
$NaBH_4$
H_3COOC
H_3COOC
OHC
O CH_3

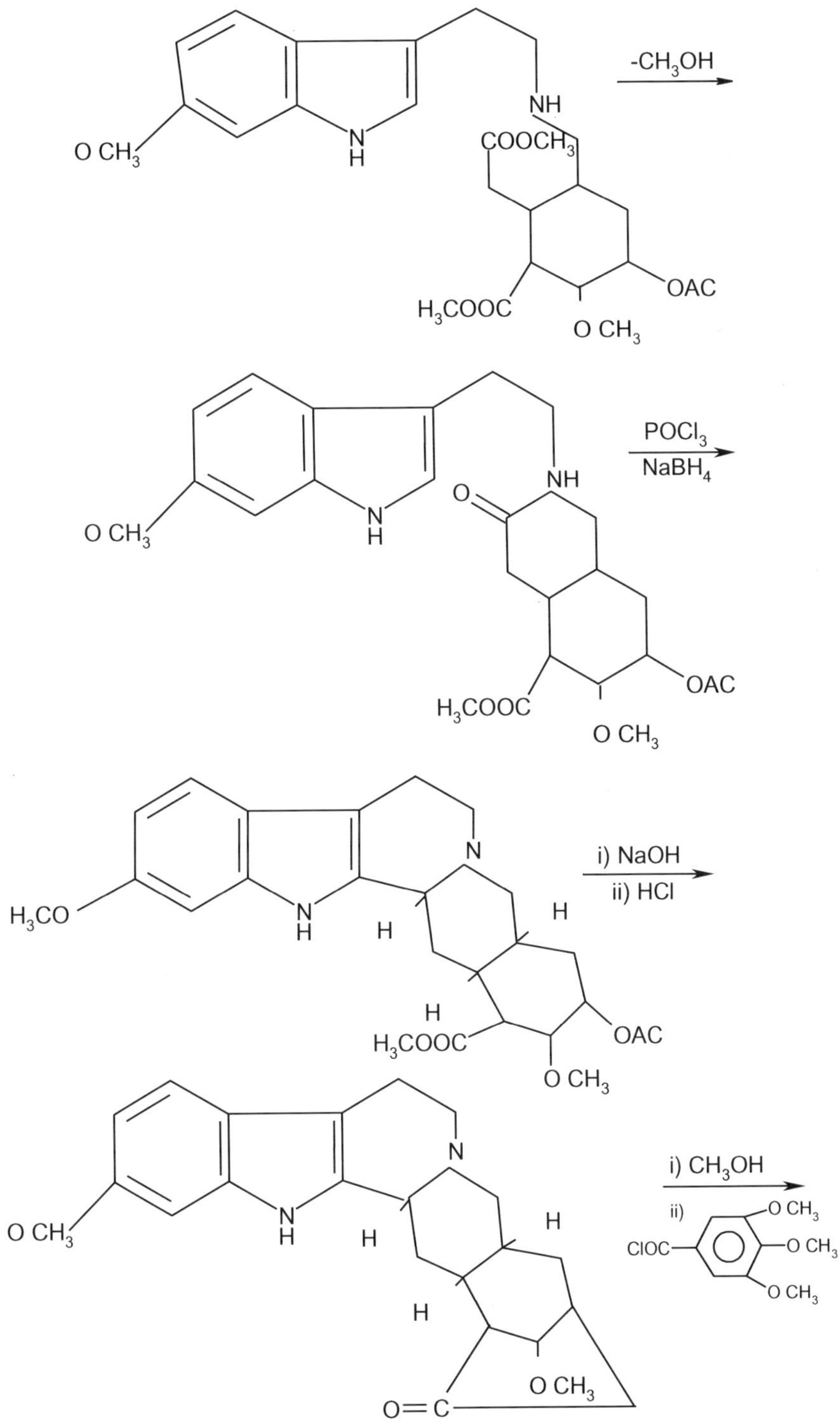

Isoreserpic acid lactone

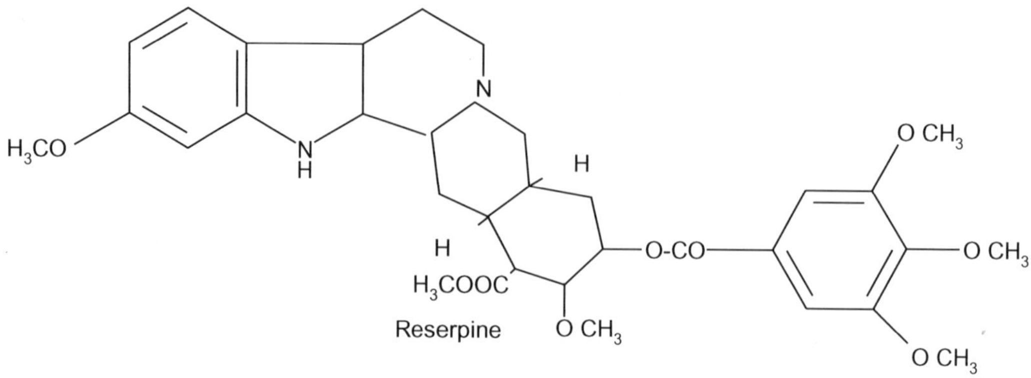

Reserpine

MORPHINE

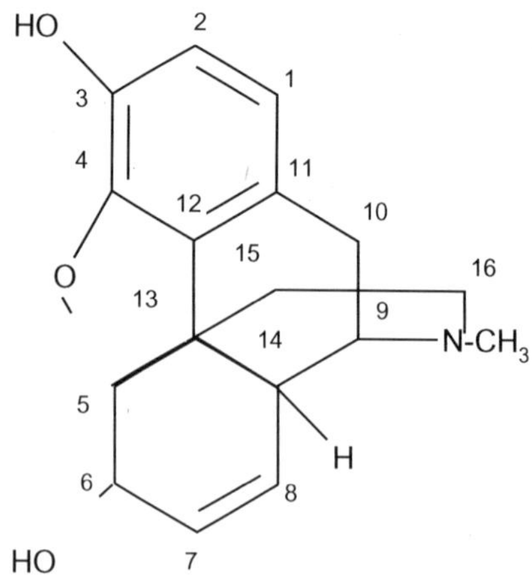

Morphine is one of the important opium alkaloid having phenanthrene nucleus. Morphine is mainly used as analgesic.

Constitution of Morphine

1. **Molecular formula of morphine is $C_{17}H_{19}NO_3$**
2. **Nature of the nitrogen atom.**

   Morphine adds one molecule of methyl iodide to form Quaternary salt, which leads to the presence of tertiary nitrogen atom.
3. **Presence of two hydroxyl groups.**

   Morphine on acetylation or benzoylation gives diacetyl or dibenzoyl derivative indicate the presence of two hydroxyl groups.

$$C_{17}H_{17}NO(OH)_2 \xrightarrow[\text{acetylation}]{2CH_2COCl} C_{17}H_{17}NO(OCOCH_3)_2 + 2HCl$$

Morphine

$$C_{17}H_{17}NO(OH)_2 \xrightarrow[\text{Benzoylation}]{2C_6H_5COCl} C_{17}H_{17}NO(OCOC_6H_5)_2 + 2HCl$$

4. Nature of the hydroxyl group

Morphine shows colouration with $Fecl_3$ and soluble in aqueous sodium hydroxide to form monosodium salt, it indicates the presence of phenolic hydroxyl group.

On treatment with halogen acids, mophine forms monohalogeno product, indicate the presence of alcoholic hydroxyl group.

5. Nature of third oxygen atom

Unreactivity of third oxygen atom and degradation product of morphine shows third oxygen atom must be in ether linkage.

6. Presence of Ethylenic bond

When codeine is subjected to reduction by palladium it takes up one molecule of hydrogen, suggesting that both codeine and morphine contain one ethylenic bond.

7. Presence of Phenanthrene nucleus

Morphine undergoes distillation with zinc dust yield Phenanthrene.

8. Presence of a cyclic teritary base system

Codeine when subjected to exhaustive methylation yield α-codeimethine -$C_{19}H_{23}NO_3$ as its molecular formula contains one more -CH_2 than codeine itself and the nitrogen atom remains intact ie not lost.

$$\underset{\text{Codeine}}{C_{18}H_{21}NO_3} \xrightarrow{CH_3I} C_{19}H_{24}NO_3I \xrightarrow{\text{alkali}} \underset{\alpha\text{ - codeimethine}}{C_{19}H_{23}NO_3}$$

All these changes are correspond to Hofmann degradation of N- methyl piperidine, the Nitrogen atom must be present in the ring

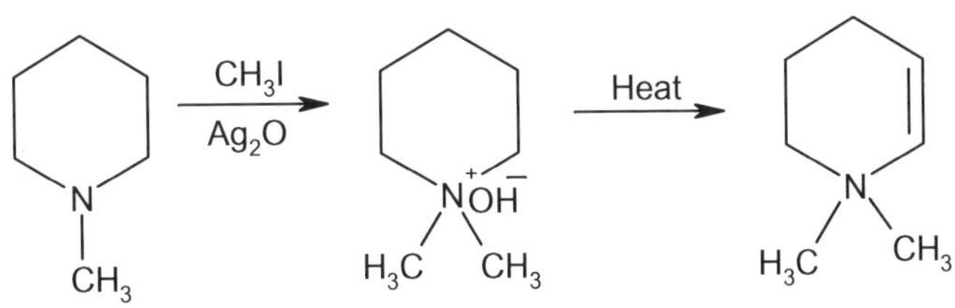

N-methylpiperidine

9. Formation of Morphol to know position of Oxygen

α-codeimethine isomerise to β-codeimethine by heating with alkali. α or β isomer when treated with methyl iodide followed by alkali, methyl morphenol is formed-which on heating with hydrobromic acid gives morphenol, which on reduction with sodium and alcohol gives Morphol

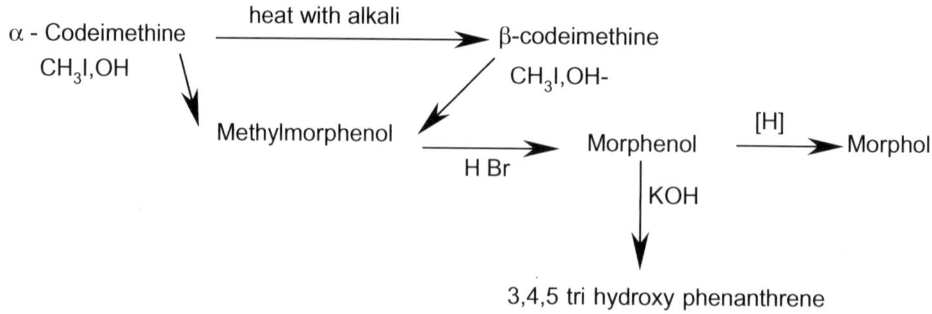

Formation of morphol and morphenol indicate oxygen function present as one phenolic at C_3 and ether linkage between C_4 and C_5.

10. Position of secondary alioholic group at C_6 of phenanthrene

Codeine methiodide on heating with Ac_2O-$AcON_a$ gives 3-methoxy -4-acetoxy phenanthrene.

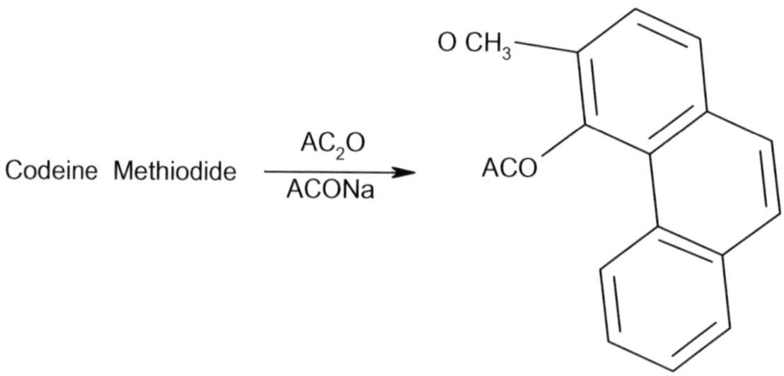

3-methoxy - 4 - acetoxy phenanthrene

but, codeinone methiodide heating with AC_2O-AcONa gives 3-methoxy -4-acetoxy phenanthrene.

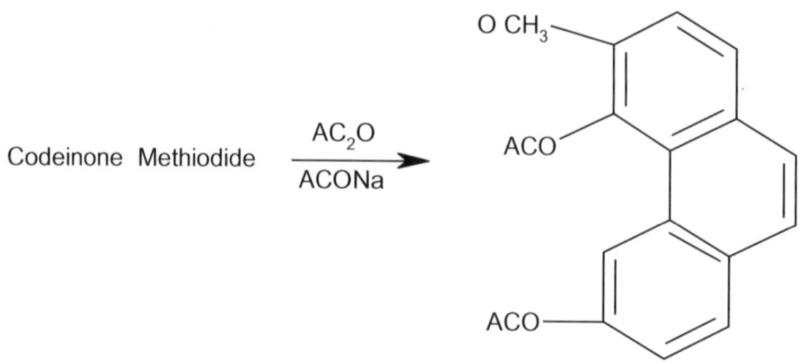

3-methoxy - 4,6- diacetoxy phenanthrene

So in the codeinone ketone group undergo enolization that is why acetoxy group in 6th positiion of product. It indicates 3rd oxygen is present as secondary alcoholic group at C_6 of the phenanthrene.

11. Point of attachment of -CH_2-CH_2-NMe chain

Codeine on oxidation give hydroxy codeine which undergo Hoffman degradation to give keto codeimethane which on heating with acetic anhydride give methoxy diacetoxy Phenanthrene. Which on oxidation give methoxy acetoxy phenan throquinone.

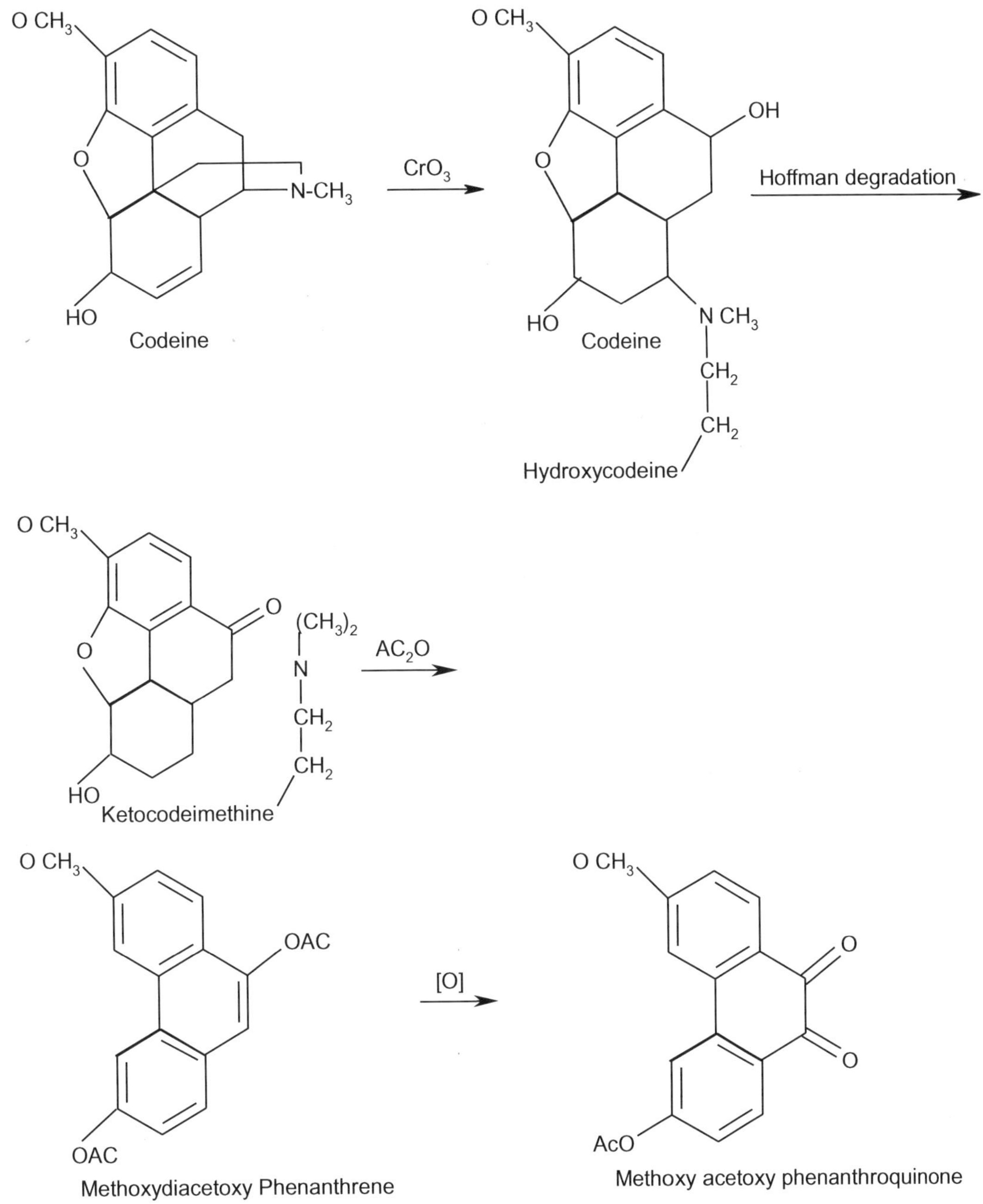

In the last step one acetyl group is lost indicating that one of the two acetoxyl groups in methoxy diacetoxy phenanthrene must be present at C_9 or C_{10}. There fore ketonic group in ketocodeimethine and hydroxyl group in hydroxy codeine must be at C_9 or C_{10}. The exact point of linkage at C_9 established by its synthesis.

12. Synthesis of Morphine

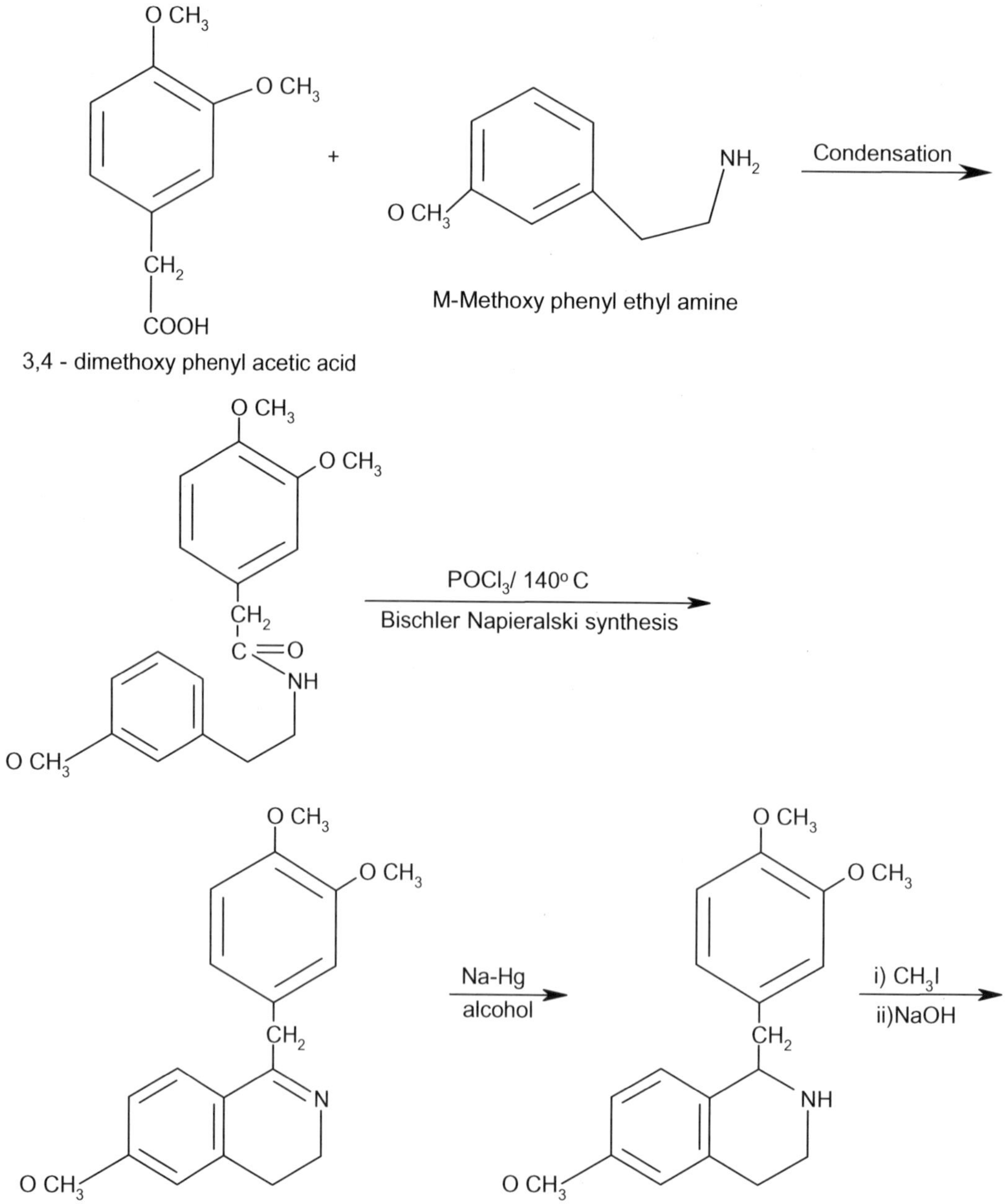

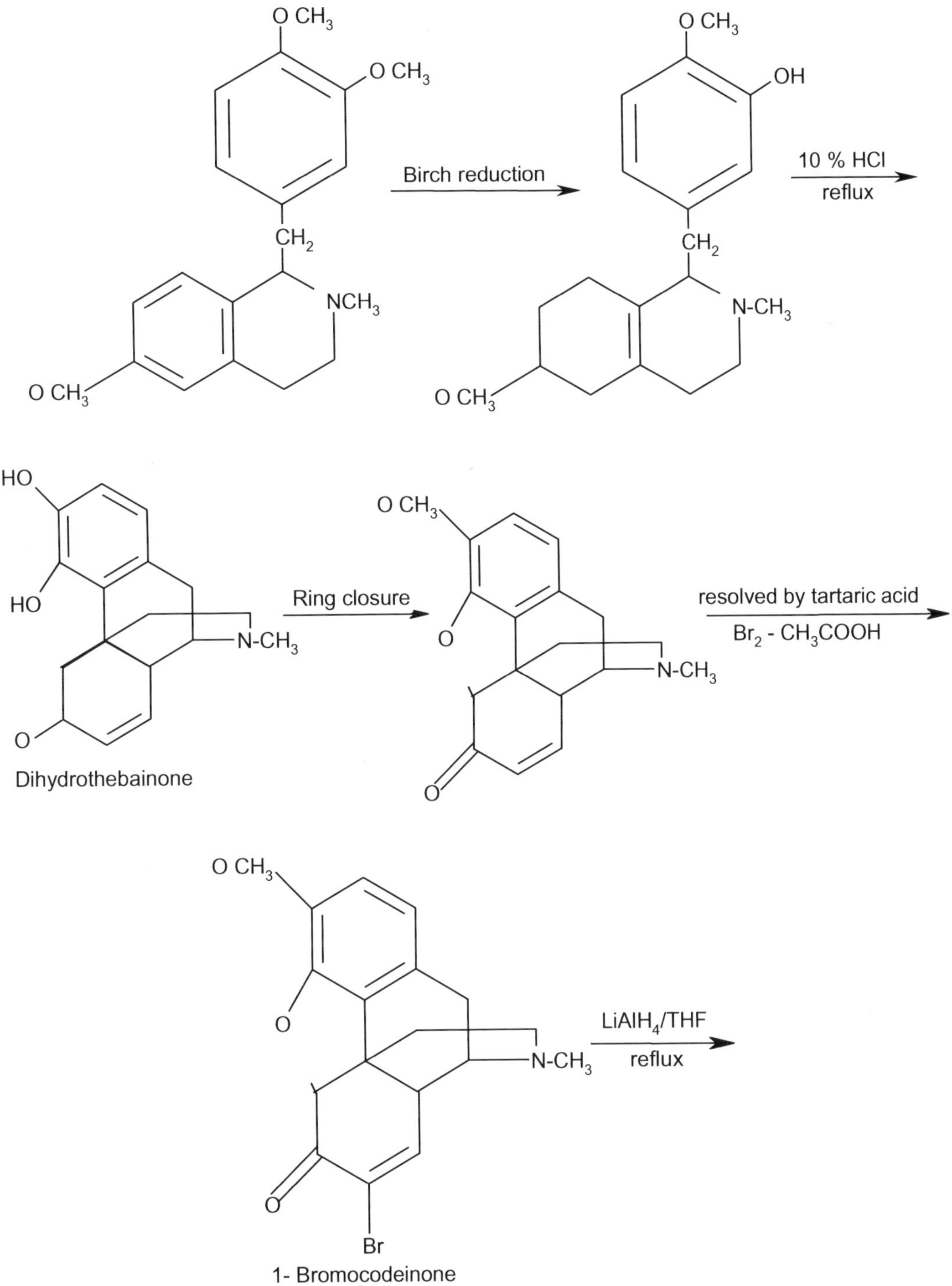
O CH3
O CH3
CH2
NCH3
O CH3
Birch reduction
O CH3
OH
CH2
N-CH3
O CH3
10 % HCl
reflux
HO
HO
N-CH3
O
Dihydrothebainone
Ring closure
O CH3
O
N-CH3
O
resolved by tartaric acid
Br2 - CH3COOH
O CH3
O
N-CH3
O
Br
1- Bromocodeinone
LiAlH4/THF
reflux

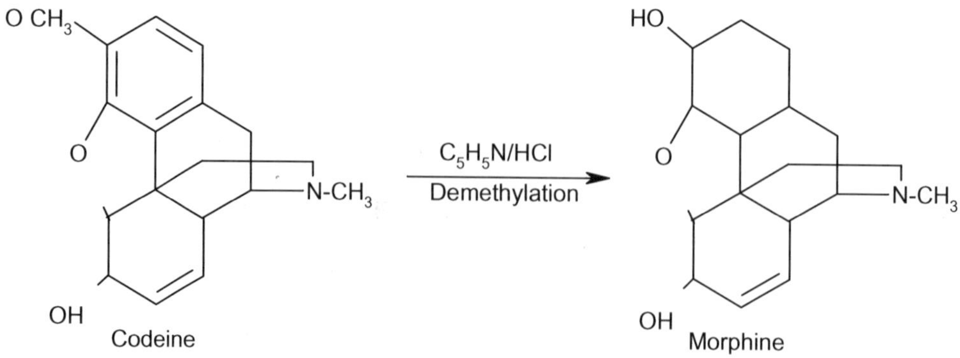

PAPAVERINE

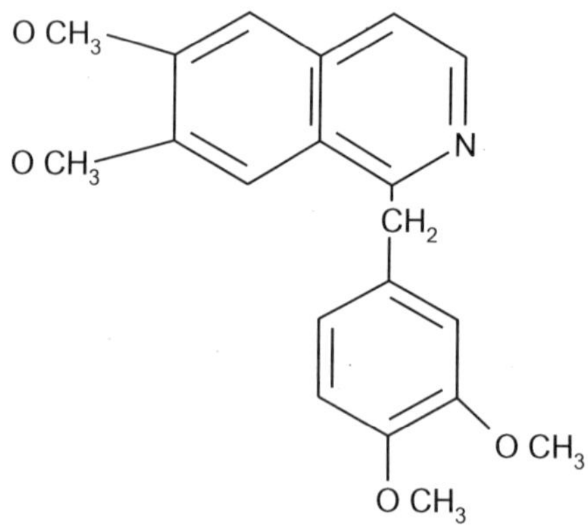

Papaverine is an isoquinoline alkaloid mainly occuring in opium .It slightly produce sleep.

Constitution

1. **Molecular formula of papaverine is $C_{20}H_{21}NO_4$**
2. **Nature of Nitrogen atom**

   Papaverine adds on one molecule of methyl iodide to form a quaternary iodide, indicate nitrogen must be in tertiary state.
3. **Presence of four methoxyl groups**

   Presence of four methoxyl group determined by zeisels method. The demethylated product is known as papaveroline.

$$\underset{\text{Papaverine}}{C_{20}H_{21}NO_4} + 4\,HI \longrightarrow 4\,CH_3I + \underset{\text{Papaveroline}}{C_{16}H_{13}NO_4}$$

4. **Presence of methylene group**

   Papaverine when oxidised with cold dil. Perman ganate papaverine converted into a secondary alcohol -namely papaverinol which on vigorous oxidation converted to a ketone namely papaveraldine. This oxidation process indicates the presence of methylene group.

$$(C_{19}H_{19}NO_4)CH_2 \xrightarrow{[O]} (C_{19}H_{19}NO_4)CHOH \xrightarrow{[O]} (C_{19}H_{19}NO_4)CO$$

Papaverine — Papaverinol — Papaveraldine

Papaverine when oxidised by hot concentrated premanganate broken into veratric acid, Metahemipinic acid, Pyridine -2,3,4 tricarboxylic acid and 6,7-dimethoxy isoquinoline -1-carboxylic acid so constitution of these compounds can give evidence for the structure of papaverine.

(a) Veratric acid

Veratric acid on decarboxylation gives veratrole which is a o-dimethoxy benzene, therefore veratric acid is dimethoxy benzoic acid. It can be confirmed by its synthesis.

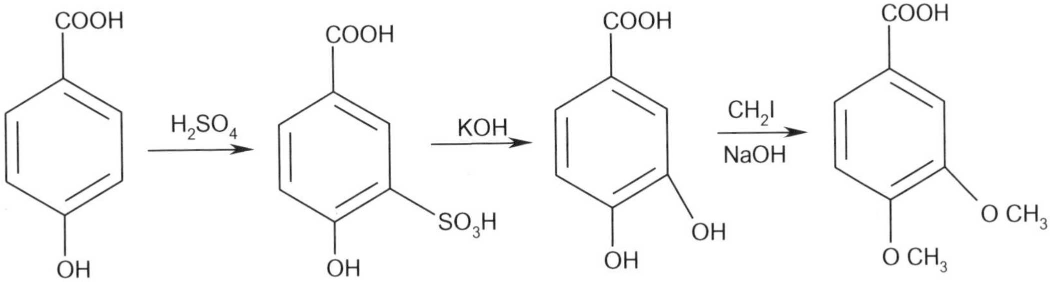

Veratric acid

(b) Metahemipinic acid

When it is decarboxylated by heating with calcium oxide veratrole is formed. Thus metaheminic acid contains two methoxyl groups in ortho-position since it forms anhydride, when heated with acetic anhydride, is possible only when carboxyl group are in ortho position. Metahemipinic acid permits the formation of only one monoester therefore metahemipinic acid is

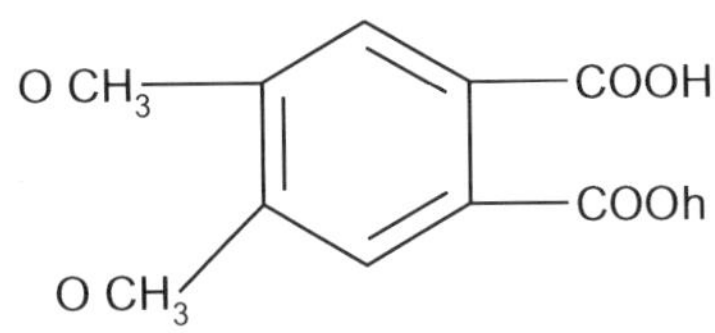

(c) Pyridine -2,3,4-tricarboxylic acid

Presence of three carboxylic acids determined as usual. On decarboxylation gives pyridine. Structure is confirmed by its formation from lepidine by oxidation.

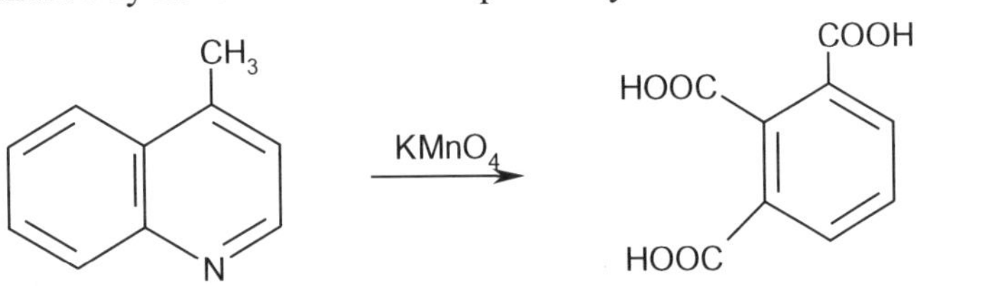

lepidine — Pyridine- 2,3,4 tricarboxylic acid

(d) 6,7-Dimethoxy isoquinoline -1-Carboxylic acid

Presence of two methoxyl group and one carboxylic acid determined as usual. Oxidation of

6,7-Dimethoxy isoquinoline-1-carboxylic acid produces pyridine -2,3,4 tricarboxylic acid. On decarboxylation by calcium oxide 6,7-Dimethoxy isoquinoline -1- carboxylic acid converted to dimethoxy isoquinoline which on oxidation give metahemipinic acid.

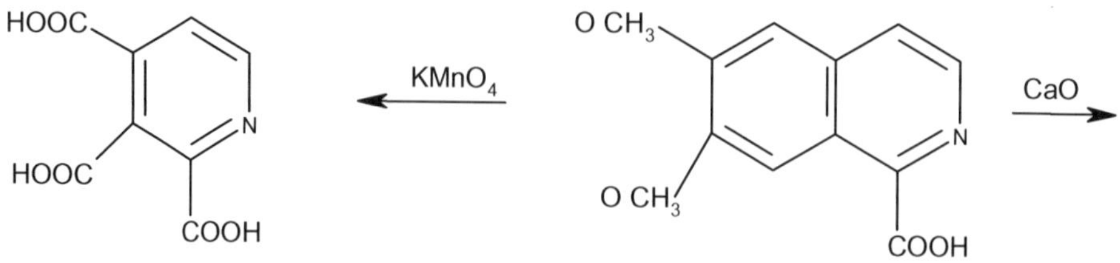

Pyridine-2,3,4 -tricarboxylic acid

6,7 -dimethoxy-isoquinoline 1 -carboxylic acid

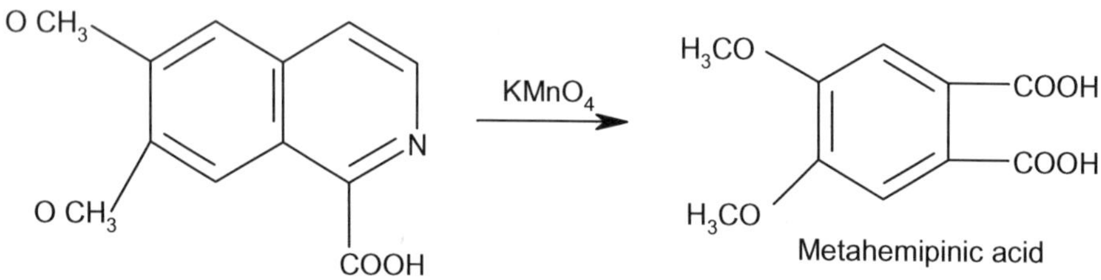

Metahemipinic acid

All above a,b,c and d accounts for structure of papaverine as

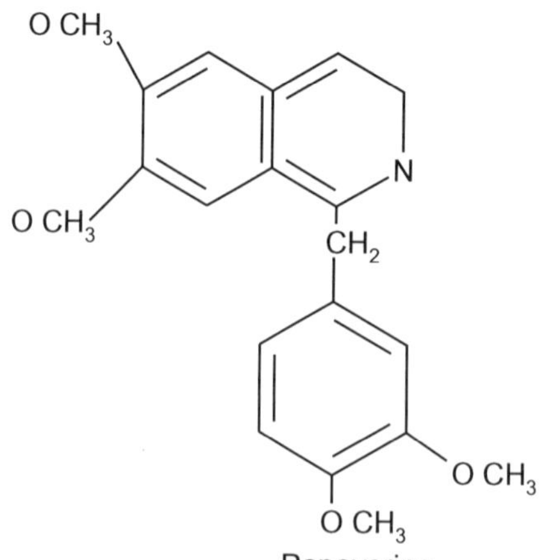

Papaverine

Finally structure of papaverine can be confirmed by its synthesis. It involves two steps. I[st] step include synthesis of homoveratryl amine and homoveratroyl chloride.

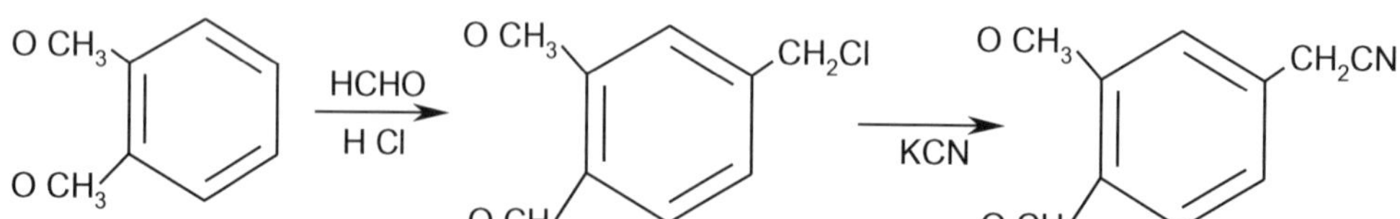

Veratrol

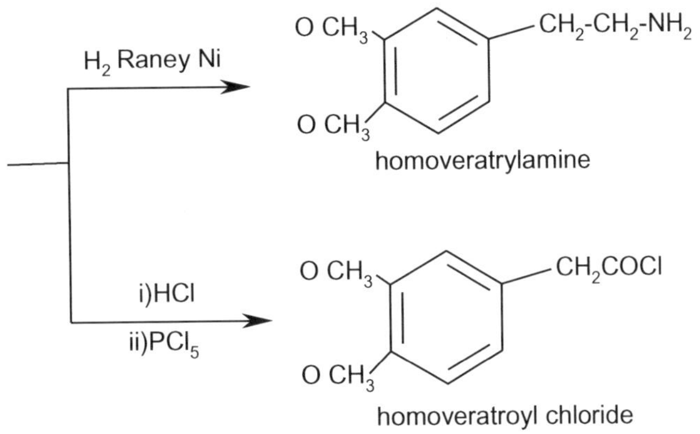

Second step involves condensaton of Homoveratryl amine and Homoveratroyl chloride.

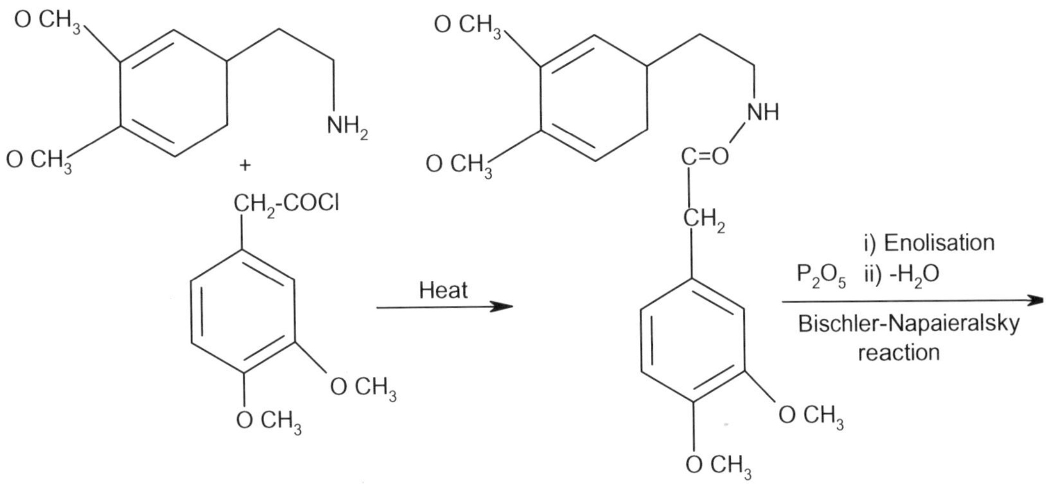

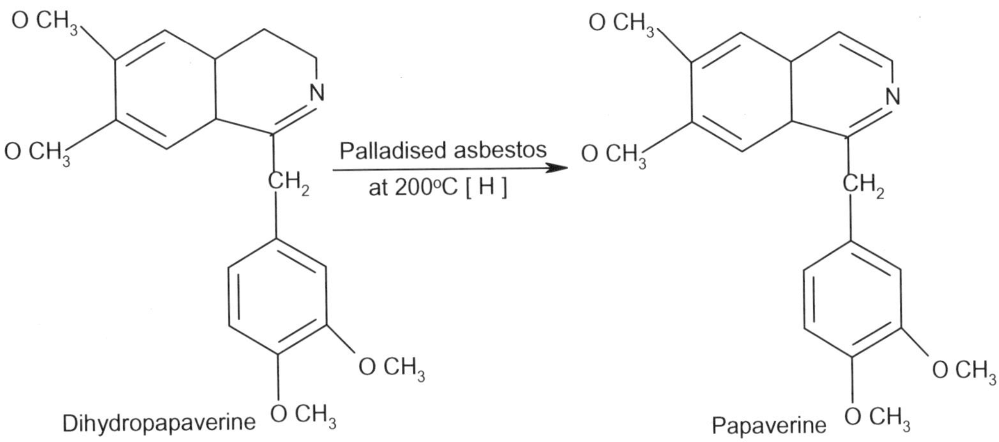

EPHEDRINE

$$C_6H_5CHOH\ (CH_3)\ NHCH_3$$

Ephedrine mainly occurs in genus Ephedra. It is mainly used to treat hay fever and in bronchial asthma.

Constitution

1. **Molecular formula of Ephedrine is $C_{10}H_{15}NO$**
2. **Presence of benzene ring with only one side chain**

   Ephedrine on oxidation give benzoic acid, indicating the presence of Benzene nucleus with one side chain.

$$C_6H_5CHOHCH\ (CH_3)NHCH_3 \xrightarrow{[O]} C_6H_5COOH$$

3. **Presence of secondary amine**

   Ephedrine on reaction with nitrous acid, forms nitroso compound indicating the presence of secondary amine.
4. **Presence of Hydroxyl group**

   On benzoylation Ephedrine forms dibenzoyl derivative indicating that one hydroxyl group must be present. One benzoyl group is accounted for imino group.
5. **Possible Structure of Ephedrine**

   When Ephedrine is heated with hydrochloric acid forms methylamine and propiophenone.

$$C_{10}H_{15}NO \xrightarrow{H\,Cl} CH_3NH_2 + C_6H_5COCH_2CH_3$$

This reaction suggests either of the following structure for ephedrine.

$$\underset{\text{I}}{C_6H_5CHOHCH_2CH_2NHCH_3} \quad \text{or} \quad \underset{\text{II}}{C_6H_5CHOH\underset{\substack{|\\ NHCH_3}}{C}HCH_3}$$

Among this structure II undergo hydramine fission to form propiophenone when heated with hydrochloric acid. Again it is supported by only structure II undergo Hofmann exhaustive methylation to give 1,2-methyl phenyl-ethylene oxide. Therefore structure II is considered as Ephedrine. Finally it is Confirmed by its synthesis.

Synthesis of Ephedrine

By the catalytic reduction of 1-phenyl propane-, 2-dion (benzoyl acetyl) in the presence of methylamine in methanol gives Ephedrine

$$C_6H_5COCOCH_3 + CH_3NH_2 \longrightarrow C_6H_5COC\ (=NCH_3)CH_3 \xrightarrow{H_2\text{-pt}} \underset{\text{(I) ephedrine}}{C_6H_5CHOHCH(CH_3)NHCH_3}$$

ERGOT ALKALOID

Ergotamine is one of the important alkaloid obtaining from a filamentous fungus Claviceps purpurea. It mainly acts on uterus and vasomotor centre. Most of the ergot alkaloids constitute isomeric pairs like ergotamine & ergotaminine; ergosine and ergosinine.

Ergotamin

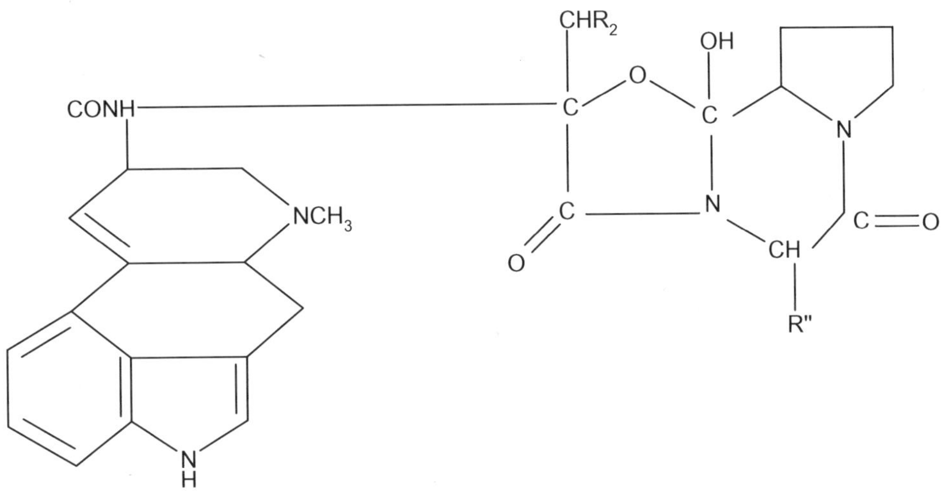

Constitution

1. **Molecular formula of ergotamine is $C_{33}H_{35}N_5O_5$**

Alkaline hydrolysis on ergotamine produces Lysergic acid and non-lysergic acid moiety. Components in non-lysergic acid moiety are α-hydroxy alanine, l-Phenylalanine and d-proline.

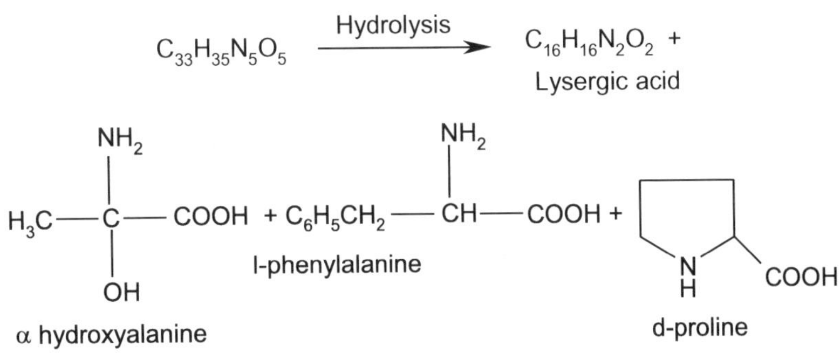

Structure of Lysergic Acid

1. **Molecular formula of lysergic acid is $C_{16}H_{16}NO_2$**
2. **Presence of carboxylic group, >NH and NcH_3 and a double bond determined as usual.**

3. Presence of indole and naphthalene nucleus.

On potassium hydroxide fusion, dihydrolysergic acid yields 3,4-dimethyl indole,1-methyl -5 aminonaphthalene and methylamine.

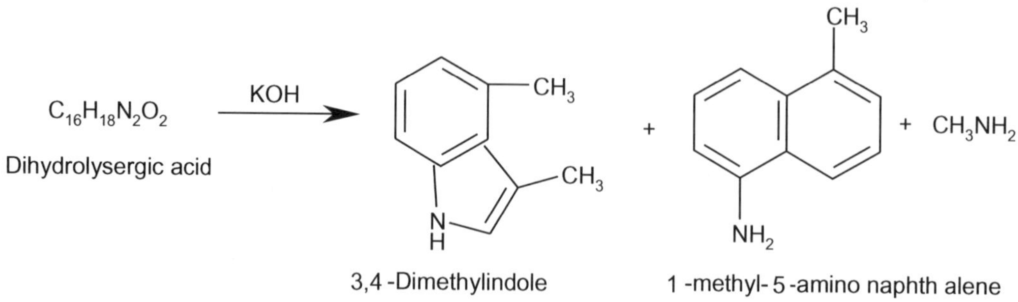

Formation of these products indicates the presence of Indole and naphthalene nulei in lysergic acid.

4. Presence of Quinoline nucleus

Lysesgic acid on oxidation with nitric acid gives a tricarboxylic acid which on distillation with soda lime yields Quinoline suggesting that lysergic acid posses a quinoline nucleus.

5. Presence of additional double band between C_9 and C_{10} or C_5 and C_{10}

UV spectra of lysergic and isolysergic acids with that of dihydrolysergic acid indicated that additional double bond of lysergic and isolysergic acid is present in between C_9 and C_{10} or C_5 and C_{10}. When lysergic acid is heated, newly formed double bond in the product is found to be in conjugation with already present double bond, it confirms double bond in lysergic acid must be between C_9 and $C_{10.}$

6. Position of carboxylic group

Carboxylic group in lysergic acid is found to be at C_8 as it behaves like a β-amino acid.

All above reactions suggests, lysergic acid have the structural formula as follows;

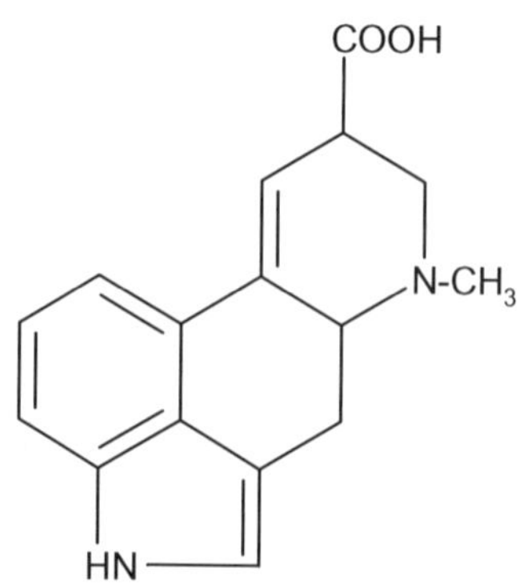

Lysergic acid

Finally structure of lysergic acid confirmed by its synthesis.

Synthesis of Lysergic Scid

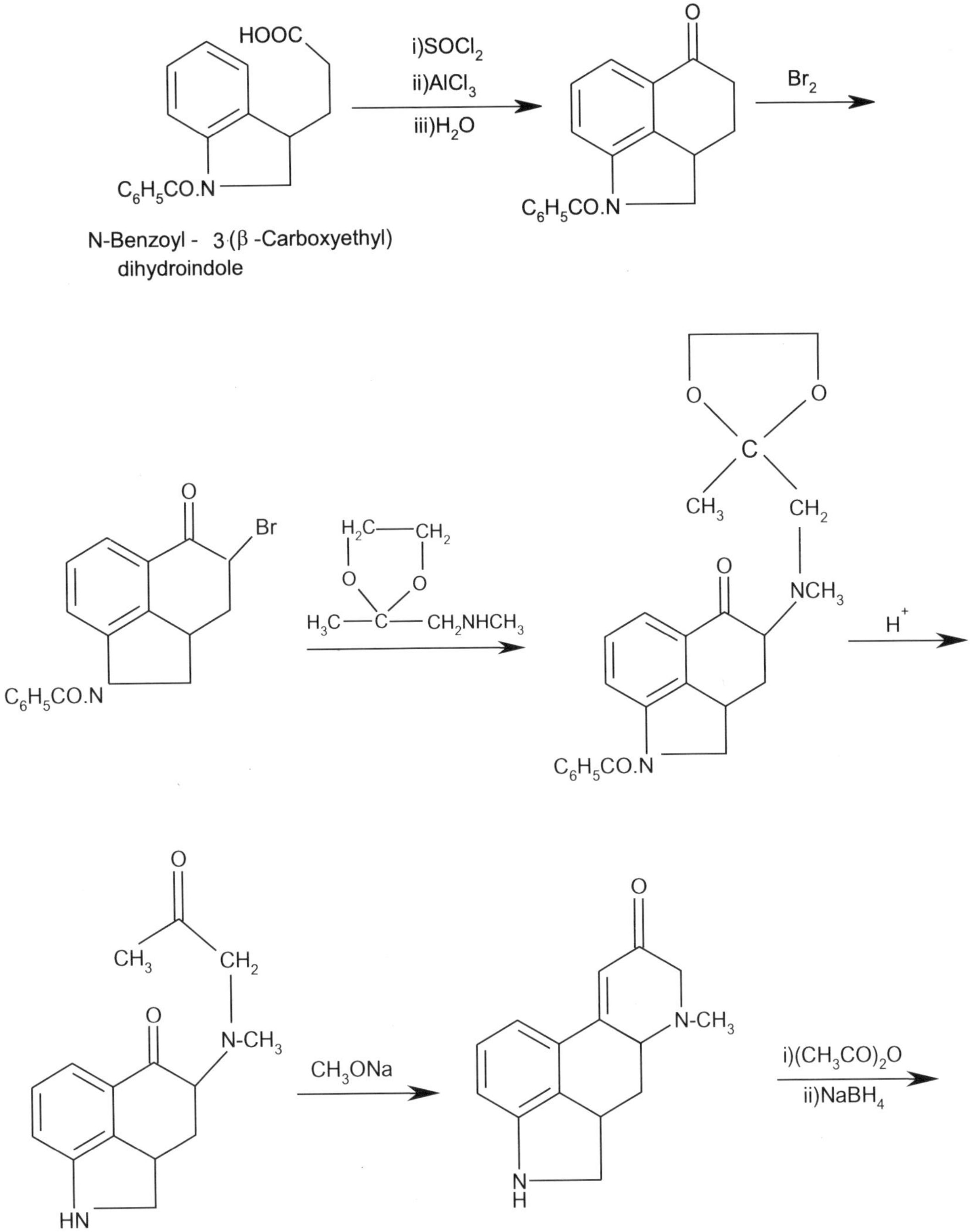

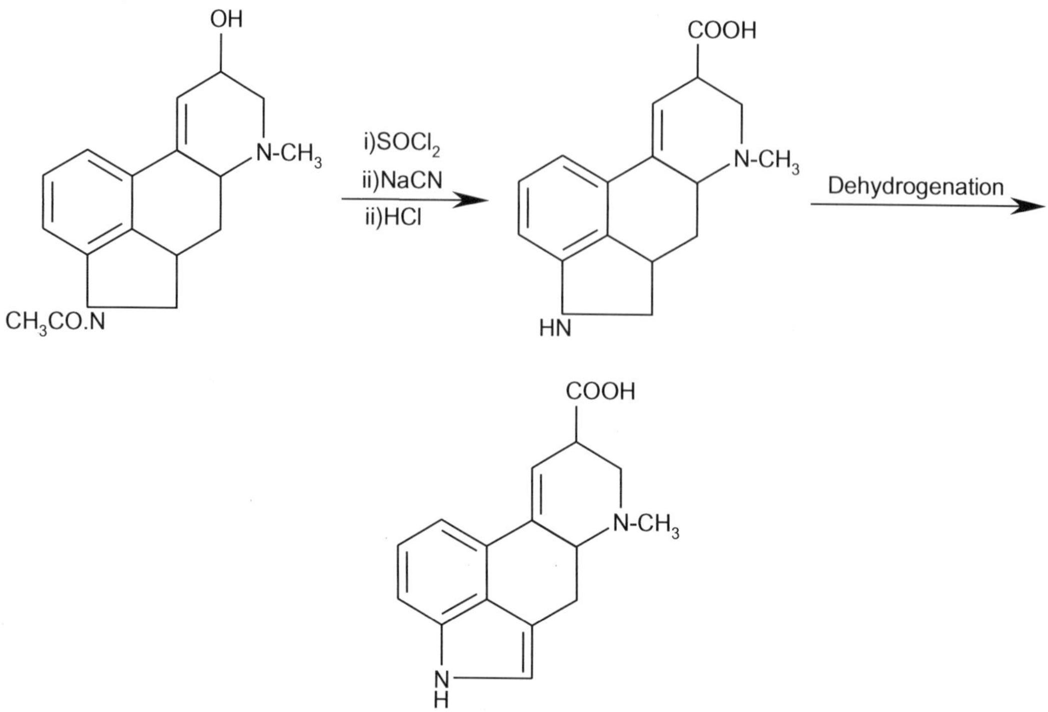

± Lysergic acid

Structure of Non-lysergic Acid Moiety

(a) Presence of peptide bond

Hydrolysis of ergotamine to lysergic acid, d-proline, phenylalanine and pyruvic acid indicate that alkaloid contain peptide bond. d-proline and phenylalanine are found to be present as such in the alkaloid.

(b) Exact structure of non-lysergic acid moiety can be drawn on the following basis

Nature of amino acids

(b_1) Non-lysergic acid moiety neither have free carboxyl group nor amino group indicate, amino acids present are in the form of cyclic structure.

(b_2) Position of peptide linkage.

On mild alkaline hydrolysis gives lysergic acid-amide instead of lysergic acid indicate peptide linkage present in between lysergic acid carboxyl and the α-hydroxy α-amino acid moiety.

(b_3) Sequence of amino acids.

Dihydro ergotamine with hydrazine gives dihydro lysergic acid hydrazide and propionyl -L-phenylalanyl-L- proline. Dihydroergotamine with alkali in alcohol gives lysergic acid and pyruvoyl -L- phenyl- alanyl -L- proline. These reactions indicate sequence of amino acids in ergotamine is pyruvic acid - phenylalanine - proline.

Thus the structure of non-lysergic acid can be proposed as.

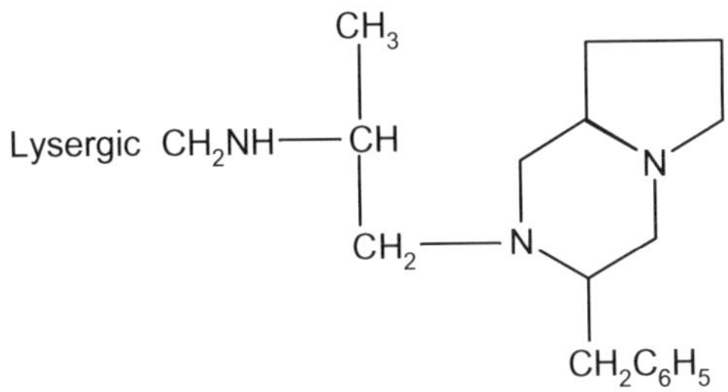

So the complete structure of Ergotamine can be written as;

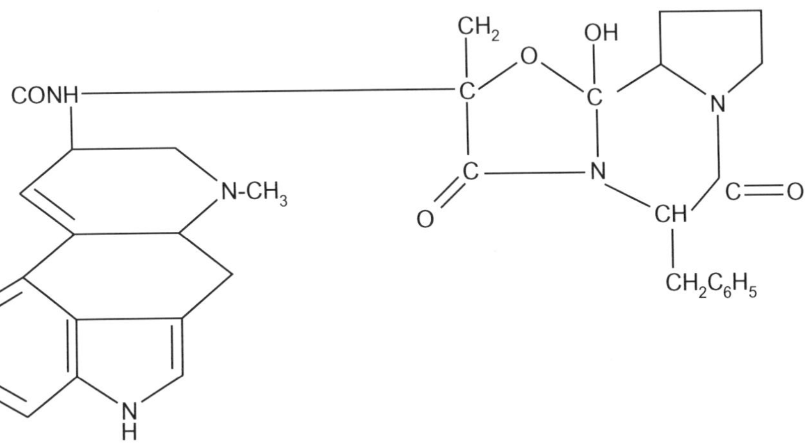

Finally structure of Ergotamine confirmed by its synthesis.

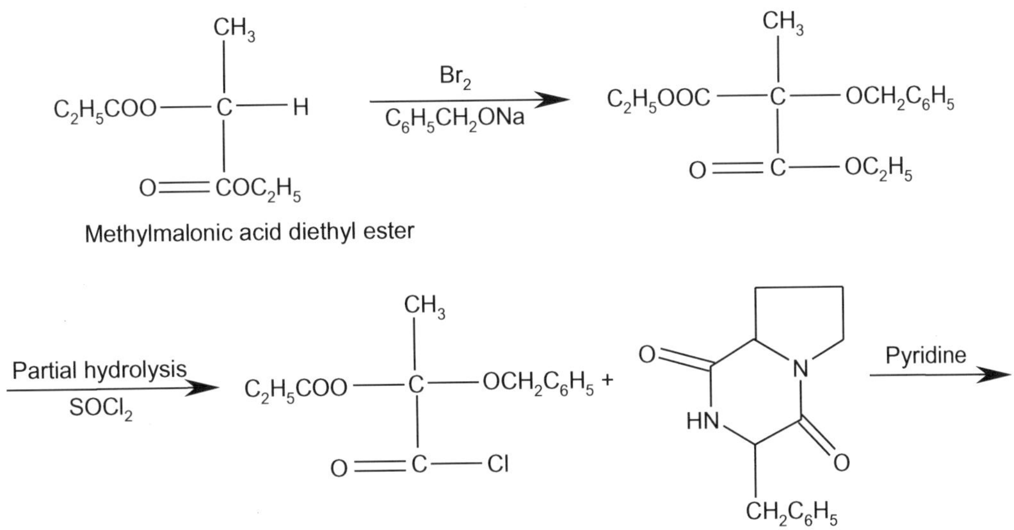

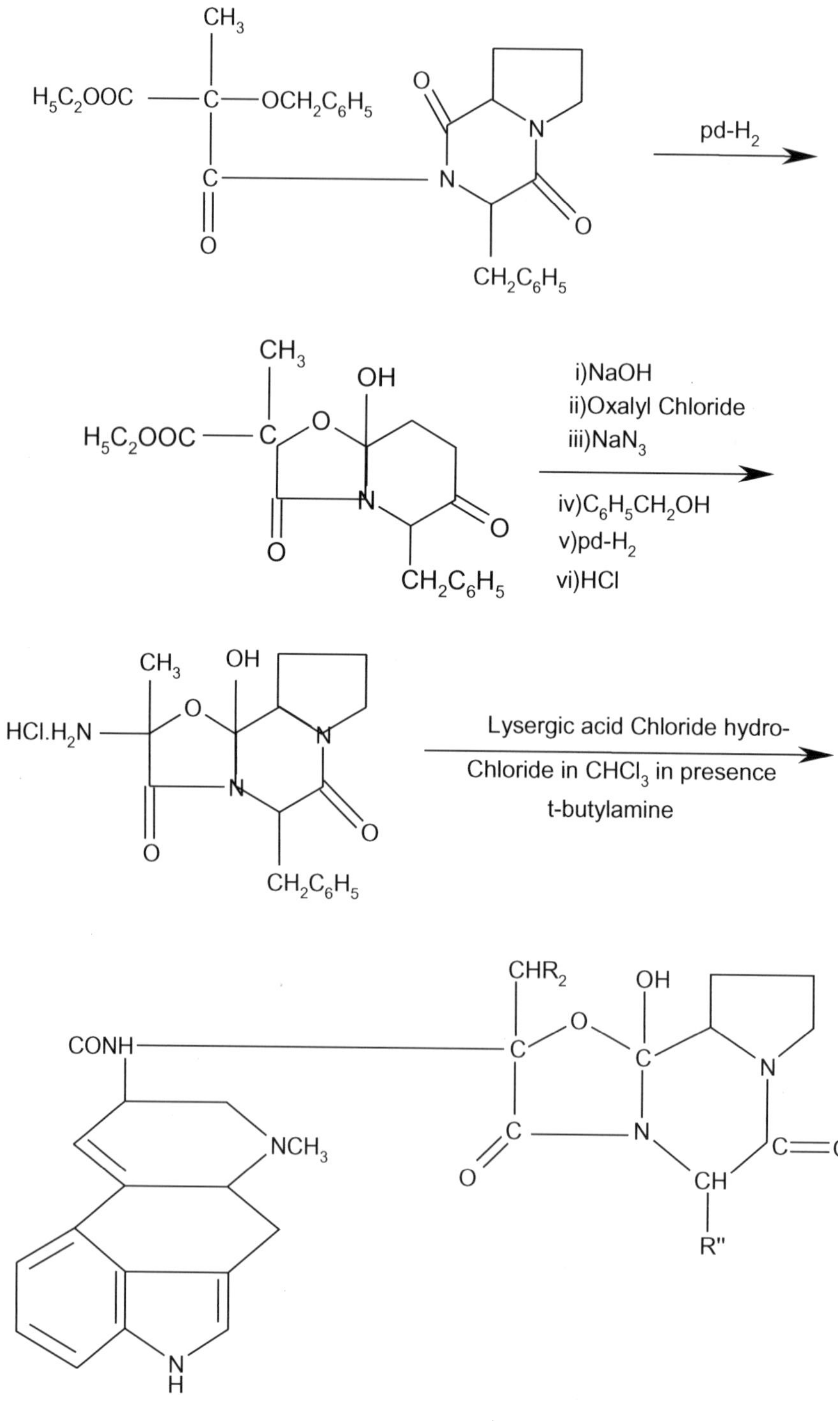

CH3
H5C2OOC
C
OCH2C6H5
O
N
pd-H2
C
N
O
O
CH2C6H5
CH3
OH
i)NaOH
ii)Oxalyl Chloride
iii)NaN3
H5C2OOC
C
O
N
O
iv)C6H5CH2OH
v)pd-H2
vi)HCl
O
CH2C6H5
CH3
OH
HCl.H2N
O
N
Lysergic acid Chloride hydro-
Chloride in CHCl3 in presence
t-butylamine
N
O
O
CH2C6H5
CHR2
OH
CONH
C
O
C
N
NCH3
C
N
C=O
O
CH
R''
N
H

VINCA ALKALOIDS

Vinca alkaloids are mainly present in catharanthus plants. Important alkaloids are vincrisine and vinblastine. Both of them are used as anti cancer drugs.

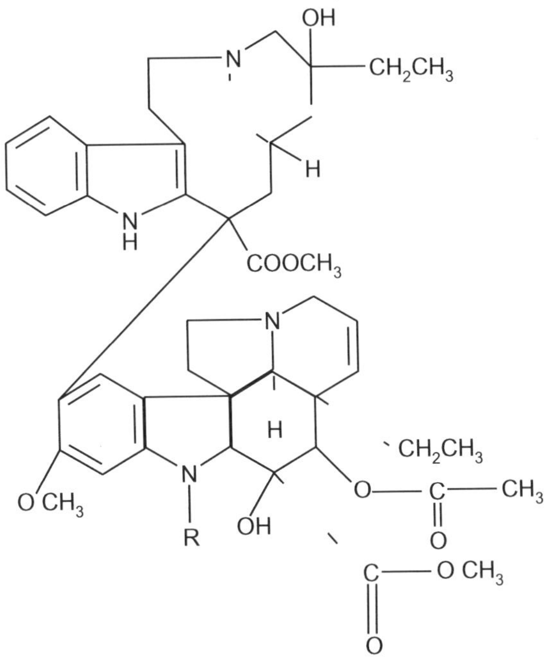

Vinblastine R=CH_3

Vincristine R=CHO

Chemistry of Vinca Alkaloids

Identification test:

$$\text{Vinca alkaloid} \xrightarrow[H_3PO_4]{FeCl_3 \text{ in}} \begin{cases}\text{Pink Colour (Vincristin)} \\ \text{Violet Colour (Vinblastin)} \\ \text{Yellow Colour (Catharanthin)}\end{cases}$$

It is a dimeric indole.

Structural composition

1. **Molecular formula of vinblastin is $C_{46}H_{58}N_4O_9$.**
2. **Presence of methyl group**

   Presence of methyl group determined by Herzig - Mayer method (reaction with hydrogen iodide at 300°C)
3. **Presence of methoxyl group determined by zeisel's method.**
4. **Presence of Ester**

   Vinca alkaloids on hydrolys is gives acids. It forms a dicarbo methoxy diacetyl mono hydrazide. It indicates the presence of CH_3 group and hydroxyl group at 4th position.

PURINES

Purines are cyclic diureides. Pyramidine ring fused with an imidazole ring in purine nucleus.

URIC ACID

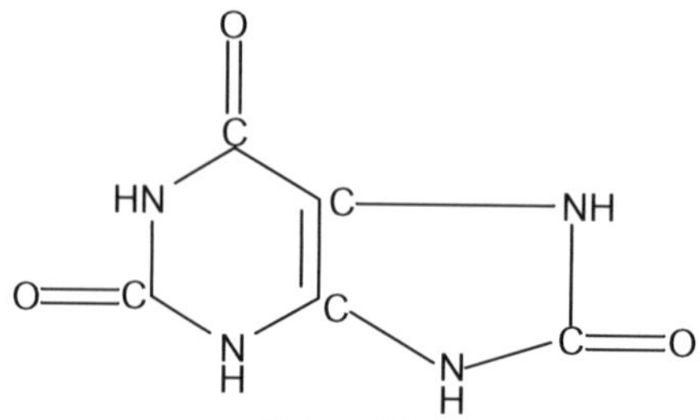

Uric acid

In human body Uric acid is formed as a metabolic product of purines which in turn are formed by the hydrolysis of nucleoproteins. Uric acid exhibits keto-enol tauto merism.

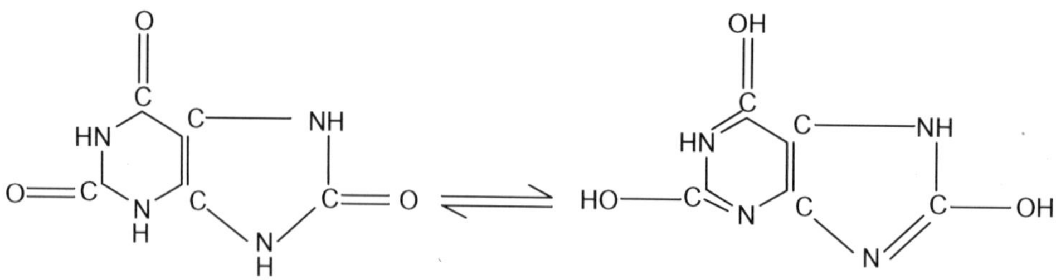

Keto - form   Enolic form

Uric acid can be alkylated by means of methyliodide, alkaline methyl sulphate or diazomethane. Depending upon the nature of alkylating agent, product may be mono, di, tri or tetra methyl uric acids. Mild oxidation of uric acid by nitric acid produces alloxan and urea.

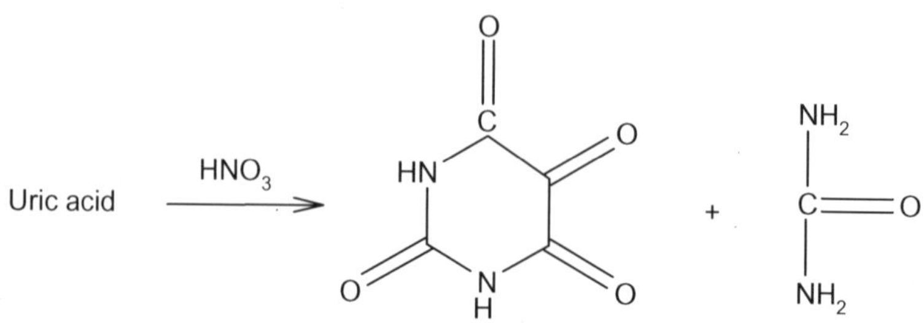

Alloxan   Urea

Vigorous oxidation of uric acid by alkaline $KMnO_4$ give allantoin and carbondioxide.

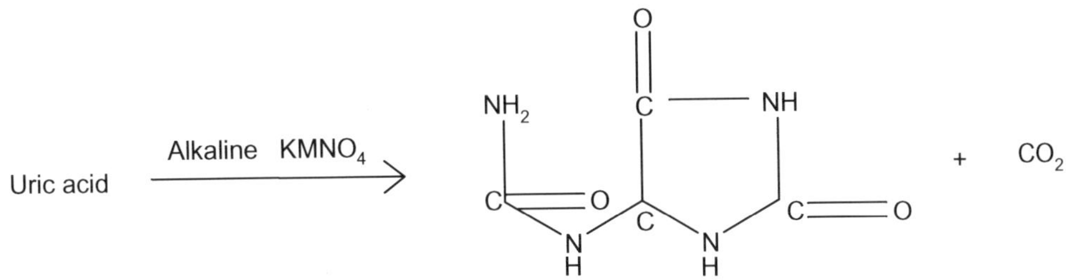

Allantoin

Uric acid on electro lytic reduction in presence of Sulphuric acid gives purine.

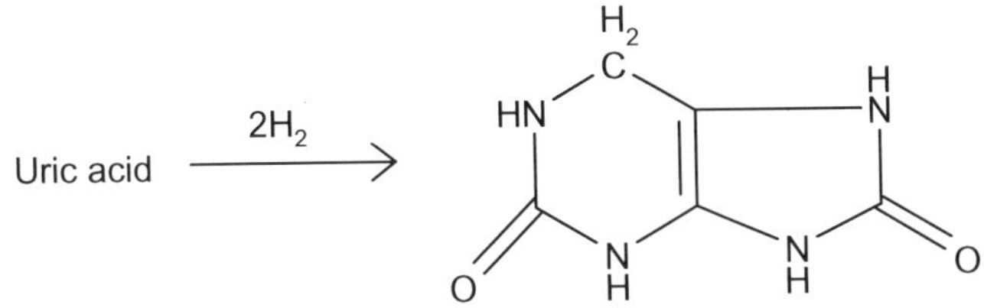

Purone

Uric acid on treatment with concentrated nitric acid followed by the addition of ammonia gives ammonium salt of purpuric acid -known as murexide.

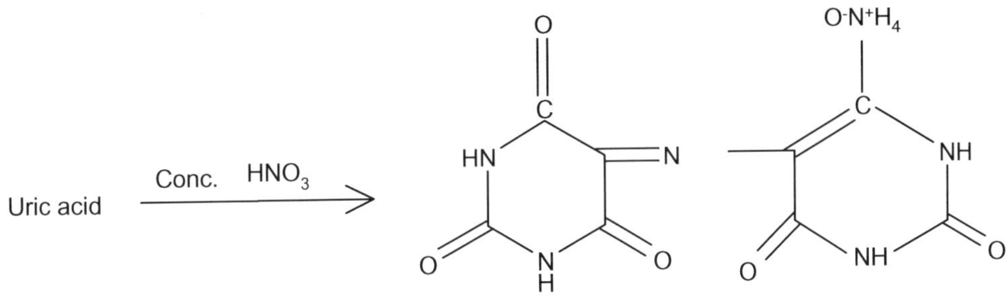

Murexide

Uric acid is otherwise known as 2,6,8-trihydroxy purine .

Constitution of uric acid

1. Molecular composition of uric acid is $C_5H_4N_4O_3$.
2. Presence of pyrimidine nucleus.
   Uric acid on mild oxidation gives alloxan from uric acid indicate the presence of pyrimidine nucleus.
3. Presence of imidazole nucleus.
   Uric acid on vigorous oxidation gives allantoin and CO_2.

Structrural Confirmation of Allantoin

Molecular composition of allantoin is found to be $C_4H_6N_4O_3$.

Allantoin on mild oxidation by nitric acid yield parabanic acid and urea.

$$\underset{\text{Allantoin}}{C_4H_6N_4O_3} \xrightarrow[{[O]}]{HNO_3} \underset{\text{Parabanic acid}}{C_3H_2N_2O_3} + \underset{\text{Urea}}{NH_2\text{-}\overset{\overset{O}{||}}{C}\text{-}NH_3}$$

Since parabanic acid is an oxalyl urea, which on hydrolysis gives. Oxalic acid and Urea. Formation of parabanic acid from allantoin-which is from uric acid indicate, both of them have imidazole nucleus. Structure of parabanic acid can be confirmed by its synthesis from oxalyl chloride and urea.

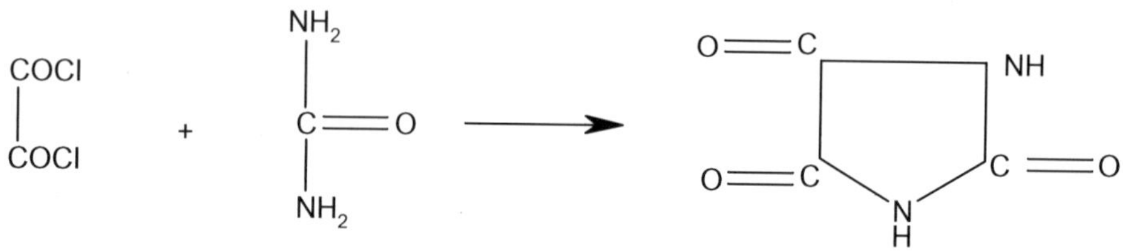

Oxalyl chloride Urea Parabanic acid

Linkage of parabanic acid with urea.

Allantoin on reduction with hydriodic acid at 100⁰ forms Urea and hydantoin.

$$\underset{\text{Allantoin}}{C_4H_6N_4O_3} \xrightarrow[HI]{[H]} \underset{\text{Hydantoin}}{C_3H_4N_2O_2} + \underset{\text{Urea}}{NH_2 - CO - NH_2}$$

Since hydantoin gives glycine, ammonia and CO_2 on hydrolysis the structure of Hydantoin must be as follows,

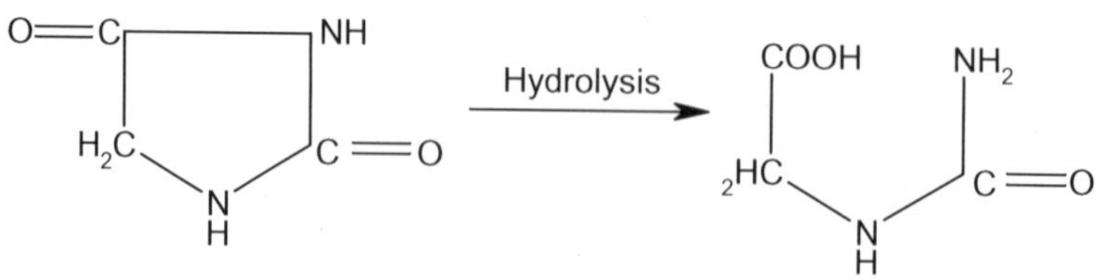

Hydantoin Hydantoic acid

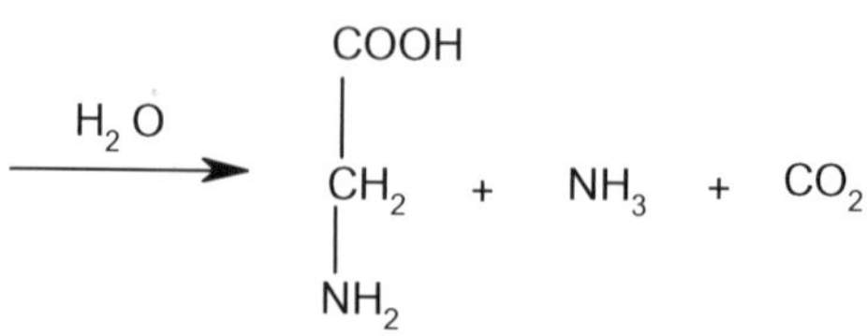

Glycine

Structure of Hydantoin can be confirmed by its synthesis.

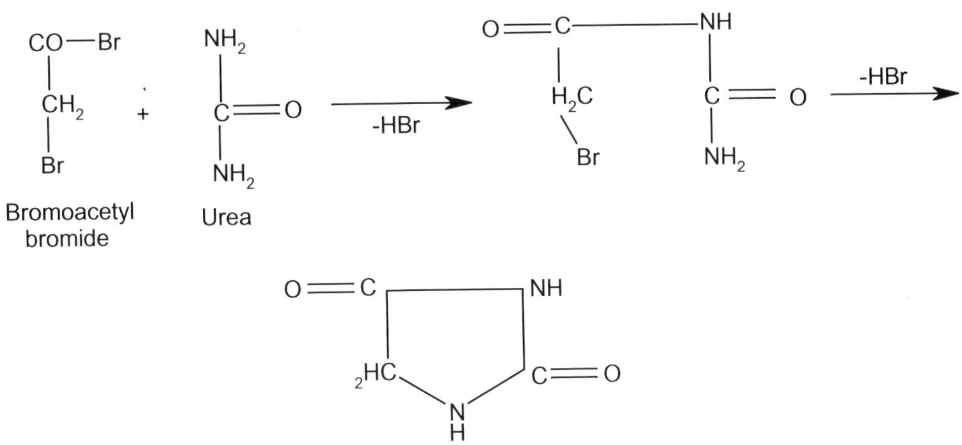

Bromoacetyl bromide

Urea

Hydantoin

Bromoacetyl Bromide Urea

Under different conditions allantoin gives Hydantoin & parabanic acid. Both have difference only in one carbon atom (marked by asterick). So that carbon atom is considered as point of attachment of Urea. So the structure of allantoin can be drawn as follows.

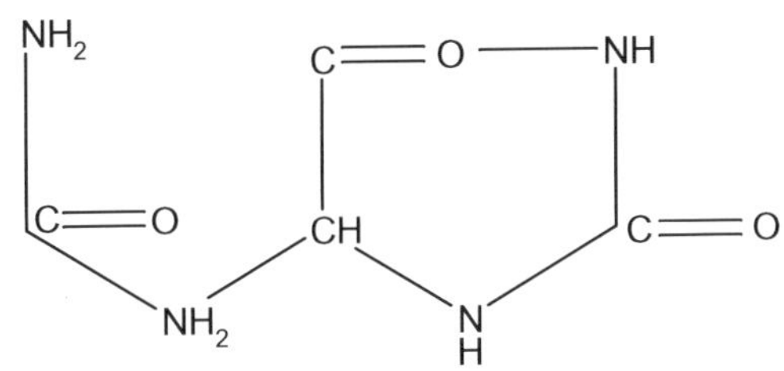

Allantoin

Strutre of allantion can be confirmed by its synthesis.

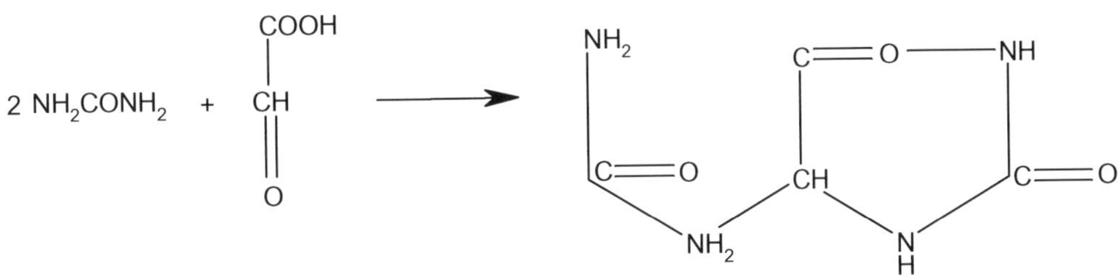

Urea Glyoxalic acid Allantoin

From all above facts structure of uric acid can be any of the following;

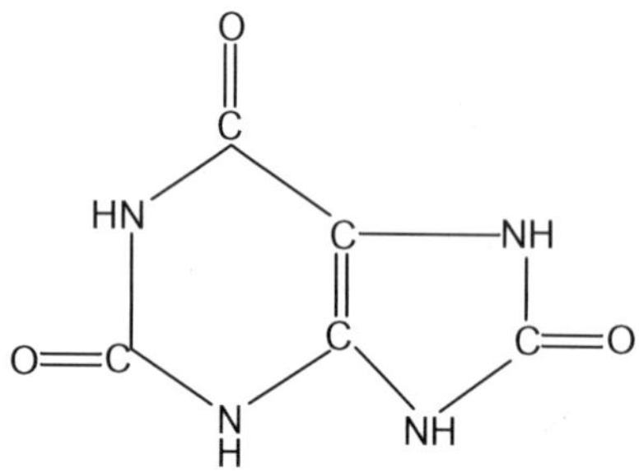

Medicus formula

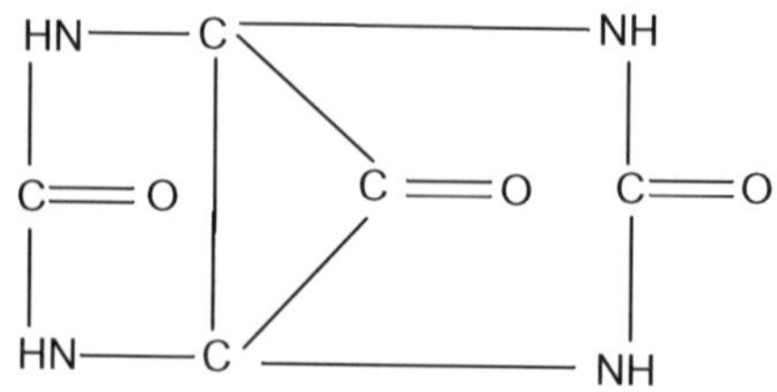

Fittig formula

Finally the structure of uric acid is found to be as medicus formula by synthesis.

Traube's Synthesis

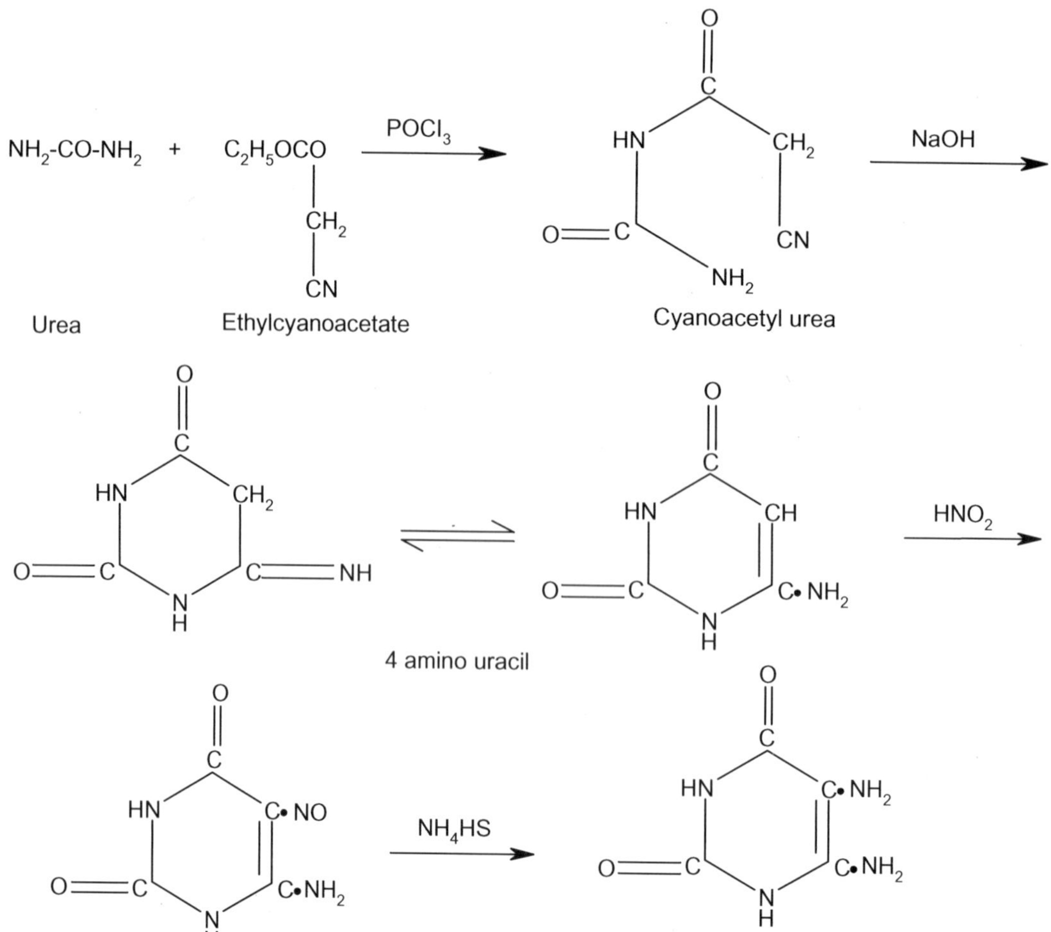

Urea

Ethylcyanoacetate

Cyanoacetyl urea

4 amino uracil

4,5 - diamino uracil

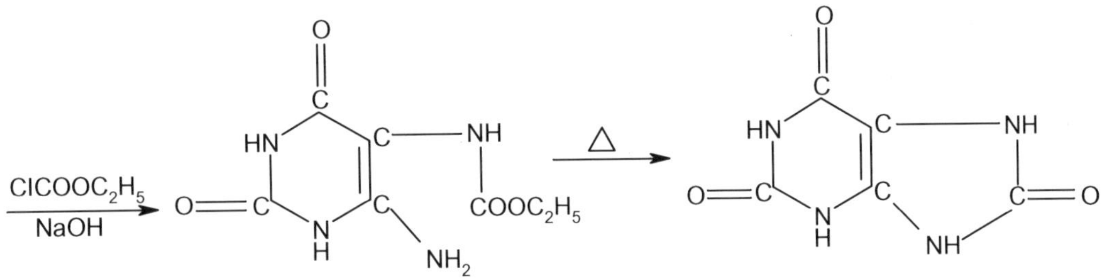

Urethane Uric acid

Baeyer - Fischer Synthesis

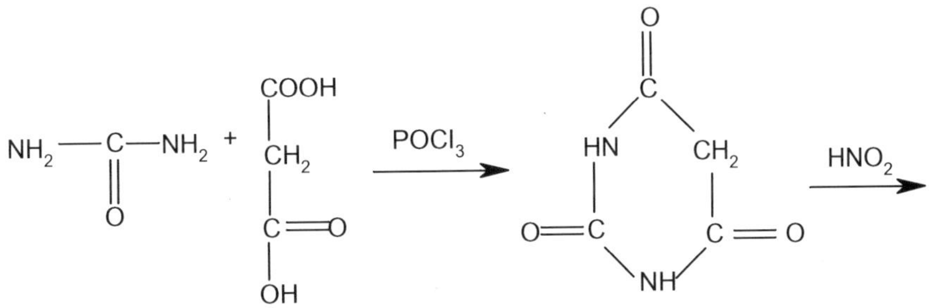

Urea Malonic acid Barbituric acid

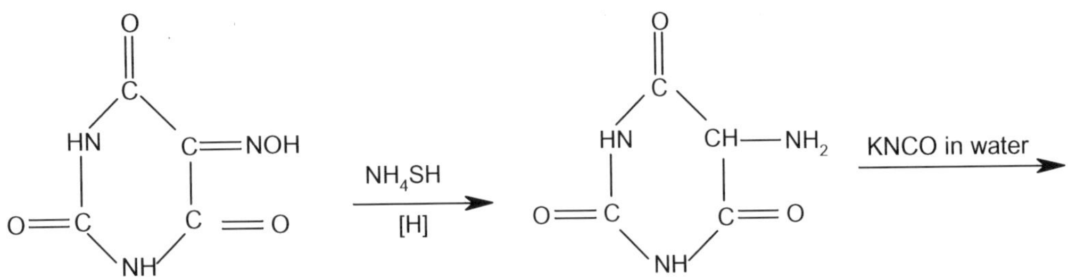

Violuric acid Uramil

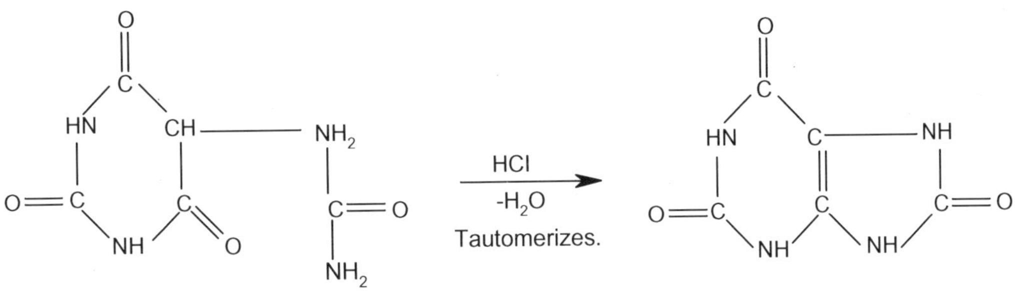

Pseudo uric acid Uric acid

CAFFEINE

Caffeine is chemically 1,3.7-trimethyl xanthine or 1,3,7 trimethyl -2,6-dihydroxy purine. Medicinally caffeine is used as its citrate or hydrochloride as diuretic and a heart and nerve stimulant.

Constitution of Caffeine

1. **Molecular composition of caffeine is $C_8H_{10}N_4O_2$**
2. **Presence of three methyl groups**

   By herzig method that is on heating with hydroiodic acid at 200°C, gives three moles of methyl iodide indicating the presence of three methyl groups.

$$\text{-N.CH}_3 \xrightarrow[200^{\circ}\text{C}]{\text{HI}} \text{-NH} + \text{CH}_3\text{I} \xrightarrow{\text{AgNO}_3} \text{AgI}\downarrow$$

3. **Presence of Uric acid skeleton**

   Caffeine on oxidation with potassium chlorate in hydrochloric acid solution gives 1,3 -dimethyl alloxan and monomethyl urea, which suggests the presence of uric acid skeleton in caffeine.

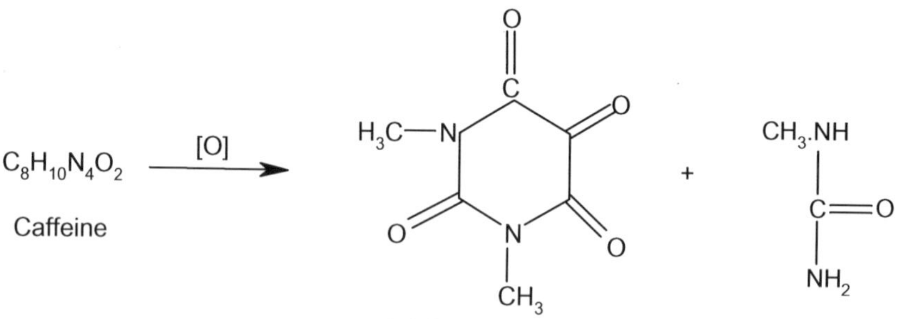

1,3-Dimethyl alloxan   Monomethyl urea

4. **Position of methyl groups**

   Formation of 1,3-Dimethyl alloxan suggests, two of the three methyl groups are in first and thrid position.Caffeine on vigorous oxidation gives sym -dimethyl oxamide ($CH_3NH.CO.CO NHCH_3$) indicating third methyl group is at 7th position.

   So the structure of caffeine can be proposed as follows;

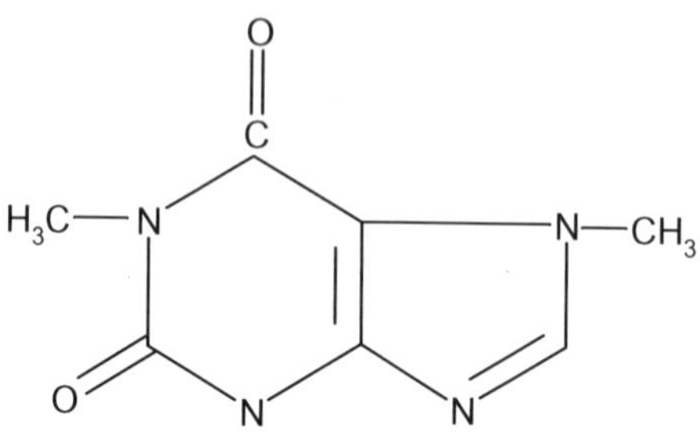

Caffeine

Finally the structure of caffeine can be confirmed by its synthesis.

Fischer's Synthesis for Caffeine

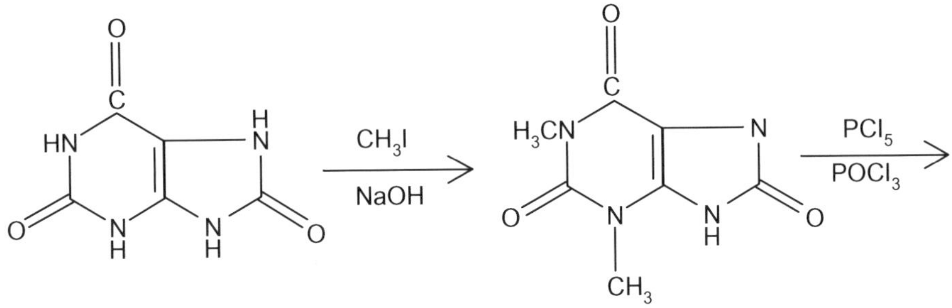

Uric acid 1,3,7 - Trymethyl uric acid

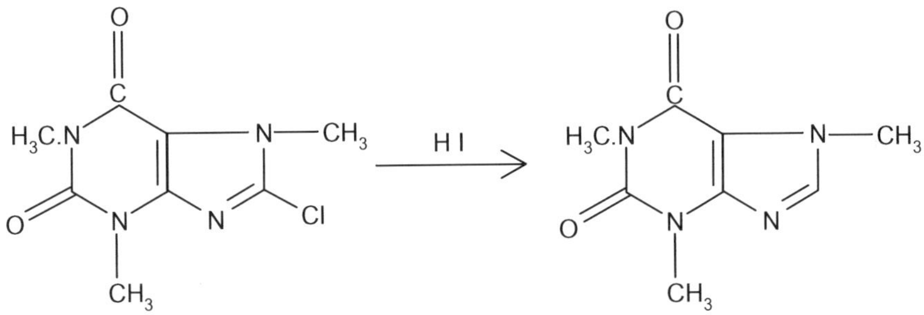

Chloro caffeine Caffeine

Traube's Synthesis of Caffeine

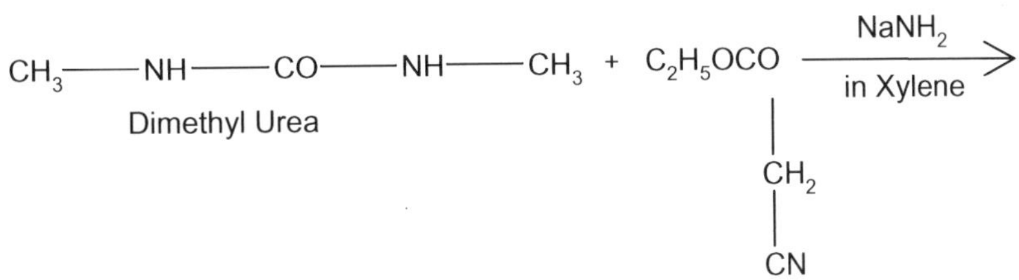

Dimethyl Urea Ethylcyanoacetate

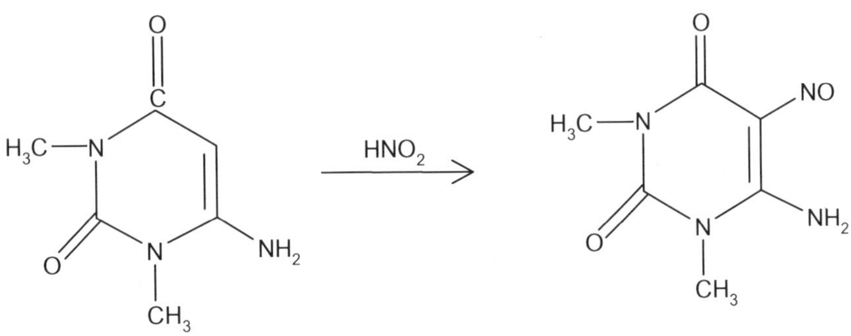

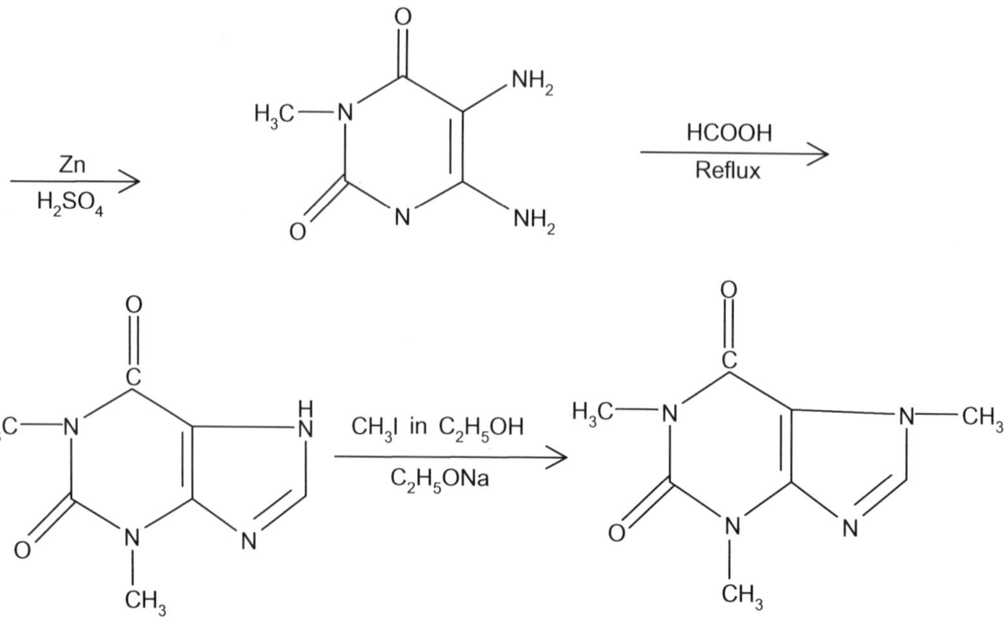

Theophylline   Caffeine

THEOBROMINE

Theobromine is chemically 3,7-Dimethyl xanthine. It is medicinally used as diuretic.

Consitution of Theobromine

1. **Molecular composition of Thebromine is $C_7H_8N_4O_2$**
2. **Presence of two methyl groups**

   By Herzig method theobromine found to have two methyl groups.
3. **Presence of uric acid skeleton**

   Theobromine on oxidation with potassium chlorate in Hydrochloric acid gives monomethyl alloxan and monomehtyl urea indicating the presence of uric acid skeleton.
4. **Position of methyl groups**

   Formation of monomethyl alloxan and monomethyl urea indicate one of the methyl groups present in pyrimidine ring (alloxan) and other in imidazole ring (Urea). On methylation Silver salt of theobromine gives caffeine indicating methyl group in imidazole is present at 7th position. Theobromine can be made from 3 or 7-methyl uric acid, but not from 1-methyl uric acid indicate methyl group in pyrimidine is at 3rd position.

   So the structure of theobromine can be drawn as follows;

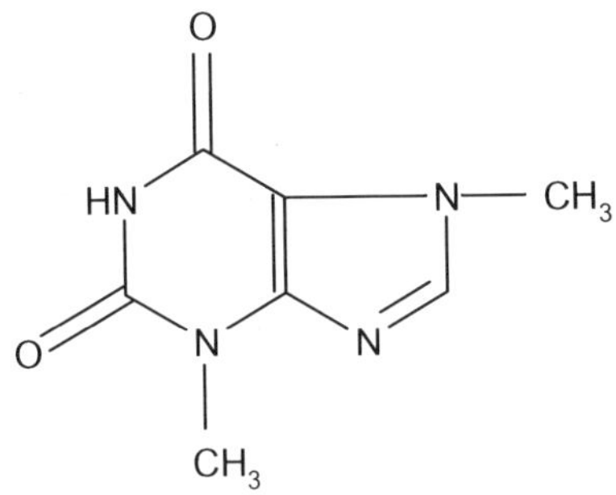

Finally structure of theobromine can be confirmed by its synthesis.

Fischer's Synthesis of Theobromine

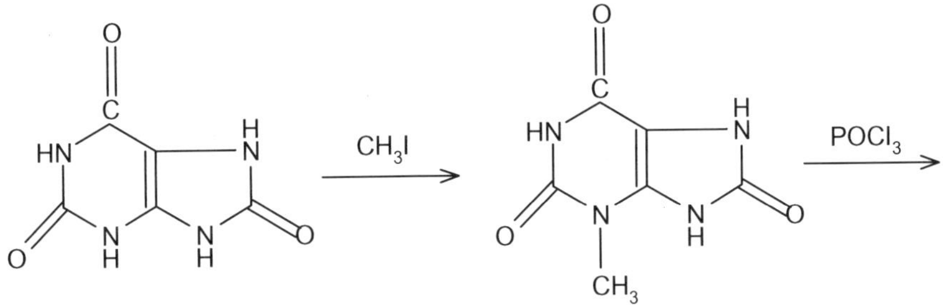

Uric acid   3 - Methyl uric acid.

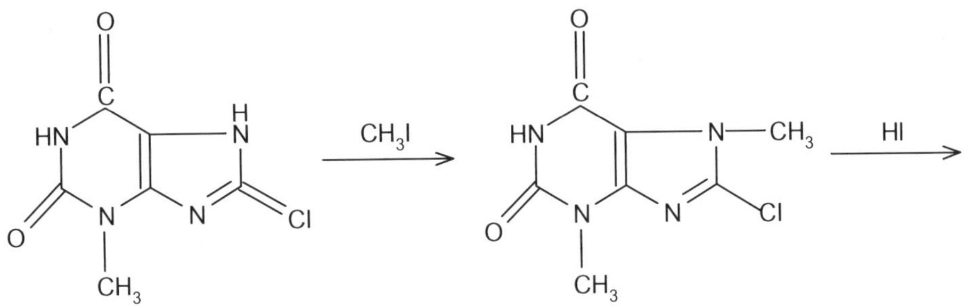

Uric acid

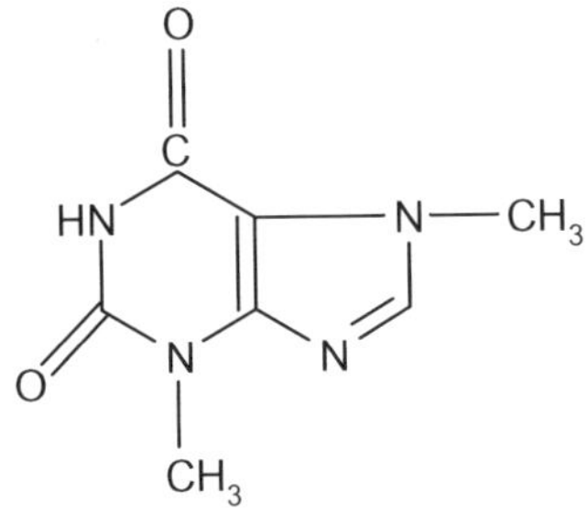

Theobromine

Traube's Synthesis for Theobromine

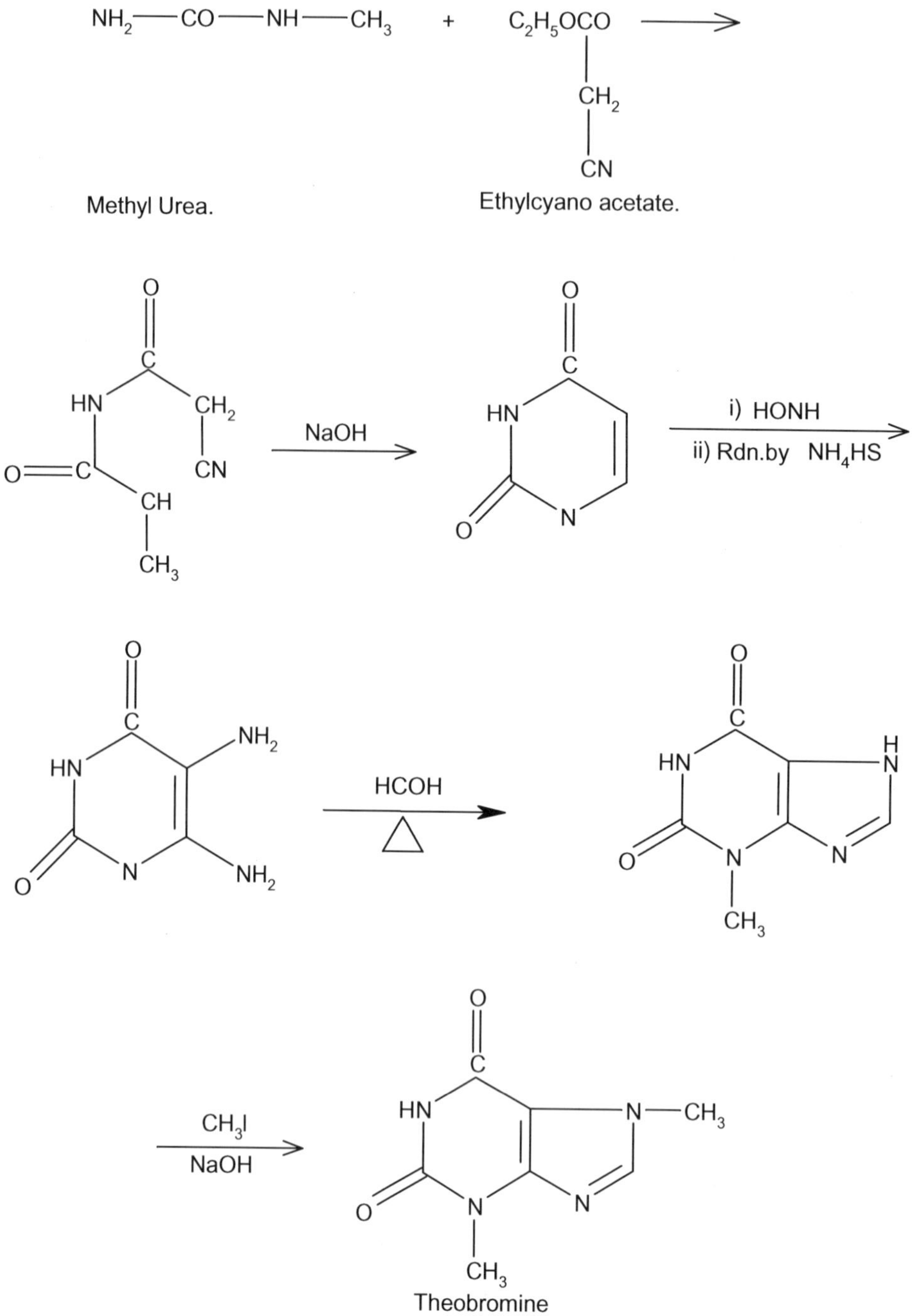

THEOPHYLLINE

Theophylline chemically is 1,3 Dimethylxanthine. Medicinally it is used as diuretic. It is quite similar to that of Theobromine. Only the difference is position of one of the methyl group.

Instead of one methyl group in theobromine is at 7th, in theophylline one methyl group is at 1st position, which can be proved by its synthesis from 1-methyl uric acid.

Remainig all can be elucidated as did in the theobromine. In this behalf structure of Theophylline can be drawn as follows.

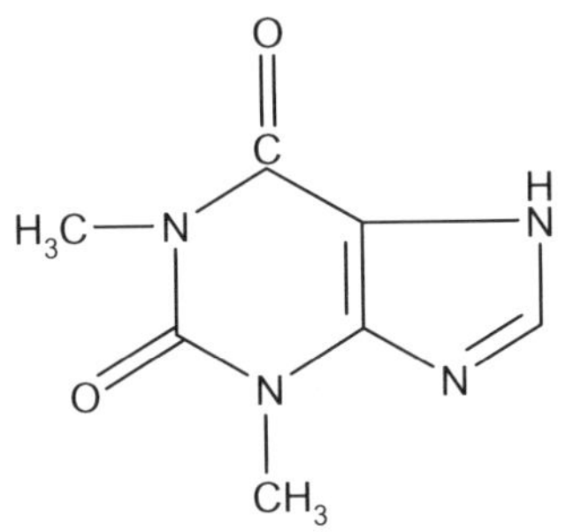

Theophylline

Finally the structure of Theophylline can be confirmed by its synthesis.

Fischer's Synthesis for Theophylline

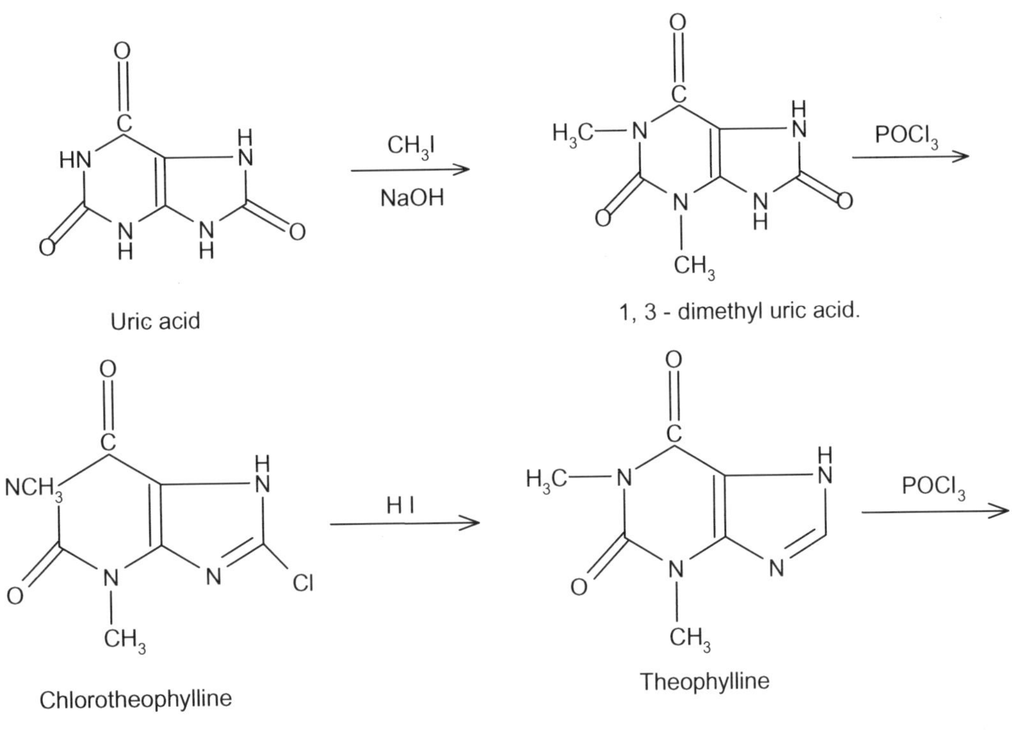

Traube's Synthesis of Theophylline

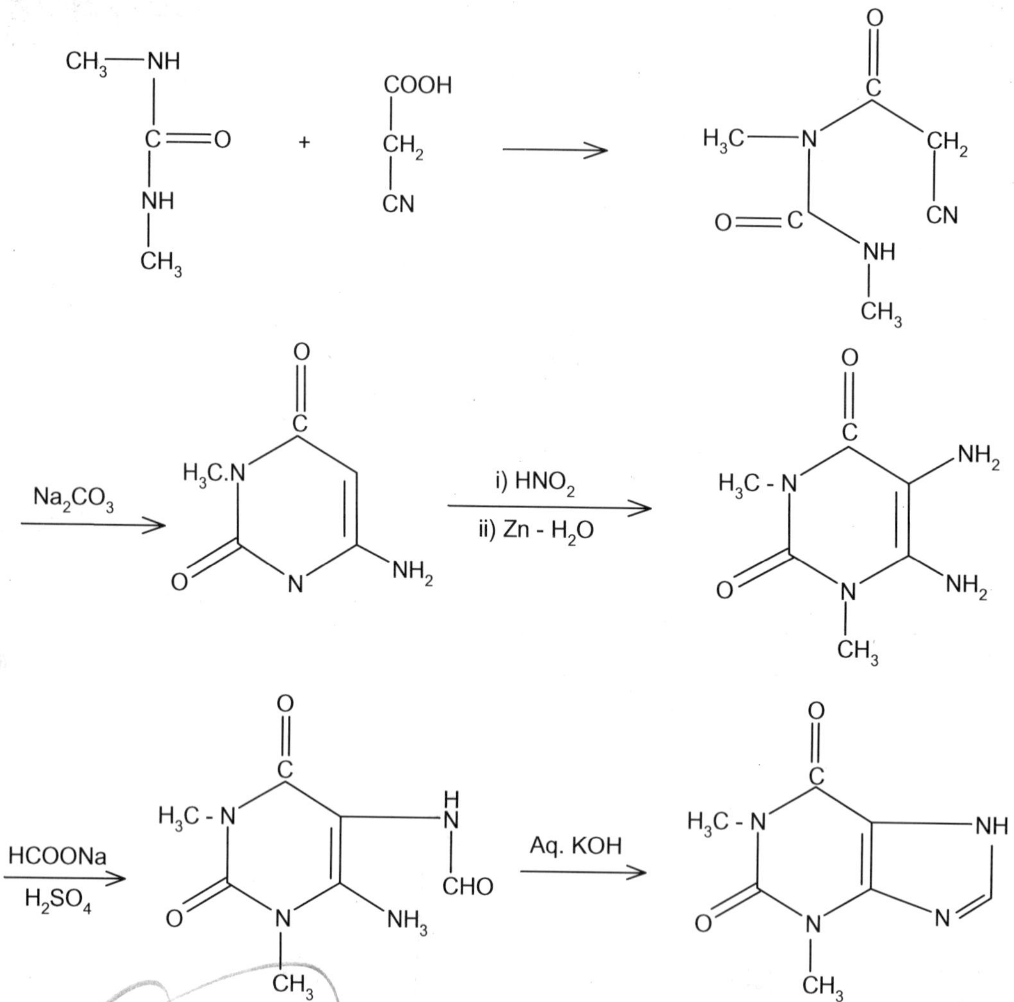

Theophylline